Critical Care MCQs
Problem-based Learning

Critical Care MCQs
Problem-based Learning

Editors

Kapil Gangadhar Zirpe
MBBS MD (Chest) FICCM FCCM FSNCC
Head
Department of Neuro-Trauma Intensive Care Unit
Grant Medical Foundation
Ruby Hall Clinic
Pune, Maharashtra, India

Subhal Bhalchandra Dixit
MD (Medicine) FCCM FICCM FICP
Director
Department of Critical Care ICU
Sanjeevan and MJM Hospital
Pune, Maharashtra, India

Atul Prabhakar Kulkarni
MD (Anesthesiology) FISCCM PGDHHM FICCM
Professor and Head
Division of Critical Care Medicine
Department of Anesthesiology, Critical Care and Pain
Tata Memorial Hospital
Homi Bhabha National Institute
Mumbai, Maharashtra, India

Associate Editors

Khalid Ismail Khatib
MD (Med) FICCM FICP
Professor
Department of Medicine
Smt. Kashibai Navale Medical College
Pune, Maharashtra, India

Harish Mallapura Maheshwarappa
MBBS MD DNB IDCCM DM (Critical Care) EDICM (Dublin)
Consultant-In-charge (Academics)
Department of Critical Care Medicine
Mazumdar Shaw Medical Centre
Narayana Health City
Bengaluru, Karnataka, India

Foreword
Yatin Mehta

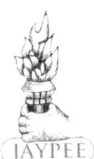

JAYPEE BROTHERS MEDICAL PUBLISHERS
The Health Sciences Publisher
New Delhi | London

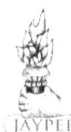 **Jaypee Brothers Medical Publishers (P) Ltd.**

Headquarters
Jaypee Brothers Medical Publishers (P) Ltd
EMCA House, 23/23-B
Ansari Road, Daryaganj
New Delhi 110 002, India
Landline: +91-11-23272143, +91-11-23272703
+91-11-23282021, +91-11-23245672
Email: jaypee@jaypeebrothers.com

Corporate Office
Jaypee Brothers Medical Publishers (P) Ltd
4838/24, Ansari Road, Daryaganj
New Delhi 110 002, India
Phone: +91-11-43574357
Fax: +91-11-43574314
Email: jaypee@jaypeebrothers.com

Overseas Office
JP Medical Ltd.
83, Victoria Street, London
SW1H 0HW (UK)
Phone: +44 20 3170 8910
Fax: +44 (0)20 3008 6180
Email: info@jpmedpub.com

Website: www.jaypeebrothers.com
Website: www.jaypeedigital.com

© 2024, Jaypee Brothers Medical Publishers

The views and opinions expressed in this book are solely those of the original contributor(s)/author(s) and do not necessarily represent those of editor(s) or publisher of the book.

All rights reserved. No part of this publication may be reproduced, stored or transmitted in any form or by any means, electronic, mechanical, photocopying, recording or otherwise, without the prior permission in writing of the publishers.

All brand names and product names used in this book are trade names, service marks, trademarks or registered trademarks of their respective owners. The publisher is not associated with any product or vendor mentioned in this book.

Medical knowledge and practice change constantly. This book is designed to provide accurate, authoritative information about the subject matter in question. However, readers are advised to check the most current information available on procedures included and check information from the manufacturer of each product to be administered, to verify the recommended dose, formula, method and duration of administration, adverse effects and contraindications. It is the responsibility of the practitioner to take all appropriate safety precautions. Neither the publisher nor the author(s)/editor(s) assume any liability for any injury and/or damage to persons or property arising from or related to use of material in this book.

This book is sold on the understanding that the publisher is not engaged in providing professional medical services. If such advice or services are required, the services of a competent medical professional should be sought.

Every effort has been made where necessary to contact holders of copyright to obtain permission to reproduce copyright material. If any have been inadvertently overlooked, the publisher will be pleased to make the necessary arrangements at the first opportunity.

Inquiries for bulk sales may be solicited at: jaypee@jaypeebrothers.com

Critical Care MCQs: Problem-based Learning

First Edition: **2024**

ISBN: 978-93-5696-310-8

Contributors

Abhijit Deshmukh
MBBS Diploma in TB and Chest Diseases IDCCM
Consultant Incharge
Department of Critical Care Medicine
Neuro-Trauma Unit
Ruby Hall Clinic
Pune, Maharashtra, India

Aditya Kumar Bang
MBBS DNB (Emergency Medicine) CTCCM EDIC
Junior Consultant
Department of Critical Care Medicine
Neuro-Trauma Unit
Ruby Hall Clinic
Pune, Maharashtra, India

Akshat Trivedi MD
Senior Resident
Department of Critical Care Medicine
King George's Medical College
Lucknow, Uttar Pradesh, India

Anirban Bhattacharjee MD DM IDCCM EDIC
Consultant
Department of Critical Care Medicine
Intensive Care Unit (ICU)
Nemcare Superspeciality Hospital
Guwahati, Assam, India

Ankit Purohit
MBBS MD DrNB (Critical Care Medicine)
Consultant
Department of Critical Care Medicine
Manipal Hospitals
New Delhi, India

Anuj M Clerk
MD (Medicine) FNB (Critical Care) IDCCM FIECMO
European Diploma (Intensive Care)
Director
Department of Critical Care
Sunshine Global Hospital, Surat, Gujarat, India

Anuja Pandit MBBS MD DM
Assistant Professor
Department of Onco-Anesthesia, Onco-Critical
Care, and Palliative Medicine
All India Institute of
Medical Sciences
New Delhi, India

Arshad Ayub MBBS MD EDAIC EDRA
Associate Professor
Department of Anesthesia
All India Institute of Medical Sciences
New Delhi, India

Atul Prabhakar Kulkarni
MD (Anesthesiology) FISCCM PGDHHM FICCM
Professor and Head
Division of Critical Care Medicine
Department of Anesthesiology,
Critical Care and Pain
Tata Memorial Hospital
Homi Bhabha National Institute
Mumbai, Maharashtra, India

Balaji Kannamani
MBBS MD DNB DM (Critical Care Medicine)
Associate Consultant
Department of Critical Care Medicine
Manipal Hospitals
New Delhi, India

Balkrishna D Nimavat
MBBS MD DNB (Anesthesiology) IDCCM FNB EDIC EDAIC
(Critical Care)
Consultant
Department of Critical Care
Sir HN Reliance Hospital
Mumbai, Maharashtra, India

Budhaditya Chattopadhyay DEM MEM (SEMI)
Associate Consultant
Department of Emergency Medicine
Accident and Emergency Medicine Unit
PD Hinduja Hospital and Medical Research Centre
Mumbai, Maharashtra, India

Carol D'Silva
MD (Anesthesiology) FNB (Critical Care) EDIC
Associate Professor
Department of Critical Care Medicine
St John's Medical College Hospital
Bengaluru, Karnataka, India

Charu Mahajan MD DM
Additional Professor
Department of Neuroanesthesiology and Critical Care
All India Institute of Medical Sciences
New Delhi, India

Deven Juneja DNB FNB EDIC FCCM
Director
Department of Critical Care Medicine
Max Super Speciality Hospital
New Delhi, India

Dhruva Chaudhry MD (Medicine) DM (PCCM)
Senior Professor and Head
Department of Pulmonary and Critical Care Medicine
Pandit Bhagwat Dayal Sharma Post Graduate Institute of Medical Sciences
Rohtak, Haryana, India

Dipali A Taggarsi
MBBS MD (Anesthesia) DM (Critical Care)
Associate Professor
Department of Critical Care Medicine
St John's Medical College Hospital
Bengaluru, Karnataka, India

Ganesh KM
DNB (Anesthesiology) FNB (Critical Care Medicine)
Associate Consultant
Medical Intensive Care Unit (MICU)
Fortis Hospital
Bengaluru, Karnataka, India

Harish Mallapura Maheshwarappa
MBBS MD DNB IDCCM DM (Critical Care) EDICM (Dublin)
Consultant-In-charge (Academics)
Department of Critical Care Medicine
Mazumdar Shaw Medical Centre
Narayana Health City
Bengaluru, Karnataka, India

Harshal Tukaram Pandve MBBS MD
Professor and Head
Department of Community Medicine
PCMC's Postgraduate Institute
Yashwantrao Chavan Memorial Hospital
Pune, Maharashtra, India

Harshavardhan Rangappa Kuri MBBS DNB
FIECMO DM-3rd year SR (Critical Care Medicine)
Senior Resident
Department of Critical Care Medicine
All India Institute of Medical Sciences
Jodhpur, Rajasthan, India

Hemanshu Prabhakar MD PhD FSNCC (Hon)
Professor
Department of Neuroanesthesiology and Critical Care
All India Institute of Medical Sciences
New Delhi, India

Impashree CM MS (OBG)
Consultant
Department of Obstetrics and Gynecology
Parency IVF Center
Bengaluru, Karnataka, India

Indu Kapoor MD
Additional Professor
Department of Neuroanesthesiology and Critical Care
All India Institute of Medical Sciences
New Delhi, India

Jignesh Shah MD DNB IFCCM EDIC
Professor
Department of Critical Care Medicine
Bharati Vidyapeeth (Deemed to be University)
Medical College
Pune, Maharashtra, India

Contributors vii

Jitin Sharma MBBS MD (Anesthesiology)
Senior Consultant
Department of Critical Care Medicine
BLK Superspeciality Hospital
New Delhi, India

Jyothi Geetha Mohankumar
MD (Respiratory Medicine) DNB (Pulmonary Medicine)
Second Year DM Fellow
Department of Pulmonary and Critical Care Medicine
Pandit Bhagwat Dayal Sharma Post Graduate Institute of Medical Sciences
Rohtak, Haryana, India

Kanwalpreet Sodhi DA DNB IDCCM EDIC FICCM
Director and Head
Department of Critical Care
Deep Hospital
Ludhiana, Punjab, India

Kapil Gangadhar Zirpe
MBBS MD (Chest) FICCM FCCM FSNCC
Head
Department of Neuro-Trauma
Intensive Care Unit
Grant Medical Foundation
Ruby Hall Clinic
Pune, Maharashtra, India

Karun Mahesh KP MD (General Medicine)
Assistant Professor
Department of General Medicine
Chandramma Dayananda Sagar Institute of Medical Education and Research (CDSIMER)
Ramanagara, Karnataka, India

Khalid Ismail Khatib MD (Medicine) FICCM FICP
Professor
Department of Medicine
Smt. Kashibai Navale Medical College
Pune, Maharashtra, India

Khusrav Bajan MD EDIC
Head
Department of Critical Care and Emergency Medicine
PD Hinduja Hospital and Medical Research Centre
Mumbai, Maharashtra, India

Kushal Rajeev Kalvit
MD (Medicine) DM (Critical Care Medicine)
Assistant Professor
Department of Anesthesiology, Critical Care and Pain
Tata Memorial Hospital
Mumbai, Maharashtra, India

Madhava Reddy D
DNB (Anesthesiology) FNB (Critical Care) EDIC
Associate Consultant
Department of Critical Care Medicine
Medanta—The Medicity
Gurugram, Haryana, India

Manender Kumar
MD PDCC (Cardiac Anesthesia and Critical Care)
Additional Director
Department of Cardiac Anesthesia and Critical Care
Fortis Hospital
Ludhiana, Punjab, India

Manu MK Varma DM (Critical Care Medicine)
Consultant
Department of Critical Care Medicine
Narayana Health City
Bengaluru, Karnataka, India

Mona Mishra MBBS MS DNB
Assistant Professor
Department of Obstetrics and Gynecology
Dr Ram Manohar Lohia (RML) Institute of Medical Sciences
Lucknow, Uttar Pradesh, India

Nandita Divekar MBBS DA (UK) FRCA FFICM DLM
Consultant
Department of Anesthesia and Critical Care
Medway NHS Trust, UK

Natesh Prabu R
MD DNB (Anesthesiology) DM (Critical Care Medicine) EDIC
Associate Professor
Department of Critical Care Medicine
St John's Medical College Hospital
Bengaluru, Karnataka, India

Nishant Agrawal MD DM
Assistant Professor
Department of Critical Care Medicine
Bharati Vidyapeeth (Deemed to be University)
Medical College
Pune, Maharashtra, India

Nithish Mukunthan MD IDCCM
Resident
Department of Critical Care Medicine
Narayana Hrudayalaya
Bengaluru, Karnataka, India

Nitika Yadav MD (Anesthesiology) DrNB
Resident
Department of Critical Care Medicine
Medanta—The Medicity
Gurugram, Haryana, India

Nitin Rai
MBBS MD (Anesthesiology, PGIMER, Chandigarh) DM
(Critical Care Medicine, AIIMS, New Delhi)
Assistant Professor
Department of Critical Care Medicine
King George's Medical University
Lucknow, Uttar Pradesh, India

PL Gautam MD DNB FICCM MNAMS
Professor and Head
Department of Critical Care
Dayanand Medical College and Hospital
Ludhiana, Punjab, India

Pradyut Bag MD IDCCM FNB EDIC
Principal Consultant
Department of Critical Care Medicine
BLK-Max Super Speciality Hospital
New Delhi, India

Prashant Nasa MD FNB EDIC FCCM
Specialist
Department of Critical Care Medicine
NMC Hospital
Dubai, UAE

Priya Gole MD (Anesthesiology) IDCCM DrNB
Resident
Department of Critical Care Medicine
Medanta—The Medicity
Gurugram, Haryana, India

Priyanka Akshay Metgud
MD (Anesthesia) IDCCM
Consultant
Department of Anesthesia and Critical care
Metgud Hospital
Belgaum, Karnataka, India

Raghavendra B Goudar
MD IDCCM IFCCM
Consultant
Department of Critical Care Medicine
Manipal Hospitals
Bengaluru, Karnataka, India

Rajesh Pande
MD PDCC (SGPGIMS) FICCM FCCM (USA)
Senior Director and Head
BLK-Max Centre of Excellence for Critical Care
BLK-Max Super Speciality Hospital
New Delhi, India

Ram Mohan Maiya GR MD
Resident
Department of Critical Care Medicine
Narayana Hrudayalaya
Bengaluru, Karnataka, India

Robert James Premkumar
MD DrNB (Critical Care Medicine)
Consultant
Department of Critical Care Medicine
Prashanth Super-Specialty Hospital
Chennai, Tamil Nadu, India

Ronak R Ankolekar
MBBS MD (Anesthesia)
DrNB Critical Care Medicine
Department of Critical Care Medicine
Narayana Hrudayalaya
Bengaluru, Karnataka, India

Sanjith Saseedharan
DA (Univ) CPS IDCCM EDIC FNCC (Israel) FIMSA
Teacher and Head
Department of Anesthesia and Critical Care
SL Raheja Hospital—A Fortis Associate
Mumbai, Maharashtra, India
President Elect—ISPEN

Saumitra Misra MD PDCC (Critical Care Medicine)
Assistant Professor
Department of Critical Care Medicine
King George's Medical University
Lucknow, Uttar Pradesh, India

Shilpushp Jagannath Bhosale
MD (Anesthesiology) DM (Critical Care Medicine)
Professor
Department of Anesthesiology
Critical Care and Pain
Tata Memorial Hospital
Homi Bhabha National Institute
Mumbai, Maharashtra, India

Shiva Kumar N
MBBS MD DM (Critical Care) DNB EDIC
Associate Consultant
Department of Critical Care
Narayana Hrudayalaya
Bengaluru, Karnataka, India

Shivangi Mishra
MBBS MD (AIIMS, New Delhi) FNB (Critical Care Medicine) EDIC
Junior Consultant
Department of Critical Care Medicine
Mazumdar Shaw Medical Centre
Bengaluru, Karnataka, India

Shrikanth Srinivasan
MBBS MD DNB FNB EDIC FICCM
Consultant and Head
Department of Critical Care Medicine
Manipal Hospitals
New Delhi, India

Srinivas Samavedam
MD DNB FRCP FNB EDIC FICCM DMLE MBA
Chief Intensivist
Department of Critical Care
TX Hospitals
Hyderabad, Telangana, India

Subhal Bhalchandra Dixit
MD (Medicine) FCCM FICCM FICP
Director
Department of Critical Care ICU
Sanjeevan and MJM Hospital
Pune, Maharashtra, India

Sudha Bala MBBS MD
Assistant Professor
Department of Community Medicine
ESIC Medical College
Hyderabad, Telangana, India

Suhail Sarwar Siddiqui MD DM EDIC
Associate Professor
Department of Critical Care Medicine
King George's Medical University
Lucknow, Uttar Pradesh, India

Sumati Verma
MD (Pediatrics) IFPCCM (Pediatric Critical Care Medicine)
Senior Resident
Department of Pediatric Critical Care
Christian Medical College
Ludhiana, Punjab, India

Sunil Karanth MD FNB EDIC FCICM (Aus/NZ)
Chairman
Department of Critical Care Medicine
Manipal Health Enterprises (P) Ltd
Consultant and Head
Department of Critical Care Medicine
Manipal Hospitals
Bengaluru, Karnataka, India

Sushil Kumar Yadav
MD (Anesthesia) FNB (Critical Care Medicine) IDCCM
IFCCM FCCU FIECMO FIECHO
Consultant Intensivist and Incharge
Department of Critical Care Medicine
Jupiter Hospital
Pune, Maharashtra, India

Syed Nabeel Muzaffar MD DM
Associate Professor
Department of Critical Care Medicine
King George's Medical University
Lucknow, Uttar Pradesh, India

Thilakchand KR
MBBS MD (Anesthesia) DrNB
DrnB Resident
Department of Critical Care Medicine
Narayana Hrudayalaya
Bengaluru, Karnataka, India

Vasudha Singhal MD FSNCC (Hon)
Senior Consultant
Department of Neuroanesthesiology and Critical Care
Medanta—The Medicity
Gurugram, Haryana, India

Vishal Raj MD (Respiratory Medicine)
Second Year DM Fellow
Department of Pulmonary and Critical Care Medicine
Pandit Bhagwat Dayal Sharma Post Graduate Institute of Medical Sciences
Rohtak, Haryana, India

Foreword

It is indeed a pleasure to write this for the landmark book edited by Drs Kapil Gangadhar Zirpe, Subhal Bhalchandra Dixit, and Atul Prabhakar Kulkarni. Indian students generally are very good at standard theoretical knowledge but tumble when it comes to a specific case scenario! This book overcomes that limitation.

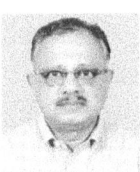

This MCQ book has almost 950+ MCQs. Each question is case based with answers, explanations, and relevant recommended references. It covers the whole spectrum of critical care including scarcely touched but important topics such as quality, patient safety, and ethics besides the clinical aspects.

This book will significantly help all students, teachers, and practitioners of critical care medicine. The editors are stalwarts in the field and have put in a lot of effort to come up with this (original MCQs are quite difficult and time-consuming to compose!). It is a must for every library/student of critical care.

Yatin Mehta
MD MNAMS FRCA FAMS FIACTA FICCM FTEE
Chairman
Medanta Institute of Critical Care and Anesthesiology
Medanta—The Medicity
Gurugram, Haryana, India
President
Sepsis Forum of India, The Simulation Society
Past President
ISCCM, IACTA, RSACP, SWAC ELSO
yatinmehta@hotmail.com

Preface

Dear Friends

It is indeed a proud moment for us. We will be releasing one of the most awaited MCQ book in the field of critical care medicine, *"Critical Care MCQs: Problem-based Learning"*. This will be third in series.

The main purpose of this book is to focus on problems that would be encountered commonly in clinical practice rather than an assessment of anyone's knowledge of trivial facts or problems that are seldom encountered. Authors have formatted majority of questions in such a way that, the clinical case scenario begins with the presentation of a problem and followed by relevant signs, symptoms, subsequent findings, etc. In essence, all the relevant information is available that is necessary for a competent candidate to answer the question. Well-constructed MCQs will test the application of medical knowledge (context-rich) rather than just the recall of information (context-free). The majority of questions are with clear directions as to what the candidate should do to answer the question. Ambiguity and the use of imprecise terms have been avoided throughout the book.

This book has 32 chapters and approximately 950+ MCQs related to critical care medicine. Emphasis has been attributed to tropical diseases, infection control, neurocritical care, quality, patient safety, ethics, hemodynamic, and mechanical ventilation. The *answers have been given for MCQs along with explanations and appropriate references at the end of every chapter.* This book is highly interactive, and the content has been so designed as to cover the syllabus of critical care medicine training courses.

This book is user-friendly and will meet the expectations of the students.

Best wishes

Kapil Gangadhar Zirpe
Subhal Bhalchandra Dixit
Atul Prabhakar Kulkarni
Khalid Ismail Khatib
Harish Mallapura Maheshwarappa

Acknowledgments

Though this was third in series, this book experience was more rewarding than I could have ever imagined.

I have to start with appreciating my awesome Editor colleagues Atul Prabhakar Kulkarni, Subhal Bhalchandra Dixit, Harish Mallapura Maheshwarappa and Khalid Ismail Khatib for guiding and giving me proper advice at every stage. Thank you so much friends.

On behalf of the Editorial Board, I sincerely appreciate the contribution of each and every author for timely completing their chapters. Everyone's contribution has added more credibility to this, *Critical Care MCQs: Problem-based Learning*. I thank for your continued trust on us and look forward to another such endeavor in the future.

I appreciate the contribution of M/s Jaypee Brothers Medical Publishers (P) Ltd, New Delhi, India. I thank Shri Jitendar P Vij (Group Chairman), Mr Ankit Vij (Managing Director), Mr MS Mani (Group President), Ms Chetna Malhotra (Senior Director—Professional Publishing, Marketing, and Business Development), Ms Pooja Bhandari (Director—Production), Ms Kritika Dua (Senior Development Editor) and Ms Suchita Gera (Development Editor) for tireless follow-up and finishing the book within the timeline.

Kapil Gangadhar Zirpe

Contents

1. **Airway Management** 1
   Shiva Kumar N, Nithish Mukunthan, Ram Mohan Maiya GR

2. **Resuscitation** 17
   Kanwalpreet Sodhi, Manender Kumar, Sumati Verma

3. **Shock** 41
   Nitin Rai, Anirban Bhattacharjee, Akshat Trivedi

4. **Mechanical Ventilation** 69
   Rajesh Pande, Pradyut Bag, Jitin Sharma

5. **Respiratory System** 90
   Harish Mallapura Maheshwarappa, Shivangi Mishra, Harshavardhan Rangappa Kuri

6. **Hemodynamic Monitoring** 111
   Harish Mallapura Maheshwarappa, Thilakchand KR, Ronak R Ankolekar

7. **Infection Control** 127
   Srinivas Samavedam

8. **Tropical Diseases** 137
   Dhruva Chaudhry, Jyothi Geetha Mohankumar, Vishal Raj

9. **Gastrointestinal System** 157
   Sushil Kumar Yadav, Priyanka Akshay Metgud

10. **Critical Care Nutrition** 175
    Sanjith Saseedharan

11. **Endocrine and Metabolism** 198
    Madhava Reddy D, Nitika Yadav, Priya Gole

12. **Neurocritical Care** 221
    Indu Kapoor, Charu Mahajan, Hemanshu Prabhakar

13. **Trauma** 241
    Khusrav Bajan, Budhaditya Chattopadhyay

14. **Cardiovascular System** 265
    Harish Mallapura Maheshwarappa, Robert James Premkumar, Ganesh KM

15. **Renal/Fluids/Electrolyte** 292
    Saumitra Misra

16. **Toxicology** 307
    Deven Juneja, Prashant Nasa

17. **Obstetric Critical Care** 333
    Manu MK Varma, Karun Mahesh KP, Impashree CM

18. **End of Life/Transplant** 344
    Nishant Agrawal, Jignesh Shah

19. **Oncology/Hematology** 363
    Shilpushp Jagannath Bhosale, Atul Prabhakar Kulkarni

20. **Thromboembolism** 385
    Kushal Rajeev Kalvit

21. **Postoperative Care** 404
    Suhail Sarwar Siddiqui, Arshad Ayub, Anuja Pandit

22. **Sepsis and Antimicrobial Stewardship** 432
    Natesh Prabu R, Carol D'Silva, Dipali A Taggarsi

23. **Neuromonitoring** 449
    Vasudha Singhal

24. **Pharmacotherapeutics** 466
    Khalid Ismail Khatib

25. **Physical Disorders (Drowning, Electrocution, Altitude and Depth Related, Temperature Related, and Rhabdomyolysis)** 483
    Sunil Karanth, Raghavendra B Goudar

26. **High-resolution Computed Tomography and Magnetic Resonance Imaging** 498
    Aditya Kumar Bang

27. **X-rays (Chest/Abdomen)** 536
    Khalid Ismail Khatib, Abhijit Deshmukh

28. **Approach for Acid–Base Disorders and Blood Gas Analysis** 550
    Balkrishna Nimavat

29. **Ultrasonography** 564
    Shrikanth Srinivasan, Balaji Kannamani, Ankit Purohit

30. **Electrocardiogram** 582
    Syed Nabeel Muzaffar, Saumitra Misra

31. **Quality, Medication Errors, and Research** 612
    Anuj Clerk, Nandita Divekar, PL Gautam

32. **Research Methodology** 629
    Harshal Tukaram Pandve, Sudha Bala, Khalid Ismail Khatib

CHAPTER

Airway Management

Shiva Kumar N, Nithish Mukunthan, Ram Mohan Maiya GR

Q.1. A 25-year-old boy had a road traffic accident while riding a two-wheeler with high velocity, he is brought to the hospital, his Glasgow Coma Scale (GCS) is E1V1M3 and is gasping, blood pressure (BP) is 100/70 mm Hg, heart rate is 120 beats/min, and oxygen saturation (SpO_2) is 87% on room air. A hard cervical collar is placed to stabilize the C spine. With regards to secure a definitive airway in this patient, which of the following statements is false?
   a. Manual inline stabilization causes worsening of laryngoscopic view.
   b. Use of videolaryngoscopy reduces the risk of failed intubation.
   c. Flexible bronchoscopy-guided intubation is better than videolaryngoscopy for intubation in this patient for intubation.
   d. Jaw thrust produces less spinal movement compared to chin lift.

Ans. c

Explanation: Manual inline stabilization maneuver increases the CL grade and worsens the laryngoscopic view; videolaryngoscopy has been found to increase success of intubation with advantage of reduced neck mobilization compared to conventional direct laryngoscopy. The jaw thrust maneuver produces less spinal movement and is recommended compared to chin lift for opening and maintaining a collapsed airway with suspected spinal cord injury. Videolaryngoscopy is better and has high success compared to flexible bronchoscopy and is recommended in this patient.

Suggested Reading
   1. Wiles MD. Airway management in patients with suspected or confirmed traumatic spinal cord injury: a narrative review of current evidence. Anaesthesia. 2022;77:1120-8.

Q.2. A 50-year-old man had a road traffic accident during which the car steering has collided with his neck in high velocity. He is being shifted to intensive care unit (ICU) for further care. He is conscious and oriented, he is complaining of severe pain in the front of neck, and he has no other injuries. His heart rate is 100 beats/min, BP is 120/90 mm Hg, and he has swelling over the neck and palpatory crepitus over the anterior neck. His saturation is 92% on 8-L oxygen face mask. His swelling over the neck is gradually increasing and is complaining of hoarseness of

voice. His respiratory rate is 34 breaths/min. Which of the following is the next best method to manage this patient?
a. Shift the patient for CT scan of head and neck and then plan further management of airway.
b. Secure patient's airway by rapid sequence intubation and direct laryngoscopy.
c. Perform an awake surgical tracheostomy in the operation theater.
d. Perform a percutaneous tracheostomy in the ICU.

Ans. c

Explanation: This patient has sustained blunt trauma of neck. He is in the ICU, he has sustained no other injuries, there is subcutaneous emphysema, and he is at a risk of airway compromise. Blunt neck injury involves damage to tracheal cartilages, also has risk of vascular injury, and airway may get obstructed if not secured early. Securing airway in blunt trauma neck is a challenge and requires teamwork—intensivist, anesthesiologist, and head and neck surgeon. Bag and mask ventilation may worsen subcutaneous emphysema if there is tracheal injury. Emergency front-of-neck access like percutaneous tracheostomy is not recommended as the extent of airway injury is not known and a blind front-of-neck access may distort already injured laryngeal structures. Computed tomography (CT) evaluation of the neck is recommended when patient is stable and airway is secured, this patient has already compromised airway and securing the airway is the priority than doing a CT scan. Rapid sequence intubation and fiberoptic-guided intubation can be performed only in patients with impending airway compromise; this patient is tachypneic but maintaining saturation with oxygen. Hence, the best method is to perform an awake surgical tracheostomy under local anesthesia in the operation theater. Surgical tracheostomy has an added advantage to assess the tracheal structures for extent of injury.

Suggested Reading
1. Shilston J, Evans DL, Simons A, Evans DA. Initial management of blunt and penetrating neck trauma. BJA Educ. 2021;21(9):329-3.

Q.3. A 36-year-old policeman was involved in a gun fight, he has sustained gunshot injury to the neck, he is hemodynamically stable, he has an open wound in the neck with minimal bleeding, he is conscious but not able to vocalize and air leak is present over the neck, and he is in respiratory distress. All of the following are true regarding management of this patient, except.
a. Zone 1 injuries are highly fatal and will need surgical exploration.
b. Cricoid pressure should not be given in this patient.
c. Try to insert a tracheostomy tube in the site of injury and ventilate from it.
d. Intubation with rapid sequence induction and fiberoptic intubation.

Ans. c

Explanation: This patient has a penetrating neck injury. Any penetrating neck injury involving breach of platysma requires surgical exploration. The neck is divided into 3 zones. Zone 1 involves the area with major blood vessels including carotids, hence injury to them carries high mortality. Cricoid pressure is not recommended while intubation as the risk of further airway cartilage increases with it. The best method to secure this patient's airway is rapid sequence induction and guided by fiberoptic intubation as this allows assessment of further any injury in the trachea and aids placement of endotracheal tube further distal to the site of injury. Inserting a tracheostomy tube blindly to this injured area is not advised as it may increase chances of further cartilage injury.

Suggested Reading
1. Shilston J, Evans DL, Simons A, Evans DA. Initial management of blunt and penetrating neck trauma. BJA Educ. 2021;21(9):329-35.

Q.4. Which among the following four methods of preoxygenation in patients with severe hypoxemia provides higher saturation during intubation?
   a. Facemask
   b. High-flow nasal cannula (HFNC)
   c. OPTINIV
   d. Noninvasive ventilation (NIV)

Ans. c

Explanation: OPTINIV is a combination of use of HFNC and NIV. An RCT conducted by Jaber et al. concluded that the OPTINIV method of preoxygenation is a method where combination of HFNC and NIV is used for preoxygenation followed by intubation with reduced rates of desaturation and adverse events during intubation. The NIV provided positive end-expiratory pressure (PEEP) and pressure support and the HFNC provided the high flows needed for apneic oxygenation as well.

Suggested Reading
1. Jaber S, Monnin M, Girard M, Conseil M, Cisse M, Carr J, et al. Apnoeic oxygenation via high-flow nasal cannula oxygen combined with non-invasive ventilation preoxygenation for intubation in hypoxaemic patients in the intensive care unit: the single-centre, blinded, randomised controlled OPTINIV trial. Intensive Care Med. 2016;42:1877-87.

Q.5. A 65-year-old obese lady is admitted to the ICU with diagnosis of severe community-acquired pneumonia and acute respiratory distress syndrome (ARDS). Her SpO_2 is 78% with 15 L oxygen, respiratory rate is 35 breaths/min, heart rate is 130 beats/min, and BP is 120/87 mm Hg; she is very drowsy. Also on evaluation, her mouth opening is <3 cm, she also has history of obstructive sleep apnea (OSA). The ICU doctor decides to intubate her, which of the following is not recommended as per guidelines for intubation in critically ill?
   a. Two operators for intubation.
   b. Use of stylet for intubation.
   c. Use of direct laryngoscopy with metallic blade.
   d. Use of videolaryngoscopy.
   e. Rapid sequence induction.

Ans. c

Explanation: According to airway management algorithm in ICU, the recommendations are to assess MACOCHA score. In this patient, the score is >3. Presence of two operators, use of rapid sequence intubation, and use of stylet are recommended. If the MACOCHA score is >3, the intubation is recommended to be performed with a videolaryngoscopy as it increases chances of success. In case of failed intubation, the algorithm recommends use of laryngeal mask and then to proceed for cricothyroidotomy.

Suggested Reading
1. De Jong A, Myatra SN, Roca O, Jaber S. How to improve intubation in the intensive care unit. Update on knowledge and devices. Intensive Care Med. 2022;48:1287-98.

Q.6. **A 25-year-old boy admitted with severe traumatic brain injury had undergone a percutaneous tracheostomy 3 days back in view of need of prolonged ventilation. He developed a tube block and suction catheter was not able to be passed inside the tube, he was desaturating and tidal volume delivery on the ventilator was not adequate. The ICU doctor decided to change the tracheostomy tube. Which of the following statements with regards to management of this patient is not correct?**
   a. A same sized new tracheostomy tube should be used.
   b. A tube exchanger must be used, and new tube must be railroaded on the tube exchanger.
   c. Routine tracheostomy tube change must be done after 3 days in the ICU to prevent tube block.
   d. If tube change is unsuccessful and airway is lost, emergent intubation with oral tracheal route must be done.

Ans. c

Explanation: Change of tracheostomy tube in an emergency setting is a challenge in the ICU. In this patient, the stoma is still not matured and risk of passing the new tube in a false track is higher with potential loss of airway. Always a tube exchanger must be used to railroad the new tube. Same sized tube must be used or a smaller sized tube. Routine change of tubes is not recommended in the ICU. First tube change can be planned after 7-14 days when the stoma is matured, and complications are less. If during a tube change the airway is lost, immediate oral tracheal intubation must be performed and later the tracheostomy tube can be inserted.

Suggested Reading
1. White AC, Kher S, O'Connor HH. When to change a tracheostomy tube. Respir Care. 2010;55(8):1069-75.

Q.7. **All of the followings are true for usage of ultrasound in airway management in the ICU, except:**
   a. For performing percutaneous tracheostomy.
   b. For assessment of vocal cords movement.
   c. For assessment of difficult airway.
   d. Confirmation of endotracheal tube postintubation.
   e. Used in penetrating neck trauma to assess extent of airway injury.

Ans. e

Explanation: Use of airway ultrasound is for various reasons. It is used for performing percutaneous tracheostomy—assessment of blood vessels and real time entry of needle into trachea, confirmation of endotracheal intubation, and assessment of neck for soft tissue to aid in difficult airway. It is also used to look at vocal cord movements in suspected vocal cord palsy. CT neck is a modality used to assess extent of injury in penetrating neck injury and presence of subcutaneous air limits usage of ultrasound in such settings.

Suggested Reading
1. Diaz-Tormo C, Rodriguez-Martinez E, Galarza L. Airway ultrasound in critically ill patients: A narrative review. J Ultrasound Med. 2022;41(6):1317-27.

Q.8. All are true with respect to hypotension postintubation in a critically ill patient, except:
 a. Use of drugs like propofol is common cause of hypotension postintubation.
 b. Use of a fluid bolus before intubation reduces incidence of postintubation hypotension.
 c. Loss of sympathetic tone and hypovolemia are major factors causing hypotension postintubation.
 d. Hypotension postintubation is related to poor outcomes.

Ans. b

Explanation: Hypotension postintubation is associated with poor outcomes in prior studies. Use of fluid bolus prior to intubation did not reduce incidence of hypotension postintubation in randomized controlled trial (RCT) by Ven der ven et al. Optimization of preload and early use of vasopressors during intubation reduces chances of postintubation hemodynamic collapse.

Suggested Reading
1. Van der Ven WH, Vlaar APJ, Veelo DP. Fluid bolus administration and cardiovascular collapse in critically ill patients undergoing tracheal intubation. JAMA. 2022;328(20):2070.

Q.9. All are true with regarding airway ultrasound, except:
 a. The thyroid cartilage is seen as a large V-shaped structure.
 b. The tracheal cartilages are seen as string of pearl in long-axis view.
 c. Visualization of endotracheal tube cuff is easy.
 d. Cricothyroid membrane is seen as hyperdense line.

Ans. c

Explanation: Visualization of the endotracheal tube cuff is difficult as it is filled with air. The tube is visualized as two parallel lines or railroad sign. Visualization can be improved if cuff is filled with saline.

Suggested Reading
1. Diaz-Tormo C, Rodriguez-Martinez E, Galarza L. Airway ultrasound in critically ill patients: A narrative review. J Ultrasound Med. 2022;41(6):1317-27.

Q.10. With respect to postextubation stridor in the ICU, all of the following statements are true except:
   a. Airway trauma and prolonged intubation are risk factors.
   b. Noninvasive ventilation should be used to manage postextubation stridor.
   c. Cuff leak test can be performed to assess risk for postextubation stridor.
   d. Heliox, nebulized adrenaline, and steroids are used for management.
   e. It can develop up to 24 hours after extubation.

Ans. b

Explanation: NIV use for management in postextubation stridor is not recommended as it has shown to increase mortality by delaying intubation in various studies. Early intubation may be indicated instead of use of NIV.

Suggested Reading
   1. Smith SE, Newsome AS, Hawkins WA. An argument for the protocolized screening and management of postextubation stridor. Am J Respir Crit Care Med. 2018;197(11):1503-5.

Q.11. All are components of MACOCHA scoring system, except:
   a. Mallampati score III or IV
   b. Limited mouth opening <3 cm
   c. Coma
   d. Morbid obesity

Ans. d

Explanation: MACOCHA scoring system is a simplified scoring system used at the bedside in critical care for prediction of difficult intubation. It has 7 variables broadly categorized under 3 subheadings with total score of 12. Score between 0 and 3 has low risk, 4 and 7 has moderate risk, and 8 and 12 has high risk of intubation.

Factors related to the patient:
- *Mallampati score III or IV:* 5
- *Obstructive apnea syndrome:* 2
- *Reduced mobility of cervical spine:* 1
- *Limited mouth opening <3 cm:* 1

Factors related to pathophysiology:
- *Coma:* 1
- *Severe hypoxia:* 1

Factors related to operator:
- *Nonanesthetist:* 1

Suggested Reading
   1. De Jong A, Molinari N, Terzi N, Mongardon N, Arnal JM, Guitton C, et al. Early identification of patients at risk for difficult intubation in the intensive care unit: Development and validation of the MACOCHA score in a multicenter cohort study. Am J Respir Crit Care Med. 2013;187(8):832-9.

Q.12. A 40-year-old man with morbid obesity and chronic obstructive pulmonary disease (COPD) presented to ICU with the complaints of breathlessness and desaturation.

He was initially managed with NIV but later planned for intubation as he became drowsier. After preoxygenation and induction with anesthetic agents, facemask ventilation was unsuccessful. What is the immediate next step of management?
a. Insert supraglottic airway to maintain O_2 and call for help.
b. Continue rescue facemask ventilation till help arrives.
c. Give a single attempt of tracheal intubation.
d. Directly go for emergency cricothyroidotomy.

Ans. c

Explanation: As per All India Difficult Airway Association (AIDAA) 2016 guidelines for tracheal intubation in ICU, if facemask ventilation fails and if SpO_2 >95%, then a single attempt of tracheal intubation may be given before putting a SAD.

Suggested Reading
1. Myatra SN, Shah A, Kundra P, Patwa A, Ramkumar V, Divatia JV, et al. All India Difficult Airway Association 2016 guidelines for the management of unanticipated difficult tracheal intubation in adults. Indian J Anaesth. 201;60(12):885-98.

Q.13. During preoxygenation for induction, all are the components of "safe apnea", except:
a. Maximal denitrogenation
b. Adequate CO_2 washout
c. Adequate functional residual capacity (FRC)
d. Minimizing shunt

Ans. b

Explanation: Ideally patients are preoxygenated for 4 minutes by making them breathe 100% O_2. This provides the window for "safe apnea". It includes three important components, first is an adequate reservoir to draw oxygen during apnea which is FRC, next is maximizing oxygen in that reservoir which is denitrogenation, and last is minimizing shunt thereby availability of that reservoir to re saturate hemoglobin.

Suggested Reading
1. Natt B, Mosier J. Airway management in the critically ill patient. Curr Anesthesiol Rep. 2021;11(2):116-27.

Q.14. What is the value of shock index, above which there is a strong prediction of postintubation hypotension?
a. 0.4
b. 0.6
c. 0.8
d. 1.0

Ans. c

Explanation: Shock index is calculated by heart rate/systolic blood pressure. An elevated shock index of >0.8 preintubation is a specific marker for postintubation hypotension. However, it is not very sensitive. In any patient with shock index >0.8 preintubation, it is advisable to resuscitate the patient with fluids or start inotropes before inducing.

Suggested Reading
1. Heffner AC, Swords DS, Nussbaum ML, Kline JA, Jones AE. Predictors of the complication of postintubation hypotension during emergency airway management. J Crit Care. 2012;27(6):587-93.

Q.15. Work of breathing is least with which type of humidifier?
 a. Heated humidifiers (HHs).
 b. Heat moist exchangers (HMEs).
 c. Heat moist exchanger filter (HMEF).
 d. No increase in work of breathing with any humidifiers.

Ans. a

Explanation: All humidifiers offer resistance and dead space during ventilation, which in turn increase work of breathing. The resistance of HH is 0.5 cmH$_2$O/L/s, HME is 1.57 cmH$_2$O/L/s, and HMEF is 2.8 cmH$_2$O/L/s. Similarly, the dead space offered by HH is zero, HME is 60 mL, and HMEF is 100 mL. Based on these values, the work of breathing is least with HH.

Suggested Reading
1. Iotti GA, Olivei MC, Palo A, Galbusera C, Veronesi R, Comelli A, et al. Unfavorable mechanical effects of heat and moisture exchangers in ventilated patients. Intensive Care Med. 1997;23(4):399-405.
2. Rathgeber J, Kazmaier S, Penack O, Züchner K. Evaluation of heated humidifiers for use on intubated patients: a comparative study of humidifying efficiency, flow resistance, and alarm functions using a lung model. Intensive Care Med. 2002;28(6):731-9.

Q.16. With regards to HME filter for ventilator patients, which of the following statements is not true?
 a. Changing HME when it is visibly soiled.
 b. Changing HME when there is overcondensation of moisture.
 c. Routine change after 48 hours of ventilation.
 d. HME does not require to be changed routinely.

Ans. b

Explanation: Routine change of HME is not recommended. There is no cut off on when to change the HME. There is no consensus on after how many hours in ICU the HME to be changed, HME can be changed after about 48–72 hours of use or when visibly soiled or due to overcondensation of moisture.

Suggested Reading
1. American Association for Respiratory Care; Restrepo RD, Walsh BK. Humidification during invasive and noninvasive mechanical ventilation: 2012. Respir Care. 2012;57(5):782-8.

Q.17. A 68-year-old male, known case of COPD on home oxygen therapy, presented with cough with expectoration and breathlessness. On examination, he was conscious but drowsy, his respiratory rate (RR) was 48 breaths/min, SpO_2 was 86% with 10 L nonrebreather mask (NRBM), and BP was 130/70 mm Hg. Arterial blood gas (ABG) showed pH—7.38, pO_2—92, pCO_2—80, and HCO_3—36. What is the immediate step for management?
   a. Intubate the patient.
   b. Send cultures, start broad-spectrum antibiotics, and continue on NRBM with 15 L O_2 flow.
   c. Connect to NIV.
   d. Connect to HFNC with 60 L flow, 100% FiO_2

Ans. c

Explanation: The patient is suffering from acute exacerbation of COPD secondary to a new infection. His ABG is showing respiratory acidosis and NIV would be most beneficial in such situation. Multiple RCTs and meta-analysis have proven that there is level-1 evidence for the use of NIV in acute exacerbation of COPD with respiratory acidosis, cariogenic pulmonary edema, and respiratory failure in immunocompromised host. The contraindications for NIV are impeding cardiac arrest, risk of aspiration, poor mental status, inability to clear secretions, and altered facial morphology where NIV mask cannot obtain a tight seal. HFNC does not improve hypercapnia; hence, it is not an indication here.

Suggested Reading
1. Brochard L, Mancebo J, Wysocki M, Lofaso F, Conti G, Rauss A, et al. Noninvasive ventilation for acute exacerbations of chronic obstructive pulmonary disease. N Engl J Med. 1995;333(13):817-22.
2. Liu YJ, Zhao J, Tang H. Non-invasive ventilation in acute respiratory failure: a meta-analysis. Clin Med (Lond). 2016;16(6):514-23.

Q.18. A 90-year-old female, known case of dementia and Parkinson's, on treatment for past 6 years and bedridden for past 1 year, now presented with the complaints of respiratory distress for past 1 week. On evaluation, she was confused to time and place but oriented to person, slightly agitated and pushing off the face mask, her BP was 100/60 mm Hg, HR was 110 beats/min, SpO_2 was 90% with facemask at 6 L, and RR was 28 breaths/min. ABG showed pH—7.40, pO_2—of 70, pCO_2—34, and HCO_3—27. What is the next step of management?
   a. Connect to HFNC.
   b. Connect to NIV.
   c. Change to nonrebreathing mask with high O_2.
   d. Intubate the patient.

Ans. a

Explanation: The patient is hypoxic and agitated and noncompliant to facemask. Initiating an HFNC would be the most appropriate next step of management. It delivers humidified oxygen in high flow rates thereby minimizing entrapment of room air. As the flow rates are high, it can overcome the high inspiratory flow rate generated by the patients during respiratory failure. As it is supplying humidified oxygen, it also helps in clearing mucus. Every 10 L/min increase in flow rate in HFNC adds a PEEP of 0.7 cmH$_2$O, hence works like a continuous positive airway pressure (CPAP) to some extent. Various studies have proven the benefit of HFNC in hypoxic respiratory failure on par with NIV in intubation rates and decrease in 90-day mortality. Compliance to HFNC would be comparatively better compared to NIV in such agitated patients.

Suggested Reading
1. Frat JP, Thille AW, Mercat A, Girault C, Ragot S, Perbet S, et al. High-flow oxygen through nasal cannula in acute hypoxemic respiratory failure. N Engl J Med. 2015;372(23):2185-96.

Q.19. A 56-year-old male chronic smoker, known case of COPD, presented with cough with copious sputum along with breathlesness. On arrival, he was conscious and oriented, his RR was 30 breaths/min, SpO$_2$ was 90% with 10 L O$_2$ with nonrebreathing mask, BP was 110/70 mm Hg, and HR was 110 beats/min. ABG done showed pH—7.40, pCO$_2$—40, pO$_2$—70, and HCO$_3$—26. Chest X-ray was done and it showed the following picture. What is the next best step of management for this ICU patient?

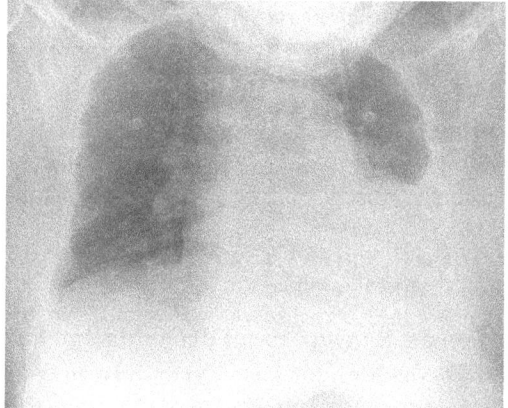

a. Initiate NIV
b. Left pigtail insertion
c. Bronchoscopy
d. Collect cultures, start antibiotics

Ans. c

Explanation: Based on the X-ray, the patient has got a left lung collapse due to mucus plug secondary to acute exacerbation of COPD and that is the main reason for hypoxia. Though initiating NIV would give relief for his respiratory distress, it is not a definitive management. X-ray shows shift of trachea to same side of collapse hence not an effusion so no role for pigtail. The definitive management would be to do immediate bronchoscopy and clear the mucus plug. It can also additionally help in collecting BAL sample for culture sensitivity for this patient.

Suggested Reading
1. Du Rand IA, Blaikley J, Booton R, Chaudhuri N, Gupta V, Khalid S, et al. British Thoracic Society guideline for diagnostic flexible bronchoscopy in adults: accredited by NICE. Thorax. 2013;68 (Suppl 1):i1-i44.

Q.20. Predictors of successful NIV initiation in patients with respiratory failure are all, except:
a. Intact dentition
b. Lower APACHE score
c. Improvement of gas exchange
d. Poor neurological status

Ans. d

Explanation:
The followings are the predictors of success for NIV initiation:
- Lower APACHE scores
- Less air leakage
- Improvement in ABG, HR, and RR in initial 2 hours of initiation
- Good neurological status
- $PaCO_2$ between 45 and 92 mm Hg
- Intact dentition

Suggested Reading
1. Spoletini G, Nicholas SH. Non-invasive positive-pressure ventilation. In: Webb A, Angus D, Finfer S, Gattinoni L, Singer M (Eds). Oxford Textbook of Critical Care, 2nd edition. Oxford, United Kingdom: Oxford University Press; 2016.

Q.21. A 32-year-old lady presented to emergency room with 3 days history of fever, burning micturition, and altered sensorium. In the emergency room, complete blood count revealed leukocytosis, urine routine showed picture of probable urosepsis, and renal function revealed normal creatinine with hypomagnesemia. She was given IV magnesium, amikacin, calcium, and other resuscitative measures. After few minutes, she developed respiratory distress and showed hypoxia, ECG revealed ventricular tachycardia for which IV amiodarone or lidocaine was given and endotracheal intubation was done with anesthetic agent and intravenous rocuronium 1.2 mg/kg body weight. 2 hours postintubation, no spontaneous efforts were noticed. Which of following drugs is not the possible cause for prolonged neuromuscular blockade.
a. Calcium
b. Amikacin
c. Magnesium
d. Lidocaine

Ans. a

Explanation: Many drugs can enhance the neuromuscular block produced by nondepolarizing muscle relaxants. These include volatile anesthetics, aminoglycoside antibiotics, magnesium, intravenous local anesthetics, furosemide, dantrolene, calcium channel blockers, and lithium. Calcium does not enhance neuromuscular blockade and, in fact, it actually antagonizes the effects of magnesium. In patients with hyperparathyroidism and hypercalcemia, there is a decreased sensitivity to nondepolarizing muscle relaxants and shorter durations of action.

Suggested Reading
1. Miller RD, Eriksson LI, Fleisher LA, Wiener-Kronish JP, Cohen NH, Young WL. Miller's Anesthesia, 8th edition. Amsterdam: Elsevier; 2015. pp. 980-3.

Q.22. A 35-year-old male patient had met with a road traffic accident, he had minimal subarachnoid hemorrhage (SAH) in frontal sulci and right clavicle fracture. His GCS was E3VtM5, in view of severe agitation and for tube tolerance, he was started on injection propofol infusion at 100 mg/h. All of the following could develop as complication during course of ICU stay if propofol infusion is continued, except:
   a. Pancreatitis
   b. Hyperlipidemia
   c. Metabolic acidosis
   d. Adrenal suppression

Ans. d

Explanation: Long-term infusion of propofol causes propofol infusion syndrome, which includes metabolic acidosis and includes rhabdomyolysis. Hyperlipidemia may occur with prolonged infusions, hence a close watch for hyperlipidemia especially if patient is on total parenteral infusion must be considered. Pancreatitis is also known complication of prolonged infusion of propofol. Adrenal suppression is a side effect of etomidate and not seen with propofol.

Suggested Reading
1. Brunton LL, Chabner BA, Knollmann BC. Goodman & Gilman's The Pharmacological Basis of Therapeutics, 12th edition. China: McGraw Hill Medical; 2011. pp. 536-7.
2. Miller RD, Pardo M. Basics of Anaesthesia, 6th edition. Philadelphia, PA: Elsevier; p. 671.

Q.23. A 50-year-old man met with a road traffic accident and brought to emergency room with severe traumatic brain injury. A decision of emergency rapid sequence endotracheal intubation was planned. Which of the following diseases is likely to require an increased dose of succinylcholine for neuromuscular blockade?
   a. Myasthenia gravis
   b. ARDS
   c. Polytrauma
   d. Huntington's chorea

Ans. a

Explanation: Succinylcholine acts at the acetylcholine receptors on the muscle. Myasthenia gravis is a condition where there is reduced number of acetylcholine receptors, hence an increased dose of succinylcholine will be required to cause muscle paralysis. Other conditions mentioned including Huntington's chorea have no effect on the number of acetylcholine receptors.

Suggested Reading
1. Fleisher LA. Anaesthesia and Uncommon Diseases, 6th edition. Philadelphia, PA: Saunders; 2012. pp. 264-5; 313-6; 574.

2. Marschall K, Hines RL. Stoelting's Anaesthesia and Co-Existing Disease, 6th edition. Philadelphia, PA: Saunders/Elsevier; 2012; pp. 247; 444; 448-52.

Q.24. A 33-year-old lady with 3 days history of fever, cough with expectoration, and breathing difficulty presents to the emergency room with severe respiratory distress and type-1 respiratory failure. A diagnosis of ARDS is made. Emergency endotracheal intubation was done using injection fentanyl, injection thiopentone sodium, and injection succinylcholine followed by injection atracurium. Postinduction monitor shows hypertension, tachycardia, and she throws an episode of seizure. Urine collected was found to be red to brown in color. The most possible drug to cause the manifestations could be:
a. Fentanyl
b. Thiopentone sodium
c. Atracurium
d. Succinylcholine

Ans. b

Explanation: Acute intermittent porphyria is a condition which presents with seizures, rhabdomyolysis. In this patient, it was triggered with barbiturate drugs (thiopentone sodium).

Suggested Reading
1. Barash PG, Cullen BF, Stoelting RK, Cahalan MK, Stock MC, Ortega R. Clinical Anesthesia, 7th edition. Philadelphia, PA: Lippincott Williams and Wilkins; 2013. pp. 624-5.
2. Marschall K, Hines RL. Stoelting's Anesthesia and Co-Existing Disease, 6th edition. Philadelphia, PA: Saunders; 2012. p. 308.

Q.25. A 34-year-old female met with road traffic accident following which she developed fracture in right frontal bone and fracture of body of C2 cervical vertebrae. During the post-trauma day 1, patient was noticed to have weakness of all four limbs, with shallow pattern of breathing. On day 10 of ward stay, patient developed an episode of fever, severe respiratory distress, and was shifted to ICU. A suspicion of aspiration pneumonitis was made. Patient was found to be tachycardic and she has severe respiratory distress with normal blood pressure. A decision of intubation was made, and injection fentanyl followed by propofol, succinylcholine, and atracurium was given. Shortly after the intubation, however, the patient was noted to develop a wide-complex dysrhythmia. Which of the following could be the possible cause in this patient?
a. Hypokalemia
b. Hypermagnesemia
c. Hypercalcemia
d. Hyperkalemia

Ans. d

Explanation: Succinylcholine-induced hyperkalemia has been described with a variety of conditions, including upper motor nerve injuries (e.g., spinal cord injury), lower motor nerve injuries (e.g., Guillain–Barré syndrome), prolonged chemical denervation, disuse atrophy, direct muscle trauma or inflammation, muscular dystrophies, burns, and sepsis. Upregulation and denervation seem to change the constituent subunits of the acetylcholine receptor, resulting in a longer duration of channel opening, and contribute to the hyperkalemia. In this patient, due to spinal cord injury-associated denervation, upregulation of acetylcholine has caused hyperkalemia.

Suggested Reading
1. Hines RL, Marschall K. Stoelting's Anesthesia and Co-Existing Disease, 5th edition. Philadelphia, PA: Saunders; 2009. pp. 240-2.
2. Miller RD. Miller's Anesthesia, 6th edition. Philadelphia: Elsevier; 2005. pp. 489-90.
3. Stoelting RK, Hillier SC. Pharmacology and Physiology in Anesthetic Practice, 4th edition. Philadelphia: Lippincott Williams & Wilkins; 2005. pp. 220-1.

Q.26. **A 45-year-old male patient with diabetes and hypertension presents to the emergency room with the complaints of fever and necrotizing fasciitis of left leg. He is also a case of coronary artery disease on regular antiplatelets and other medications with EF of 20%. 15 minutes postpresentation to emergency room, he develops severe respiratory distress and hypotension. After fluid bolus and inotrope agents initiation, a decision of endotracheal intubation is made. The emergency room resident gives injection fentanyl, injection etomidate, and injection rocuronium and performs endotracheal intubation. Which of the complications is less likely?**
a. Nausea and vomiting
b. Pain on injection
c. Adrenal suppression
d. None

Ans. c

Explanation: Etomidate is an inducing agent used for rapid sequence intubation. The incidence of hypotension is less compared to other agents. It is associated with risk of adrenal suppression.

Suggested Reading
1. Ray DC, McKeown DW. Effect of induction agent on vasopressor and steroid use, and outcome in patients with septic shock. Crit Care. 2007;11:R56.
2. Miller RD. Miller's Anaesthesia, 6th edition. Philadelphia: Elsevier; 2005. p. 354.

Q.27. **A 70-year-old male patient, a known case of seizure disorder and bronchial asthma, presented to the emergency room with an episode of seizure. On asking about the history, he was found to have missed a dose of routine antiepileptic. He was given injection lorazepam, oxygen through facemask, levetiracetam, and seizures settled after the initial measures. 5 minutes later, the patient had a second episode of seizure and a repeat dose of lorazepam was given and a decision of endotracheal intubation was taken by the emergency room doctor. A plan of giving injection fentanyl, injection propofol, and succinylcholine was made and endotracheal intubation was performed. Postintubation after 8 minutes, injection atracurium was given IV and plan to shift the patient to ICU was made. The bedside sister comes running saying that the patient is now having tachycardia, hypotension,**

and ventilator is alarming high peak airway pressure. What would be our next immediate step in management?
   a. Extubate the patient.
   b. Give another dose of lorazepam and antiepileptic.
   c. IV fluids and injection adrenaline
   d. Repeat dose of atracurium

Ans. c

Explanation: Anaphylactic reaction can range from mild reaction to severe anaphylactic shock and death. Signs and symptoms include flushing, urticaria, hypotension, tachycardia, bronchospasm, and cardiac arrest, but silent chest and impending cardiac arrest are rare events. Epinephrine is the most useful drug as it is effective in both bronchospasm and cardiovascular collapse. Anaphylaxis to atracurium has been reported. Anaphylactic reaction may take several hours to resolve and the patient must be closely observed and managed symptomatically until stable. Antihistamines and corticosteroids are usually administered once the acute phase is over. Every patient with suspected anaphylactic reaction should be investigated with skin pinprick test, radioimmunoassays, etc. to identify the responsible drugs.

Suggested Reading
   1. Siler JN, Mager JG. Atracurium: Hypotension, tachycardia and bronchospasm. Anaesthesiology. 1985;62:645-6.

Q.28. A 29-year-old female with COVID-19 pneumonia and moderate ARDS is planned for a surgical tracheostomy. Which of the following measures is not helpful in preventing droplet infection?
   a. Preoperative positioning of cuff at the level of vocal cord
   b. Negative pressure room
   c. Good plane of sedation and paralysis
   d. Using a transparent film above tracheal rent during withdrawal

Ans. a

Explanation: Tracheostomy in a COVID patient poses risk of drop transmission during the procedure. Various strategies are described to reduce droplet spread: use of negative pressure room, adequate sedation, neuromuscular blockade to prevent coughing, and a transparent film placed on the incision while withdrawing the tube. The endotracheal tube to be withdrawn and cuff to be repositioned below the vocal cord to prevent air leak.

Q.29. Which of the following is a technique of percutaneous tracheostomy?
   a. Frova technique
   b. Fantoni's translaryngeal tracheostomy
   c. Griggs technique
   d. All of the above

Ans. d

Suggested Reading

1. Mehta C, Mehta Y. Percutaneous tracheostomy. Ann Card Anaesth. 2017; 20(Supplement): S19-S25.

Q.30. A 29-year-old male patient is brought to the hospital with history of road traffic accident following two-wheeler versus four-wheeler head-on collision. On arrival, his GCS was very low with crepitus present on multiple facial regions. Bleeding was noted from nose and ear. In order to protect the airway, the emergency room resident decides to intubate the patient but fails to do so after following the difficult airway algorithm, he realizes that he is in a CICO/cannot oxygenate situation and consultant plans for emergency surgical cricothyrotomy. Which of the following is complication of the procedure?
a. Bleeding
b. Unintentional tracheostomy
c. Passage of the tube into an extratracheal location
d. All of the above

Ans. d

Explanation: All of the above are complications of a surgical cricothyroidotomy.

Suggested Reading

1. McKenna P, Desai NM, Tariq A, Morley EJ. (2023). Cricothyrotomy. [online] Available from: https://www.ncbi.nlm.nih.gov/books/NBK537350/. [Last accessed May, 2023]

CHAPTER 2

Resuscitation

Kanwalpreet Sodhi, Manender Kumar, Sumati Verma

A-TYPE QUESTIONS

Q.1. While providing basic life support to adult cardiac arrest victim, after the placement of an advanced airway such as laryngeal mask airway:
a. The compression: ventilations ratio remains the same, i.e., 30:2.
b. As there is second rescuer available, the compression:ventilation ratio changes to 15:2.
c. The compression:ventilation ratio changes to 1:1.
d. There is no ratio; the compressor continues with the compressions and the other rescuer provides ventilation at 10 breaths/min.

Ans. d

Explanation: According to the American Heart Association (AHA) and International Liaison Committee on Resuscitation (ILCOR) cardiopulmonary resuscitation (CPR) 2020 guidelines, the compressions and ventilation are done independently and ratio is 30:2, whether there is single or double rescuer. But after the placement of advanced airway (either endotracheal tube or supraglottic device), there is no ratio between compressions and ventilation. In such case, the person doing compression continues chest compression uninterruptedly for a period of 2 minutes at the rate of 100–120 compressions/min and the person performing ventilation continues to deliver breaths at the rate of 10 breaths/min through advanced airway. After 2 minutes, the pulse check is to be performed.

Suggested Reading
1. Merchant RM, Topjian AA, Panchal AR, Cheng A, Aziz K, Berg KM, et al.; on behalf of the Adult Basic and Advanced Life Support, Pediatric Basic and Advanced Life Support, Neonatal Life Support, Resuscitation Education Science, and Systems of Care Writing Groups. Part 1: executive summary: 2020 American Heart Association Guidelines for Cardiopulmonary Resuscitation and Emergency Cardiovascular Care. Circulation. 2020;142(Suppl 2): S337-57.
2. Panchal AR, Bartos JA, Cabañas JG, Donnino MW, Drennan IR, Hirsch KG, et al.; on behalf of the Adult Basic and Advanced Life Support Writing Group. Part 3: adult basic and advanced life support: 2020 American Heart Association Guidelines for Cardiopulmonary Resuscitation and Emergency Cardiovascular Care. Circulation. 2020;142(Suppl 2):S366-S468.

Q.2. Which of the following is not an inclusion criterion for extracorporeal cardiopulmonary resuscitation (eCPR)?
  a. Witnessed cardiac arrest
  b. Aortic valve incompetence
  c. Presence of reversible cause of cardiac arrest
  d. Arrest to extracorporeal membrane oxygenation (ECMO) flow <60 minutes "low-flow interval"
  e. Arrest to first CPR (no-flow interval) <5 minutes, i.e., bystander CPR

Ans. b

Explanation: Extracorporeal cardiopulmonary resuscitation (eCPR) is defined as the rapid initiation of venoarterial ECMO during CPR in patients who have a sudden, witnessed cessation of cardiac mechanical activity. eCPR is indicated in patients with witnessed cardiac arrest having a reversible cause of arrest, those undergoing continuous CPR, with no response to conventional CPR. According to Extracorporeal Life Support Organization (ELSO) guidelines, potential inclusion criteria for eCPR include:
- Age <70 years
- Witnessed cardiac arrest
- Arrest to first CPR (no-flow interval) <5 minutes (i.e., bystander CPR)
- Initial cardiac rhythm of VF/pulseless VT/pulseless electrical activity (PEA)
- Arrest to ECMO flow <60 minutes "low-flow interval"
- End-tidal carbon dioxide ($ETCO_2$) >10 mm Hg (1.3 kPa) during conventional CPR before cannulation for ECMO
- Intermittent return of spontaneous circulation (ROSC) or recurrent VF
- Absence of previously known life-limiting comorbidities, e.g., end-stage heart failure/chronic obstructive pulmonary disease/end-stage renal failure/liver failure/terminal illness
- No known aortic valve incompetence

In the out-of-hospital cardiac arrest scenarios, other potential indications for eCPR are accidental hypothermia and poisoning due to sedative and/or cardiotoxic drugs. Contraindications for eCPR include concomitant major trauma, end-stage terminal illness or significant medical comorbidities, uncontrolled hemorrhage or recent cerebral hemorrhage, uncontrolled coagulopathy, unsuccessful CPR with no ROSC for 30 minutes or if DNR orders are there and any other potential contraindications for ECMO perse such as acute aortic valve insufficiency.

Suggested Reading
1. Kumar KM. ECPR-extracorporeal cardiopulmonary resuscitation. Indian J Thorac Cardiovasc Surg. 2021;37(Suppl 2):294-302.
2. Mishra RC, Sodhi K, Prakash KC, Kapoor PM. Extracorporeal Cardiopulmonary Resuscitation. ISCCM Manual of RRT and ECMO in ICU, 1st edition. New Delhi: Jaypee Brothers Medical Publisher; 2020.
3. Pappalardo F, Montisci A. What is extracorporeal cardiopulmonary resuscitation? J Thorac Dis. 2017;9:1415-9.

4. Richardson AC, Tonna JE, Nanjayya V, Nixon P, Abrams DC, Raman L, et al. Extracorporeal cardiopulmonary resuscitation in adults. Interim Guideline Consensus Statement from the Extracorporeal Life Support Organization. ASAIO J. 2021;67(3):221-8.

Q.3. During resuscitation of a 6-year-old child in cardiac arrest with asystole, appropriate doses of epinephrine are provided every 3–5 minutes. The rationale for epinephrine administration in cardiac arrest is:
   a. Epinephrine decreases systemic vascular resistance.
   b. Epinephrine decreases myocardial contraction.
   c. Epinephrine increases coronary artery perfusion.
   d. Epinephrine decreases myocardial oxygen consumption.

Ans. c

Explanation: At resuscitative doses of epinephrine, the α-adrenergic receptor effect predominates, increasing systemic vascular resistance in addition to increasing cardiac output. The α-adrenergic mediated vasoconstriction of epinephrine increases aortic diastolic pressure and thus coronary perfusion pressure which is a critical determinant of successful resuscitation.

Suggested Reading
1. Jayashree M, Kulgod V, Sharma AK. IAP ALS Handbook, Second edition. IAP National Publication House, New Delhi: Indian Academy of Pediatrics; 2020.
2. Panchal AR, Bartos JA, Cabañas JG, Donnino MW, Drennan IR, Hirsch KG, et al.; on behalf of the Adult Basic and Advanced Life Support Writing Group. Part 3: adult basic and advanced life support: 2020 American Heart Association Guidelines for Cardiopulmonary Resuscitation and Emergency Cardiovascular Care. Circulation. 2020;142 (Suppl 2): S366-S468.
3. Shaffner DH, Nichols DG. Rogers' Textbook of Pediatric Intensive Care, 5th edition. Philadelphia: Lippincott Williams and Wilkins; 2015.

Q.4. You are resuscitating an adult cardiac arrest victim and performing 4th set of compressions. Your associate who had gone to activate EMS comes back with an automated external defibrillator (AED). What should be your next action?
   a. You continue with chest compressions and ventilations and apply the AED after completion of five cycles of compressions:ventilation.
   b. You stop compressions and apply AED, as the priority is to assess the rhythm.
   c. You continue with chest compressions and the associate applies the AED pads and tells you to stop compressions to check for rhythm.
   d. Your associate applies AED pads during compressions and you check for the rhythm after completion of five cycles of compressions:ventilation.

Ans. c

Explanation: Ventricular fibrillation (VF) is the most common cause of adult cardiac arrest. With every passing minute, the chances of reverting to organized rhythm decrease by 7%. The only effective treatment of VF is rapid defibrillation as soon as possible. Automated external defibrillator (AED) analyzes the heart rhythm: whether shockable or nonshockable and gives voice prompts to deliver DC shock in case of shockable rhythm. When AED is brought to the scenario, the priority is to analyze the heart rhythm and AED pads should be applied promptly. But at the same time, the cornerstone of effective CPR is to minimize interruptions in chest compressions. So, it is advisable to attach the AED pads while chest compressions are going on and pause for rhythm check once the pads have been applied.

Suggested Reading
1. Panchal AR, Bartos JA, Cabañas JG, Donnino MW, Drennan IR, Hirsch KG, et al.; on behalf of the Adult Basic and Advanced Life Support Writing Group. Part 3: adult basic and advanced life support: 2020 American Heart Association Guidelines for Cardiopulmonary Resuscitation and Emergency Cardiovascular Care. Circulation. 2020;142 (Suppl 2):S366-S468.

Q.5. Which is the most common presenting rhythm in a pediatric patient in cardiac arrest?
 a. Asystole
 b. Bradycardia
 c. Torsades de Pointes
 d. Ventricular fibrillation

Ans. a

Explanation: Asystole is the most common presenting rhythm in a pediatric patient who presents in cardiac arrest (CA), seen in 25–70% of victims. Bradycardia and pulseless electrical activity (PEA) are other common rhythms, while ventricular arrest rhythm, ventricular fibrillation (VF), or pulseless ventricular tachycardia (VT) is infrequent, being reported in 10–14% of the pediatric patients with in-hospital CA. Systemic disturbances, such as hypoxia, acidosis, sepsis, and hypovolemia, often precede the arrest and lead to asystole rhythm.

Suggested Reading
1. Nadkarni VM, Larkin GL, Peberdy MA, Carey SM, Kaye W, Mancini ME, et al. First documented rhythm and clinical outcome from in-hospital cardiac arrest among children and adults. JAMA. 2006;295:50-7.
2. Shaffner DH, Nichols DG. Rogers' Textbook of Pediatric Intensive Care, 5th edition. Philadelphia: Lippincott Williams and Wilkins; 2015.
3. Zimmerman JJ, Rotta AT. Fuhrman & Zimmerman's Pediatric Critical Care, 6th edition. Philadelphia: Elsevier; 2021.

Q.6. What is the most accurate method of confirmation of correct placement of advanced airway?
 a. Plethysmography to watch for rise in SpO_2
 b. Continuous waveform capnography
 c. 5-point chest auscultation
 d. Quantitative capnometry

Ans. b

Explanation: Continuous waveform capnography is the most accurate method of confirmation of correct placement of advanced airway. Literature has shown 100% specificity with waveform capnography for confirming endotracheal tube (ETT) position during cardiac arrest. It provides visual waveform analysis and the numerical value of exhaled end-tidal carbon dioxide (EtCO$_2$). EtCO$_2$ is also an important parameter to analyze the quality of chest compressions. EtCO$_2$ values remaining consistently below 10 mm Hg are poor prognostic indicator for ROSC. Quantitative capnometry only provides numerical value of EtCO$_2$ that may be misleading as during esophageal intubation, first few breaths may continue to have EtCO$_2$ due to the presence of gastric air, thereby giving false positive value. Plethysmography providing SpO$_2$ values has no role during cardiac arrest scenario. 5-point auscultation may be misleading in detecting correct placement of advanced airway.

Suggested Reading
1. Mohamed BA. Airway management during cardiopulmonary resuscitation. Curr Anesthesiol Rep. 2022;12(3):363-72.
2. Panchal AR, Bartos JA, Cabañas JG, Donnino MW, Drennan IR, Hirsch KG, et al.; on behalf of the Adult Basic and Advanced Life Support Writing Group. Part 3: adult basic and advanced life support: 2020 American Heart Association Guidelines for Cardiopulmonary Resuscitation and Emergency Cardiovascular Care. Circulation. 2020;142 (Suppl 2):S366-468.
3. Sandroni C, De Santis P, D'Arrigo S. Capnography during cardiac arrest. Resuscitation. 2018;132:73-7.
4. Sheak KR, Wiebe DJ, Leary M, Babaeizadeh S, Yuen TC, Zive D, et al. Quantitative relationship between end-tidal carbon dioxide and CPR quality during both in-hospital and out-of-hospital cardiac arrest. Resuscitation. 2015;89:149-54.

Q.7. With regard to targeted temperature management (TTM), which of the following is incorrect?
a. Cardiac arrest patients do not benefit from lowering temperatures, targeting hypothermia at 32°C for 12–24 hours.
b. Routine use of prehospital cooling with rapid infusion of cold intravenous fluids is beneficial in comatose patients after return of spontaneous circulation (ROSC).
c. Active prevention of fever <37.5°C for at least 72 hours is recommended in postcardiac arrest patients who remain comatose.
d. During postresuscitation TTM, surface or endovascular temperature lowering techniques can be used.

Ans. b

Explanation: European Resuscitation Council and European Society of Intensive Care Medicine guidelines 2021 on postresuscitation care recommend targeted temperature management (TTM) for adults after either out-of-hospital or in-hospital cardiac arrest (OHCA or IHCA) with any initial rhythm who remain unresponsive after ROSC, maintaining a target temperature at a constant value between 32 and 36°C for at least 24 hours; using surface or endovascular temperature lowering techniques avoiding fever (>37.7°C) for at least 72 hours after ROSC in patients who remain in coma and not using any prehospital intravenous cold fluids to initiate hypothermia.

Suggested Reading
1. Nolan JP, Sandroni C, Böttiger BW, Cariou A, Cronberg T, Friberg H, et al. European Resuscitation Council and European Society of Intensive Care Medicine guidelines 2021: post-resuscitation care. Intensive Care Med. 2021;47:369-421.

2. Panchal AR, Bartos JA, Cabañas JG, Donnino MW, Drennan IR, Hirsch KG, et al.; on behalf of the Adult Basic and Advanced Life Support Writing Group. Part 3: adult basic and advanced life support: 2020 American Heart Association Guidelines for Cardiopulmonary Resuscitation and Emergency Cardiovascular Care. Circulation. 2020;142 (Suppl 2):S366-468.

Q.8. An 8-year-old boy presents to emergency after being struck by a vehicle while riding his bike. He was awake and complaining of neck pain immediately after the accident but is somnolent with sonorous respirations on examination in the emergency. His oxygen saturation is 89% and heart rate is 50 beats/min. What are the most appropriate initial steps in assessment and management for this patient?
  a. Evaluate-identify-intervene; STAT head CT scan
  b. Evaluate-identify-intervene; intubation
  c. First impression; focused assessment with sonography for trauma (FAST) examination to evaluate for pericardial fluid
  d. First impression; cardiopulmonary resuscitation

Ans. d

Explanation: Pediatric Advanced Life Support (PALS) recommends a systematic approach in such scenario, similar to both advanced cardiac life support (ACLS) and advanced trauma life support (ATLS). First impression followed by evaluate-identify-intervene (which includes primary assessment, secondary assessment, and diagnostic tests) constitutes the algorithmic steps in the PALS algorithm. The algorithm starts with a first impression to help determine whether or not the patient is in imminent danger, either of cardiac or respiratory failure. Patients who are conscious or unconscious, but breathing can progress to the evaluate-identify-intervene step in the algorithm. Patients who are not breathing adequately but have a pulse greater than 60 beats/min should undergo rescue breathing. Patients with a pulse <60 beats/min should undergo CPR. Evaluate-identify-intervene are components of the primary assessment and secondary assessment and guide the choice of diagnostic testing. The primary assessment follows the primary survey in ATLS: Airway, Breathing, Circulation, Disability, Exposure. An oxygen saturation that is <90% indicates that respiratory support is needed. In the pediatric population, a heart rate <60 beats/min suggests cardiac failure, and CPR should be initiated.

Suggested Reading
1. de Caen AR, Berg MD, Charmides L, Gooden CK, Hickey RW, Scott HF, et al. Part 12: Pediatric Advanced Life Support: 2015 American Heart Association Guidelines Update for Cardiopulmonary Resuscitation and Emergency Cardiovascular Care. Circulation. 2015;132(18 Suppl 2):S52 6-42.
2. Jayashree M, Kulgod V, Sharma AK. IAP ALS Handbook, Second edition. IAP National Publication House, New Delhi: Indian Academy of Pediatrics; 2020.
3. Topjian AA, Raymond TT, Atkins D, Chan M, Duff JP, Joyner Jr BL, et al.; on behalf of the Pediatric Basic and Advanced Life Support Collaborators. Pediatric Basic and Advanced Life Support: 2020 American Heart Association Guidelines for Cardiopulmonary Resuscitation and Emergency Cardiovascular Care. Circulation. 2020;142:S469-523.

Q.9. As a part of EMS team, you arrive at the scenario and find an unconscious, unresponsive adult. You try to palpate for the carotid pulse and look for any signs of respiration. There are no signs of normal respiration, but you are unsure about presence of carotid pulse. What should you do next?
   a. Start immediately with chest compressions.
   b. You should look for the carotid pulse on the other side for 5-10 seconds.
   c. You should immediately start with rescue breaths and try to palpate the carotid after 2 rescue breaths.
   d. You should start with bag and mask ventilation and look for carotid pulse after 2 minutes.

Ans. a

Explanation: All healthcare providers providing CPR must check carotid pulse within 5-10 seconds. They have to check the carotid pulse on the same side on which are standing/kneeling. The healthcare providers must feel for a definitive pulse and if you cannot find a definitive carotid pulse within 10 seconds, you should proceed immediately with chest compressions.

Suggested Reading
1. Panchal AR, Bartos JA, Cabañas JG, Donnino MW, Drennan IR, Hirsch KG, et al.; on behalf of the Adult Basic and Advanced Life Support Writing Group. Part 3: adult basic and advanced life support: 2020 American Heart Association Guidelines for Cardiopulmonary Resuscitation and Emergency Cardiovascular Care. Circulation. 2020;142(Suppl 2):S366-468.

Q.10. You arrive at the scenario of an adult cardiac arrest and upon attaching the monitor, you find the following rhythm on ECG monitor. What should be your next action?

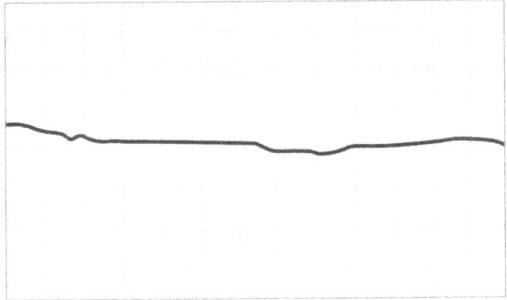

   a. Start with chest compressions immediately.
   b. Start chest compressions and prepare for defibrillation.
   c. Check for other differentials for the flat line ECG like lead placement, ECG gain, etc..
   d. Announce to terminate the resuscitative efforts.

Ans. c

Explanation: The rhythm in the provided ECG is asystole for which the intervention required is chest compressions followed by administration of epinephrine as in asystole/PEA limb of adult cardiac arrest ACLS algorithm. Whenever this rhythm is detected, before proceeding further, it is important to differentiate true asystole from false asystole. For this, flat line protocol should be performed. In this, firstly, all the ECG leads connections on patient's body and the monitor should be confirmed. Thereafter, it should be checked that correct lead has been selected on the monitor and it is not showing paddle mode. Another important maneuver to be done is increasing the size/gain of ECG, to rule out fine ventricular fibrillation, that may otherwise show as asystole, but may become prominent when ECG gain is increased. It is important to differentiate asystole from VF since the treatment protocols are entirely different and VF is a favorable rhythm than asystole as it denotes presence of some ATP in the myocardium, the treatment of which is immediate defibrillation which can revert the rhythm to organized rhythm.

Suggested Reading
1. Jordan MR, Lopez RA, Morrisonponce D. Asystole. [online] Available from https://www.ncbi.nlm.nih.gov/books/NBK430866/. [Last accessed May, 2023]
2. Panchal AR, Bartos JA, Cabañas JG, Donnino MW, Drennan IR, Hirsch KG, et al.; on behalf of the Adult Basic and Advanced Life Support Writing Group. Part 3: adult basic and advanced life support: 2020 American Heart Association Guidelines for Cardiopulmonary Resuscitation and Emergency Cardiovascular Care. Circulation. 2020;142(Suppl 2):S366-468.

Q.11. **A 6-year-old female suffers a cardiac arrest in pediatric ward. She is in ventricular fibrillation. The team is struggling with venous access. Full CPR is in progress. The patient is intubated. What is the recommended next intervention?**
a. A precordial thump
b. Administration of emergency drugs via the endotracheal tube (ETT)
c. Intraosseous access as a route of drug delivery
d. Amiodarone after the fourth DC shock

Ans. c

Explanation: The role of precordial thump is de-emphasized and should not be attempted unless the arrest was witnessed and current monitored. Delivery of drugs via tracheal tube is no longer recommended as per the guidelines. Both adult and pediatric resuscitation guidelines recommend that if intravenous access cannot be achieved, drugs should be immediately administered via the intraosseous (IO) route. IO cannulation provides access to a noncollapsible venous plexus, enabling drug delivery similar to that achieved by central venous access. Amiodarone 5 mg/kg (in children) is recommended immediately after third shock and may be repeated up to maximum three doses for refractory VF or pulseless VT.

Suggested Reading
1. Jayashree M, Kulgod V, Sharma AK. IAP ALS Handbook, Second edition. IAP National Publication House, New Delhi: Indian Academy of Pediatrics; 2020.
2. Panchal AR, Bartos JA, Cabañas JG, Donnino MW, Drennan IR, Hirsch KG, et al.; on behalf of the Adult Basic and Advanced Life Support Writing Group. Part 3: adult basic and advanced life support: 2020 American Heart Association Guidelines for Cardiopulmonary Resuscitation and Emergency Cardiovascular Care. Circulation. 2020;142(Suppl 2): S366-468.

3. Topjian AA, Raymond TT, Atkins D, Chan M, Duff JP, Joyner Jr BL, et al.; on behalf of the Pediatric Basic and Advanced Life Support Collaborators. Pediatric Basic and Advanced Life Support: 2020 American Heart Association Guidelines for Cardiopulmonary Resuscitation and Emergency Cardiovascular Care. Circulation. 2020;142:S469-523.

Q.12. Which of the following is not a component of good team dynamics during CPR?
  a. Draw continuous attention to decisions about differential diagnoses.
  b. Give drugs without verbally confirming the order with the team leader.
  c. Suggest an alternative drug or dose in a confident manner.
  d. Ask for a new task or role if you are unable to perform your assigned task because it is beyond your level of experience or competence.

Ans. b

Explanation: For an effective CPR, a very high-performance team is needed with a leader to organize the efforts of the group and making sure everything is done at the right time in the right way by monitoring and integrating individual performance of team members who perform the skills efficiently as per their scope of practice. The components of effective team dynamics include clear roles and responsibility, clear messages, knowing your limitations, constructive interventions, knowledge sharing, summarizing and reevaluating, closed-loop communications, and mutual respect. Verbal confirmation is important for the closed-loop communication.

Suggested Reading
1. American Heart Association. Effective high performance team dynamics. [online] Available from https://ebooks.heart.org/contentresolver/epub/50044708/OEBPS/Part3.html. [Last accessed May, 2023]

Q.13. During cardiac arrest in pregnancy, which is not true?
  a. Oxygenation and airway management should be prioritized during resuscitation.
  b. Fetal monitoring should always be undertaken during cardiac arrest in pregnancy.
  c. Targeted temperature management (TTM) for pregnant women who remain comatose after resuscitation from cardiac arrest is recommended.
  d. During TTM of pregnant patient, it is recommended that the fetus be continuously monitored for bradycardia as a potential complication, and obstetric and neonatal consultation should be sought.

Ans. b

Explanation: Recommendations for managing cardiac arrest in pregnancy were reviewed in the 2020 AHA CPR Guidelines. Airway, ventilation, and oxygenation are priorities in pregnancy due to an increase in maternal metabolism, a decrease in functional reserve capacity due to the gravid uterus, and the risk of fetal hypoxemia and the associated brain injury. Evaluation of the fetal heart may distract the performer from necessary resuscitation elements and is not helpful during maternal cardiac arrest. Pregnant women who survive cardiac arrest should receive TTM just as any other survivors would, with consideration for the status of the fetus that may remain in utero, thereby needing continuous fetal monitoring.

Suggested Reading
1. Jeejeebhoy FM, Zelop CM, Lipman S, Carvalho B, Joglar J, Mhyre JM, et al. Cardiac Arrest in Pregnancy: A Scientific Statement from the American Heart Association. Circulation. 2015;132:1747-73.
2. Panchal AR, Bartos JA, Cabañas JG, Donnino MW, Drennan IR, Hirsch KG, et al.; on behalf of the Adult Basic and Advanced Life Support Writing Group. Part 3: adult basic and advanced life support: 2020 American Heart Association Guidelines for Cardiopulmonary Resuscitation and Emergency Cardiovascular Care. Circulation. 2020;142(Suppl 2):S366-468.

For questions 14–16:
You are a team leader of the ACLS team in the scenario of adult cardiac arrest. The victim is unresponsive, not breathing, and has a nondefinitive carotid pulse. The initial rhythm found on ECG monitor is following:

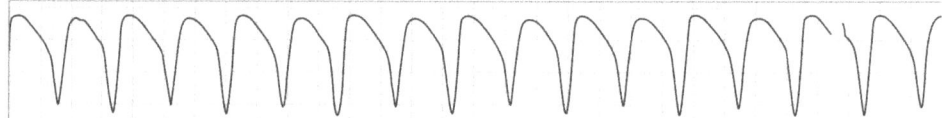

Q.14. What should be the immediate action taken by your team?
a. Immediate cardioversion with 100 Joules.
b. Continue chest compressions with ventilations and reassess the rhythm after 2 minutes.
c. Try to look for the causes such as 5Hs and 5Ts.
d. Immediate defibrillation and start chest compressions.

Ans. d

Explanation: The given scenario is adult cardiac arrest with pulseless ventricular tachycardia. Immediate intervention required in this case is rapid defibrillation with high-energy current. It is recommended to use device-specific energy, which is usually 120–200 Joules and 360 Joules in case of biphasic and monophasic defibrillator, respectively. The delivery of DC shock must be immediately followed by good-quality chest compressions and no rhythm check should be done immediately after delivery of shock. Considering differential diagnoses is important which should go side by side, but the first and immediate intervention in this case is rapid defibrillation and immediate resumption of chest compressions.

Suggested Reading
1. Panchal AR, Bartos JA, Cabañas JG, Donnino MW, Drennan IR, Hirsch KG, et al.; on behalf of the Adult Basic and Advanced Life Support Writing Group. Part 3: adult basic and advanced life support: 2020 American Heart Association Guidelines for Cardiopulmonary Resuscitation and Emergency Cardiovascular Care. Circulation. 2020;142(Suppl 2): S366-468.

Q.15. After 2 minutes of DC shock and continued CPR, the rhythm on the monitor remains the same. What should you do now?
a. Give 2–3 stacked DC shocks and look for the rhythm change.

b. Give 3 stacked DC shocks of increasing energy and start chest compressions.
c. Give only one shock of preferably higher energy and look for the change in rhythm and administer 1 mg of epinephrine and amiodarone.
d. Give only one shock of preferably higher energy; start with chest compressions immediately; and administer 1 mg epinephrine.

Ans. d

Explanation: According to AHA cardiac arrest algorithm, after the delivery of 1st shock and 2 minutes of CPR, rhythm check is recommended. When there is no change in rhythm from previous one, like in this case where rhythm is again pulseless VT, no pulse check should be performed. Another unsynchronized DC shock is to be given. The energy of shock may be higher than the previous one. There are studies showing that stacked shock strategy or double sequential external defibrillation was superior to a single shock strategy for successful defibrillation and better resuscitation outcomes in treating shockable rythms but the strategy has not been included in the guidelines. Immediately after the delivery of shock, no rhythm or pulse check is to be done and chest compressions must be started as soon as the shock is delivered. The drug recommended at this time is epinephrine in the dosage of 1 mg rapid IV/IO push followed by 20 mL of saline and raising the extremity while chest compressions are going on. The epinephrine can be repeated after every 3–5 minutes.

Suggested Reading
1. Cheskes S, Dorian P, Feldman M, McLeod S, Scales DC, Pinto R, et al. Double sequential external defibrillation for refractory ventricular fibrillation: the DOSE VF pilot randomized controlled trial. Resuscitation. 2020;150:178-84. doi: 10.1016/j.resuscitation.2020.02.010
2. Kim S, Jung WJ, Roh YI, Kim TY, Hwang SO, Cha KC. Comparison of Resuscitation Outcomes Between 2- or 3-Stacked Defibrillation Strategies with Minimally Interrupted Chest Compression and the Single Defibrillation Strategy: A Swine Cardiac Arrest Model. J Am Heart Assoc. 2021;10:e021250. https://doi.org/10.1161/JAHA.121.021250
3. Panchal AR, Bartos JA, Cabañas JG, Donnino MW, Drennan IR, Hirsch KG, et al.; on behalf of the Adult Basic and Advanced Life Support Writing Group. Part 3: adult basic and advanced life support: 2020 American Heart Association Guidelines for Cardiopulmonary Resuscitation and Emergency Cardiovascular Care. Circulation. 2020;142(Suppl 2): S366-468.

Q.16. After giving 2 shocks and continued high-quality CPR, there is no change in rhythm. What is your next action?
a. Immediate defibrillation followed by chest compressions and administration of amiodarone or lignocaine.
b. Immediate defibrillation followed by chest and administration of second dose of 1 mg of epinephrine.
c. Continue with high-quality chest compressions without defibrillation as defibrillation is unlikely to help now.
d. Announce for termination of resuscitative efforts.

Ans. a

Explanation: According to AHA cardiac arrest ACLS algorithm, when there is no change in rhythm from VF/pulseless VT even after delivery of 2 shocks and high-quality basic life support (BLS), the next action is delivery of one unsynchronized high-energy defibrillatory shock. This is to be followed by immediate resumption of chest compressions. The drug recommended at this stage is amiodarone or lignocaine rapid IV/IO push followed by 20 mL of saline after 3-5 minutes and raising the extremity. The first dose of amiodarone is 300 mg, which can be repeated as second dose of 150 mg. The first dose of lignocaine is 1.0-1.5 mg/kg and subsequent second dose is 0.5-0.75 mg/kg. At all these times, there should be ongoing efforts to look for and treat any reversible causes like 5Hs and 5Ts [hypovolemia, hypoxia, hydrogen ion (acidosis), hypo-/hyperkalemia, hypothermia, tension pneumothorax, cardiac tamponade, toxins, pulmonary thrombosis, and coronary thrombosis].

Suggested Reading
1. Panchal AR, Bartos JA, Cabañas JG, Donnino MW, Drennan IR, Hirsch KG, et al.; on behalf of the Adult Basic and Advanced Life Support Writing Group. Part 3: adult basic and advanced life support: 2020 American Heart Association Guidelines for Cardiopulmonary Resuscitation and Emergency Cardiovascular Care. Circulation. 2020;142(Suppl 2):S366-468.

Q.17. Which of the following statements regarding temperature regulation in postresuscitation care is true?
a. Fever (temperature >37.5°C) should be aggressively treated.
b. Continuous temperature monitoring is not required.
c. Therapeutic hypothermia has shown beneficial effects and is recommended for all patients who remain comatose after ROSC.
d. Fever after ROSC is associated with good neurological outcome.

Ans. a

Explanation: Guidelines on postresuscitation care recommend TTM for adults after either out-of-hospital or in-hospital cardiac arrest (OHCA or IHCA) with any initial rhythm who remain unresponsive after ROSC, maintaining a target temperature at a constant value between 32 and 36°C for at least 24 hours; avoiding fever (>37.7°C) for at least 72 hours after ROSC in patients who remain in coma. Postresuscitation fever and hyperglycemia have been associated with worse neurological outcomes and must be strictly avoided. For infants and children (1 day old to <18 years) remaining comatose after OHCA or IHCA, the recommendations are either 2 days of initial continuous hypothermia (32-34°C) followed by normothermia for 3 days or maintaining normothermia (36-37.5°C), strictly avoiding hyperthermia. TTM-2 trial has convincingly shown no benefit of hypothermia as compared to normothermia.

Suggested Reading
1. Dankiewicz J, Cronberg T, Lilja G, Jakobsen JC, Levin H, Ullén S, et al.; for the TTM2 Trial Investigators. Hypothermia versus normothermia after out-of-hospital cardiac arrest. N Engl J Med. 2021;384:2283-94.
2. Jayashree M, Kulgod V, Sharma AK. IAP ALS Handbook, Second edition. IAP National Publication House, New Delhi: Indian Academy of Pediatrics; 2020.

3. Nolan JP, Sandroni C, Böttiger BW, Cariou A, Cronberg T, Friberg H, et al. European Resuscitation Council and European Society of Intensive Care Medicine guidelines 2021: post-resuscitation care. Intensive Care Med. 2021;47:369-421.
4. Panchal AR, Bartos JA, Cabañas JG, Donnino MW, Drennan IR, Hirsch KG, et al.; on behalf of the Adult Basic and Advanced Life Support Writing Group. Part 3: adult basic and advanced life support: 2020 American Heart Association Guidelines for Cardiopulmonary Resuscitation and Emergency Cardiovascular Care. Circulation. 2020;142(Suppl 2):S366-468.
5. Topjian AA, Raymond TT, Atkins D, Chan M, Duff JP, Joyner BL, et al.; on behalf of the Pediatric Basic and Advanced Life Support Collaborators. Part 4: pediatric basic and advanced life support: 2020 American Heart Association Guidelines for Cardiopulmonary Resuscitation and Emergency Cardiovascular Care. Circulation. 2020;142(Suppl 2):S469-523.

Q.18. Which of the following is not a recognized complication of therapeutic hypothermia?
a. Coagulopathy
b. Sepsis
c. Renal failure
d. Pneumonia
e. Hyperglycemia

Ans. c

Explanation: Therapeutic hypothermia has been trailed in the management of postcardiac arrest syndrome, traumatic brain injury, and neonatal encephalopathy. Increased rates of bleeding, pneumonia, sepsis, hyperglycemia, hypokalemia, and myocardial dysfunction with associated hemodynamic instability and dysrhythmias have been reported with its use. There is no evidence to suggest an independent link of hypothermia to worsening renal function.

Suggested Reading
1. Luscombe M, Andrzejowski JC. Clinical application of induced hypothermia. Contin Educ Anaesth Crit Care Pain. 2006;6(1):23-7.
2. Nolan JP, Morley PT, Vanden Hoek TL, Hickey RW, Kloeck WG, Billi J, et al. Therapeutic hypothermia after cardiac arrest: an advisory statement by the advanced life support task force of the International Liaison Committee on Resuscitation. Circulation. 2003;108(1):118-21.
3. Scirica BM. Therapeutic hypothermia after cardiac arrest. Circulation. 2013;127:244-50.

Q.19. Which among the following is not a predictor of poor neurological outcomes postresuscitation?
a. Bilateral absent pupillary reflexes at ≥72 hours after ROSC.
b. Low serum neuron-specific enolase (NSE) values at 48-72 hours after ROSC.
c. An unreactive malignant EEG pattern (burst suppression and status epilepticus) after rewarming.
d. Bilateral absence of N20 component of somatosensory evoked potentials (SSEP) wave after rewarming.

Ans. b

Explanation: Postresuscitation, the most robust predictors for prediction of poor neurological outcomes include bilaterally absent pupillary reflexes at ≥72 hours after ROSC and/or a bilaterally absent N20 SSEP wave after rewarming. If none of these signs is present, less robust predictors include the presence of high serum NSE values at

48–72 hours after ROSC, early (<48 hours) status myoclonus, absent corneal reflex at 72 hours, an unreactive malignant EEG pattern (burst suppression and status epilepticus) after rewarming, and the presence of diffuse ischemic injury on brain CT within 24 hours after ROSC or on brain MRI at 2–5 days after ROSC; and combining at least two of these predictors is suggested.

Suggested Reading

1. Sandroni C, D'Arrigo S, Nolan JP. Prognostication after cardiac arrest. Crit Care. 2018;22:150.

Q.20. A young 30-year-old female presents to the emergency room (ER) with complaint of palpitations for last half an hour. She gives history of similar complaints in the past. She is having the following rhythm on the monitor with blood pressure of 96/50 mm Hg and SpO$_2$ of 95%. Which of the following statements regarding the management of this patient is true?

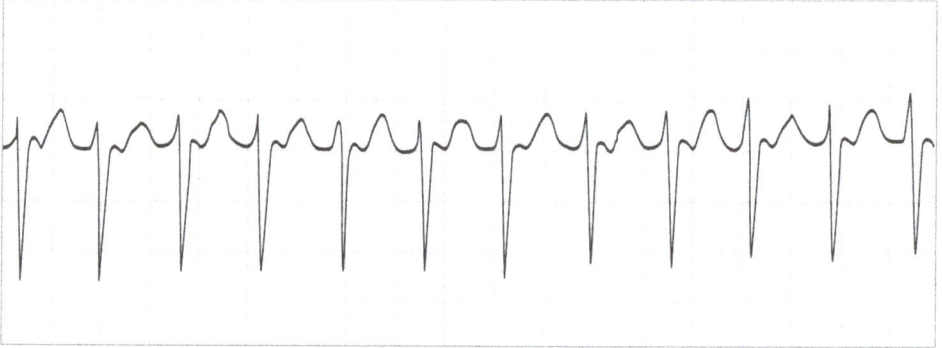

a. Oxygen by facemask should be started as soon as possible.
b. Synchronized cardioversion should be performed immediately.
c. Vagal maneuvers like carotid sinus massage should be attempted.
d. Doing carotid sinus massage on both sides may increase the chances of success.
e. Intravenous adenosine in dose of 3 mg should be administered and flushed immediately.

Ans. c

Explanation: The given scenario is a classical presentation of paroxysmal supraventricular tachycardia (PSVT). In such cases, patient's vital signs are monitored and 12-lead ECG should be done if available. Oxygen should only be given if the patient is hypoxemic with SpO$_2$ <94%. Patient should be watched for signs of hemodynamic instability, i.e., persistent tachyarrhythmias causing hypotension (systolic blood pressure <90 mm Hg), acutely altered mental status, signs of shock, ischemic chest discomfort, or acute heart failure. If any of these signs are present, immediate synchronized cardioversion should be performed considering sedation. Cardioversion is to be done with the device-specific recommended energy to minimize first shock excess. In addition, intravenous adenosine 6 mg should be given as rapid IV push followed by saline flush. In refractory cases, higher energy cardioversion with addition of antiarrhythmic drugs with expert consultation is advised. But in case the patient is hemodynamically stable, like in the current scenario, the vagal maneuver should be tried. Carotid sinus massage, only on one side of the patient, should be performed. Care should be taken for bradycardia and possibility of any atheromatous plaque migration from the carotid arteries leading on to stroke. In narrow complex SVT, rapid IV push of adenosine followed by saline flush can be given. First dose of adenosine is 6 mg followed by second dose of 12 mg if needed.

Suggested Reading
1. Panchal AR, Bartos JA, Cabañas JG, Donnino MW, Drennan IR, Hirsch KG, et al.; on behalf of the Adult Basic and Advanced Life Support Writing Group. Part 3: adult basic and advanced life support: 2020 American Heart Association Guidelines for Cardiopulmonary Resuscitation and Emergency Cardiovascular Care. Circulation. 2020;142(Suppl 2):S366-468.

Q.21. Looking at the literature on targeted temperature management, which is false?
a. TTM-1 trial compared target temperatures of 33 and 36°C in out-of-hospital cardiac arrest (OHCA) patients with shockable or nonshockable rhythms.
b. Hypothermia After Cardiac Arrest (HACA) trial compared target temperatures of 32 and 34°C with normal temperature in out-of-hospital cardiac arrest (OHCA) patients with shockable rhythms.
c. HYPERION trial compared target temperatures of 32 and 34°C in out-of-hospital cardiac arrest (OHCA) patients.
d. TTM-2 trial compared target temperatures of 33 and 37.5°C in patients with shockable or nonshockable rhythms.

Ans. c

Explanation

Study	Number of patients	Intervention	Cardiac arrest setting	Rhythm	Outcomes
HACA	275	32–34°C vs. normothermia for 24 hours	IHCA/OHCA	Shockable	Favorable neurological outcome at 6 months (55% vs. 39%)
TTM-1	950	33°C vs. 36°C for 28 hours	OHCA	Shockable and nonshockable	Death or unfavorable neurological outcome at 6 months (50% vs. 48%)
HYPERION	584	33°C vs. 36.5–37.5°C for 24 hours	IHCA/OHCA	Nonshockable	Favorable neurological outcome at 90 days (10.2% vs. 5.7%)
TTM-2	1,861	33°C vs. 37.5°C for 28 hours	–	Shockable and nonshockable	• Death or Unfavorable neurological outcome at 6 months • Arrhythmias (24% vs. 17%)

(HACA: hypothermia after cardiac arrest; IHCA: in-hospital cardiac arrest; OHCA: out-of-hospital cardiac arrest; TTM: targeted temperature management)

Suggested Reading
1. Dankiewicz J, Cronberg T, Lilja G, Jakobsen JC, Levin H, Ullén S, et al.; for the TTM2 Trial Investigators. Hypothermia versus normothermia after out-of-hospital cardiac arrest. N Engl J Med. 2021;384:2283-94.
2. Hypothermia after Cardiac Arrest Study Group. Mild therapeutic hypothermia to improve the neurologic outcome after cardiac arrest. N Engl J Med. 2002;346:549-56.
3. Lascarrou J, Merdji H, Le Gouge A, Colin G, Grillet G, Girardie P, et al.; for the CRICS-TRIGGERSEP Group. Targeted temperature management for cardiac arrest with nonshockable rhythm. N Engl J Med. 2019;381:2327-37.
4. Nielsen N, Wetterslev J, Cronberg T, Erlinge D, Gasche Y, Hassager C, et al. Targeted temperature management at 33°C versus 36°C after cardiac arrest. N Engl J Med. 2013;369:2197-206.

K-TYPE QUESTIONS

Q.22. A young 30-year-old male vehicular accident trauma victim is brought to the emergency. He is unconscious, unresponsive with doubtful feeble carotid pulse, and is not breathing. The ECG monitor shows following rhythm. Which of the following statements are true?

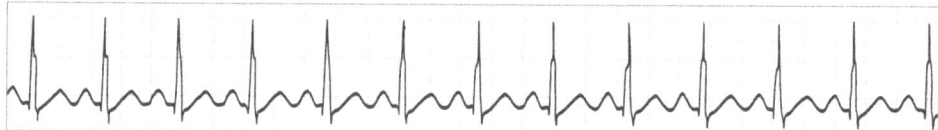

a. There is no immediate need to start CPR but one should search for differential diagnoses of tachycardia and treat them.
b. The patient is considered to be in cardiac arrest and managed according to PEA arm of ACLS arrest algorithm.
c. The patient should be looked for any signs of bleeding, tension pneumothorax, or pericardial tamponade.
d. During CPR of this patient, after 2 minutes of CPR, there is no need to check carotid pulse again if there is same rhythm on the monitor.
e. Epinephrine should be avoided as it may aggravate tachycardia.

Ans. a: F; b: T; c: T; d: F; e: F

Explanation: The shown rhythm on ECG is sinus tachycardia. But as the patient is unconscious, unresponsive, not breathing, and with no definitive carotid pulse, the victim is assumed to be in cardiac arrest. In cardiac arrest, presence of any organized rhythm with the absence of pulse is termed as pulseless electrical activity (PEA). The management of PEA is to be done according to asystole/PEA arm of AHA ACLS cardiac arrest algorithm. It mandates starting of BLS with high-quality chest compressions and effective ventilation. An important consideration is to find out any reversible cause leading to PEA, e.g., in this patient, with the history of trauma, one should look for the signs of hypovolemia, cardiac tamponade, or tension pneumothorax (particularly in steering wheel injury) or hypothermia, etc. While managing PEA, one has to check for the carotid pulse after every 2 minutes of CPR, as there is a possibility of presence of pulse even when the rhythm remains the same. As recommended in AHA ACLS algorithm, epinephrine in the dose of 1 mg IV/IO is to be administered as soon as possible. Also, consider advanced airway insertion to rule out any possibility of hypoxia/hypercarbia.

Suggested Reading
1. Panchal AR, Bartos JA, Cabañas JG, Donnino MW, Drennan IR, Hirsch KG, et al.; on behalf of the Adult Basic and Advanced Life Support Writing Group. Part 3: adult basic and advanced life support: 2020 American Heart Association Guidelines for Cardiopulmonary Resuscitation and Emergency Cardiovascular Care. Circulation. 2020;142 (Suppl 2):S366-468.

Q.23. Regarding survival with extracorporeal cardiopulmonary resuscitation (eCPR), which of the following statements are true?
a. The absolute time from sudden cardiac arrest to initiation of eCPR has no significant effect on outcomes.
b. Literature shows survival benefit as well as favorable neurological outcomes with eCPR.
c. eCPR performed in catheterization laboratory has shown worse prognosis than in other hospital locations.
d. eCPR has shown survival benefit in patients with initial nonshockable rhythm like PEA.

Ans. a: T; b: T; c: F; d: T

Explanation: Most of the guidelines recommend that eCPR should be implemented within 60 minutes of collapse but literature has shown that the absolute time from time of sudden cardiac arrest to initiation of eCPR has no significant effect on outcomes. Literature has shown good functional outcomes in up to 30–40% of cardiac arrest patients with eCPR, especially when performed in the in-hospital setting. A meta-analysis of nine studies reported increased 30-day survival by 13% and favorable neurological outcomes by 14% with eCPR as compared to standard ACLS. One study has reported a 48% 3-month survival with intact neurological function with the use of eCPR in OHCA ventricular fibrillation (VF) patients. Jaski et al. showed that eCPR performed in the catheterization laboratory was associated with significantly better long-term survival than in other hospital locations (50% *vs.* 15%), most likely due to immediate availability of ECLS equipment and skilled personnel in the catheterization laboratory. In nonshockable initial rhythms, mostly PEA, favorable neurological and survival outcomes have been shown in patients receiving eCPR, but with asystole as the initial cardiac arrest rhythm, eCPR has been reported to be futile.

Suggested Reading
1. Bartos JA, Carlson K, Carlson C, Raveendran G, John R, Aufderheide TP, et al. Surviving refractory out-of-hospital ventricular fibrillation cardiac arrest: Critical care and extracorporeal membrane oxygenation management. Resuscitation. 2018;132:47-55.
2. Fagnoul D, Combes A, De Backer D. Extracorporeal cardiopulmonary resuscitation. Curr Opin Crit Care. 2014;20:259-65.

3. Jaski BE, Ortiz B, Alla KR, Smith SC, Glaser D, Walsh C, et al. A 20-year experience with urgent percutaneous cardiopulmonary bypass for salvage of potential survivors of refractory cardiovascular collapse. J Thorac Cardiovasc Surg. 2010;139:753-57.
4. Mishra RC, Sodhi K, Gupta V, Prakash KC. Extracorporeal Cardiopulmonary Resuscitation. ISCCM Manual of RRT and ECMO in ICU, 2nd edition. New Delhi: Jaypee Brothers Medical Publisher; 2023.
5. Nakashima T, Noguchi T, Tahara Y, Nishimura K, Ogata S, Yasuda S, et al. Patients with refractory out-of-cardiac arrest and sustained ventricular fibrillation as candidates for extracorporeal cardiopulmonary resuscitation—Prospective multi-center observational study. Circ J. 2019;83:1011-8.
6. Ouweneel DM, Schotborgh JV, Limpens J, Sjauw KD, Engström AE, Lagrand WK, et al. Extracorporeal life support during cardiac arrest and cardiogenic shock: a systematic review and meta-analysis. Intensive Care Med. 2016;42(12):1922-34.
7. Pabst D, Brehm CE. Is pulseless electrical activity a reason to refuse cardiopulmonary resuscitation with ECMO support? Am J Emerg Med. 2018;36(4):637-40.
8. Patricio D, Peluso L, Brasseur A, Lheureux O, Belliato M, Vincent JL, et al. Comparison of extracorporeal and conventional cardiopulmonary resuscitation: a retrospective propensity score matched study. Crit Care. 2019;23:27.
9. Richardson AC, Tonna JE, Nanjayya V, Nixon P, Abrams DC, Raman L, et al. Extracorporeal cardiopulmonary resuscitation in adults. Interim Guideline Consensus Statement from the Extracorporeal Life Support Organization. ASAIO J. 2021;67(3):221-8.

Q.24. The following are appropriate for the resuscitation of the average 4-year-old child:
a. Size 5 cuffed endotracheal tube.
b. In the case of witnessed ventricular fibrillation, synchronized defibrillation at 64 Joules
c. In a cardiac arrest, 160 µg adrenaline, IO or IV.
d. Lorazepam 1.6 mg/kg IV for emergency treatment of convulsions.
e. Atropine 640 µg for emergency treatment of bradycardia suspected to be due to vagal overactivity.

Ans. a: T; b: F; c: T; d: F; e: F

Explanation: In pediatric resuscitation, most drugs, fluids, and equipment are used on a weight basis. It is important to determine a child's weight as soon as possible and if weighing the child is impractical, weight can be estimated using formulae:

0–12 months	Weight (kg) = (0.5 × age in months) + 4
1–5 years	Weight (kg) = (2 × age in years) + 8
6–12 years	Weight (kg) = (3 × age in years) + 7

Estimated patient's weight in the present case = 16 kg [(2 × 4) + 2]

Both cuffed and uncuffed tubes are suitable for an infant or child undergoing emergency intubation, but cuffed tubes, if available, are preferred. The size of the endotracheal tube can be estimated using various formulae like:

Internal diameter (mm) = Age/4 + 4 (uncuffed); Age/4 + 3.5 (cuffed)
Length of tube (cm) = Age/2 +12

Although the presenting rhythm for most pediatric arrests is nonshockable, should the child have a shockable rhythm, 4 J/kg is the energy selection of asynchronous DC shock (64 Joules).

In a cardiac arrest situation, the dose of adrenaline is 0.1 mL/kg or 0.01 mg/kg of 1:10,000 dilution (10 µg/kg = 160 µg), administered either intravenously or intraosseously.

Five minutes after a seizure has started, a benzodiazepine should be administered. If intravenous access is secured, preferred is intravenous lorazepam 100 µg/kg, if not, buccal midazolam (0.5 mg/kg) or rectal diazepam (0.5 mg/kg) should be given.

If a child presents in shock with bradycardia and vagal activity is suspected, 20 µg/kg (= 320 µg) atropine should be administered.

Suggested Reading
1. Samuels M, Wieteska S. Advanced Life Support Group. Advanced Paediatric Life Support. The Practical Approach, 5th edition. Oxford, UK: Wiley-Blackwell; 2005.
2. Topjian AA, Raymond TT, Atkins D, Chan M, Duff JP, Joyner Jr BL, et al.; on behalf of the Pediatric Basic and Advanced Life Support Collaborators. Pediatric Basic and Advanced Life Support: 2020 American Heart Association Guidelines for Cardiopulmonary Resuscitation and Emergency Cardiovascular Care. Circulation. 2020;142:S469-523.

Q.25. A 70-year-old female with history of coronary artery disease has a witnessed cardiac arrest. She undergoes 15 minutes of resuscitation with ROSC but remains comatose. Which of the following treatments for postresuscitation care are most likely to improve outcome for this patient?
a. 100% FiO_2 for at least 24 hours.
b. Permissive hypotension to avoid using vasopressors.
c. Hypothermia between 32 and 34°C for 24 hours.
d. Glycemic control with RBS goal <180 mg/dL.
e. Normocarbia with a $PaCO_2$ between 35 and 40 mm Hg.

Ans. a: F; b: F; c: F; d: T; e: T

Explanation: The tenets of postcardiac arrest care include targeted temperature management (TTM), hemodynamic and ventilation optimization, immediate coronary perfusion with percutaneous coronary intervention, glycemic control, and neurologic care.

The 2020 ACLS guidelines do not recommend lowering of body temperatures, but only preventing hyperthermia. In the previous guidelines, it was recommended that all comatose (i.e., lacking meaningful response to verbal commands) adult patients with ROSC after cardiac arrest should undergo TTM, with a target temperature between 32 and 34°C maintained constantly for at least 24 hours. This recommendation was based on studies of TTM which compared cooling to temperatures between 32 and 34°C with no well-defined TTM and found improvement in neurologic outcome for those in whom hypothermia was induced. But after TTM-2 trial, this practice has been abandoned and no longer recommended.

There are multiple goals related to hemodynamic and ventilation optimization in postcardiac arrest patients. Based on the ACLS guidelines, patients should receive the lowest possible FiO_2 to maintain an SpO_2 of 94% or greater. Permissive hypercapnia may be most appropriate in patients with acute lung injury while maintenance of normocarbia is warranted with cerebral edema. With regards to hemodynamic goals, the ACLS guidelines recommend maintaining a mean arterial pressure of 65 mm Hg or greater. In patients who have suspected coronary artery occlusion as the source of cardiac arrest, coronary reperfusion is warranted after ROSC. There is a strong association between high blood glucose after resuscitation from cardiac arrest and poor neurological outcome. European Resuscitation Council (ERC) recommends maintaining blood glucose at ≤180 mg/dL (10 mmol/L) and avoiding hypoglycemia following ROSC. Strict glucose control in adult patients with ROSC after cardiac arrest increases the risk of hypoglycemia.

Suggested Reading
1. Nakashima R, Hifumi T, Kawakita K, Okazaki T, Egawa S, Inoue A, et al. Critical care management focused on optimizing brain function after cardiac arrest. Circ J. 2017;81(4):427-39.
2. Nolan JP, Sandroni C, Böttiger BW, Cariou A, Cronberg T, Friberg H, et al. European Resuscitation Council and European Society of Intensive Care Medicine guidelines 2021: post-resuscitation care. Intensive Care Med. 2021;47:369-421.
3. Panchal AR, Bartos JA, Cabañas JG, Donnino MW, Drennan IR, Hirsch KG, et al.; on behalf of the Adult Basic and Advanced Life Support Writing Group. Part 3: adult basic and advanced life support: 2020 American Heart Association Guidelines for Cardiopulmonary Resuscitation and Emergency Cardiovascular Care. Circulation. 2020;142 (Suppl 2):S366-468.

Q.26. Regarding use of vasopressin during cardiac arrest, which is true?
a. There is no role of vasopressin in cardiac arrest according to AHA ACLS 2020 guidelines.
b. Vasopressin increases the myocardial oxygen demand.
c. Vasopressin causes intense vasoconstriction across different vascular beds.
d. Meta-analyses have shown mortality benefits with vasopressin in in-hospital cardiac arrest.

Ans. a: T; b: F; c: F; d: F

Explanation: With enough evidence from literature, vasopressin has been abandoned for use during cardiac arrest as per the latest 2020 AHA ACLS guidelines. Due to absence of β-adrenergic activity, vasopressin does not increase myocardial oxygen demand. Vasopressin has differential vasoconstrictive effects in different vascular beds in the body: direct action on V1 receptors leading to more intense vasoconstriction in skin, gastrointestinal tract, skeletal muscles, and fatty tissue as compared to the coronaries and the renal vascular bed while it causes vasodilation in the cerebral vasculature. Meta-analyses have not shown mortality benefits with vasopressin in in-hospital cardiac arrest victims.

Suggested Reading
1. Abdelazeem B, Awad A, Manasrah N, et al. The effect of vasopressin and methylprednisolone on return of spontaneous circulation in patients with in-hospital cardiac arrest: a systematic

review and meta-analysis of randomized controlled trials. J Am Coll Cardiol; 79 (9_Supplement): 1645. https://doi.org/10.1016/S0735-1097(22)02636-5
2. Aung K, Htay T. Vasopressin for Cardiac Arrest: A systematic Review and Meta-analysis. Arch Intern Med. 2005;165(1):17-24.
3. Holmberg MJ, Issa MS, Moskowitz A, Morley P, Welsford M, Neumar RW, et al.; International Liaison Committee on Resuscitation Advanced Life Support Task Force Collaborators. Vasopressors during adult cardiac arrest: A systematic review and meta-analysis. Resuscitation. 2019;139:106-21.
4. Mishra RC, Myatra SN, Govil D, Todi S. Use of Vasopressin during cardiac arrest. Critical Care Update, 5th edition. New Delhi: Jaypee Brothers Medical Publisher; 2023.
5. Panchal AR, Bartos JA, Cabañas JG, Donnino MW, Drennan IR, Hirsch KG, et al.; on behalf of the Adult Basic and Advanced Life Support Writing Group. Part 3: adult basic and advanced life support: 2020 American Heart Association Guidelines for Cardiopulmonary Resuscitation and Emergency Cardiovascular Care. Circulation. 2020;142(Suppl 2):S366-468.

Q.27. **An old man aged 70 years is wheeled into the emergency with complaints of chest heaviness. The monitor shows the following ECG rhythm. His blood pressure is 84/50 mm Hg and SpO$_2$ is 95%. He is having cold and clammy skin and starts feeling dizzy. He gives the past history of type-2 diabetes mellitus and hypertension and was on regular medication. Which of the following statements are true in managing this patient?**

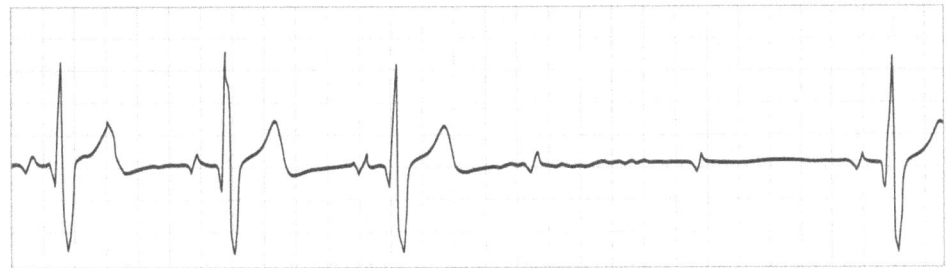

a. Rapid defibrillation with DC shock should be done as soon as possible.
b. Intravenous atropine 0.6 mg should be administered.
c. Transcutaneous pacing should be started if available.
d. Dopamine/epinephrine infusions should be started.
e. Patient should be monitored and observed with no immediate intervention required.

Ans. a: F; b: T; c: T; d: T; e: F

Explanation: The shown rhythm in the ECG is bradycardia with second degree type-2 AV block (Mobitz type-2 block). This is a dangerous rhythm that leads to significant reduction in cardiac output and can lead to complete heart block. The underlying cause in this case may be acute coronary syndrome, probably affecting the right coronary artery leading to ischemia of the conduction system and/or inferior wall of the heart. According to AHA ACLS adult bradycardia algorithm, primary ABCD survey (airway, breathing, circulation, and drugs) should be performed. Airway should be kept patent and oxygen should be administered if hypoxemic (SpO$_2$ <94%). ECG, blood pressure, and SpO_2 should be monitored and IV access should be obtained. 12-lead ECG should be done and toxicological and hypoxemic causes (5 Hs and 5 Ts) should be considered. Patient should be watched for signs of hypotension, acutely altered mental status, shock, ischemic chest discomfort, and acute heart failure. If none of these signs are present, patient should be monitored and observed continuously. But if any of these signs are present, like in this scenario, where the patient is having hypotension with cold clammy skin and dizziness, immediate intervention is necessary. Intravenous atropine in the dose of 0.6–1 mg should be administered although this drug may not help in second degree type-2 or higher AV blocks. Atropine can be repeated every 3–5 minutes up to a maximum dose of 3 mg. In case atropine is ineffective, transcutaneous pacing should be started. Dopamine infusion (5–20 µg/kg/min) or epinephrine infusion (2–10 µcg/min) can be started and titrated to patient's response. Expert cardiology consultation should be sought and transvenous pacing should be considered.

Suggested Reading
1. Panchal AR, Bartos JA, Cabañas JG, Donnino MW, Drennan IR, Hirsch KG, et al.; on behalf of the Adult Basic and Advanced Life Support Writing Group. Part 3: adult basic and advanced life support: 2020 American Heart Association Guidelines for Cardiopulmonary Resuscitation and Emergency Cardiovascular Care. Circulation. 2020;142 (Suppl 2):S366-468.

Q.28. A healthy 18-year-old footballer is posted for surgery for an ingrowing toenail. Upon examination, he was found to have pulse rate of 40/min. Rest of his vital signs were within normal limits. ECG was done that showed the following rhythm. The next line of action/actions should be following:

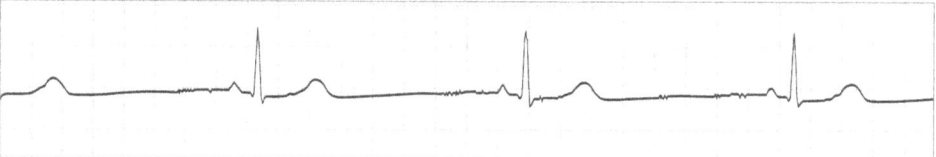

a. Immediately administer intravenous atropine.
b. Prepare for standby transcutaneous/transvenous pacing.
c. Postpone the surgery and consider expert consultation.
d. No intervention required and proceed for surgery.
e. Start intravenous fluids and administer intravenous epinephrine 1 mg.

Ans. a: F; b: F; c: F; d: T; e: F

Explanation: The shown rhythm is sinus bradycardia. The presence of sinus bradycardia or first degree AV block is a common finding in athletes, players and muscular men. According to AHA ACLS adult bradycardia algorithm, it is important to assess appropriateness for the clinical condition. The young boy in the current scenario is an otherwise healthy footballer with no signs and symptoms due to the underlying bradycardia. So, in this case, no active intervention to evaluate and treat bradycardia is needed. The boy can proceed with surgery without the need of any intervention.

Suggested Reading

1. Panchal AR, Bartos JA, Cabañas JG, Donnino MW, Drennan IR, Hirsch KG, et al.; on behalf of the Adult Basic and Advanced Life Support Writing Group. Part 3: adult basic and advanced life support: 2020 American Heart Association Guidelines for Cardiopulmonary Resuscitation and Emergency Cardiovascular Care. Circulation. 2020;142 (Suppl 2):S366-468.

Q.29. Which of the following regarding CPR in pregnancy are true?
 a. Modify CPR by a manual left uterine displacement to relieve the pressure of the enlarged uterus on the abdominal aorta and the inferior vena cava.
 b. Hands are placed over the lower half of the sternum, just as with CPR for any other adult.
 c. AED use is the same as with any adult victim with no modification of placement of electrode pads or of electric shock is recommended.
 d. Compressions are given to a depth of 2.5 inches, at the rate of 120 per minute.

Ans. a: T; b: T; c: T; d: F

Explanation: As per recommendations by American Heart Association (AHA) for CPR during pregnancy, the patient should be placed in a full left lateral decubitus position to relieve aortocaval compression (Class I; Level of Evidence C). The rescuer should place the heel of one hand on the center (middle) of the victim's chest (the lower half of the sternum) and the heel of the other hand on top of the first so that the hands overlap and are parallel (Class IIa; Level of Evidence C). Previous guidelines recommended placing the hands slightly higher on the sternum in the pregnant patient, but there is no scientific data to support this recommendation. The recommended defibrillation protocol is the same in the pregnant patient as in the nonpregnant patient. There is no modification of the recommended application of electric shock during pregnancy (Class I; Level of Evidence C). Chest compressions should be performed at a rate of at least 100 per minute at a depth of at least 2 inches (5 cm), allowing full recoil before the next compression, with minimal interruptions, and at a compression–ventilation ratio of 30:2 (Class IIa; Level of Evidence C).

Suggested Reading

1. Jeejeebhoy FM, Zelop CM, Lipman S, Carvalho B, Joglar J, Mhyre JM, et al. Cardiac Arrest in Pregnancy: A Scientific Statement from the American Heart Association. Circulation. 2015;132:1747-73.
2. Panchal AR, Bartos JA, Cabañas JG, Donnino MW, Drennan IR, Hirsch KG, et al.; on behalf of the Adult Basic and Advanced Life Support Writing Group. Part 3: adult basic and advanced life support: 2020 American Heart Association Guidelines for Cardiopulmonary Resuscitation and Emergency Cardiovascular Care. Circulation. 2020;142(Suppl 2): S366-468.

Q.30. A woman aged 60 years is brought to emergency in midnight with complaints of breathlessness. She is a known case of type-2 diabetes mellitus and hypertension on regular medications. She gives history of fever for last 5 days and was at home taking some antipyretics. Her ECG shows the following rhythm. Her blood pressure is 106/62 mm Hg, temperature is 101°F, and SpO$_2$ is 92%. On auscultation of chest,

she is found to have bronchial breathing in left lower region that is confirmed by the chest X-ray. Line of management of this patient will be:

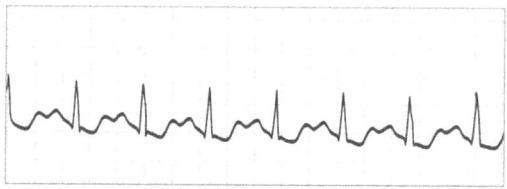

a. Start oxygen by facemask and nebulize with ipratropium bromide.
b. Send complete blood count and blood ± sputum culture and start intravenous antibiotics as per local antimicrobial flora.
c. Start antipyretic maneuvers such as intravenous paracetamol and wet sponging of the extremities.
d. Drugs like beta blocker or calcium channel blocker can be administered to control rate.
e. Attach defibrillation pads to the patient's chest so that no time is wasted if the patient needs defibrillation.

Ans. a: T; b: T; c: T; d: F; e: F

Explanation: The given rhythm is sinus tachycardia. According to AHA ACLS adult tachycardia algorithm, patient should be monitored for any signs and symptoms of low cardiac output due to the presence of underlying tachycardia. It is also important to note whether tachycardia is causing the signs and symptoms or the tachycardia is due to some underlying cause. In the presence of the later scenario, it is prudent to identify and treat the underlying cause. No treatment is usually needed to treat the tachycardia per se. In the given scenario, there are possibly underlying chest infection and fever which are causing all the signs and symptoms. Thus, the patient should be treated with nebulizers, oxygen, antipyretic maneuvers, and systemic antibiotics as per the local guidelines.

Suggested Reading
1. Panchal AR, Bartos JA, Cabañas JG, Donnino MW, Drennan IR, Hirsch KG, et al.; on behalf of the Adult Basic and Advanced Life Support Writing Group. Part 3: adult basic and advanced life support: 2020 American Heart Association Guidelines for Cardiopulmonary Resuscitation and Emergency Cardiovascular Care. Circulation. 2020;142 (Suppl 2):S366-468.

CHAPTER 3

Shock

Nitin Rai, Anirban Bhattacharjee, Akshat Trivedi

Q.1. A 54-year-old male, chronic smoker, diabetic, hypertensive, and benign prostatic hyperplasia (BPH), presented to emergency department with complaints of burning micturition, difficulty in passing urine, and high-grade fever for 5 days (T_{max} = 104.5°C). On examination, he had respiratory rate of 35 breaths/min, blood pressure of 90/55 mm Hg, and heart rate of 140 beats/min. The patient was slightly drowsy but responded to painful stimuli. Respiratory and cardiovascular examination was unremarkable with no obvious focal neurological deficit. What would be the next step in management?
   a. Screen the patient using quick sequential organ failure assessment (qSOFA) + measure lactate + fluid administration of 30 mL/kg body weight.
   b. Screen the patient using qSOFA + measure lactate + fluid administration of 30 mL/kg body weight + antibiotics administration.
   c. Screen the patient using qSOFA + measure lactate + fluid administration of 30 mL/kg body weight + antibiotics administration + paired blood cultures.
   d. Screen the patient using systemic inflammatory response syndrome (SIRS) and qSOFA + measure lactate + fluid administration 30 mL/kg body weight resuscitation + antibiotics administration + paired blood cultures.

Ans. d

Explanation: qSOFA identifies patients with poor outcome or suspected infection. Positive qSOFA alarms the possibility of sepsis but given the poor sensitivity, it is advisable not to use qSOFA as a single screening tool. For screening purpose, combining multiple tools is a better approach.

Surviving sepsis campaign (SSC) bundles were revised from 6- to 3-h bundles in 2015. The guidelines published in 2018 state that this resuscitation bundle treatment should be initiated within 1 hour of the emergency department (ED) triage time or the earliest chart annotation if presenting from another care venue. The 1-h bundle is composed of the following five elements: (1) measuring the lactate level, (2) obtaining blood culture prior to administration of antibiotics, (3) administering broad-spectrum antibiotics, (4) beginning rapid administration of 30 mL/kg crystalloid fluid for hypotension or lactate ≥4 mmol/L, and (5) administering vasopressors if the patient is hypotensive during or after fluid resuscitation to maintain mean arterial pressure (MAP) at ≥65 mm Hg within 1 hour from sepsis recognition. The fixed dose of 30 mL/kg in all patients stems from three large interventional trials: the PROMISE, PROCESS, and ARISE trials where the volumes of prerandomization fluid given to patients were approximately 30 mL/kg ideal body weight.

Suggested Reading
1. Levy MM, Evans LE, Rhodes A. The surviving sepsis campaign bundle: 2018 update. Intensive Care Med. 2018;44:925-8.
2. Seymour CW, Liu VX, Iwashyna TJ, Brunkhorst FM, Rea TD, Scherag A, et al. Assessment of clinical criteria for sepsis: for the third international consensus definitions for sepsis and septic shock (Sepsis-3). JAMA. 2016;315(8):762-74.

Q.2. A 66-year-old, 75-kg male was found unconscious in a park. On examination, he had a large abscess over left foot. No reliable history was found. His heart rate (HR) was 156 bpm, respiratory rate (RR) was 34 breaths/min, MAP was 45 mm Hg, and oxygen saturation (SpO_2) was 92% on 15 LPM oxygen. He received 2.5 L of Ringer's lactate. His MAP improved to 56. Which of the following is true regarding fluid management?
a. Starch/colloids can be used as initial resuscitation fluid.
b. Balanced crystalloid compared to saline reduce reduced 90-day mortality.
c. Fluid resuscitation should be guided by dynamic over static markers of resuscitation.
d. Normalizing of lactate and capillary refill time (CRT) has no relevance in fluid resuscitation.

Ans. c

Explanation: The surviving sepsis campaign (SSC) recommendation to "rapidly administer a minimum of 30 mL/kg (ideal body weight) crystalloid for hypotension or lactate ≥4 mmol/L" is a "strong recommendation, with a low quality of evidence". Indeed, this strong recommendation is based largely on expert opinion with minimal supporting clinical data. In addition to the lack of credible data demonstrating the benefit of such a strategy, recent studies have demonstrated the potential harms with such an approach. Furthermore, results from experimental, observational, and randomized clinical studies strongly suggest improved outcomes with a more restrictive approach to fluid resuscitation.

The *SSC* recommends against using starches for initial resuscitation. Albumin may be used for patients who received large volumes of crystalloids. Regarding the choice of fluids for resuscitation, evidence is more in favor of balanced salt solution (BSS) over crystalloid without evident effect on mortality. The most recently published BaSICS trial showed no difference in 90-day mortality between Plasma-Lyte and 0.9% sodium chloride in 11,000 adult intensive care patients.

The SMART trial involving 15,000 adult intensive care unit (ICU) patients in 2018 showed a reduction in a composite outcome of death, new renal replacement therapy, and persistent renal dysfunction at 30 days, with balanced crystalloid use. The SPLIT trial in 2015 compared Plasma-Lyte to 0.9% sodium chloride in 2,278 critically ill patients. There was no difference in the primary outcome of proportion of patients with an acute kidney injury.

Dynamic markers of fluid responsiveness such as stroke volume variation, pulse pressure variation, and passive leg raise test have better diagnostic accuracy compared with static techniques. Additionally, only approximately 50% of patients with septic shock will demonstrate fluid responsiveness by significant increase in stroke volume in response to a fluid bolus.

Moreover, calculation of maintenance fluid therapy after the initial 30 mL/kg administration should again be guided by dynamic markers of fluid responsiveness and measuring stroke volume and cardiac output. For adults with sepsis or septic shock, the adequacy of fluid resuscitation strategies should target decrease in elevated serum lactate levels or normalization of capillary refill time (CRT). The ANDROMEDA-SHOCK trial compared CRT normalization versus lactate clearance as resuscitation strategy. Targeting CRT has no effect on mortality, but CRT targeted during resuscitation is physiologically plausibility, cost-effective, and easy to adopt in clinical routine practice.

Suggested Reading
1. Fleischmann-Struzek C, Mellhammar L, Rose N, Cassini A, Rudd KE, Schlattmann P, et al. Incidence and mortality of hospital- and ICU-treated sepsis: results from an updated and expanded systematic review and meta-analysis. Intensive Care Med. 2020;46(8):1552-62.
2. Hernandez G, Ospina-Tascón GA, Damiani LP, Estenssoro E, Dubin A, Hurtado J, et al. Effect of a resuscitation strategy targeting peripheral perfusion status vs serum lactate levels on 28-day mortality among patients with septic shock: the ANDROMEDA-SHOCK Randomized Clinical Trial. JAMA. 2019;321(7):654-64.

Q.3. A 23-year-old male with a known chronic kidney disease (on maintenance hemodialysis, with last session done a day prior to presentation) presented with shortness of breath, bilateral lower limb pitting edema, and cough with low-grade fever for past 7 days. On examination, his vitals were stable. Initial laboratory tests were sent and results awaited. Decision was made to start the antibiotics. Which of the following statements is true?
   a. Antimicrobials should be started immediately, ideally within 1 hour of presentation.
   b. Defer antimicrobials while closely monitoring the patient.
   c. Complete rapid investigation and if concern for infection persists, administer antibiotics within 3 hours.
   d. Immediately take up the patient for hemodialysis.

Ans. c

Explanation: Delivering antibiotics in sepsis/septic shock is an important intervention. The mortality reduction with early antimicrobials is strongest in patients with septic shock; however, there is a weaker association in sepsis patients without shock. This patient presented with dyspnea and cough, possibly secondary to fluid overload. However, presence of fever points toward possible sepsis.

While possibility of fluid overload and requirement of dialysis still exist, sepsis should be ruled out at the onset and in absence of pending concerns over infectious etiology after thorough rapid assessment, history, and clinical examination, the plan to initiate dialysis can be taken. For this case, in lines with the new surviving sepsis guidelines, a rapid workup of infectious versus noninfectious etiologies should be undertaken within 3 hours, while closely monitoring the patient and if concern for infection persists, antibiotics should be administered. But time to administer antibiotics should not exceed 3-5 hours from hospital admission/sepsis recognition as mortality may increase, as suggested by various observational studies.

Suggested Reading
1. Alam N, Oskam E, Stassen PM, Exter PV, van de Ven PM, Haak HR, et al. Prehospital antibiotics in the ambulance for sepsis: a multicentre, open label, randomised trial. Lancet Respir Med. 2018;6(1):40-50.
2. Seymour CW, Gesten F, Prescott HC, Friedrich ME, Iwashyna TJ, Phillips GS, et al. Time to treatment and mortality during mandated emergency care for sepsis. N Engl J Med. 2017;376(23):2235-44.

Q.4. A 58-year-old male gentleman with a diagnosed case of chronic obstructive pulmonary disease (COPD) and carcinoma rectum (on chemotherapy via chemo port inserted in right subclavian vein) has presented with acute onset shortness of breath, fever, and yellow-colored sputum production for 1 week. After initial stabilization with noninvasive ventilation and bronchodilators, the patient was planned to receive antimicrobials. Initial chest X-ray revealed right-sided lobar pneumonia. There is in addition a past history of exacerbation of COPD 2 months back where patient was admitted and received IV medications. In line with current case scenario, which is the appropriate antimicrobial choice?
a. Piperacillin–tazobactam
b. Piperacillin–tazobactam + Levofloxacin + Linezolid + Gentamycin
c. Piperacillin–tazobactam + Levofloxacin + Gentamycin
d. Piperacillin–tazobactam + Levofloxacin + Linezolid

Ans. d

Explanation: The decision to start empirical antibiotics against methicillin-resistant *Staphylococcus aureus* (MRSA) depends on presence of risk factors. Risk factors for MRSA infections are past history of MRSA infection/colonization, recurrent skin infections/chronic wounds, recent intravenous antibiotics, recent hospital admissions, presence of invasive devices like dialysis catheter or long-term chemotherapy port, hemodialysis recipients, and severity of illness. A delay of >24–48 hours for antibiotics administration in patients with proven MRSA infection is associated with increased mortality. However, extreme caution should be taken because administration of anti-MRSA antibiotics to patients without MRSA infection is associated with higher mortality. This patient received recent IV antibiotics during his past hospital stay and also harbors a chemotherapy port mandating anti-MRSA therapy initiation as an appropriate step.

It is recommended that the use of dual gram-negative coverage should be based on risk of multi-drug resistant (MDR) pathogens. Such risk factors include infection/colonization with MDR pathogen in preceding year, hospital-acquired infections, use of broad-spectrum antibiotic in the last 90 days, use of selective digestive decontamination, etc. History of IV antibiotics during last hospitalization places this patient in a high-risk category of MDR infection, hence dual gram-negative coverage is recommended here. A combination of dual gram-negative coverage piperacillin-tazobactam + levofloxacin along with anti-MRSA cover and linezolid is the most appropriate empirical antimicrobial choice.

Suggested Reading
1. Callejo-Torre F, Eiros Bouza JM, Olaechea Astigarraga P, Coma Del Corral MJ, Palomar Martínez M, Alvarez-Lerma F, et al. Risk factors for methicillin-resistant *Staphylococcus aureus* colonisation or infection in intensive care units and their reliability for predicting MRSA on ICU admission. Infez Med. 2016;24(3):201-9.
2. Gasch O, Camoez M, Domínguez MA, Padilla B, Pintado V, Almirante B, et al. Predictive factors for early mortality among patients with methicillin-resistant *Staphylococcus aureus* bacteraemia. J Antimicrob Chemother. 2013;68(6):1423-30.
3. Rottier WC, Bamberg YR, Dorigo-Zetsma JW, van der Linden PD, Ammerlaan HS, Bonten MJ. Predictive value of prior colonization and antibiotic use for third-generation cephalosporin-resistant enterobacteriaceae bacteremia in patients with sepsis. Clin Infect Dis. 2015;60(11):1622-30.

Q.5. Which of the following is not true about vasoactive agents in septic shock?
   a. Norepinephrine is the first-line agent over other vasopressors.
   b. Adrenaline is the second line of vasopressor.
   c. Vasopressin should be started when the dose of norepinephrine is 0.25–0.5 µg/kg/min.
   d. Selepressin is a potential noncatecholamine vasopressor alternative to norepinephrine.

Ans. b

Explanation: Norepinephrine is the first-line agent in septic shock. It is α-1 and β-1 adrenergic receptors agonist, producing vasoconstriction and rise in MAP with minimal effect on heart rate.

At higher dose of noradrenaline (0.25–0.5 µg/kg/min) maximum number of alpha 1 receptors are already saturated, hence it is advisable to use a drug of different catagory with different mechanism of action. Vasopressin is the preferred drug in such cases.

Vasopressin is produced in the hypothalamus. It is an endogenous peptide hormone, and its dose is not titrated to response, but rather administered at a fixed dose of 0.03 units/min in septic shock. Catecholamine-sparing effect of vasopressin has been demonstrated in two large trials—VANISH and VASST trials. The threshold for adding vasopressin to norepinephrine varies between studies and remains unclear. It is suggested to start vasopressin when the dose of norepinephrine is 0.25–0.5 µg/kg/min.

Selepressin is selective V1 agonist which acts by stimulating vascular smooth muscle producing vasoconstriction. However, unlike vasopressin, it has no effect on V1b and V2 receptors like release of corticosteroid and nitric oxide, increased procoagulant activity, and fluid retention. Selepressin (dose: 2.5 ng/kg/min) is a potential noncatecholamine vasopressor alternative to norepinephrine.

Suggested Reading
1. Avni T, Lador A, Lev S, Leibovici L, Paul M, Grossman A. Vasopressors for the treatment of septic shock: systematic review and meta-analysis. PLoS One. 2015;10(8):e0129305.
2. Gordon AC, Mason AJ, Thirunavukkarasu N, Perkins GD, Cecconi M, Cepkova M, et al. Effect of early vasopressin vs norepinephrine on kidney failure in patients with septic shock: the VANISH randomized clinical trial. JAMA. 2016;316(5):509-18.
3. Ukor IF, Walley KR. Vasopressin in vasodilatory shock. Crit Care Clin. 2019;35(2):247-61.

Q.6. A 35-year-old female visited the emergency department with pain abdomen in epigastric region. Ultrasonogram (USG) examination of abdomen showed features suggestive of acute pancreatitis due to gallstone disease. 1 week after admission, she started developing shortness of breath progressively associated with fall in saturation to 60% on nasal prongs. Chest X-ray showed bilateral diffuse lung opacities. Arterial blood gas on high-flow nasal cannula at 60 L/min and fraction of inspired oxygen (FiO_2) of 1.0:

pH	7.32
PO_2	55
PCO_2	45
HCO_3	22
BE	−3.1
Lactate	1.3

A decision was made to intubate and mechanically ventilate the patient. Which of the following is the best ventilator strategy for this patient?
a. Tidal volume 8 mL/kg body weight, high positive end-expiratory pressure (PEEP), plateau pressure <30 cmH_2O, prone ventilation of 8-hour duration, and routine recruitment maneuver.
b. Tidal volume 6 mL/kg body weight, high PEEP, plateau pressure <30 cmH_2O, prone ventilation of 16-hour duration, and avoiding routine recruitment maneuver.
c. Tidal volume 6 mL/kg body weight, high PEEP, plateau pressure <35 cmH_2O, prone ventilation of 16-hour duration, and routine recruitment maneuver.
d. Tidal volume 6 mL/kg body weight, high PEEP, plateau pressure <30 cmH_2O, prone ventilation of 8-hour duration, and avoiding routine recruitment maneuver.

Ans. b

Explanation: It is recommended to use lung-protective strategies for patients with acute respiratory distress syndrome (ARDS). A large trial comparing tidal volumes of 6 mL/kg with 12 mL/kg predicted body weight (PBW) in ARDS patients showed 9% absolute decrease in mortality. Tidal volume should be lowered even with plateau pressures ≤30 cmH_2O because lower plateau pressures were associated with reduced hospital mortality.

Mortality reduction is observed when low-tidal volume is combined with limited plateau pressure. A large international observational study (LUNGSAFE) also reported the importance of limiting plateau pressure by demonstrating its correlation with mortality. Therefore, it is recommended to keep the upper limit for plateau pressure to <30 cmH$_2$O.

Adopting open lung ventilation approach by applying high PEEP in ARDS patients may open lung units and help in improving gas exchange and increasing PaO$_2$. In patients with moderate or severe ARDS (PaO$_2$/FiO$_2$ ≤200 mm Hg), higher PEEP is associated with reduced mortality. The optimal method for selecting PEEP is not clear. PEEP titration can be done bedside by measuring thoracopulmonary compliance with the aim of achieving lowest driving pressure or best compliance. Other options are use of a PEEP/FiO$_2$ titration table, esophageal pressure-guided PEEP titration, using pressure volume loop, etc.

Severe hypoxemia patients may benefit from recruitment maneuvers in combination with higher PEEP, but the evidence to support its routine use in all ARDS patients is limited, so it is recommended for only moderate-to-severe refractory ARDS. Moreover, "traditional" recruitment maneuver like sustained continuous PEEP (e.g., 30–40 cmH$_2$O for 30–40 seconds) is preferred over "nontraditional" approach where lung recruitment with incremental followed by decremental PEEP levels is done titrating to achieve best respiratory static compliance or oxygen saturation.

The use of prone compared with supine position within the first 36 hours of intubation, when performed for >12 hours a day, showed improved survival in ARDS and a PaO$_2$/FiO$_2$ ratio <200. Neuromuscular blocking agents (NMBAs) in ARDS help in improving chest wall compliance, preventing respiratory asynchrony, decreasing the work of breathing, and reducing peak airway pressures. Surviving sepsis guidelines suggest intermittent neuromuscular blocking agent boluses over continuous infusion. ROSE trial result demonstrated that continuous neuromuscular blocking agent infusion did not reduce mortality when compared with a light sedation strategy with intermittent neuromuscular blocking agent boluses.

Suggested Reading
1. Brower RG, Matthay MA, Morris A, Schoenfeld D, Thompson BT, Wheeler A; Acute Respiratory Distress Syndrome Network. Ventilation with lower tidal volumes as compared with traditional tidal volumes for acute lung injury and the ARDS. N Engl J Med. 2000;342:1301-8.
2. Fan E, Wilcox ME, Brower RG, Stewart TE, Mehta S, Lapinsky SE, et al. Recruitment maneuvers for acute lung injury: a systematic review. Am J Respir Crit Care Med. 2008;178:1156-63.
3. Laffey JG, Bellani G, Pham T, Fan E, Madotto F, Bajwa EK, et al. Potentially modifiable factors contributing to outcome from acute respiratory distress syndrome: The LUNG SAFE study. Intensive Care Med. 2016;42:1865-76.
4. National Heart, Lung, and Blood Institute PETAL Clinical Trials Network; Moss M, Huang DT, Brower RG, Ferguson ND, Ginde AA, et al. Early neuromuscular blockade in the acute respiratory distress syndrome. N Engl J Med. 2019;380:1997-2008.

Q.7. A 77-year-old male, postcoronary artery bypass graft (CABG), with a baseline left ventricular ejection fraction of 25%, is admitted to ICU following repair of perforated peritonitis. He continues to have high-grade fever (maximum temperature = 103.6°C), tachycardia of 130 beats/min, and hypotension (BP = 78/43 mm Hg) on noradrenaline infusion of 0.8 μg/kg/min. 1.5 L of

Plasma-Lyte was given, but his blood pressure remained low for next 8 hours. Which is the next optimal strategy for this patient?
a. Increase noradrenaline infusion dose to 1.0 μg/kg/min.
b. Give 500 mL further fluid bolus as assess hemodynamic response.
c. Add IV hydrocortisone as 50 mg intravenously every 6 hours.
d. Add adrenaline.

Ans. c

Explanation: Steroids in sepsis should be reserved for those patients who are refractory to fluids and vasopressors. Rationale for steroids in sepsis includes reversal of relative adrenal insufficiency, reversal of inflammatory overactivity, "reprogramming" of the immune response, improved response to catecholamines, deactivation of nitric oxide synthase, improved cardiac tolerance of bacterial endotoxin, improved retention of resuscitation fluid, and repair of the endothelial glycocalyx. The commonly used corticosteroid in adult patients with septic shock is hydrocortisone given at a dose of 50 mg IV every 6 hours or as continuous infusion. It is suggested to initiate corticosteroid when dose of norepinephrine/epinephrine is ≥0.25 μg/kg/min for at least 4 hours after the initiation.

This patient being nonresponsive to fluid bolus, further fluid is less likely to be useful. Moreover, a conservative/restrictive fluid strategy should be employed with baseline left ventricular ejection fraction of 25%. When norepinephrine is used at higher concentrations, the α-1 receptors are already saturated and start to get downregulated. In this case, use of drugs which target different receptor is advisable, hence vasopressin is more adequate choice/second-line agent in this scenario.

The CORTICUS and ADRENAL trial showed no improvement in mortality; however, APROCCHSS study and multiple other meta-analyses showed accelerated resolution of shock and increase vasopressor-free days.

Suggested Reading
1. Akinaga J, Lima V, Kiguti LR, Hebeler-Barbosa F, Alcántara-Hernández R, García-Sáinz JA, et al. Differential phosphorylation, desensitization, and internalization of α1A-adrenoceptors activated by norepinephrine and oxymetazoline. Mol Pharmacol. 2013;83:870-81.
2. Annane D, Renault A, Brun-Buisson C, Megarbane B, Quenot JP, Siami S, et al.; CRICSTRIGGERSEP Network. Hydrocortisone plus fludrocortisone for adults with septic shock. N Engl J Med. 2018;378:809-18.
3. Rygård SL, Butler E, Granholm A, Møller MH, Cohen J, Finfer S, et al. Low-dose corticosteroids for adult patients with septic shock: a systematic review with meta-analysis and trial sequential analysis. Intensive Care Med. 2018;44:1003-16.
4. Venkatesh B, Finfer S, Cohen J, Rajbhandari D, Arabi Y, Bellomo R, et al.; ADRENAL Trial Investigators and the Australian-New Zealand Intensive Care Society Clinical Trials Group. Adjunctive glucocorticoid therapy in patients with septic shock. N Engl J Med. 2018;378:797-808.

Q.8. Which of the following statements is true for a patient with septic shock?
a. Polymyxin B hemoperfusion is a useful adjunct for recovery of septic shock.
b. Use of intravenous (IV) immunoglobulins is recommended.

c. Stress ulcer prophylaxis is suggested.
d. Use of vitamin C does not reduce mortality.

Ans. c

Explanation: Substantial uncertainty exits regarding any beneficial effect of polymyxin B hemoperfusion. Polymyxin B hemoperfusion is not cost-effective and availability is limited. Recently performed sensitivity analyses also observed occurrence of undesirable side effects. So, for adults with sepsis or septic shock, using polymyxin B hemoperfusion is not recommended.

Sepsis/septic shock is a condition of hyperinflammation and immune suppression. However, high-quality studies are lacking, which examine the effect of intravenous immunoglobulins (IVIg) on the outcomes in sepsis/septic shock. So, use of intravenous (IV) immunoglobulins is not recommended.

Vitamin C has anti-inflammatory properties. But multiple studies including an analysis of seven randomized controlled trials (RCTs) and two additional RCTs of vitamin C versus placebo reported no reduced mortality or difference of other outcomes like of time alive and vasopressor-free days. There is a weak recommendation against using vitamin C in sepsis/septic shock.

Stress ulcers develop in gastrointestinal (GI) tract of critically ill patients and are associated with significant morbidity and mortality. There is a modest reduction in gastrointestinal hemorrhage with the use of stress ulcer prophylaxis (SUP). Patients with risk factors for clinically important GI bleeding (coagulopathy, shock, and chronic liver disease) are particularly benefited from SUP.

Suggested Reading
1. Fujii T, Luethi N, Young PJ, Frei DR, Eastwood GM, French CJ, et al.; VITAMINS Trial Investigators. Effect of vitamin C, hydrocortisone, and thiamine vs hydrocortisone alone on time alive and free of vasopressor support among patients with septic shock: The VITAMINS randomized clinical trial. JAMA. 2020;323:423-31.
2. Krag M, Marker S, Perner A, Wetterslev J, Wise MP, Schefold JC, et al.; SUP-ICU trial group. Pantoprazole in patients at risk for gastrointestinal bleeding in the ICU. N Engl J Med. 2018;379:2199-208.
3. Moskowitz A, Huang DT, Hou PC, Gong J, Doshi PB, Grossestreuer AV, et al.; ACTS Clinical Trial Investigators. Effect of ascorbic acid, corticosteroids, and thiamine on organ injury in septic shock: The ACTS randomized clinical trial. JAMA. 2020;324:642-50.
4. Zhou F, Peng Z, Murugan R, Kellum JA. Blood purification and mortality in sepsis: A meta-analysis of randomized trials. Crit Care Med. 2013;41:2209-20.

Q.9. Blood transfusion is an important adjunct in sepsis/septic shock. Which of the following statements is true regarding blood transfusion practices in such scenario?
a. Restricted transfusion protocol is associated with reduced mortality.
b. Liberal transfusion is associated with lower mortality and ischemic events.
c. A restrictive transfusion strategy includes a hemoglobin trigger of 8 g/dL.
d. Restrictive transfusion strategy is preferred over liberal strategy.

Ans. d

Explanation: TRISS trial (Transfusion Requirements in Septic Shock) compared a transfusion threshold of 7 g/dL versus 9 g/dL in patients with septic shock in ICU. There were a similar 90-day mortality, use of life support, and ischemic events in both the groups. TRICC trial (Transfusion requirements in Critical Care) compared transfusion threshold of 7 g/dL versus 10 g/dL in euvolemic ICU patients. There was a similar 30-day mortality in both the groups. TRICOP trial (Transfusion Requirements in Critically Ill Oncologic Patients) compared liberal (Hb threshold <9 g/dL) or restrictive strategy (Hb threshold <7 g/dL) in adult cancer patients with septic shock. 28-day mortality rate in the liberal group was 45% versus 56% in the restrictive group with similar ICU and hospital length of stay. But 90-day mortality was lower in liberal group (59%) compared with restrictive group (70%). Based on the trials performed, restrictive transfusion strategy typically involves an Hb concentration transfusion trigger of 7 g/dL.

Suggested Reading

1. Bergamin FS, Almeida JP, Landoni G, Galas FRBG, Fukushima JT, Fominskiy E, et al. Liberal versus restrictive transfusion strategy in critically ill oncologic patients: The transfusion requirements in critically ill oncologic patients randomized controlled trial. Crit Care Med. 2017;45:766-73.
2. Hébert PC, Wells G, Blajchman MA, Marshall J, Martin C, Pagliarello G, et al. A multicenter, randomized, controlled clinical trial of transfusion requirements in critical care. N Eng J Med. 1999;340:409-17.
3. Holst LB, Haase N, Wetterslev J, Wernerman J, Guttormsen AB, Karlsson S, et al.; TRISS Trial Group; Scandinavian Critical Care Trials Group. Lower versus higher hemoglobin threshold for transfusion in septic shock. N Engl J Med. 2014;371:1381-91.

Q.10. **A 62-year-old female presented with altered mental status, hypotension, diminished pulses, dyspnea, peripheral edema, jugular venous distention, and orthopnea. The patient is a known case of acute coronary syndrome on dual antiplatelets. A clinical suspicion of cardiogenic shock (CS) is made. Which of the following definitions is consistent with the diagnosis of CS?**

   a. SBP <90 mm Hg for <30 minutes or supportive intervention to maintain SBP >90 mm Hg.
   b. SBP <90 mm Hg with appropriate fluid resuscitation without clinical and laboratory evidence of end-organ damage.
   c. MAP >70 mm Hg or SBP >100 mm Hg after adequate fluid resuscitation (at least 1 L of crystalloids or 500 mL of colloids).
   d. SBP <90 mm Hg for >30 minutes or vasopressor support to maintain SBP >90 mm Hg and hemodynamic criteria: CI <2.2 and PCWP >15 mm Hg.

Ans. d

Explanation: The clinical criteria for the diagnosis of cardiogenic shock based on the SHOCK (Should We Emergently Revascularize Occluded Coronaries For Cardiogenic Shock) and the IABP-SHOCK II (Intra-aortic Balloon Pump in Cardiogenic Shock II) trials were defined by systolic blood pressure (SBP) <90 mm Hg for >30 minutes, use of mechanical or pharmacologic support to maintain SBP >90 mm Hg, urine

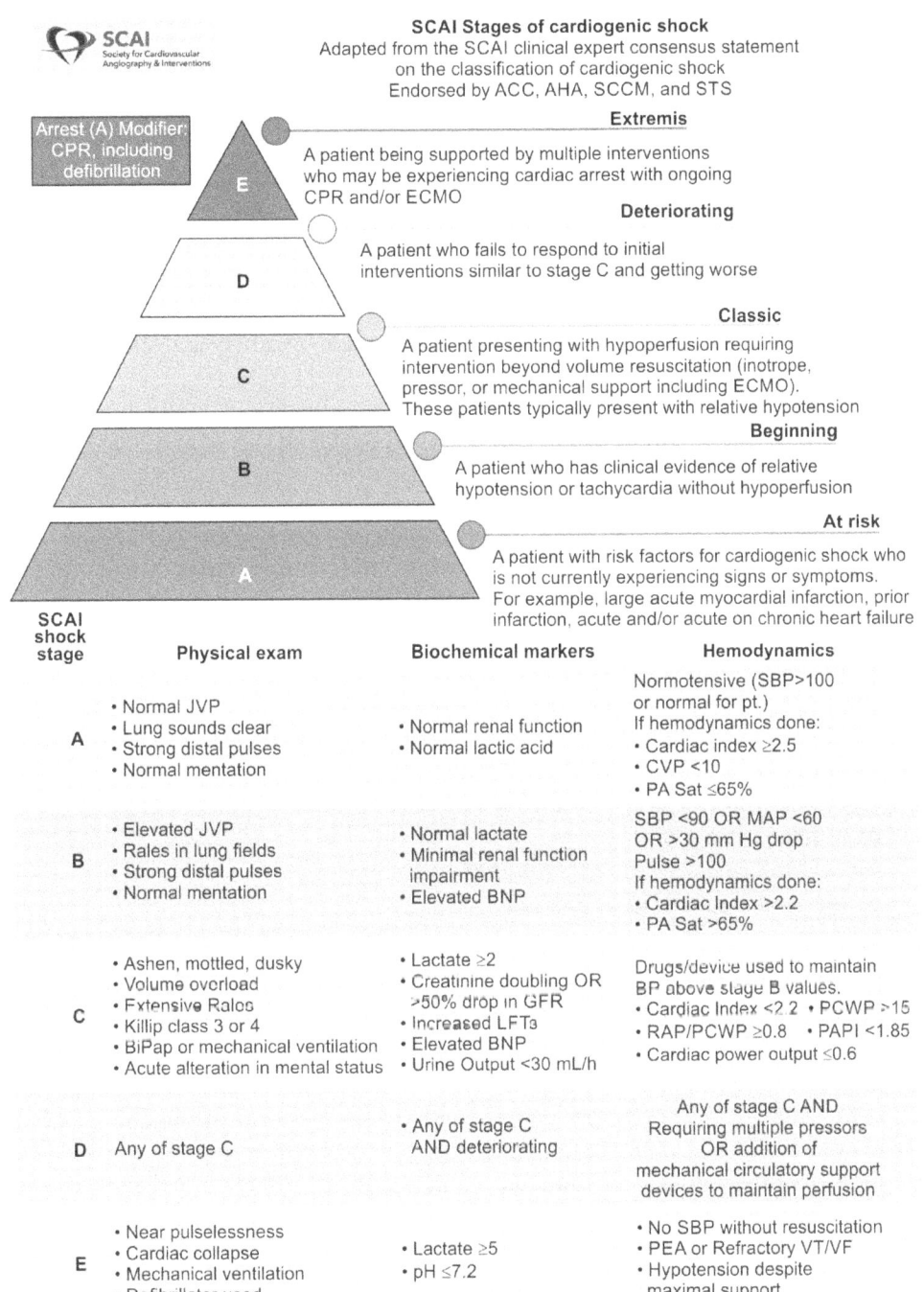

(BNP: brain natriuretic peptide; CPR: cardiopulmonary resuscitation; CVP: central venous pressure; ECMO: extracorporeal membrane oxygenation; GFR: glomerular filtration rate; JVP: jugular venous pressure; LFT: liver function test; MAP: mean arterial pressure; PCWP: pulmonary capillary wedge pressure; RAP: right atrial pressure; SBP: systolic blood pressure)

output <30 mL/hour, cardiac index (CI) <2.2 L/min/m^2, pulmonary capillary wedge pressure (PCWP) >15 mm Hg, and lactate >2 mmol/L.

The 2016 European Society of Cardiology Heart Failure guidelines include clinical criteria along with hemodynamic criteria in the definition of cardiogenic shock: SBP <90 mm Hg despite appropriate fluid resuscitation with clinical and laboratory evidence of end-organ damage. Clinical criteria were defined as cold extremities, oliguria, altered mental status change, and narrow pulse pressure, and laboratory abnormalities included metabolic acidosis, elevated serum lactate, and elevated creatinine.

The Society for Angiography and Cardiovascular Interventions (SCAI) has recently proposed a classification system for cardiogenic shock encompassing clinical, biochemical, and hemodynamic parameters to guide treatment and classify outcomes.

Suggested Reading
1. Baran DA, Grines CL, Bailey S, Burkhoff D, Hall SA, Henry TD, et al. SCAI clinical expert consensus statement on the classification of cardiogenic shock. Catheter Cardiovasc Interv. 2019;94:29-37.
2. Hochman JS, Buller CE, Sleeper LA, Boland J, Dzavik V, Sanborn TA, et al. Cardiogenic shock complicating acute myocardial infarction–etiologies, management and outcome: a report from the SHOCK trial registry. Should we emergently revascularize occluded coronaries for cardiogenic shock? J Am Coll Cardiol. 2000;36:1063-70.

Q.11. A 62-year-old diabetic, known case of chronic kidney disease (CKD) on maintenance hemodialysis, presented with chest pain and dyspnea for last 7 days, with acute worsening of dyspnea over last 1 day. On examination, he was found to have Beck's triad. Bedside POCUS revealed a large pericardial effusion causing compression of right ventricle. The components of Beck's triad are all, except:
a. Hypotension
b. Muffled heart sound
c. Low-voltage QRS complexes on ECG
d. Elevated jugular venous pressure

Ans. a

Explanation: Cardiac tamponade is the term given to hemodynamic instability caused by compression of cardiac chambers by increased pericardial pressure due to accumulation of fluid, blood, or gas in pericardium. Beck's triad was described by American cardiothoracic surgeon Claude Beck as the presence of hypotension, muffled heart sounds on auscultation, and a raised jugular venous pressure (JVP). ECG often shows low-voltage complexes and pulsus paradoxus, i.e., inspiratory fall in SBP of more than 10 mm Hg during spontaneous breathing, may be seen. The diagnosis is made by echocardiography showing variable amount of pleural effusion with compression of right ventricular outflow tract in early diastole, and/or right atrium at end diastole. Treatment is urgent pericardiocentesis with hemodynamic management with fluid resuscitation and vasopressor infusions.

Suggested Reading
1. Mekontso Dessap A, Chew MS. Cardiac tamponade. Intensive Care Med. 2018;44(6):936-9.
2. Sternbach G. Claude Beck: cardiac compression triads. J Emerg Med. 1988;6(5):417-9.

Q.12. A 55-year-old female was admitted in ward with community-acquired pneumonia and mild hypoxemia requiring oxygen by nasal cannula. She is a known case of breast cancer with lungs and bone metastases. She is on enoxaparin for a known deep venous thrombosis in right femoral vein. Patient developed new onset hypotension in ward and has been transferred to ICU with altered sensorium. On admission to ICU, she is mildly febrile, with heart rate of 150 beats/min, respiratory rate of 35 breaths/min, and blood pressure of 80/60 mm Hg. She is drowsy but arousable and has distended neck veins with clear chest. ECG shows sinus tachycardia. The next most appropriate step in management should be:
  a. Initial fluid resuscitation with point-of-care ultrasound assessment of shock.
  b. Pan cultures followed by broad-spectrum antibiotic administration.
  c. CT pulmonary angiography should be done to rule out pulmonary embolism.
  d. D-dimer levels should be sent to rule out pulmonary embolism.

Ans. a

Explanation: The differential diagnoses for the new onset shock include acute pulmonary embolism (PE), septic shock, and acute decompensated heart failure. Initial management includes initial fluid resuscitation while evaluating the cause of shock, 1-hour sepsis bundle should be followed if sepsis is one of the differential diagnoses. A rapid ultrasound in shock (RUSH) protocol can give important clues about possible diagnoses, and appropriate therapy can be given without losing time. Computed tomography pulmonary angiography (CTPA) should be performed to diagnose PE if transthoracic echocardiography shows features of RV dysfunctions. Clinical probability of PE is determined in hemodynamically stable patients as per clinical gestalt or prediction rules before deciding whether a CTPA is needed to rule out PE. D-dimer should not be used to rule out PE in patients with moderate-to-high probability of PE. Because of its high negative predictive value in patients at low risk of PE, it is used to rule out PE in this category of patients.

Suggested Reading
1. Konstantinides SV, Meyer G, Becattini C, Bueno H, Geersing GJ, Harjola VP, et al.; ESC Scientific Document Group. 2019 ESC Guidelines for the diagnosis and management of acute pulmonary embolism developed in collaboration with the European Respiratory Society (ERS). Eur Heart J. 2020;41(4):543-603.
2. Seif D, Perera P, Mailhot T, Riley D, Mandavia D. Bedside ultrasound in resuscitation and the rapid ultrasound in shock protocol. Crit Care Res Pract. 2012;2012:503254.

Q.13. A 56-year-old gentleman, a known diabetic, presented with sudden onset chest pain and shortness of breath. A diagnosis of anterolateral wall ST-elevation myocardial infarction (STEMI) was made, and the patient underwent percutaneous coronary intervention (PCI). During the procedure, patient's BP decreased to 80/40 mm Hg and he was intubated in view of acute pulmonary edema leading to acute hypoxaemic respiratory failure. Regarding management of cardiogenic shock,

which of the following is the least preferred agent in the management of cardiogenic shock:
a. Norepinephrine
b. Dopamine
c. Dobutamine
d. Levosimendan

Ans. b

Explanation: Norepinephrine is the vasopressor of choice in the management of cardiogenic shock. Dobutamine can be used in combination with norepinephrine to improve cardiac contractility. In the subgroup of patients with cardiogenic shock in SHOCK II randomized control trial, dopamine use as first-line inotrope was associated with higher mortality and increased arrhythmogenicity compared to norepinephrine. Levosimendan infusion without bolus may also be used as an alternative to dobutamine in combination with norepinephrine, especially in patients who were on beta-blockers.

Suggested Reading
1. McDonagh TA, Metra M, Adamo M, Gardner RS, Baumbach A, Böhm M, et al. 2021 ESC Guidelines for the diagnosis and treatment of acute and chronic heart failure. Eur Heart J. 2021;42(36):3599-726.

Q.14. A patient of urosepsis and septic shock is on norepinephrine infusion at 1 µg/kg/min and vasopressin infusion at 0.04 units/kg/h. His MAP is 45 mm Hg. He is not fluid responsive. The following are appropriate course of actions, except:
a. Increase norepinephrine dose to 1.5 µg/kg/min.
b. Increase vasopressin infusion rate to 0.05 U/kg/h.
c. Add hydrocortisone 50 mg IV every 6 hourly.
d. Add epinephrine infusion.

Ans. b

Explanation: Vasopressin is a nonapeptide hormone produced by paraventricular and supraoptic nuclei of hypothalamus and secreted by posterior pituitary. It acts as a noncatecholamine vasoconstrictor by its action on V1 receptors in vascular smooth muscles. It is also known as antidiuretic hormone because of its action on V2 receptors in renal collecting ducts causing reabsorption of free water. During septic shock, there is an initial increase in vasopressin levels followed by vasopressin deficiency. The sensitivity of V1 receptors increases in vasoplegic shock. The vasopressin is administered at a dose of 0.01–0.04 units per kilogram per hour. Doses higher than 0.04 U/kg/h may be associated with coronary and mesenteric ischemia and skin necrosis and are, therefore, avoided. Besides vasoconstriction, vasopressin reduces pulmonary hypertension, has immunomodulatory property, and may reduce endothelial permeability and edema formation.

Escalation of norepinephrine dose, addition of epinephrine, and administration of steroid are all acceptable strategies as per surviving sepsis guidelines.

Suggested Reading
1. Ukor IF, Walley KR. Vasopressin in vasodilatory shock. Crit Care Clin. 2019;35(2):247-61.

Q.15. A 20-year-old boy presented with altered sensorium and hypotension. He has warm peripheries and flushed face. He is hypoxemic and tachypneic. Auscultation of chest reveals bilateral crepitations. Clinical features point toward distributive shock. All of the following are causes of distributive shock, except:
   a. Toxic shock syndrome
   b. Anaphylactic shock
   c. Septic shock
   d. Spinal shock

Ans. d

Explanation: Neurogenic shock is caused by loss of sympathetic tone due to spinal cord injury leading to vasodilation and decreased cardiac contractility. Spinal shock, on the other hand, is the temporary loss of neurological reflexes distal to the site of spinal cord injury. Anaphylaxis, sepsis, and toxic shock syndrome are all causes of vasodilatory or distributive shock. Other rare causes of distributive shock are adrenal crisis, MIS-C, and drug overdoses (barbiturates, antihypertensives, etc.).

Suggested Reading
   1. Narayan S, Petersen TL. Uncommon etiologies of shock. Crit Care Clin. 2022;38:429-41.

Q.16. You have administered 1.5 L of crystalloid to a patient in septic shock. The MAP is still less than 65 mm Hg and you want to decide if you should administer further intravenous fluid. You decide to administer a fluid challenge by administering 200 mL of crystalloid over 10 minutes and monitoring response. The following are positive target response that indicate fluid responsiveness, except:
   a. Increase in SV by 10% on Vigileo–FloTrac
   b. Increase in VTI by 10% on transthoracic echocardiography
   c. Increase in pulse pressure by 10%
   d. Increase in CVP by 10%

Ans. d

Explanation: Fluid administration can be useful in increasing cardiac output and oxygen delivery in fluid-responsive patients. In fluid unresponsive patients, fluid can hamper oxygen delivery by hemodilution and can lead to edema formation. Fluid challenge is performed to understand if the patient is fluid responsive or not. The considerations for fluid challenge can be described with TROL mnemonic: Type of fluid, Rate of administration, Objective and Limit. Increase in any direct or surrogate estimate of cardiac output, viz., velocity time integral, end-tidal CO_2, etc., can be used as a positive response to fluid challenge. Increase in filling pressures, viz., PCWP, E/E' ratio, and central venous pressure (CVP), indicates fluid nonresponsiveness and acts as indicators to limit fluid challenge.

Suggested Reading
   1. Vincent JL, Cecconi M, De Backer D. The fluid challenge. Crit Care. 2020;24(1):703.

Q.17. Which of the following is most closely related to systemic vascular resistance?
   a. Systolic blood pressure
   b. Diastolic blood pressure
   c. Mean arterial pressure
   d. Central venous pressure

Ans. b

Explanation: According to Ohm's law:

$$\text{Pressure} = \text{Flow} \times \text{Resistance}$$

From a hemodynamic point of view, flow is the cardiac output and resistance is systemic vascular resistance. Therefore:

$$\text{Pressure} = \text{CO} \times \text{SVR} = \text{SV} \times \text{HR} \times \text{SVR}$$

During systole, stroke volume (SV) ejected from left ventricle distends proximal arterial conduit, generating pressure proportional to SV and indirectly proportional to the capacitance of the arterial walls. Therefore:

$$\text{SBP} = \text{SV} \div \text{Capacitance}$$

During diastole, the stored SV in distended proximal arteries fills peripheral arterioles, leading to decay of pressure from SBP to diastolic blood pressure (DBP), depending on the systemic vascular resistance (SVR) and capacitance. Therefore, low DBP means low SVR and/or capacitance.

Decreased SV is usually associated with low SBP and normal-to-low pulse pressure. Decreased SVR usually leads to decreased SVR and widened pulse pressure.

Suggested Reading
1. McLean AW, Gunnerson KJ, Chawla LS. Low systemic arterial blood pressure. In: Vincent JL, Abraham E, Moore FA, Kochanek PM, Fink MP (Eds). Textbook of Critical Care, 7th edition. Philadelphia, PA: Elsevier; 2017. pp. 24-6.

Q.18. The FALLS (Fluid Administration Limited by Lung Sonography) protocol of point-of care ultrasound in acute circulatory shock is as follows:

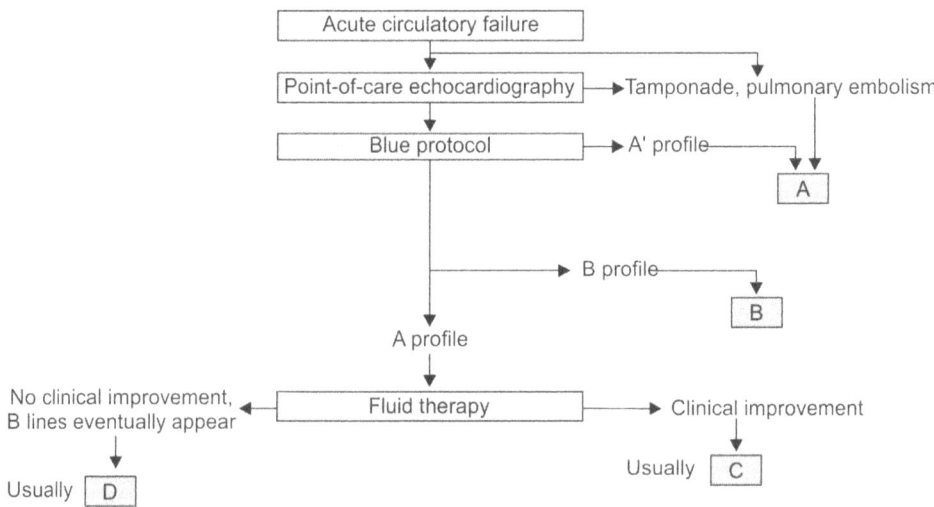

Which of the following are appropriate labels for the flowchart:
a. A: Hypovolemic shock; B: Septic shock; C: Obstructive shock; D: Cardiogenic shock
b. A: Septic shock; B: Obstructive shock; C: Cardiogenic shock; D: Hypovolemic shock

c. A: Cardiogenic shock; B: Septic shock; C: Hypovolemic shock; D: Obstructive shock
d. A: Obstructive shock; B: Cardiogenic shock; C: Hypovolemic shock; D: Septic shock

Ans. d

Explanation: The FALLS protocol (Fluid Administration Limited by Lung Sonography) uses point-of-care echocardiography and lung ultrasound to identify the different etiology of shock as mentioned in the algorithm above. First, the point-of-care echocardiography is done to rule out cardiac tamponade and right heart enlargement, which are potential causes of obstructive shock. Then, bedside lung ultrasound in emergency (BLUE) protocol is done. Abolished lung sliding with underlying A lines (A' profile) indicates the possibility of tension pneumothorax which is another cause of obstructive shock. If lung sliding is present, absence of B lines rules out left cardiogenic shock. Fluid boluses are administered with repeat lung ultrasonography. Good clinical improvement usually indicates hypovolemic shock. Absence of improvement and eventual accumulation of B lines usually indicates septic shock. One potential limitation of this protocol is that an initial lung disorder may generate a B-profile on admission, which can complicate the interpretation of ultrasound findings.

Suggested Reading
1. Lichtenstein D. FALLS-protocol: lung ultrasound in hemodynamic assessment of shock. Heart Lung Vessel. 2013;5(3):142-7.

Q.19. The following is a graphical representation of hemodynamic profile before and after administration of drugs A, B, and C. Identify the drugs correctly.

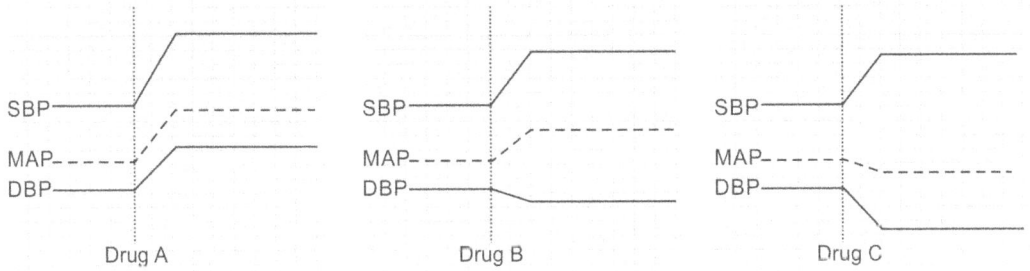

a. A: Norepinephrine; B: Epinephrine; C: Isoprenaline
b. A: Epinephrine; B: Isoprenaline; C: Norepinephrine
c. A: Isoprenaline; B: Norepinephrine; C: Epinephrine
d. A: Norepinephrine; B: Isoprenaline; C: Adrenaline

Ans. a

Explanation: The main hemodynamic effect of norepinephrine (NE) is dose-dependent arterial and venous vasoconstriction by α-adrenergic stimulation. The positive inotropic and chronotropic effects of β1 stimulation are generally counterbalanced by the increased afterload and reflex vagal response to increased peripheral vascular resistance. Therefore, NE usually leads to increase in SBP, DBP, and MAP with variable effect on pulse pressure. Epinephrine increases cardiac output by its action of β1 receptors, thereby increasing SBP and MAP. However, epinephrine in low dose causes β2-mediated vasodilation in skeletal muscles and may lead to nonimprovement or even decrease in DBP. Isoprenaline is a pure β1 and β2 receptor agonist and increases heart rate and cardiac output. However, it can lead to decrease in mean arterial and diastolic blood pressure with β2-mediated vasodilation.

Suggested Reading
1. Givertz MM, Fang JC. Approach to the patient with hypotension and hemodynamic instability. In: Irwin RS, Rippe JM (Eds). Irwin and Rippe's Intensive care medicine, 7th edition. Philadelphia (PA): Lippincott Williams and Wilkins; pp. 307-17.

Q.20. A 70-year-old gentleman was being treated in medicine ward for urinary tract infection. He was shifted to ICU in view of hypotension and worsening mentation. His BP was 84/59 mm Hg and HR was 140 beats per min. 2-L crystalloid was administered, and noradrenaline infusion was started at 0.1 μg/kg/min. Central venous catheter (CVC) and arterial lines were inserted and blood gas analyses of arterial and central venous samples were done and presented below:

	ABG	CVBG
pH	7.31	7.27
PaO_2	120	25
$PaCO_2$	33	42
HCO_3A	15.8	–
SO_2	99%	45%
Lactate	12	–

(ABG: arterial blood gas; CVBG: central venous blood gas)

From the above information, the following are true regarding patient's shock, except:
a. Low $ScvO_2$ indicates DO_2/VO_2 mismatch.
b. Venoarterial PCO_2 gap is high, indicating inadequate macro- or microcirculatory flow.
c. Critical oxygen delivery is lower in septic shock compared to normal individuals.
d. Further fluid bolus may improve perfusion in this patient.

Ans. c

Explanation: The fundamental abnormality of shock state is impairment of oxidative metabolism resulting in cellular and organ failures. This usually happens because of inadequate oxygen delivery to tissue, either due to less oxygen content or inadequate global blood flow or as a result of maldistribution of microcirculatory blood flow.

In a normal state, the global delivery of oxygen (DO_2) far exceeds the oxygen consumption (VO_2). At this point, VO_2 is independent of oxygen delivery and cardiac output (given in below **Figure 1**). As DO_2 decreases, VO_2 remains same by increasing oxygen extraction ratio (O_2ER), i.e., the ratio of $VO_2:DO_2$ from a normal level of 25% to a maximum level of 80%. The increase in oxygen extraction is clinically evident as a

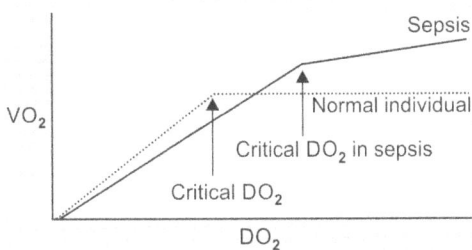

Fig. 1: Relation between delivery of oxygen (DO_2) and oxygen consumption (VO_2) in sepsis and normal individual.

decrease in mixed and central venous oxygen saturation. When oxygen extraction is maximized, a critical level of oxygen delivery (DO_2 crit) is reached below which VO_2 decreases proportionally to DO_2, and anaerobic metabolism ensues. This is the point from where the lactate levels increase significantly. The maximal oxygen extraction is less in altered states of sepsis and, therefore, critical oxygen delivery and anaerobic metabolism ensue at a higher DO_2 level.

Therefore, the markers of tissue dysoxia (impaired oxidative metabolism) include lactate and $ScvO_2$. Impairment of blood flow leads to accumulation of tissue CO_2 content. A stagnation or microcirculatory flow, either due to global decrease in cardiac output or microcirculatory flow abnormalities, leads to increase in venous partial pressure of CO_2 and consequent widening of venoarterial PCO_2 gap. A va-PCO_2 gap of more than 6 mm Hg usually indicates poor perfusion. Therefore, our patient with a PCO_2 gap of 9 mm Hg may benefit from augmentation of cardiac output with further fluid challenge.

Suggested Reading
1. Astiz ME. Pathophysiology and Classification of Shock States. In: Vincent JL, Abraham E, Moore FA, Kochanek PM, Fink MP (Eds). Textbook of Critical Care, 7th edition. Philadelphia, PA: Elsevier; 2017. pp. 617-22.
2. Ltaief Z, Schneider AG, Liaudet L. Pathophysiology and clinical implications of the venoarterial PCO_2 gap. Crit Care. 2021;25:318.

Q.21. A 56-year-old gentleman was shifted to your ICU from cardiac catheterization laboratory following primary PCI for anterior-wall myocardial infarction (MI). The patient has been placed on IABP counterpulsation for cardiogenic shock. The following are true regarding IABP counterpulsation, except:
 a. The augmented end-diastolic pressure is lower than unassisted end-diastolic pressure.
 b. Presence of blood in helium line indicates balloon rupture.
 c. Aortic regurgitation is an absolute contraindication to placement of IABP.
 d. The use of IABP is associated with reduction of mortality in patients of acute myocardial infarction with cardiogenic shock in the recent multicenter RCT.

Ans. d

Explanation: Intra-aortic balloon counterpulsation provides hemodynamic support to patients with heart failure. The procedure of "balloon counterpulsation" involves introducing an 8–9.5-Fr double lumen catheter with a 25–50-mL balloon toward its tip into the descending aorta through femoral or brachial approach. The balloon is inflated at closure of aortic valve and deflated at opening of aortic valve in the beginning of systole. The counterpulsation causes diastolic augmentation of aortic root pressure, and reduction of systolic and end-diastolic arterial pressures. Reduction of systolic pressure leads to reduction of afterload and improvement of stroke volume and myocardial oxygen demand.

The IABP insertion is contraindicated in aortic regurgitation as it increases the magnitude of regurgitation. IABP is contraindicated in suspected or known aortic dissection. It should be avoided in patients with severe peripheral artery disease.

Complications of IABP insertion are vascular (limb ischemia, thrombosis, aortic dissection or rupture, and bleeding), mechanical (balloon rupture, embolization, and inadequate inflation), infections, or related to anticoagulation. Presence of blood in helium line is an indicator of balloon rupture and requires prompt removal.

The IABP-SHOCK trial was a multicenter, open-label, randomized controlled trial that randomized 600 patients with cardiogenic shock complicating acute myocardial infarction undergoing early revascularization to intra-aortic balloon counterpulsation or no intra-aortic balloon counterpulsation. There was no difference in 30-day mortality or any secondary outcomes. The study had high crossover rate, with 10% of patients in control group subsequently had IABP insertion.

Suggested Reading
1. Thiele H, Zeymer U, Neumann FJ, Ferenc M, Olbrich HG, Hausleiter J, et al. Intra-aortic balloon support for myocardial infarction with cardiogenic shock. N Engl J Med. 2012;367(14):1287-96.
2. Trost JC, Hillis LD. Intra-aortic balloon counterpulsation. Am J Cardiol. 2006;97(9):1391-8.

Q.22. In the patient mentioned in previous question, regarding choice of vasoactive medications in acute heart failure, which of the following medication is least likely to increase myocardial oxygen demand?
a. Norepinephrine
b. Milrinone
c. Dobutamine
d. Levosimendan

Ans. d

Explanation: Norepinephrine increases afterload by its activity on α receptors. Also, it has positive inotropic action by its effect of β receptors. All β agonists increase myocardial oxygen demand. Milrinone is a phosphodiesterase inhibitor that increases cyclic adenosine monophosphate (cAMP) concentration inside cardiomyocytes and vascular smooth muscle cells. It is a positive inotrope and chronotrope and vasodilator. It causes less increase in myocardial oxygen demand and tachycardia compared to β agonists. Levosimendan improves actin–myosin crossbridge formation rate by stabilizing the calcium–troponin C conformation. This mechanism leads to an increase in contractility without impairment of diastolic relaxation or increase in myocardial oxygen demand. Levosimendan also has weak phosphodiesterase inhibition activity. It also causes vasodilation by opening ATP-sensitive K^+ channels in vascular smooth muscle.

Suggested Reading
1. Felker GM, Teerlink JR. Diagnosis and Management of Acute Heart Failure. In: Libby P, Bonow RO, Mann DL, Tomaselli GF, Bhatt DL, Solomon SD (Eds). Braunwald's Heart Disease: A Textbook of Cardiovascular Medicine, 12 edition. Philadelphia, PA: Elsevier; 2022. pp. 946-74.
2. Pathak A, Lebrin M, Vaccaro A, Senard JM, Despas F. Pharmacology of levosimendan: inotropic, vasodilatory and cardioprotective effects. J Clin Pharm Ther. 2013;38(5):341-9.

Q.23. A 72-year-old gentleman has been brought in with alleged history of road traffic accident and blunt abdominal trauma. He is in profound hemorrhagic shock not responding to initial fluid bolus. Patient is on oral apixaban for permanent atrial fibrillation. The following are acceptable measures for reversal of apixaban, except:
a. Hemodialysis
b. Oral activated charcoal
c. Tranexamic acid
d. Andexanet alfa

Ans. a

Explanation: With the increasing popularity of newer oral anticoagulants (NOACs), the number of patients with life-threatening bleed who are on NOACs is increasing. NOACs usually have shorter half-lives compared to warfarin. They are direct thrombin inhibitors (dabigatran) and direct factor Xa inhibitors (rivaroxaban, apixaban, and edoxaban).

The following strategy can be applied for patients on NOACs presenting with life-threatening bleeding:
- Immediate discontinuation of drugs along with other general measures including blood transfusions in all patients.
- Oral activated charcoal, in case of recent last dose (2-4 hours).
- Antifibrinolytic agents such as tranexamic acid.
- Specific antidotes may be needed in major bleeding wherein the risk of bleeding far outweighs thrombosis-related complications.
  - *Dabigatran:* Idarucizumab. If unavailable, use prothrombin complex concentrate (PCC) or activated PCC (aPCC).
  - *Factor Xa inhibitors:* Andexanet alfa. If unavailable, use PCC or aPCC.
- Dabigatran is dialyzable, but factor Xa inhibitors are not removed by hemodialysis.

Suggested Reading
1. Tomaselli GF, Mahaffey KW, Cuker A, Dobesh PP, Doherty JU, Eikelboom JW, et al. 2020 ACC Expert Consensus Decision Pathway on Management of Bleeding in Patients on Oral Anticoagulants: A Report of the American College of Cardiology Solution Set Oversight Committee. J Am Coll Cardiol. 2020;76(5):594-622.

Q.24. A young male presented to the trauma ER after a high-velocity motor vehicle accident. He has sustained traumatic brain injury (TBI) with multiple contusions and blunt abdominal trauma with high-grade splenic laceration. Regarding resuscitation of shock in this patient, the fluid of choice will be:
a. Normal saline
b. Ringer's lactate
c. 5% human albumin
d. Hydroxyethyl starch solution

Ans. a

Explanation: Isotonic 0.9% saline may be a better option than mildly hypotonic balanced crystalloids in patients of TBI at risk of cerebral edema. Subgroup analysis of BASICS study found less 90-day mortality rate in the saline group compared to the balanced solution group. As per the latest Advanced Trauma Life Support (ATLS) guidelines, crystalloid administration should be limited to initial 1 L and a damage control resuscitation is advocated. A patient not responding to initial 1 L bolus should receive blood transfusion. Human albumin is not advisable in patients with brain trauma, as its use has been found to be associated with increased mortality in the subgroup of patients with TBI in the SAFE study. The probable reason may be related to the hypotonic carrier of albumin rather than albumin itself. However, the lack of evidence of definite superiority as a resuscitative fluid and potential harm make albumin an unpopular option in TBI. Hydroxyethyl starch has fallen out of favor due to possibility of worsening kidney functions and coagulopathy. An excellent review of fluid resuscitation in critically ill patients is recommended in the first reference below.

Suggested Reading
1. Finfer S, Myburgh J, Bellomo R. Intravenous fluid therapy in critically ill adults. Nat Rev Nephrol. 2018;14(9):541-57.
2. SAFE Study Investigators; Australian and New Zealand Intensive Care Society Clinical Trials Group; Australian Red Cross Blood Service; George Institute for International Health; Myburgh J, Cooper DJ, et al. Saline or albumin for fluid resuscitation in patients with traumatic brain injury. N Engl J Med. 2007;357(9):874-84.
3. Zampieri FG, Machado FR, Biondi RS, Freitas FGR, Veiga VC, Figueiredo RC, et al. Effect of intravenous fluid treatment with a balanced solution vs 0.9% saline solution on mortality in critically ill patients: The BaSICS Randomized Clinical Trial. JAMA. 2021;326(9):818-29.

Q.25. A 20-year-old female, ASA-PS 1, is undergoing laparoscopic cholecystectomy. Immediately after administration of antibiotics, she develops profound hypotension and her oxygen saturation drops. Her peak airway pressure increases, and diffuse wheeze and crepitations are found on chest auscultation. The drug of choice for management of shock in this patient is:
a. Norepinephrine
b. Epinephrine 1 mg IM
c. Vasopressin
d. Epinephrine 100 µg IV boluses

Ans. d

Explanation: Perioperative anaphylaxis is an immediate life-threatening event with a mortality rate of approximately 4%. The most commonly involved agents include antibiotics followed by neuromuscular blocking agents. Other agents that may trigger anaphylaxis include dyes, latex, chlorhexidine, etc. Clinical manifestations are acute onset of hypotension, often associated with mucocutaneous signs, bronchospasm with increased airway pressures, and gastrointestinal signs. In extreme cases, sudden cardiac arrest may occur. The severity of clinical manifestations is classified by Ring and Messmer classification. The treatment includes stoppage of all ongoing medications—epinephrine and liberal intravenous fluid administration. As patient already has IV access in situ in perioperative settings, intravenous boluses of 100–200 µg epinephrine, starting with lower dose, are administered and repeated every 1–2 minutes. Epinephrine infusion can also be started at a rate from 0.05 to 0.5 µg/kg/min if shock is not resolving or recurrent after three boluses. Inhaled salbutamol is used to treat bronchospasm. Glucagon is used in patients with refractory shock who were on β blockers. Other drugs commonly used without much evidence of benefit include steroid, antihistamines, and sugammadex.

Suggested Reading
1. Dewachter P, Savic L. Perioperative anaphylaxis: pathophysiology, clinical presentation and management. BJA Educ. 2019;19(10):313-20.

Q.26. A 29-year-old pregnant lady presented with acute shortness of breath. On examination, she was found to be tachypneic and tachycardiac. She is normotensive. Auscultation of chest is unremarkable. Serum D-dimer is high and a diagnosis of PE is suspected. The next investigation to be performed is:
a. 2D-echocardiography
b. Compression proximal venous duplex ultrasound
c. CT pulmonary angiography
d. V/Q lung scan

Ans. b

Explanation: In a pregnant lady suspected to have PE (based on clinical prediction rules with/without D-dimer), venous compression ultrasound (CUS) should be initially done to avoid unnecessary irradiation. Further imaging (CTPA or perfusion lung scan) needs to be done only if CUS does not show a proximal deep venous thrombosis (DVT).

Suggested Reading
1. Konstantinides SV, Meyer G, Becattini C, Bueno H, Geersing GJ, Harjola VP, et al. 2019 ESC Guidelines for the diagnosis and management of acute pulmonary embolism developed in collaboration with the European Respiratory Society (ERS). Eur Heart J. 2020;41(4):543-603.

Q.27. A 76-year-old male presents with acute-onset epigastric pain, shortness of breath, and sweating. On evaluation, the patient had anterolateral territory ST elevation on ECG. The patient was planned for coronary angiography. Screening 2D-echocardiography showed regional wall motion abnormality in anterior wall with left ventricle ejection fraction of 25%. Intra-aortic balloon counterpulsation (IABP) was planned before taking up the patient for angiography. Which of the following is true regarding intra-aortic balloon counterpulsation in this patient?
a. The use of IABP is associated with reduction of mortality in patients of acute myocardial infarction with cardiogenic shock.
b. IABP leads to reduction of left ventricular afterload, leading to leftward shift of pressure–volume curve.
c. IABP insertion is class-1 recommendation in this patient.
d. Helium-filled balloon of IABP is placed just distal (around 1 cm) to left subclavian artery.

Ans. b

Explanation: Intra-aortic counterpulsation has been widely used since its introduction to cardiovascular practice in 1967. It functions by augmentation of diastolic blood pressure and reduction of left ventricular afterload, leading to leftward shift of pressure-volume curve using a helium-filled balloon placed just distal (around 1 cm) to left subclavian artery. The inflation and deflation of the balloon are synchronized with cardiac mechanical activity by using either a continuous ECG or an invasive arterial waveform.

The use of IABP in cardiogenic shock was supported by European Society of Cardiology (ESC) in year 2008 as Class-1, Level-C recommendation based on its beneficial effects on hemodynamic, renal functions, and overall reduction in mortality. But, the whole perspective changed after results of IABP-Shock II trial in 2012 and this now recommends it as Class 3, Level B in management of acute heart failure due to myocardial infarction.

However, some recent literatures contradict the neutral results of IABP-Shock II in managing cardiogenic shock. A retrospective study of 193 patients admitted with cardiogenic shock (70% attributed to acute coronary syndrome) compared 30-day mortality between groups receiving "early" (within 1 hour) and "late" institution of IABP. Mortality was less in early group (24%) in comparison to late (49%).

The IABP use in cardiac surgery holds its ground and is supported by German S3 guidelines, which recommend that hemodynamically stable patients with high-risk cardiac surgery should be implanted a preoperative IABP even before induction of anesthesia (Grade B Recommendation, Level of evidence 1b). IABP proves to be more physiological in producing a pulsatile blood flow to organs during cardiopulmonary bypass (CPB).

Suggested Reading
1. Gul B, Bellumkonda L. Usefulness of intra-aortic balloon pump in patients with cardiogenic shock. Am J Cardiol. 2019;123:750-6.
2. Heringlake M, Berggreen AE, Paarmann H. Still a place for aortic counterpulsation in cardiac surgery and patients with cardiogenic shock? Crit Care. 2021;25:309.
3. Pilarczyk K, Bauer A, Boening A, von der Brelie M, Eichler I, Gohrbandt B, et al. S3-guideline: recommendations for intra-aortic balloon pumping in cardiac surgery. Thorac Cardiovasc Surg. 2015;63(Suppl 2):S131-96.
4. Thiele H, Zeymer U, Neumann FJ, Ferenc M, Olbrich HG, Hausleiter J, et al. Intra-aortic balloon support for myocardial infarction with cardiogenic shock. N Engl J Med. 2012;367:1287-96.

Q.28. A 52-year-old female presented with hypotension, diminished pulses, and jugular venous distention with normal oxygen saturation orthopnea. The patient is a known case of acute coronary syndrome (inferior-wall MI) with left ventricular ejection fraction of 35%. Blood gases showed central venous oxygen saturation (ScVO$_2$) of 55%, and central venous-to-arterial carbon dioxide partial pressure difference (ΔPCO$_2$) was 9%. Which is the optimal end point for fluid resuscitation in this scenario?
 a. Fluid should not be administered to this patient.
 b. ScVO$_2$ of <70% and ΔPCO$_2$ of >6%

c. ScVO$_2$ of >70% and ΔPCO$_2$ of >6%
d. ScVO$_2$ of >70% and ΔPCO$_2$ of <6%

Ans. d

Explanation: Cardiogenic shock is not merely a state of reduced cardiac output, rather it involves multiorgan dysfunction, vasodilation, and systemic inflammatory response. As per the SHOCK trial, acute myocardial infarction presenting as left ventricular dysfunction is the leading cause of cardiogenic shock (80%). Patients presenting with inferior-wall MI and RV dysfunction show a good hemodynamic response to fluid resuscitation, but it can be potentially detrimental in cases of noninferior-wall MI, where increasing LV preload can further stress the failing heart or even in cases of RV dysfunction but occurring due to structural causes such as severe ARDS or pulmonary embolism. However, end point of resuscitation is necessary in both the situations.

Increase in cardiac output >10% with preload augmentation either by a fluid challenge or by performing passive leg raising (PLR) test is the gold standard for defining fluid responsiveness. Stroke volume and volume responsiveness assessment by Swan-Ganz pulmonary artery catheter is no longer preferred due to invasiveness and presence of rather noninvasive and reliable techniques like left ventricle outflow tract velocity time integral (LVOT-VTI). Stroke volume variation (SVV) and pulse pressure variation (PPV) are more feasible, but require sinus rhythm along with mechanical ventilation with tidal volume of 8 mL/kg body weight. Recent literature also supports rise in end-tidal carbon dioxide (EtCO$_2$) as a marker of fluid responsiveness. A rise of ≥2 mm Hg after 1 minute of PLR was associated with fluid responsiveness with a sensitivity of 75% and a specificity of 70% in a study done by Toupin et al. Central venous oxygen saturation (ScVO$_2$) of <70% may indicate reduced cardiac output, anemia, hypoxemia, or increased oxygen extraction by tissues in state of shock as a result of fall in DO$_2$ (delivery of oxygen to peripheral tissues). Central venous-to-arterial carbon dioxide partial pressure difference (ΔPCO$_2$) is also a marker of reduced cardiac output and peripheral hypoperfusion. In patients in cardiogenic or vasodilatory shock, without signs of global hypoxia or anaerobic metabolism, ΔPCO$_2$ can be used to reflect organ perfusion status. COA gap of >6 is an indicator of stagnation of CO$_2$ in the venous system during initial phases. Later, its rise is also attributed to the anaerobic metabolism due to hypoxic hypoxia. It also implies that inotropy will help in improving the shock at this point. The closure of this gap can also be used as an indicator of adequate resuscitation along with reduction serum lactic acid levels and improvement of ScVO$_2$.

Suggested Reading
1. Hochman JS, Buller CE, Sleeper LA, Boland J, Dzavik V, Sanborn TA, et al. Cardiogenic shock complicating acute myocardial infarction—etiologies, management and outcome: a report from the SHOCK Trial Registry. J Am Coll Cardiol. 2000;36(3 Suppl 1):1063-70.
2. Memon AR, Ansari MI, Shaikh SA, Abubakar J, Karim M, Salahuddin N. Fluid resuscitation in cardiogenic shock: an assessment of responsiveness and outcome. J Ayub Med Coll Abbottabad. 2021;33(3):471-4.

Q.29. Which of the following is inotrope of choice in cardiogenic shock?
a. Levosimendan
b. Norepinephrine
c. Milrinone
d. Dobutamine

Ans. b

Explanation: Cardiogenic shock is a state of profound myocardial depression leading to reduction in cardiac output, in turn causing reduced mean arterial pressure, further reducing coronary perfusion causing myocardial ischemia and depression. This stimulates sympathetic nervous system as a protective response causing increase in heart rate and systemic vasoconstriction at the expense of increased myocardial oxygen demand. However, there is often peripheral vasodilation as a result of activation of proinflammatory pathways. All this pathophysiology needs to be addressed with continuous hemodynamic monitoring and frequent assessment to manage a patient with cardiogenic shock.

Inotropes (dopamine, dobutamine, milrinone, and levosimendan) and vasopressors (norepinephrine, epinephrine, vasopressin, and phenylephrine) are the cornerstone of medical management of cardiogenic shock. Vasopressors are class IIb/c and class IIb/b recommended by the European Society of Cardiology guidelines in the management of cardiogenic shock. The American Heart Association (AHA) recommends norepinephrine as the vasopressor of choice in many patients as it is associated with fewer arrhythmias. However, no single drug can be labeled as the optimal first-line vasoactive drug due to the heterogeneity in the etiology of cardiogenic shock. The European Society of Cardiology 2017 guidelines for the management of acute myocardial infarction causing cardiogenic shock patients with ST elevation recommend norepinephrine as a vasopressor of choice in hypotensive patients with insufficient organ perfusion pressures (class IIb) based on a study done by De Backer et al., showing lower rate of cardiac arrhythmia and lower mortality when compared to dopamine. For augmentation of cardiac contractility (class IIb), inotropes like dobutamine may be given simultaneously to norepinephrine. In 2021, a prospective, double-blind randomized trial (CAPITAL DOREMI) compared 192 patients admitted in intensive care unit with cardiogenic shock with respect to in-hospital death from any cause, TIA, cardiovascular, or renal event. They were randomized into milrinone or dobutamine cohort, the conclusion was—no significant difference between the two drugs was found. Another CAPITAL DOREMI2 study is a multicenter, double-blind, randomized, placebo-controlled trial which began recruitment in March 2022. It is anticipated that the trial will be completed over a 3-year period at multiple centers across North America. It is aimed at comparing dobutamine and milrinone with placebo in cases of cardiogenic shock admitted to intensive care unit.

Suggested Reading
1. Mathew R, Di Santo P, Jung RG, Marbach JA, Hutson J, Simard T, et al. Milrinone as compared with dobutamine in the treatment of cardiogenic shock. N Engl J Med. 2021;385(6):516-25.

2. Shankar A, Gurumurthy G, Sridharan L, Gupta D, Nicholson WJ, Jaber WA, et al. A clinical update on vasoactive medication in the management of cardiogenic shock. Clin Med Insights Cardiol. 2022;16:11795468221075064.
3. Van Diepen S, Katz JN, Albert NM, Henry TD, Jacobs AK, Kapur NK, et al. Contemporary management of cardiogenic shock: a scientific statement from the American Heart Association. Circulation. 2017; 136(16):e232-68.

Q.30. Which of the following is true regarding Impella (cardiac assist device) in cardiogenic shock?
a. Impella can provide 4.0–5.0 L/min of cardiac output.
b. Impella device was not associated with lower 30-day mortality compared with IABP.
c. Impella results in an increase in mean arterial pressure and cardiac output, improved systemic perfusion, and increased coronary flow.
d. All of the above.

Ans. d

Explanation: The Impella device is a catheter-based miniaturized ventricular assist device. Using a retrograde femoral artery access, it is placed in the left ventricle across the aortic valve. The device pumps blood from left ventricle into ascending aorta and helps to maintain a systemic circulation at an upper rate between 2.5 and 5.0 L/min. The most common indications for using the Impella device are in the treatment of acute myocardial infarction complicated by cardiogenic shock and to facilitate high-risk coronary angioplasty. Other indications include the treatment of cardiomyopathy with acute decompensation, postcardiotomy shock, and off-pump coronary bypass surgery.

The Impella 5.0/LD can be placed directly into the proximal aorta via an end-to-end anastomotic conduit. All models are placed across the aortic valve using fluoroscopic or echocardiographic guidance. The pigtail shape of the catheter facilitates crossing of the aortic valve and promotes a stable position. Once in a satisfactory position within the LV, the Impella catheter is connected distally to a portable mobile console that displays invasive pressures with the actual revolutions per minute of the pump, thus guiding the correct positioning of the device. Once activated, the Impella continuously draws blood from the LV via the inlet port and then expels it into the ascending aorta via the outlet port. The Impella can provide 4.0–5.0 L/min. In comparison, the ability of the IABP to augment cardiac output is very modest, no more than 0.5 L/min. By continuously drawing blood from the LV, the Impella unloads the LV, thereby decreasing LV work and myocardial oxygen demand. In addition, by delivering large volumes of blood to the aorta, Impella operation results in an increase in mean arterial pressure and cardiac output, resulting, in turn, in improved systemic perfusion and increased coronary flow. Finally, Impella leads to a decrease in pulmonary wedge pressure and a secondary reduction in right ventricular afterload.
- IMPRESS TRIAL 2 retrospective analysis of patients with AMI-CS: The use of an Impella device was not associated with lower 30-day mortality compared with

matched patients from the IABP-SHOCK II trial treated with an IABP or medical therapy.
- PROTECT II TRIAL 3 (A Prospective, Randomized Clinical Trial of Hemodynamic Support with Impella 2.5 versus Intra-Aortic Balloon Pump in Patients Undergoing High-Risk Percutaneous Coronary Intervention): The 30-day incidence of major adverse events was not different for patients with IABP or Impella 2.5 hemodynamic support. However, trends for improved outcomes were observed for Impella 2.5-supported patients at 90 days.

Suggested Reading
1. Neill WW, Kleiman NS, Moses J, Henriques JP, Dixon S, Massaro J, et al. A prospective, randomized clinical trial of hemodynamic support with Impella 2.5 versus intra-aortic balloon pump in patients undergoing high-risk percutaneous coronary intervention: the PROTECT II study. Circulation. 2012;126(14):1717-27.
2. Schrage B, Ibrahim K, Loehn T, Werner N, Sinning JM, Pappalardo F, et al. Impella support for acute myocardial infarction complicated by cardiogenic shock. Circulation. 2019;139(10):1249-58.

CHAPTER 4

Mechanical Ventilation

Rajesh Pande, Pradyut Bag, Jitin Sharma

Q.1. The determinants of mechanical Ti (inspiratory time) in pressure support ventilation (PSV) mode of ventilation include all the following, except:
   a. Inspiratory trigger
   b. Level of pressure support
   c. Cycling off percentage
   d. Respiratory system mechanics

Ans. a

Explanation: The determinants of mechanical Ti in PSV include patient efforts [muscle pressure (P_{mus})], level of pressure support, cycling off percentage set by operator and the respiratory system mechanics. Therefore, mechanical Ti in PSV is modified by several other variables, independent of neural Ti, and there is a significant risk for expiratory asynchronies due to premature or delayed cycling off.

Suggested Reading
1. Proklou A, Karageorgos, Vaproidi K. The potential risk of pressure support ventilation. In: Vincent JL (Ed). Annual Update in Intensive Care and Emergency Medicine 2023. Cham: Springer; 2023. p. 1006.

Q.2. The determinants of tidal volume during PSV include all of the following, except:
   a. Patient effort
   b. Set level of pressure support by ventilator
   c. Inspiratory time
   d. Inspiratory flow

Ans. d

Explanation: The tidal volume delivered in each PSV assisted breath is determined by patient effort (Pmus), set level of pressure support, inspiratory time as determined by cycling off criteria and the respiratory system mechanics.

Suggested Reading
1. Proklou A, Karageorgos, Vaproidi K. The potential risk of pressure support ventilation. In: Vincent JL (Ed). Annual Update in Intensive Care and Emergency Medicine 2023. Cham: Springer; 2023. p. 1006.

Q.3. Which of the following modes is not a closed loop system:
   a. Adaptive support ventilation
   b. Pressure support ventilation
   c. Pressure regulated volume support (PRVC)
   d. Volume support

Ans. b

Explanation: The term "closed-loop control" refers to the use of a feedback signal to adjust the output of a system. Ventilators use closed-loop control to maintain consistent pressure and flow waveforms in the face of changing patient/system conditions. This is accomplished by using the output as a feedback signal that is compared to the operator-set input. The difference between the two is used to drive the system toward the desired output.

Suggested Reading
1. Chatburn RL, Cabodevila EM. Closed-loop control of mechanical ventilation: description and classification of targeting schemes. Respir Care. 2011;56(1):85-98.

Q.4. In which mode of ventilation is only the pressure support level adjusted automatically to achieve the target tidal volume?
a. Volume support (VS)
b. VAPS (volume-assured pressure support)
c. MMV (mandatory minute ventilation)
d. APRV (airway pressure release ventilation)

Ans. a

Explanation: Volume support is a hybrid mode-variable pressure support. This closed loop variant of PSV adjusts the inspiratory pressure assist level within set limits to provide desired tidal volume. This mode is beneficial for patients who can initiate their own breaths but require additional support to achieve adequate ventilation.

Suggested Reading
1. Abbasi S, Alikiaii B, Kashefi P, Haddadzadegan N. Comparison of volume support, volume-assured pressure support, and spontaneous modes in postoperative early extubated patients. Adv Biomed Res. 2022;11:99.

Q.5. When a patient does not breathe spontaneously on the APRV mode of ventilation, the pressure-time scalar resembles like that of which of the following mode?
a. Bilevel ventilation
b. Pressure control-synchronized intermittent mandatory ventilation
c. Pressure-controlled inverse ratio ventilation (PCIRV)
d. Volume-controlled continuous mandatory ventilation (VC-CMV)

Ans. c

Explanation: Airway pressure release ventilation is a spontaneously breathing mode used in ARDS patients with hypoxemic respiratory failure and uses a much longer inspiratory time and a very short expiratory time (0.4–0.6 seconds). The inverse ratio ranges from 1:5 to 1:9. In case the patient stops breathing, the mode works like pressure control ventilation (PCV) with extreme inverse I:E ratio and may be detrimental to the patient.

Suggested Reading
1. Habashi NM. Other approaches to open-lung ventilation: airway pressure release ventilation. Crit Care Med. 2005;33(Suppl 3):S228-40.

Q.6. The incidence of VAP may be reduced by employing which of the following procedures?
   a. Proper handwashing
   b. More frequent ventilator circuit change
   c. Use of prophylactic appropriate antibiotics
   d. Closed suction system

Ans. a

Explanation: Change of ventilator circuit is recommended only when it is visibly soiled or contaminated. There is no role of prophylactic antibiotics in ventilated patients for prevention of pneumonia. Closed and open suction techniques are similar in relation to incidence of VAP, however closed suction prevents loss of positive end-expiratory pressure (PEEP) and desaturation in high-risk patients. Hand hygiene compliance reduces microbial concentration and reduces VAP.

Suggested Reading
   1. Hellyer TP, Ewan V, Wilson P, Simpson AJ. The Intensive Care Society recommended bundle of interventions for the prevention of ventilator-associated pneumonia. J Intensive Care Soc. 2016;17(3):238-43.

Q.7. Inverse ratio ventilation (IRV) is accomplished mainly by:
   a. Decreasing the VT
   b. Increasing the inspiratory flow rate
   c. Increase mean airway pressure
   d. Decreasing the peak inspiratory pressure (PIP)

Ans. c

Explanation: In conventional pressure controlled inverse ratio ventilation (PC-IRV), the patient is paralyzed, sedated, and the ventilator is set in the PCV mode with reversal of the I:E ratio. The inspiratory phase is much longer and the area under the pressure time scalar increases significantly with increase in mean alveolar pressure, resulting in better oxygenation.

Suggested Reading
   1. Marcy TX, Marini J. Inverse ratio ventilation in ARDS. Chest. 1991;100:494-504.

Q.8. Which statement is false regarding mean airway pressure?
   a. High I:E ratio increase mean airway pressure.
   b. In volume-controlled ventilation (VCV) mean airway pressure is higher compared to PCV.
   c. PEEP is the main determinant of mean airway pressure.
   d. A decelerating flow waveform pattern shown to increase mean airway pressure.

Ans. b

Explanation: Mean airway pressure (MAP) is the average pressure in the airways during mechanical ventilation. By maintaining an adequate MAP, ventilation can be optimized to improve oxygenation and support lung function. The MAP is determined by several factors during mechanical ventilation that include inspiratory time—a longer inspiratory time increases the mean airway pressure, inspiratory flow rate—a higher flow rate results in a faster rise in pressure and thus increases the mean airway pressure, PEEP—higher levels of PEEP increase the baseline pressure and raise MAP. Higher PIP also results in increased MAP. Similarly a higher respiratory rate decreases the time available for expiration, leading to an increased MAP. In addition, decreased compliance or increased resistance can also result in higher MAP.

In VCV the MAP is primarily influenced by the inspiratory time, inspiratory flow rate, and PEEP, whereas PCV uses a decelerating flow pattern, and the flow rate decreases as inspiration progresses, resulting in a longer inspiratory time. This longer inspiratory time allows for a higher MAP to be maintained since the pressure is sustained for a longer duration.

Suggested Reading
1. Marini JJ, Ravenscraft SA. Mean airway pressure: physiologic determinants and clinical importance-part 2. Crit Care Med. 1992;20(11):1604-16.

Q.9. All statements regarding time constant in mechanical ventilation are true, except:
a. The time constant mathematically corresponds to the product of resistance and compliance.
b. ARDS alveoli have a shorter time constant.
c. Longer time constant suggests that the alveoli fill and empty slowly.
d. One time constant (τ) indicates the time required to achieve 86.5% of the maximum volume variation when applying constant pressure to the respiratory system under muscular relaxation.

Ans. d

Explanation: Time constant refers to the response time of the respiratory system; the time constant (TC) is determined by the product of respiratory system compliance (Crs) and resistance (Rrs). One time constant quantifies the time taken for the lung volume to reach approximately 63% of its final value. A shorter time constant (ARDS alveoli) indicates a more rapid response of the respiratory system, whereas a longer time constant (COPD) suggests a slower response. Complete lung emptying or filling typically requires approximately 5-time constants.

Suggested Reading
1. Shevade MS. Time constant: what do we need to know to use it? Indian J Respir Care. 2019;8:4-7.

Q.10. All the statements regarding driving pressure in mechanical ventilation are true, except:
a. Driving pressures correlate with global lung strain.
b. Driving pressure can be expressed as the ratio between V_T and respiratory system compliance.

c. Driving pressure >14 cmH$_2$O was associated with an increased risk of hospital mortality in patients with moderate and severe ARDS.
d. Driving pressure predicts mortality irrespective of TV and PEEP in severe ARDS patients.

Ans. d

Explanation: Driving pressure is the difference between plateau pressure and PEEP. Amato's seminal work has shown that like low tidal volume and P$_{plat}$ <30 cmH$_2$O, the driving pressure >14 is also associated with higher mortality in ventilated ARDS patients.

Suggested Reading
1. Amato MBP, Meade MO, Slutsky AS, Brochard L, Costa EL, Schoenfeld DA, et al. Driving pressure and survival in the acute respiratory distress syndrome. N Engl J Med. 2015;372:747-55.

Q.11. A 50-year-old woman presents to the emergency department with 5 days of fevers and progressive dyspnea and is admitted to the intensive care unit (ICU). She is intubated in view of increasing respiratory distress, and chest X-ray following intubation demonstrates bilateral patchy opacities and interstitial markings throughout all lung fields, without any effusions. Her upper respiratory biofire is positive for influenza A. Her bedside echocardiogram reveals a left ventricular ejection fraction of 50% with otherwise normal findings. Her ventilator settings are volume control, tidal volume (VT) 425 mL, respiratory rate (RR) 18 breaths/minute, FiO$_2$ 1.0, and positive end expiratory pressure (PEEP) 8 cmH$_2$O. An initial arterial blood gas (ABG) is pH 7.30 PCO$_2$ 46 mm Hg and PO$_2$ 70 mm Hg. Which of the following therapies has been best shown to improve the survival of such patients?
a. Titration of PEEP with recruitment maneuver to optimize lung compliance.
b. Use of intravenous steroids
c. Use of inhaled pulmonary vasodilator for severe hypoxemia
d. Ventilation at a TV of 6 mL/kg of ideal body weight (IBW)
e. Frusemide infusion to maintain a negative fluid balance

Ans. d

Explanation: This patient is presenting with severe ARDS, as defined by the Berlin criteria—onset within 1 week or presentation, bilateral opacities on imaging, edema not fully explained by cardiogenic etiology, and PaO$_2$: FiO$_2$ ratio of <100. The ARDSNet trial demonstrated a significant mortality benefit with lung protective, low-TV ventilation (6 mL/kg IBW). Diuresis to an even fluid balance increases ventilator-free days in patients with ARDS but has not been found to have a mortality benefit. Similarly, while inhaled nitric oxide and PEEP titration may improve oxygenation, neither intervention has been demonstrated to improve survival. Although steroids are recommended for severe CAP if shock is present, their use has not shown any mortality benefits in viral severe community-acquired pneumonia (sCAP) due to influenza, severe acute respiratory syndrome (SARS), and Middle East respiratory syndrome (MERS).

Suggested Reading
1. ARDS Definition Task Force; Ranieri VM, Rubenfeld GD, Thompson BT, Ferguson ND, Caldwell E, et al. Acute respiratory distress syndrome: the Berlin definition. JAMA. 2012;307(23):2526-33.
2. Gebistorf F, Karam O, Wetterslev J, Afshari A. Inhaled nitric oxide for acute respiratory distress syndrome (ARDS) in children and adults. Cochrane Database Syst Rev. 2016;(6):CD002787.
3. Martin-Loeches I, Torres A, Nagavci B, Aliberti S, Antonelli M, Bassetti M, et al. ERS/ESICM/ESCMID/ALAT guidelines for the management of severe community-acquired pneumonia. Intensive Care Med. 2023;4:1-18.
4. The Acute Respiratory Distress Syndrome Network. Ventilation with lower tidal volumes as compared with traditional tidal volumes for acute lung injury and the acute respiratory distress syndrome. N Engl J Med. 2000;342:1301-8.

Q.12. A 54-year-old woman has been intubated for 4 days for community-acquired pneumonia. She is placed on a spontaneous breathing trial on ventilator settings of pressure support of 6 cmH$_2$O, PEEP of 6 cmH$_2$O, and FiO$_2$ of 0.3. What is the most accurate explanation of how breaths are cycled on this ventilator mode?
a. Breaths are initiated based on a set respiratory rate and I/E ratio.
b. Breaths are terminated when a target volume is reached.
c. Breaths are terminated when inspiratory flow decreases to a set percentage of peak inspiratory flow.
d. Breathes are initiated based on diaphragmatic inspiratory effort.
e. Breaths are terminated when a peak inspiratory flow is reached.

Ans. c

Explanation:

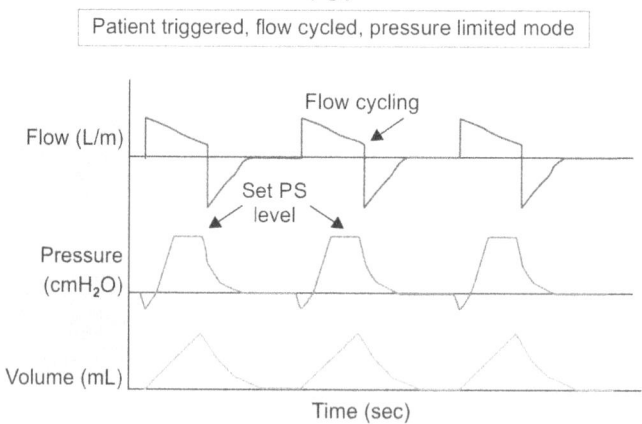

(PSV: pressure support ventilation)

Pressure support ventilation is a ventilator mode that relies completely on patient-triggered breaths. In this mode, the ventilator will cycle between two different pressures (PEEP and pressure support). PEEP will be the remaining pressure at the end of exhalation, and pressure support is the pressure above the PEEP that the ventilator will administer during each breath for support of ventilation. Pressure support breaths are cycled from inspiratory to expiratory when the patient's inspiratory flow reaches a set percentage of the peak inspiratory flow, often 25% of peak inspiratory flow by default (answer C is correct). Pressure assist-control, a form of continuous mandatory ventilation, cycles based on a set inspiratory time (answer A is incorrect). Volume assist-control, a form of continuous mandatory ventilation, cycles when a breath reaches a target TV, the time for which is dictated by an inspiratory flow rate (answer B is incorrect). Neurally assisted ventilation coordinates inspiratory support with diaphragmatic muscular effort (answer D is incorrect). There are no modes that are terminated by reaching a peak inspiratory flow (answer E is incorrect).

Suggested Reading
1. Gentile MA. Cycling of the mechanical ventilator breath. Respir Care. 2011;56(1):52-62.
2. Mora Carpio AL, Mora JI. Ventilator management. In: StatPearls [Internet]. Treasure Island (FL): StatPearls Publishing; 2023.

Q.13. All of the following are described as weaning failure, except:
a. Failed spontaneous breathing trial (SBT)
b. Reintubation and/or resumption of ventilatory support within 48 hours following successful extubation
c. Death within 48 hours following extubation
d. Requirement of noninvasive ventilation (NIV) postextubation

Ans. d

Explanation: Weaning success is defined as extubation and the absence of ventilatory support 48 hours following the extubation. Weaning failure is defined as one of the followings: (1) failed SBT; (2) reintubation and/or resumption of ventilatory support following successful extubation; or (3) death within 48 hours following extubation. The term *weaning in progress* is used for the patients who are extubated but remain supported by NIV.

Suggested Reading
1. Boles JM, Bion J, Connors A. Weaning from mechanical ventilation. Eur Respir J. 2007; 29:1033-56.
2. Chawla R, Varma V, Sharma R. (2012). Weaning. In: Chawla R, Todi S (Eds). ICU Protocols. India: Springer; 2012.

Q.14. A 36-year-old man was injured in a high-speed motor vehicle accident. On arrival in the emergency room, his Glasgow Coma Scale (GCS) score is 7, and he is immediately intubated. Injuries include a subdural hematoma and subarachnoid hemorrhage, as well as diffuse axonal injury, multiple nondisplaced rib fractures on left side, left pulmonary contusions, grade 2 splenic injury managed conservatively. On post-trauma 7, his GCS score is 11T, and he qualifies for extubation. Which of the following criteria for extubation is best supported by literature?
a. PaO_2/FiO_2 >300
b. Vital capacity >10 mL/kg

c. Cuff leak
d. Successful 30-minute spontaneous breathing trial
e. Maximal inspiratory pressure <-25 cmH$_2$O

Ans. d

Explanation: The option with the most literature support is a successful spontaneous breathing trial (SBT). Once the primary condition that led to intubation is resolved, the patient should be transitioned to SBT before extubation. It has been shown that ICU protocol-driven extubation shortens ventilation days. For an SBT to be successful, the patient must breathe spontaneously with little or no ventilator support for at least 30 minutes without tachypnea (respiratory rate >35 breaths/minute), no oxygen desaturation below 90%, heart rate below 140 beats/minute, no systolic blood pressure fluctuations of >180 or <90 mm Hg, no anxiety, and no diaphoresis. If this is successful, the patient should be able to protect the airway without too many secretions. All the other options, although useful, are not supported by literature in and of themselves but can be used in combination with other criteria.

Suggested Reading

1. McConville JF, Kress JP. Weaning patients from the ventilator. N Engl J Med. 2012;367(23):2233-9.
2. Zein H, Baratloo A, Negida A, Safari S. Ventilator weaning and spontaneous breathing trials: an educational review. Emerg (Tehran). 2016;4(2):65-71.

Q.15. A 56-year-old male is intubated and mechanically ventilated through a size 8 cuffed endotracheal tube after an exploratory laparotomy for intestinal obstruction. The patient is shifted to ICU for postoperative care. During the course of approximately 20 minutes, his oxygen saturation as measured by pulse oximetry begins to decrease from 97 to 91%, and his end-tidal carbon dioxide increases from 36 to 52 mm Hg. A flow-volume loop displayed on the ventilator is shown below.

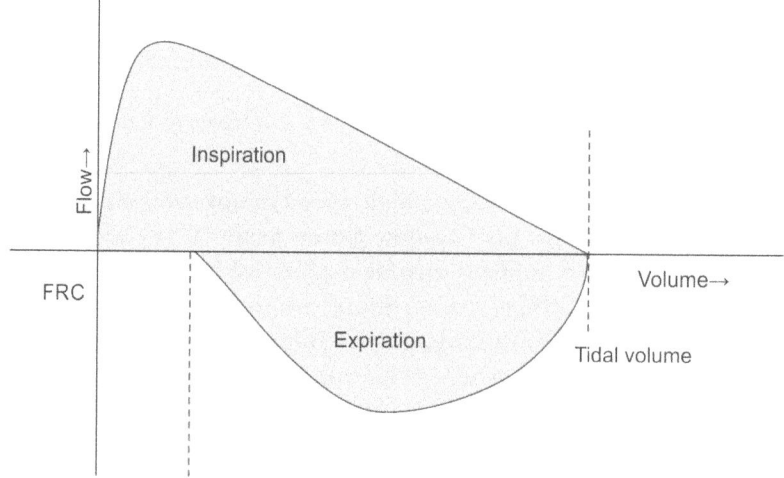

Which of the following is the most appropriate next step in management?
a. Decreasing the tidal volume delivered by the ventilator.
b. Administer inhaled bronchodilators.
c. Check whether the endotracheal tube balloon is deflated.
d. Reintubate the patient with bigger size tube.
e. Check the endotracheal tube for any blockage.

Ans. c

Explanation: The flow volume loop demonstrates a leak in the ventilator circuit. Inspired volume is greater than exhaled volume. This can be at any level in the circuit but commonly a ruptured balloon can cause a leak. In the setting of a circuit leak, decreasing the tidal volume would decrease minute volume and increase end-tidal carbon dioxide, and might worsen oxygenation by permitting alveolar collapse. Inhaled bronchodilators are not appropriate since there is no evidence of acute obstructive lung disease. Checking the endotracheal tube for any obstruction is not likely to be effective since there is no evidence of intrathoracic obstruction. Reintubating the patient might be necessary, but this would not be the next step since the cuff might require simple reinstallation of air.

Suggested Reading
1. Emrath E. The basics of ventilator waveforms. Curr Pediatr Rep. 2021;9:11-9.
3. Guntupalli KK, Bandi V, Sirgi C, Pope C, Rios A, Eshenbacher W. Usefulness of flow volume loops in emergency center and ICU settings. Chest. 1997;111(2):481-8.
2. Main E, Castle R, Stocks J, James I, Hatch D. The influence of endotracheal tube leak on the assessment of respiratory function in ventilated children. Intensive Care Med. 2001;27(11):1788-97.

Q.16. A 55-year-old woman with a history of chronic obstructive pulmonary disease presents with increasing shortness of breath over last 5 days. She is intubated in emergency room and shifted to ICU for further management. After initial stabilization on the ventilator, her oxygen saturation suddenly decreases to 80% despite a fraction of inspired oxygen of 100%. An inspiratory hold maneuver is performed which reveals the following parameters—peak inspiratory pressure 42 cmH$_2$O, plateau pressure 20 cmH$_2$O, positive end-expiratory pressure 5 cmH$_2$O. Which of the following is the most likely reason for her sudden hypoxia?
a. Decreased dynamic lung compliance, suggesting pneumothorax
b. Decreased static lung compliance, suggesting bronchospasm
c. Increased dynamic lung compliance, suggesting pneumothorax
d. Decreased dynamic lung compliance, suggesting bronchospasm
e. Increased static lung compliance, suggesting pneumothorax

Ans. d

Explanation: Static lung compliance is defined as the change in volume for a given applied pressure: Static compliance (C_{stat}) = tidal volume/[plateau pressure (P_{plat}) - positive end-expiratory pressure (PEEP)]. Common causes of decreased static lung compliance (stiff lungs) include restrictive lung diseases, pneumothorax, pleural effusion, and acute respiratory distress syndrome. Dynamic lung compliance is the compliance of the lungs during movement of air: Dynamic compliance (C_{dyn}) = tidal volume/[peak inspiratory pressure (PIP) − PEEP]. It is more directly affected by obstructive physiology, such as endotracheal tube occlusion, bronchial secretions, or bronchospasm. This patient has decreased dynamic lung compliance, demonstrated by the increase in PIP, but static lung compliance is unchanged. This suggests an obstructive process such as bronchospasm.

Suggested Reading
1. Desai JP, Moustarah F. Pulmonary compliance. In: StatPearls [Internet]. Treasure Island (FL): StatPearls Publishing; 2023.
2. Marino PL. Principles of mechanical ventilation. In: The ICU Book, 3rd edition. Philadelphia. PA: Lippincott Williams and Wilkins; 2007.

Q.17. A 74-year-old man with severe chronic obstructive pulmonary disease is admitted with severe hypoxemic respiratory failure. He is intubated and placed on volume assist control ventilation with a set TV of 400 mL (6.5 mL/kg IBW), PEEP of 8 cmH$_2$O and a respiratory rate of 30 breaths/min. When the paralytic used for intubation wears off, the patient is noted to be triggering additional spontaneous breaths with a total respiratory rate of 36 breaths/min, and his exhaled TVs vary from 100 to 800 mL. During an end-expiratory pause, his airway pressure is 18 cmH$_2$O. Which of the following is the most accurate statement regarding his ventilator settings?
   a. Because the patient is on volume control, he is receiving lung protective TVs.
   b. The patient's intrinsic PEEP is likely overestimated by the measured end-expiratory airway pressure.
   c. Changing the patient to pressure control will improve the patient's intrinsic PEEP.
   d. The patient's intrinsic PEEP is likely making it more difficult for him to trigger spontaneous breaths.
   e. Changing the patient to pressure control will provide more lung-protective TVs.

Ans. d

Explanation: The patient has evidence of intrinsic PEEP with an end-expiratory pressure that is greater than the set PEEP. In order to trigger breaths on the ventilator, or breath spontaneously, a patient needs to decrease his/her airway opening pressure and (depending on a ventilator trigger mode) create inspiratory flow. When a patient has intrinsic PEEP, he/she must overcome this PEEP to decrease his/her airway opening pressure or initiate inspiratory flow; this is the inspiratory threshold load and it increases the work of breathing both in spontaneously breathing and patients who are mechanically breathing and triggering breaths (answer D is correct). This patient is on a volume-control mode of ventilation but is asynchronous with variable exhaled TVs, which indicates "breath stacking," a type of cycle asynchrony in which patients do not fully exhale before taking their next breath. In this situation, the patient is no longer receiving the lung-protective TV that has been set despite being on a volume control mode (answer A is incorrect). If the ventilator setting were changed to pressure control, his TVs would vary with respiratory effort and therefore he would not be guaranteed to have more lung-protective TVs (answer E is incorrect). Changing the ventilator mode to pressure control will not necessarily decrease intrinsic PEEP (answer C is incorrect). The measurement of end-expiratory airway pressure often underestimates intrinsic PEEP because lung units that are slow emptying may not equilibrate with the airway opening and therefore the sickest lung units with the highest intrinsic PEEP are not fully represented by bedside measurements (answer B is incorrect).

Suggested Reading
1. Nilsestuen JO, Hargett KD. Using ventilator graphics to identify patient ventilator asynchrony. Respir Care. 2005;50(2):202-34.

Q.18. A 58-year-old man with community-acquired pneumonia is intubated in the ICU with respiratory failure. Following intubation, while paralyzed, his ventilator is set on volume assist-control, TV 450 mL, respiratory rate 14 breaths/min, FiO_2 0.7, and PEEP 8 cmH_2O. An inspiratory hold maneuver is performed, and his peak inspiratory pressure is 25 cmH_2O and plateau pressure is 18 cmH_2O. Which of the following is true regarding this patient's respiratory mechanics?
a. The patient's lung compliance is 45 mL/cmH_2O.
b. The patient's chest wall compliance is 30 mL/cmH_2O.
c. The patient's lung compliance is 10 mL/cmH_2O.
d. The patient's respiratory system compliance is 45 mL/cmH_2O.

Ans. d

Explanation: The respiratory system compliance is equal to the change in volume divided by the change in pressure. In this case, the change in volume is the TV (450 mL) and the change in pressure is the plateau pressure minus the PEEP (15 cmH_2O – 5 cmH_2O = 10 cmH_2O) (answer D is correct). Without a measure of a pleural pressure, it is not possible to separately calculate lung and chest wall compliance (answers A, B, and C are incorrect).

Suggested Reading
1. Desai JP, Moustarah F. Pulmonary compliance. In: StatPearls [Internet]. Treasure Island (FL): StatPearls Publishing; 2023.
2. Marino PL. Principles of mechanical ventilation. In: The ICU Book, 3rd edition. Philadelphia, PA: Lippincott Williams and Wilkins; 2007.

Q.19. One time constant should allow approximately what percentage of a lung unit to fill?
a. 37%
b. 100%
c. 63%
d. 86%

Ans. c

Explanation: The length of time lung units requires to fill and empty can be determined by the product of compliance (C) and resistance (R_{aw}) called a time constant. For any value of C and R_{aw}, the time constant always equals the length of time (in seconds) required for the lungs to inflate or deflate to a certain amount (percentage) of their volume. One-time constant equals the amount of time that it takes for 63% of the volume to be inhaled (or exhaled), two time constants represent that amount of time for about 86% of the volume to be inhaled (or exhaled), three time constants equal the time for about 95% to be inhaled (or exhaled), and four time constants is the time required for 98% of the volume to be inhaled (or exhaled).

After five-time constants, the lung is considered to contain 100% of tidal volume to be inhaled or 100% of tidal volume has been exhaled.

Suggested Reading
1. Cairo JM. Pilbeam's Mechanical Ventilation, 6th edition. Elsevier. 2016.

Q.20. The advantage of APRV compared with conventional ventilation is:
a. Unfamiliarity of staff with the technique
b. Improved patient-ventilator synchrony even if patient efforts are not matched with the ventilator.
c. Better CO_2 elimination in patients with increased R_{aw}
d. Augmented renal perfusion when spontaneous breathing is maintained.

Ans. d

Explanation: Airway pressure release ventilation is a form of continuous pressure support ventilation in which two pressures are set—pressure high (P high) and pressure low (P low). APRV delivers mandatory breaths through brief transition from P high to P low and then resumption of P high to avoid alveolar collapse. The amount of time spent at the higher pressure (T high) is generally 80–95% of cycle. The patient is allowed to breath spontaneously throughout the respiratory cycle, facilitating CO_2 removal. The fundamental principles underlying APRV are the provision of near continuous airway pressures with allowance of unrestricted spontaneous ventilation.

Spontaneous breathing during APRV mimics normal negative pressure ventilation. Intrathoracic pressure decreases during inspiration, augmenting systemic venous return to the heart from the abdominal organs and alleviating pressure on the pulmonary capillaries. These hemodynamic changes can improve cardiac performance and oxygen delivery at the tissue level. Compared with conventional ventilation modes that do not permit spontaneous respirations, the use of APRV has been associated with better hemodynamic profile leading to better renal perfusion.

Potential limitations of APRV will include unfamiliarity of technique, poor elimination of CO_2 in case of increased airway resistance and patient-ventilator asynchrony if patient efforts are not matched with that of ventilator.

Suggested Reading
1. Fredericks AS, Bunker MP, Gliga LA, Ebeling CG, Ringqvist JR, Heravi H, et al. Airway pressure release ventilation: a review of the evidence, theoretical benefits, and alternative titration strategies. Clin Med Insights Circ Respir Pulm Med. 2020;5;14:1179548420903297.
2. Swindin J, Sampson C, Howatson A. Airway pressure release ventilation. BJA Educ. 2020;20(3):80-8.

Q.21. A patient has been on NIV for 1 hour in the assist mode only. Ventilator settings include inspiratory positive airway pressure (IPAP) at 8 cmH$_2$O and expiratory positive airway pressure (EPAP) at 4 cmH$_2$O. Oxygen is being bled into the circuit at 4 L/minute. The patient's ABGs after 1 hour reveal pH = 7.34, PaCO$_2$ = 62 mm Hg, and PaO$_2$ = 62 mm Hg. The patient's respiratory rate is 27 breaths/minute and SpO$_2$ is 92%. There is minimal leaking around the face mask. What would be the most appropriate ventilator change to make at this time?
   a. Increase EPAP level to 8 cmH$_2$O.
   b. Decrease EPAP level to 2 cmH$_2$O.
   c. Increase IPAP level to 10 cmH$_2$O.
   d. Decrease IPAP level to 6 cmH$_2$O.

Ans. c

Explanation: During noninvasive ventilation (NIV), tidal volume (V$_t$) will depend upon the difference between inspiratory and expiratory positive airway pressure (IPAP and EPAP, respectively), provided there in minimal leak around the mask. EPAP has several potential advantages, for example, maintaining upper airway patency, preventing basal atelectasis and facilitating triggering. EPAP does, however, appear to reduce V$_t$. So in order to increase minute ventilation IPAP can be increased to increase the difference between IPAP and EPAP, which in turn will lead to increase tidal volume (V$_t$) thus decreasing the CO$_2$ levels.

Suggested Reading
1. Kinnear W, Watson L, Smith P, Johnson L, Burrows S, Colt J, et al. Effect of expiratory positive airway pressure on tidal volume during non-invasive ventilation. Chron Respir Dis. 2017;14(2):105-9.

Q.22. All of the following are recommendations for the use of NIV, except:
   a. In hospital patients with ARF, due to cardiogenic pulmonary edema
   b. To wean high risk patients from invasive mechanical ventilation as it reduces reintubation rate.
   c. To manage respiratory distress postextubation in high-risk patients.
   d. Acute exacerbation of COPD in patients with acute or acute-on-chronic respiratory acidosis (pH = 7.25-7.35)

Ans. c

Explanation: Postextubation respiratory failure requires reintubation, and is associated with more chances of developing pneumonia, prolonged ICU stay and high mortality rate. A multicenter RCT showed no difference in the rate of reintubation but there was increased intensive care mortality in NIV group as compared to standard medical treatment.

Another study found there was no difference in the rate of reintubation or hospital mortality with NIV. Subsequently a meta-analysis showed that NIV in established respiratory failure postextubation did not decrease the reintubation rate and ICU mortality compared to standard medical therapy.

Noninvasive ventilation may be used to wean high risk patients from invasive mechanical ventilation as it reduces reintubation rate. Such patients include-more than one consecutive failure of weaning trial, chronic heart failure, PaCO$_2$ >45 mm Hg after extubation, more than one comorbidity (excluding chronic heart failure), weak cough defined as airway care score values ≥8 and <12 and upper airways stridor at extubation not requiring immediate reintubation.

Studies have shown that immediate postextubation NIV use in selected high-risk population for reintubation was associated with reduction in need for reintubation and significantly decreased the ICU and hospital mortality.

A randomized controlled clinical trial (RCT) by Khilnani et al. found that NIV immediately postextubation in COPD patients was associated with less frequent need for reintubation in patients treated with NIV but no change in ICU and in-hospital stay.

Suggested Reading
1. Chawla R, Dixit SB, Zirpe KG, Chaudhry D, Khilnani GC, Mehta Y, et al. ISCCM Guidelines for the Use of Non-invasive Ventilation in Acute Respiratory Failure in Adult ICUs. Indian J Crit Care Med. 2020;24(Suppl 1):S61-S81.
2. Khilnani GC, Galle AD, Hadda V, Sharma SK. Non-invasive ventilation after extubation in patients with chronic obstructive airways disease: a randomised controlled trial. Anaesth Intensive Care. 2011;39(2):217-23.
3. Nava S, Gregoretti C, Fanfulla F, Squadrone E, Grassi M, Carlucci A, et al. Noninvasive ventilation to prevent respiratory failure after extubation in high-risk patients. Crit Care Med. 2005;33(11):2465-70.

Q.23. Which of the following can be used to describe the process where inspiratory flow ends and exhalation begins when a set time has elapsed?
   a. Pressure cycling
   b. Time triggering
   c. Time cycling
   d. Flow cycling

Ans. c

Explanation: Time cycling indicates that the mechanical ventilator breath switches from inspiration to expiration after a set time threshold is reached. This can be accomplished by setting the respiratory rate, inspiratory time, or I:E ratio. This is found in pressure-controlled ventilation mode. Flow cycling means that the expiratory valve opens after a preset reduction in peak flow occurs and is typically preset in most ventilators at 25%. It is used in pressure support ventilation.

Time triggering refers to controlled modes where the next breath starts after a preset time interval has elapsed (also called machine triggered). Pressure cycling refers to a certain change from inspiration to exhalation, once a preset pressure threshold is reached. The most common application for pressure cycling is for alarm settings.

If a patient becomes extremely asynchronous or coughs, the high-pressure alarm may be triggered and the inspiratory phase ends, resulting in exhalation.

Suggested Reading
1. Gentile MA. Cycling of the mechanical ventilator breath. Respiratory care. 2011;56(1):52-60.

Q.24. Automatic tube compensation can best be described as:
   a. Variable PS with variable inspiratory flow compensation
   b. Low-level PS with fixed flow-cycling criteria
   c. Mandatory minute ventilation
   d. Adaptive support using pressure support

Ans. a

Explanation: Automatic tube compensation (ATC) compensates for the flow-dependent pressure drop across the tracheal tube by a positive pressure support in inspiration and by a negative pressure support in expiration. ATC delivers exactly the amount of pressure required to overcome the resistive load imposed by the ET for the flow measured at the time. ATC when applied as a part of weaning compensates for any additional work of breathing implied by artificial airway. The weaning process can be usefully performed by ATC (at least as effective as PSV) but without significant hastening of the weaning process.

Suggested Reading
1. Figueroa-Casas JB, Montoya R, Arzabala A, Connery SM. Comparison between automatic tube compensation and continuous positive airway pressure during spontaneous breathing trials. Respir Care. 2010;55(5):549-54.
2. Guttmann J, Haberthür C, Stocker R, Lichtwarck-Aschoff M. Automatische Tubuskompensation (ATC) [Automatic tube compensation (ATC)]. Anaesthesist. 2001;50(3):171-80.

Q.25. A 14-year-old boy weighing 78 kg is admitted to ICU following intubation and initiation of mechanical ventilation for pneumonia associated with severe hypoxemia. His breathing pattern is dyssynchronous. Ventilator setting on assist-control volume cycled ventilation are FiO_2 0.7, tidal volume 480 mL, rate of 16 (total-assisted respiratory rate is 24), PEEP of 10 and peak inspiratory flow of 60 L/minute with a square inspiratory flow waveform. Pulse oximetry reveals a saturation of 94%. Pressure with time waveform is shown in the figure. What intervention is most likely to relieve the patient's asynchronous breathing?
   a. Increasing ventilator rate
   b. Switching to deaccelerating inspiratory flow waveform
   c. Decreasing PEEP
   d. Increasing peak inspiratory flow rate

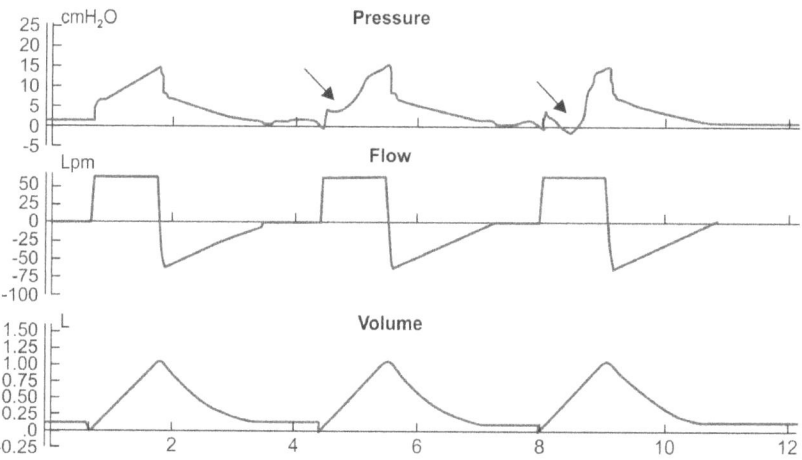

Ans. d

Explanation: The scooping pressure time scalar indicates inadequate peak inspiratory flow (flow starvation) during volume-controlled ventilation and patient ventilator asynchrony as patient is trying to compensate by making an inspiratory effort. Increasing respiratory rate would further worsen it. PEEP has no effect as it is related to flow and the situation requires an increase in the inspiratory flow.

Suggested Reading
1. Nilsestuen JO, Hargett KD. Using ventilatory graphics to identify patient ventilator asynchrony. Respir Care. 2005;50:202-4.

Q.26. **What is associated with an increase in the work of breathing in mechanically ventilated patients?**
a. Bronchodilation
b. Decreased spontaneous breathing frequency
c. Switching from controlled mechanical ventilation to assisted ventilation
d. Using a larger endotracheal tube

Ans. c

Explanation: Several factors can contribute to an increase in the work of breathing in mechanically ventilated patients including high airway resistance. High airway resistance could be because of narrowed or obstructed airways, smaller endotracheal tube size, or excessive secretions. Other factors causing increase in work of breathing include reduced lung compliance, inappropriate ventilator settings—improper ventilator settings such as inadequate tidal volume, excessive inspiratory flow, or high positive end-expiratory pressure (PEEP). These settings may not adequately support the patient's respiratory efforts or may impose additional resistance. It may also be due to respiratory muscle weakness in neuromuscular disorders or critical illness myopathy, or due to psychological factors, such as anxiety, pain, or discomfort.

In controlled mechanical ventilation, the patient does not initiate any breaths, and the ventilator delivers a full breath spending 100% energy toward work of breathing. Prolonged use of controlled modes may lead to ventilator-induced diaphragmatic dysfunction.

When a patient is switched from controlled mechanical ventilation to assist control mode, the work of breathing can vary depending on several factors, including the patient's condition and the specific settings used in each mode. The work of breathing can potentially increase when transitioning to assist control mode, if the patient's respiratory drive is low or his/her lung mechanics are compromised, he/she may rely heavily on the ventilator's support, resulting in reduced respiratory muscle activity and potentially increased work of breathing.

Adjustments in ventilator settings may be needed to optimize the balance between patient effort and ventilator support and minimize the work of breathing.

Q.27. Which of the following is not considered a benefit of APRV compared with conventional mechanical ventilation in patients with ARDS?
 a. Less circulatory interference
 b. Better gas exchange
 c. Higher PIP
 d. Improved oxygenation

Ans. c

Explanation: Airway pressure release ventilation (APRV) is a ventilation mode that combines two levels of continuous positive airway pressure (CPAP) with intermittent release phases. APRV typically has minimal circulatory interference, as the intermittent release phases allow for brief periods of lower airway pressure, which helps to reduce the potential for hemodynamic compromise compared to continuous high-pressure ventilation modes. This can be advantageous for patients with compromised cardiovascular function.

Airway pressure release ventilation can provide effective gas exchange. The prolonged periods of elevated airway pressure during the CPAP (inspiratory) phase facilitate alveolar recruitment and maintain lung volumes, promoting better oxygenation and carbon dioxide elimination. The intermittent release phases also allow for passive exhalation and the elimination of trapped gas.

The APRV mode is generally associated with lower PIP compared to traditional ventilation modes such as volume-controlled ventilation. The high pressure is generally not kept >30 cmH_2O. As it is a time-cycled mode consistent with other pressure-targeted modes of ventilation, it is affected by changes in lung compliance and/or resistance. A decrease in compliance or an increase in resistance may increase the peak inspiratory pressure. An increase in peak inspiratory pressure is undesirable and should be corrected.

Suggested Reading
 1. Daoud EG, Farag Hla, Chatburn RL. Airway pressure release ventilation: what do we know? Respir Care. 2012;57(2):282-92.

Q.28. A 23-year-old male is involved in road traffic accident. He is brought to ER with a GCS of 5. A cervical injury is also suspect and the patient is intubated with all precautions. Placement of endotracheal placement of ET is confirmed by capnography. All following options are true regarding capnography, except:
  a. Mainstream devices increase the amount of dead space added to the ventilator circuit.
  b. Helps in monitoring the severity of pulmonary disease and evaluating the response to therapy.
  c. The reliability of the contour of the capnogram is not affected by the stability of the minute volume, tidal volume, and cardiac output.
  d. The gas sampling rate from some sidestream analyzers may be high enough to cause autotriggering when flow triggering of mechanical breaths is used.

Ans. c

Explanation: Although capnography can provide valuable information about the efficiency of ventilation, as well as systemic, pulmonary, and coronary perfusion, $PaCO_2$ should be routinely determined by standard arterial blood gas analysis. Leaks in the ventilator circuit or leaks around the tracheal tube can lead to inaccurate measurements of expired CO_2. The reliability of the contour of the capnogram can also be affected by the stability of the minute volume, tidal volume, cardiac output, and CO_2 body stores. High breathing frequencies may exceed the response capabilities of the capnograph and therefore affect the integrity of the capnogram recorded. Low cardiac output may cause a false negative result when attempting to verify the endotracheal tube (ET) position in the trachea. Positioning the ET in the pharynx, as well as the presence of antacids and carbonated beverage in the stomach, can lead to false-positive results when assessing ET placement. The sampling rate of respired gases when using sidestream analyzers may be high enough to cause autotriggering when flow triggering of mechanical breaths is used. The effect is inversely proportional to the size of the patient. The gas-sampling rate can also diminish delivered tidal volume in neonates and small patients while using volume-targeted or volume-controlled ventilation.

Suggested Reading
1. Ortega R, Connor C, Kim S, Djang R, Patel K. Monitoring ventilation with capnography. N Engl J Med. 2012;367:e27.
2. Walsh BK, Crotwell DN, Restrepo RD. Capnography/capnometry during mechanical ventilation. Respir Care. 2011;56:503-9.

Q.29. The PEEP is increased on a patient receiving mechanical ventilation. The single-breath CO_2 ($SBCO_2$) curve shows a simultaneous shift to the right and an increase in the area of zone Y. This would indicate which of the following?
  a. Lung recruitment and emptying of previously collapsed alveoli
  b. Increased alveolar dead space from reduced pulmonary perfusion
  c. Decreased $PaCO_2$ from improvement in oxygenation
  d. Increase in rebreathed volume

Ans. b

Explanation: The SBCO$_2$ graph is produced by the integration of airway flow and CO$_2$ concentration; it is presented on a breath-to-breath basis. As shown in the figure, below the graph can provide information on anatomic dead space, alveolar dead space (when PaCO$_2$ is known), and CO$_2$ elimination (VCO$_2$) for each breath. If a horizontal line is drawn at the top of the curve, representing %CO$_2$ in arterial blood, three distinct regions of the curve are established.

Application of PEEP can also alter the contour of the volumetric SBCO$_2$ curve. As PEEP is increased from zero to 15 cmH$_2$O, the phase 2 portion of the curve shifts to the right because of expanding airways (increasing PEEP keeps the airways open) and reduced perfusion. The addition of PEEP can cause compression of the pulmonary capillaries and a drop in perfusion to the lungs, reducing effective perfusion to the ventilated alveoli. This change represents an increase in alveolar dead space. The slope of phase 2 decreases as well; this is a result of lower CO$_2$ concentration occurring at an identical volume point on the *x*-axis, causing a rise in PaCO$_2$.

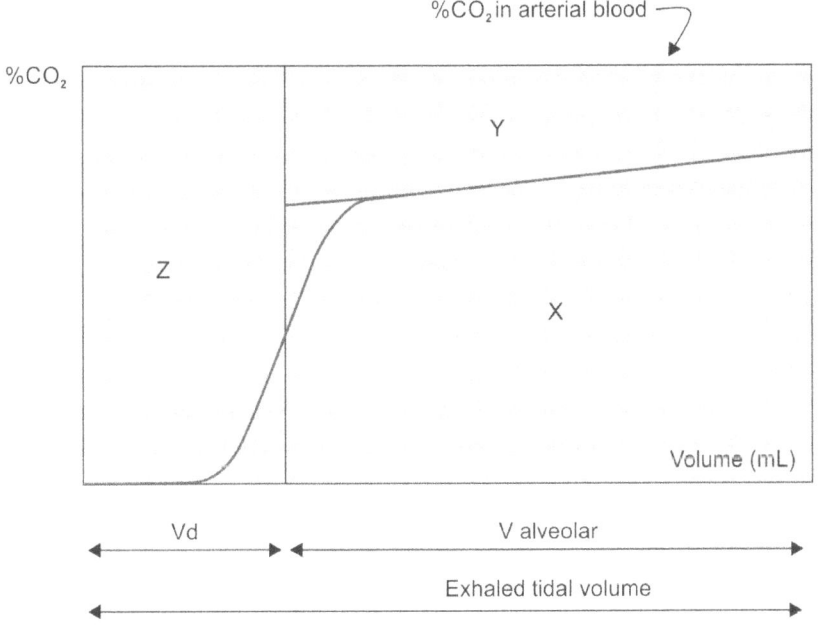

Graph of exhaled volume (X axis) versus % CO$_2$ (Y axis). A horizontal line drawn at the top of the curve represents the % CO$_2$ in arterial blood. Three distinct regions are illustrated: Area X represents actual CO$_2$ exhaled in one breath; area Y is the amount of CO$_2$ not eliminated because of alveolar dead space; and area Z is the amount of CO$_2$ not eliminated because of anatomic dead space. V, alveolar volume volume; Vd, dead space volume.
Source: Redrawn from material from Respironics, Murrysville, PA.

Suggested Reading

1. Arnold JH, Thompson JE, Arnold LW. Single breath CO$_2$ analysis: description and validation of a method. Crit Care Med. 1996;24(1):96-102.

Q.30. All of the following conditions will adversely affect pulse oximeter readings, except:
  a. Hypovolemia
  b. Methemoglobinemia
  c. Anemia
  d. Hyperbilirubinemia

Ans. d

Explanation: Pulse oximetry measures oxygen saturation by illuminating the skin and measuring changes in light absorption of oxygenated (oxyhemoglobin) and deoxygenated blood (reduced hemoglobin) using two light wavelengths—660 nm (red) and 940 nm (infrared). The ratio of absorbance at these wavelengths is calculated and calibrated against direct measurements of arterial oxygen saturation (SaO_2) to establish the pulse oximeter's measure of arterial saturation (SpO_2). Oximeters have limitations which may result in erroneous readings. Because of the sigmoid shape of the oxyhemoglobin dissociation curve, oximetry may not detect hypoxemia in patients with high arterial oxygen tension (PaO_2) levels. Conventional pulse oximeters can distinguish only two substances—reduced hemoglobin and oxyhemoglobin; it assumes that dyshemoglobins—such as carboxyhemoglobin (COHb) and methemoglobin (MetHb)—are absent studies showed that the presence of elevated levels of COHb and MetHb could affect the accuracy of SpO_2 readings. Pulse oximetry can also be affected by other conditions such as low perfusion states, dyes, anemia, nail polish, but is not affected by hyperbilirubinemia.

Suggested Reading
1. Jubran A. Pulse oximetry. Crit Care. 2015;19(1):272. https://doi.org/10.1186/s13054-015-0984-8
2. Veyckemans F, Baele P, Guillaume JE, Willems E, Robert A, Clerbaux T. Hyperbilirubinemia does not interfere with hemoglobin saturation measured by pulse oximetry. Anesthesiology. 1989;70(1):118-22.

Q.31. A 42-year-old man, who is a known case of acute asthma exacerbation, is admitted to the ICU. He is intubated, paralyzed, and mechanically ventilated. His ventilator settings are assist control/volume control, TV 400 mL, respiratory rate 18 breaths/minute, FiO_2 0.5, and PEEP 6 cmH_2O. His ABG on these settings is pH 7.30, PCO_2 56 mm Hg, and PO_2 140 mm Hg. On day 2 of his ICU stay, an end-expiratory hold maneuver is performed and his airway pressure is measured at 15 cmH_2O. Several hours later, he is noted to have progressive tachycardia, and his blood pressure has decreased from 130/90 to 78/56 mm Hg. A chest radiograph demonstrates no new finding and there is no evidence of new infiltrate or pneumothorax. What is the best next step in management?
  a. Perform an emergent bronchoscopy.
  b. Perform a needle decompression at the second intercostal space.
  c. Briefly disconnect the mechanical ventilator from the endotracheal tube.
  d. Decrease the set PEEP on the ventilator.

Ans. c

Explanation: The patient has developed hemodynamic instability as a result of intrinsic PEEP, or dynamic hyperinflation, which increases intrathoracic pressure and decreases venous return. This is a life-threatening complication that requires immediate release of trapped gas from the lungs. This is best accomplished by disconnecting the ventilator circuit for a brief period of time. Without evidence of pneumothorax on radiograph, ultrasound, or other high suspicion, a needle decompression is not warranted. Bronchoscopy is occasionally utilized to clear mucous plugging in patient with severe asthma, however this would not explain the patient's hemodynamic instability. An increase in the respiratory rate will decrease the patient's expiratory time and lead to worsening gas trapping. A decrease in the extrinsic PEEP set on the ventilator will not decrease intrinsic PEEP and will not improve this patient's hemodynamic.

Suggested Reading
1. MacIntyre NR, Cheng KC, McConnell R. Applied PEEP during pressure support reduces the inspiratory threshold load of intrinsic PEEP. Chest. 1997;111(1):188.
2. Milic-Emili J. Dynamic pulmonary hyperinflation and intrinsic PEEP: consequences and management in patients with chronic obstructive pulmonary disease. Recenti Prog Med. 1990;81(11):733-7.

Q.32. According to new global definition of ARDS all are included in new definition, except:
   a. PaO_2/FiO_2 <300 mm Hg
   b. SpO_2/FiO_2 <315 mm Hg with SpO_2 ≤97
   c. High flow nasal oxygen >30 L/minute or NIV/CPAP >5 cmH_2O end expiratory pressure
   d. Unilateral or bilateral opacities confirmed by chest X-ray, CT scan or USG with a well-trained operator

Ans. d

Explanation: The new global definition of ARDS expands upon the Berlin definition of ARDS. The four main recommendations are:
1. To include HFNO with a minimum flow rate of ≥30 L/minute or NIV/CPAP with at least 5 cmH_2O end expiratory pressure.
2. To use either PaO_2/FiO_2 ≤300 mm Hg or SpO_2/FiO_2 ≤315 mm Hg with SpO_2 <97% to identify hypoxemia.
3. To retain bilateral opacities for imaging criteria by chest X-ray and CT scan and to add USG if operator is well trained.
4. For resource variable setting, to not require PEEP, oxygen flow or specific respiratory support device to diagnose ARDS.

Suggested Reading
1. Matthay MA, Arabi Y, Arroliga AC, Bernard GR, Bersten AD, Brochard LJ, et al. A new global definition of acute respiratory distress syndrome. Am J Respir Crit Care Med. 2023;207: A6229.

CHAPTER

Respiratory System

Harish Mallapura Maheshwarappa, Shivangi Mishra, Harshavardhan Rangappa Kuri

Q.1. A 44-year-old man is admitted to the hospital with breathing difficulty, cough and fever. Computed tomography (CT) thorax was done which showed evidence of subpleural consolidation. He deteriorated rapidly needing intubation. However despite intubation and proning his oxygenation remained poor. Venovenous extracorporeal membrane oxygenation (ECMO) was initiated immediately. After initiation of ECMO, arterial blood gas (ABG) showed: pH 7.10, partial arterial carbon dioxide pressure 88 mm Hg, and partial arterial oxygen pressure 69 mm Hg. What is the next step?
a. Increase blood flow rate.
b. Increase sweep gas flow.
c. Increase tidal volume on ventilator.
d. Increase ventilatory respiratory rate.

Ans. b

Explanation: The blood flow through the ECMO circuit has very less effect on CO_2. The carbon dioxide removal rate is relatively independent of the flow. Increasing sweep gas flow rate is one of the major ways to remove CO_2. As the sweep gas removes CO_2, the tidal volume and respiratory rate on the ventilator are decreased to allow the lungs time to recover. At the time of weaning ECMO, the lungs are recruited, and the sweep gas flow titrated down.

Suggested Reading
1. Bishop MA, Moore A. Extracorporeal membrane oxygenation weaning. In: StatPearls [Internet]. Treasure Island (FL): StatPearls Publishing; 2023.

Q.2. A 40-year-old woman is admitted in the intensive care unit (ICU) after being intubated for worsening status asthmaticus. She is on inhaled and systemic corticosteroids, anticholinergic medications, bronchodilators, and intravenous (IV) magnesium. However her airway pressure, bronchospasm, and partial pressure of carbon dioxide still remain high. She is started on ketamine infusion.
How does ketamine help in bronchospasm?
a. Increased minute ventilation
b. Decreased functional residual capacity

c. Bronchodilatation
   d. Decreased pharyngeal secretions

   Ans. c

   Explanation: Ketamine is a dissociative anesthetic agent with analgesic properties. It is a vagolytic agent. It helps in expiratory flow limitation by direct smooth muscle relaxation, thereby relieving bronchospasm. Since it causes minimal respiratory depression, it preserves functional residual capacity and minute ventilation. It has no effect on pulmonary secretions.

   Suggested Reading
   1. Goyal S, Agrawal A. Ketamine in status asthmaticus: a review. Indian J Crit Care Med. 2013;17(3):154-61.

Q.3. **A 56-year-old female presented with fever, cough, and breathing difficulty for 5 days. She is a known case of chronic obstructive pulmonary disease (COPD) on regular bronchodilator therapy. On arrival her heart rate was 110/min, respiratory rate of 30/min, blood pressure of 98/56 mm Hg, and temperature of 101°F. On evaluation her ABG showed pH of 7.25 and $PaCO_2$ of 75 mm Hg. Which of the following is not included as part of severe COPD exacerbation as per GOLD COPD report 2023?**
   a. Hypercapnia >45 mm Hg and pH <7.35
   b. Respiratory rate >24/min
   c. C-reactive protein >10 mg/L
   d. Temperature >100.4°F

   Ans. d

   Explanation: Severe COPD exacerbation is defined by dyspnea visual analog scale >5, respiratory rate >24/min, heart rate >95/min, resting SaO_2 <92% breathing ambient air, CRP >10 mg/L and ABG showing PaO_2 <60 mm Hg and $PaCO_2$ >45 mm Hg with acidosis (pH <7.35).

   Suggested Reading
   1. 2023 GOLD Report. (2023). Global Initiative for Chronic Obstructive Lung Disease - GOLD. [online] Available from: https://goldcopd.org/2023-gold-report-2/ [Last accessed June, 2023].

Q.4. **A 35-year-old female, who is a known case of bronchial asthma, gets admitted with complain of breathing difficulty and tachypnea. On examination she is drowsy, with a blood pressure of 85/54 mm Hg, heart rate of 166/min in atrial fibrillation. ABG showed pH 7.1, PaO_2 of 48 mm Hg, and $PaCO_2$ of 85 mm Hg. She was subsequently intubated and put on mechanical ventilation. Which of the following shows evidence of near fatal asthma in this patient?**
   a. Presence of atrial fibrillation
   b. Hypotension
   c. $PaCO_2$ of 85 mm Hg
   d. PaO_2 of 48 mm Hg

   Ans. c

Explanation: Any feature of life-threatening bronchial asthma along with raised $PaCO_2$ and/or requiring mechanical ventilation with raised inflation pressures can be suggestive of near fatal asthma. The features of life-threatening bronchial asthma include peak expiratory flow (PEF) <33% of best or predicted, SpO_2 <92%, silent chest, cyanosis, or feeble respiratory effort, arrhythmia or hypotension, exhaustion and altered consciousness.

Suggested Reading

1. British Thoracic Society. (2020). Better lung health for all. [online] Available from: https://www.brit-thoracic.org.uk/quality-improvement/guidelines/asthma/ [Last accessed June, 2023].

Q.5. A 55-year-old male admitted with COPD exacerbation is started on beta agonist, inhaled corticosteroids, anticholinergics, and noninvasive ventilation (NIV) support. Despite these his breathing difficulty worsens and he is started on systemic corticosteroids. How do systemic corticosteroids help in COPD exacerbation?
 a. Increase forced expiratory volume in 1 second (FEV_1).
 b. Decrease requirement of invasive mechanical ventilation.
 c. Bronchodilation
 d. Reduce incidence of infection.

Ans. a

Explanation: Data from various literatures indicates that systemic corticosteroids in COPD exacerbations decrease recovery time and improve the lung function by increasing FEV_1. They also improve oxygenation, reduce risk of relapse, treatment failure, and the length of hospital stay. A prednisone-equivalent dose of 40 mg/day for 5 days is recommended. It has been seen that longer courses of oral corticosteroids in COPD exacerbations increase the risk of pneumonia and mortality.

Suggested Reading

1. 2023 GOLD Report (2023). Global Initiative for Chronic Obstructive Lung Disease - GOLD. [online] Available from: https://goldcopd.org/2023-gold-report-2/ [Last accessed June, 2023].

Q.6. A 25-year-old man was brought to emergency room (ER) after sustaining a road traffic accident. He was noticed to be having multiple facial fractures. He is drowsy, with a respiratory rate of 35 breaths/min. Arterial blood gas analysis intubation was planned to protect the airway.
 Which of the following is the best way to secure his airway?
 a. Fiberoptic nasal intubation
 b. Oral intubation with in-line cervical spine stabilization
 c. Cricothyrotomy
 d. Video laryngoscopy

Ans. b

Explanation: The patient's altered mental status is because of result of poor gas exchange or a head injury. In such patients a high index cervical spine injury or head injury should be kept. Oral intubation with manual in-line stabilization is probably the best way to secure his airway.

Oral fiberoptic intubation or video laryngoscopy is also good alternatives. Cricothyrotomy would be indicated if the patient's respiratory mechanics suddenly deteriorates and orotracheal intubation is not possible. However, for all the other three procedure as well manual in-line stabilization should be continued.

Suggested Reading
1. ACS. Advanced Trauma Life Support [Internet]. [online] Available from: https://www.facs.org/quality-programs/trauma/education/advanced-trauma-life-support/ [Last accessed June, 2023].

Q.7. A 38-year-old male is admitted with history of fever and altered sensorium. He was subsequently intubated in view of airway protection. However postintubation his oxygenation worsens, SpO_2 is 85% on 100% FiO_2, with peak inspiratory pressure of 35 on ventilator. His blood pressure is 98/58 mm Hg and heart rate 129/min, respiratory rate 35/min. CT scan is done, which shows the following image. What is the probable cause leading to the CT findings?
a. Emphysema
b. Barotrauma due to mechanical ventilation
c. Consolidation
d. Endobronchial intubation

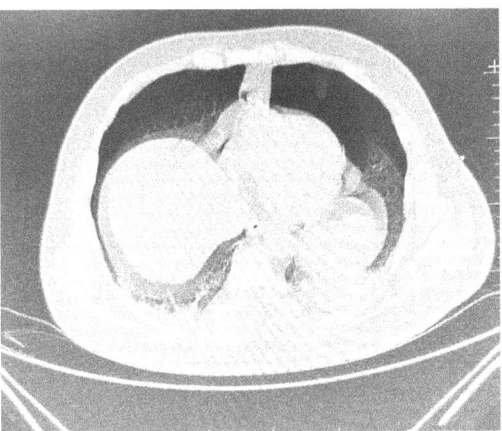

Ans. b

Explanation: Primary spontaneous pneumothorax is an abnormal accumulation of air in the space between the lungs and the chest cavity (called the pleural space) that can result in the partial or complete collapse of a lung. This type of pneumothorax is described as primary because it occurs in the absence of lung disease such as emphysema. Spontaneous means the pneumothorax was not caused by an injury such as a rib fracture. Primary spontaneous pneumothorax is likely due to the formation of small sacs of air (blebs) in lung tissue that rupture, causing air to leak into the pleural space. Air in the pleural space creates pressure on the lung and can lead to its collapse.

Suggested Reading
1. McKnight CL, Burns B. Pneumothorax. In: StatPearls [Internet]. Treasure Island (FL): StatPearls Publishing; 2023.

Q.8. A 63-year-old morbid obese woman presents to ER with breathing difficulty and lower extremity edema. Four weeks ago, as an outpatient, she had chronic hypoxemia. ABG analysis showed on outpatient basis was pH 7.37, $PaCO_2$ 65 mm Hg, and PaO_2 60 mm Hg on ambient air. In ER, arterial blood gas analysis showed: pH 7.28, $PaCO_2$ 84 mm Hg, and PaO_2 58 mm Hg with 4 L O_2 face mask. Chest X-ray (CXR) was normal. Temperature is 36.7°C (98.1°F), heart rate 83 beats/min, blood pressure 147/78 mm Hg, and respiratory rate 11 breaths/min. She is drowsy but arousable.

Which of the following strategies should be implemented first to improve her ventilator status?
a. Diuresis
b. Noninvasive ventilation
c. Nebulizer treatment
d. Invasive mechanical ventilation

Ans. b

Explanation: The patient is having obstructive sleep apnea with obesity hypoventilation syndrome. The normal pH at outpatient basis indicates chronicity of the disease. In view of chronicity of disease, the current management in this situation with a nonurgent presentation, the best method to manage is to start the patient on noninvasive ventilation and assess for responsiveness. In this urgent scenario, initiation of bi-level positive airway pressure (BiPAP) support is reasonable. In absence of response or if her condition worsens, invasive mechanical ventilation might be required. The presence of lower extremity edema and chronic hypoxemia suggests cor pulmonale. Diuretics can be helpful in long term, however, in acute setting noninvasive ventilation is the first strategy. Nebulizer treatment has no role in obesity hypoventilation syndrome.

Suggested Reading
1. Shetty S, Parthasarathy S. Obesity hypoventilation syndrome. Curr Pulmonol Rep. 2015;4(1):42-55.

Q.9. A 75-year-old man presents with a several-week history of productive cough, occasionally blood-streaked sputum, night sweats, and pleuritic chest pain. Chest CT is pending.

Which of the following is the most common radiologic manifestation of nocardiosis in nonendemic areas?
a. Cavitatory nodule
b. Centrilobular micronodules
c. Ground-glass opacity
d. Pleural effusion

Ans. a

Explanation: Nocardiosis is an opportunistic infection which mainly affects immunocompromised patients such as patients with acquired immunodeficiency syndrome (AIDS), long-term steroid use, or transplant recipients. However, nocardiosis can also be life-threatening condition in immunocompetent patients. The most frequent radiologic manifestations of nocardiosis are airspace consolidation (52.8%), and nodules (82.3%), single or multiple, that can be confused with metastatic carcinoma. Empyema can be seen in approximately one-third cases. The other common radiographic manifestation is cavitation, which is seen in both consolidation and nodules. The mortality rate is 18.75% for pulmonary nocardiosis. Death is frequent among patients who received immunosuppressive drugs. In patients with pulmonary nocardiosis, mortality rate is around 50%.

Suggested Reading
1. Chen J, Zhou H, Xu P, Zhang P, Ma S, Zhou J. Clinical and radiographic characteristics of pulmonary nocardiosis: clues to earlier diagnosis. PLoS One. 2014;9(3):e90724.

Q.10. A 45-year-old man, a known case of hypertension and diabetes mellitus, is admitted with community-acquired pneumonia which progresses to acute respiratory distress syndrome. He is test positive for H1N1 pneumonia and treatment is started with oseltamivir. His oxygenation starts improving after three cycles of proning. However, on day 7 of hospital stay, he starts developing fever, hypotension and his oxygenation worsens. What is the next step of management?
 a. CT thorax
 b. Escalation of antibiotics with at least two antipseudomonal agents
 c. Culture tracheobronchial aspirate
 d. Bronchoscopy

Ans. c

Explanation: The patient is probably developing a ventilator-associated condition (VAC). In presence of positive microbiological culture he can be diagnosed to be having ventilator-associated pneumonia. IDSA 2016 guidelines recommend use of noninvasive semiquantitative methods of culture over invasive methods for sample collection. Ventilator-associated pneumonia in presence of shock needs to be treated by at least two antipseudomonal agents along with a gram-positive cover. However, we need to culture this patient first before starting on antibiotics.

Suggested Reading
1. Kalil AC, Metersky ML, Klompas M, Muscedere J, Sweeney DA, Palmer LB, et al. Management of adults with hospital-acquired and ventilator-associated pneumonia: 2016 Clinical Practice Guidelines by the Infectious Diseases Society of America and the American Thoracic Society. Clin Infect Dis. 2016;63(5):e61-e111.

Q.11. A 21-year-old IV drug abuser presents with the history of fever for 6 days, cough, and blood-streaked sputum. On examination his heart rate is 130/min, respiratory rate is 35/min, and blood pressure is 93/49 mm Hg. CT thorax done is showing

evidence of necrotizing pneumonia. What is the expected duration of antibiotic therapy?
a. 7 days
b. 10 days
c. 14 days
d. 21 days

Ans. d

Explanation: The patient has presented with necrotizing pneumonia caused by probably gram-positive infection or most likely MRSA (methicillin-resistant *Staphylococcus aureus*). He is an IV drug abuser which increases the incidence of MRSA infections. Other risk factors for MRSA infection are influenza, prisoners, professional athletes, army recruits, men having sex with men (MSM), close contact with MRSA carrier regular sauna users, and recent antibiotic use. Guidelines recommends treatment for a period of 14–21 days for a patient with necrotizing pneumonia caused by MRSA or gram-negative bacteria.

Suggested Reading
1. Khilnani GC, Zirpe K, Hadda V, Mehta Y, Madan K, Kulkarni A, et al. Guidelines for antibiotic prescription in intensive care unit. Indian J Crit Care Med. 2019;23(Suppl 1): S1-S63.

Q.12. A 43-year-old man is admitted with malignant stroke. He was intubated for airway protection. On day 6 postintubation and mechanical ventilation, he develops fever, new infiltrates on chest X-ray, and increased endotracheal secretions. The hospital antibiogram shows an incidence of MRSA in 11% and resistant gram-negative organism in 42% isolates. What will be best choice of empiric antibiotics for the present condition?
a. Two antipseudomonal agents
b. Two antipseudomonal agent with a gram-positive cover
c. Two antipseudomonal agent with antifungal cover
d. Single antipseudomonal agent with gram-positive cover

Ans. a

Explanation: Patients with ventilator-associated pneumonia (VAP) who are at high risk of multidrug-resistant (MDR) pathogens or are being treated in ICU with a high prevalence of MRSA (>15%) and resistant gram-negative organisms (>10%), an agent active against MRSA and at least two antipseudomonal agents is recommended. Risk factors for MDR pathogens causing VAP are age >60 years, mechanical ventilation ≥7 days, previous antibiotic use within 3 months, severe sepsis or septic shock, acute respiratory distress syndrome preceding VAP, renal replacement therapy, and systemic steroid therapy.

Suggested Reading
1. Khilnani GC, Zirpe K, Hadda V, Mehta Y, Madan K, Kulkarni A, et al. Guidelines for antibiotic prescription in intensive care unit. Indian J Crit Care Med. 2019;23(Suppl 1): S1-S63.

Q.13. A 65-year-old man is admitted to the hospital with COPD exacerbation. He is intubated in the ER, and a subclavian triple-lumen catheter is placed in view of hypotension requiring vasopressors. However, despite high dose of vasopressors hypotension persists. Which of the following is most appropriate in the diagnosis of pneumothorax using ultrasound?
   a. The absence of lung sliding has more specificity and less sensitivity for pneumothorax.
   b. Lung sliding is less sensitive than chest radiography in detecting pneumothoraces in trauma patients.
   c. Artifacts in A line rules out a pneumothorax.
   d. Artifacts in B line rules out a pneumothorax.

Ans. d

Explanation: Pneumothoraces occur commonly in ICU patients, with an incidence of 6%. Lung ultrasound is most rapidly available bedside test to assess presence of pneumothorax. The absence of lung sliding has a sensitivity of 95.3% and specificity of 91.1% in diagnosing pneumothorax. However, lung sliding can be absent in patients with ARDS, emphysematous blebs, etc. Lung ultrasound has higher sensitivity and chest radiographs have higher specificity in diagnosing pneumothorax. A lines are reflections of the pleural interface while B lines are vertical lines that project from the parietal pleura to the lung parenchyma. Presence of artifacts in B lines rules out pneumothorax.

Suggested Reading
  1. Lichtenstein DA, Menu Y. A bedside ultrasound sign ruling out pneumothorax in the critically ill. Lung sliding. Chest. 1995;108(5):1345-8.

Q.14. A 65-year-old man, a known case of colon cancer on chemotherapy, presents with complain of chest pain and breathing difficulty. CT thorax done showed presence of saddle embolus in main pulmonary artery. He was thrombolyzed with alteplase. Which is the drug of choice for further anticoagulation?
   a. Enoxaparin
   b. Unfractionated heparin
   c. Apixaban
   d. Fondaprinux

Ans. a

Explanation: According to 2019 European Society of Cardiology Guidelines for management of pulmonary embolism, therapeutic anticoagulation in patient with cancer should be done with either low molecular weight heparin or rivaroxaban. However, in cases of gastrointestinal malignancy, only low molecular weight heparin is recommended in view of increased incidence of gastrointestinal bleeding with rivaroxaban. The therapy with low molecular weight heparin should be continued for a period of 6 months.

Suggested Reading
  1. Konstantinides SV, Meyer G, Becattini C, Bueno H, Geersing GJ, Harjola VP, et al. 2019 ESC Guidelines for the diagnosis and management of acute pulmonary embolism developed in collaboration with the European Respiratory Society (ERS): The Task Force for the diagnosis and management of acute pulmonary embolism of the European Society of Cardiology (ESC). Eur Heart J. 2020;41(4):543-603.

Q.15. A 33-year-old female presents with lobar pneumonia. She requires intubation and mechanical ventilation in view of worsening breathing mechanics. Feeding is initiated with a 14-French nasogastric tube. Which of the following is not a strategy to reduce ventilator-associated pneumonia during mechanical ventilation?
  a. Endotracheal tube with subglottic suction
  b. Elevate head of bed
  c. Early tracheostomy
  d. Administration of proton pump inhibitors.

Ans. d

Explanation: Approximately 5–10% patients on mechanical ventilation can develop ventilator-associated events. Ventilator-associated pneumonia can increase duration of ventilator stay and hospital stay. Recommended essential approaches for prevention of ventilator associated pneumonia are:
- Use of high flow nasal oxygen or noninvasive ventilation to avoid intubation
- Minimizing sedation
- Endotracheal tubes with subglottic secretion drainage
- Oral care with daily toothbrushing
- Early tracheostomy
- Elevation of head end of bed by 30–45°

Strategies, which are not recommended, include
- Probiotics
- Oral care with chlorhexidine
- Proton pump inhibitors
- Ultrathin polyurethane endotracheal tube cuffs
- Tapered endotracheal tube cuffs
- Automated control of endotracheal cuff pressures
- Frequent endotracheal cuff pressure monitoring

Suggested Reading
1. Klompas M, Branson R, Cawcutt K, Crist M, Eichenwald EC, Greene LR, et al. Strategies to prevent ventilator-associated pneumonia, ventilator-associated events, and nonventilator hospital-acquired pneumonia in acute-care hospitals: 2022 Update. Infect Control Hosp Epidemiol. 2022;43(6):687-713.

Q.16. A 48-year-old male with a history of alcoholic cirrhosis presents to the clinic with progressive dyspnea and cyanosis. On examination, digital clubbing is noted. He specifically tells he is more breathless on sitting and prefers to lie down to relieve his breathlessness. Arterial blood gas analysis reveals a PaO_2 of 58 mm Hg while breathing room air. The patient undergoes a contrast-enhanced echocardiography, which shows the presence of bubbles in left atrium after six heart beats. Which of the following mechanisms is primarily responsible for the development of intrapulmonary vascular dilatations in this patient?
  a. Systemic inflammation and oxidative stress
  b. Impaired hepatic clearance of vasoactive substances

c. Chronic hypoxia-induced pulmonary arterial hypertension
d. Increased bacterial translocation and toxin release leading to angiogenesis and neovascularization and release of nitric oxide and carbon monoxide

Ans. d

Explanation: In patients with hepatopulmonary syndrome (HPS), the primary mechanism responsible for the development of intrapulmonary vascular dilatations is angiogenesis and neovascularization. In chronic liver disease, there is an upregulation of angiogenic factors and growth factors that promote the formation of abnormal blood vessels within the lungs. These vessels exhibit dilation and tortuosity, leading to intrapulmonary vascular dilatations. This vascular remodeling contributes to the ventilation-perfusion mismatch and arterial hypoxemia seen in HPS. Systemic inflammation and oxidative stress, impaired hepatic clearance of vasoactive substances, and chronic hypoxia-induced pulmonary arterial hypertension may also play secondary roles in the pathogenesis of HPS, but angiogenesis and neovascularization are the primary drivers of intrapulmonary vascular abnormalities in this condition.

Suggested Reading
1. Rodríguez-Roisin R, Krowka MJ. Hepatopulmonary syndrome—a liver-induced lung vascular disorder. N Engl J Med. 2008;358(22):2378-87.
2. Soulaidopoulos S, Cholongitas E, Giannakoulas G, Vlachou M, Goulis I. Review article: Update on current and emergent data on hepatopulmonary syndrome. World J Gastroenterol. 2018;24(12):1285-98.

Q.17. What is the sign seen in this scan? It is the diagnostic of:
a. Quad sign—pleural effusion
b. Sinusoidal sign—pneumothorax
c. Thoracic spine sign—pleural effusion
d. Absent lung slide scan—pneumothorax

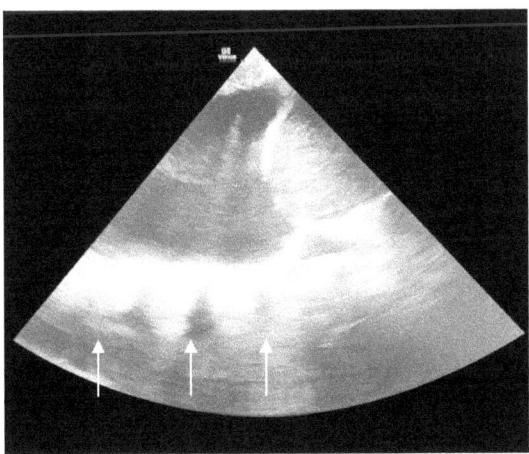

Ans. d

Explanation: The vertebral bodies just above the diaphragm line are very much indicative of pleural effects. Gross pleural effusion is easy to identify; this particularly helps in case of minimal pleural effusion with debris or clots. Fluid acts as a good condition of ultrasound waves, easily visualizing the thoracic vertebrae behind. Quad sign is seen in pleural effusion. It is defined by four lines—two rib shadows, other two by parietal pleural and visceral pleura, not seen in the image.

Sinusoidal sign is seen in pleural effusion. It is seen in M mode. It is caused by respiratory variation which decreases the distance between both the pleural linings. It might not be seen in pleural effusion associated with dense septation.

Absent pleural lung slide is seen in pneumothorax which is not shown here.

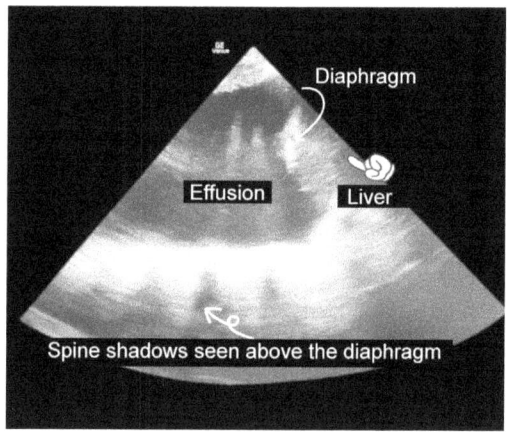

Suggested Reading
1. Ahmed AA, Martin JA, Saul T, Lewiss RE. The thoracic spine sign in bedside ultrasound. three cases report. Med Ultrason. 2014;16(2):179-81.

Q.18. A 32-year-old pregnant woman with twins at 34 weeks of gestation presents to the emergency department with shortness of breath and cough. She has a history of preterm labor and was started on a tocolytic agent, terbutaline, earlier in the day. On examination, her respiratory rate is 28 breaths/min, and auscultation reveals crackles in the bilateral lung fields. Arterial blood gas analysis shows hypoxemia and respiratory alkalosis. Chest X-ray reveals bilateral infiltrates consistent with pulmonary edema. What is the most likely cause of her symptoms?
  a. Terbutaline toxicity
  b. Amniotic fluid embolism
  c. Preeclampsia with pulmonary edema
  d. Pulmonary embolism

Ans. a

Explanation: Tocolytic-induced pulmonary edema—the clinical presentation of this patient with shortness of breath, cough, bilateral lung crackles, hypoxemia, respiratory alkalosis, and bilateral infiltrates on chest X-ray is consistent with pulmonary edema. Tocolytic agents, such as terbutaline, can rarely cause pulmonary edema as an adverse effect. Terbutaline is a beta-2 adrenergic agonist that is used to inhibit uterine contractions and delay preterm labor. However, it can lead to fluid overload and pulmonary edema in some cases. The symptoms usually resolve with discontinuation of the medication and supportive management with diuretics and NIV. Amniotic fluid embolism is characterized by the sudden onset of respiratory distress, hypotension, and coagulopathy in the setting of labor or immediately after delivery. It is a rare but potentially life-threatening condition caused by the entry of amniotic fluid into the maternal circulation. Preeclampsia with pulmonary edema is a hypertensive disorder of pregnancy characterized by hypertension, proteinuria, and end-organ dysfunction. Pulmonary edema can develop as a severe manifestation of preeclampsia, but the absence of hypertension and proteinuria in this vignette makes it less likely. Pulmonary embolism can present with sudden-onset dyspnea, pleuritic chest pain, and signs of right heart strain. Although it can occur during pregnancy, the absence of characteristic symptoms and risk factors makes it less likely in this case. Therefore, the most likely cause of the patient's symptoms is terbutaline toxicity, a known adverse effect of tocolytic agents.

Suggested Reading
1. Abbas OM, Nassar AH, Kanj NA, Usta IM. Acute pulmonary edema during tocolytic therapy with nifedipine. Am J Obstet Gynecol. 2006;195(4):e3-4.

Q.19. Which of the following is a recognized risk factor for re-expansion pulmonary edema?
   a. Advanced age
   b. Female gender
   c. Young age
   d. Shorter duration of lung collapse

Ans. c

Explanation: Re-expansion pulmonary edema is more commonly seen in younger individuals, possibly due to increased lung elasticity and higher pulmonary capillary pressures. Men have been found to be at a slightly higher risk of developing re-expansion pulmonary edema compared to women. The longer is the duration of lung collapse, the higher the risk of re-expansion pulmonary edema. Rapid re-expansion of a collapsed lung can lead to increased capillary permeability and fluid leakage into the alveoli.

Suggested Reading
1. Yoon JS, Suh JH, Choi SY, Kwon JB, Lee BY, Lee SH, et al. Risk factors for the development of reexpansion pulmonary edema in patients with spontaneous pneumothorax. J Cardiothorac Surg. 2013;8:164.

Q.20. A 58-year-old male presents to the emergency department with a 2-week history of cough, dyspnea, and hemoptysis. He also reports fatigue, joint pain, and recurrent sinus infections over the past several months. On examination, he appears pale and in respiratory distress. Lung auscultation reveals bilateral crackles. He was admitted in ICU due to his worsening dyspnea, initially was in face mask and later got intubated put on mechanical ventilation.
Laboratory investigations show anemia, elevated erythrocyte sedimentation rate (ESR), raised creatinine and urea. High index of vasculitic background was kept.

Further laboratory investigations showed—A positive c-ANCA (antineutrophil cytoplasmic antibody) with a cytoplasmic pattern. Chest X-ray shows bilateral infiltrates.

Bronchoscopy with bronchoalveolar lavage demonstrates hemosiderin-laden macrophages. What is the most likely diagnosis?

a. Granulomatosis with polyangiitis (Wegener's) with diffuse alveolar hemorrhage (DAH)
b. Goodpasture syndrome with DAH
c. Churg-Strauss syndrome with pulmonary involvement
d. Microscopic polyangiitis with pulmonary manifestations

Ans. a

Explanation: The patient's clinical presentation of cough, dyspnea, hemoptysis, fatigue, joint pain, and recurrent sinus infections, along with positive c-ANCA with a cytoplasmic pattern, is highly suggestive of granulomatosis with polyangiitis (formerly known as Wegener's granulomatosis). The presence of diffuse alveolar hemorrhage (DAH) is indicated by the bilateral crackles on lung auscultation, anemia, and the finding of hemosiderin-laden macrophages on bronchoscopy with bronchoalveolar lavage. Granulomatosis with polyangiitis is a systemic vasculitis that primarily affects the small blood vessels, including those in the lungs and kidneys. DAH is a severe manifestation of the disease, characterized by bleeding into the lungs and subsequent coughing up of blood (hemoptysis). The positive c-ANCA is consistent with the disease, although other serologic tests and a biopsy may also be performed for confirmation.

Prompt diagnosis and treatment with immunosuppressive therapy, including corticosteroids and immunosuppressive medications such as cyclophosphamide or rituximab, are crucial in managing granulomatosis with polyangiitis and preventing further complications.

Suggested Reading
1. Cartin-Ceba R, Peikert T, Specks U. Pathogenesis of ANCA-associated vasculitis. Curr Rheumatol Rep. 2012;14(6):481-93.

Q.21. A 54-year-old farmer comes with history of short breath, decreased urine output, and yellowish discoloration of eyes. On further questioning, he gives alleged history of consumption of unknown compound 4 days ago. And you notice color change in the urine after adding dithionate solution.

What is likely diagnosis?

a. Paraquat poisoning
b. Organophosphate poisoning
c. Phenol poisoning
d. Acid intake

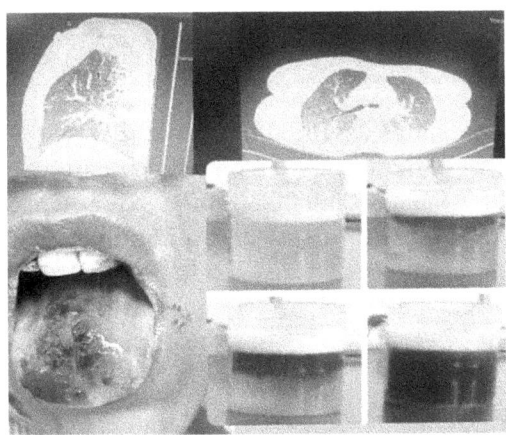

Ans. a

Explanation:

Clinical features of paraquat poisoning:
- *Gastrointestinal symptoms:* Within a few hours of ingestion, patients may experience nausea, vomiting, abdominal pain, and diarrhea. These symptoms are often accompanied by oral and throat burns due to the caustic nature of paraquat.
- *Pulmonary manifestations:* Paraquat poisoning can cause severe damage to the lungs, leading to progressive respiratory distress. Symptoms may include cough, shortness of breath, chest pain, and rapid breathing. In severe cases, pulmonary fibrosis and acute respiratory distress syndrome (ARDS) can develop, which can be fatal.
- *Renal and hepatic involvement:* Paraquat toxicity can also affect the kidneys and liver. Patients may exhibit signs of kidney dysfunction, such as decreased urine output, edema, and elevated blood urea nitrogen (BUN) and creatinine levels. Liver enzymes may be elevated, indicating hepatocellular injury.
- *Central nervous system (CNS) effects:* In some cases, paraquat poisoning can result in CNS manifestations, including confusion, seizures, and coma. These effects are typically associated with severe poisoning and often indicate a poor prognosis.
- Paraquat tongue—characteristic large ulcer over tongue is seen, with yellow necrotic base.
- Urine sodium dithionite test—sodium thionite 1% solution is prepared in 1 N sodium hydroxide. Then this solution is added to urine, sodium thionite reduces paraquat to blue color, which should be observed within a minute.

No specific treatment available, supportive care, and antioxidant therapy has been used to counteract the oxidative damage caused by paraquat. N-acetylcysteine (NAC) and vitamin C are commonly employed as antioxidants in the treatment of paraquat poisoning. There is no role of hemodialysis or hemoperfusion in removal of paraquat. Immunosuppressant therapy such as cyclophosphamide and steroid can be tried but have no much benefits.

Suggested Reading
1. Ingale PW, Shelke SN, Sundharan S, Raul NM. Importance of urine sodium dithionite test in paraquat poisoning: a case study. Int J Res Med Sci. 2015;3(1):310-11.

Q.22. A 58-year-old patient is admitted to the hospital following a brainstem lesion. On examination, the patient exhibits a respiratory pattern characterized by prolonged inhalation with a pause at full inspiration, followed by a brief exhalation. There is no associated change in the depth of respiration. Which of the following terms best describes this respiratory pattern?
  a. Cheyne-Stokes respiration
  b. Ataxic breathing
  c. Central apnea
  d. Apneustic breathing

Ans. d

Explanation: Apneustic breathing is characterized by prolonged inhalation with a pause at full inspiration, followed by a brief and inadequate exhalation. This pattern is often associated with lesions in the pons, particularly affecting the pontine respiratory centers that regulate the transition between inspiration and expiration. The prolonged inhalation phase seen in apneustic breathing suggests dysfunction in the normal termination of the inspiratory phase, resulting in the pause and inadequate exhalation.

Suggested Reading
1. Whited L, Graham DD. Abnormal respirations. In: StatPearls [Internet]. Treasure Island (FL): StatPearls Publishing; 2023.

Q.23. A 68-year-old woman admitted in an ICU after right middle cerebral artery (RMCA) infarct post-thrombolysis, her Glasgow Coma Scale (GCS) was full on admission with power 3/5 in left upper and lower limb.
A total of 4 hours later you notice the monitor screen which is shown below, her GCS dropped to 10. What is the type of respiration seen?
  a. Cheyne-Stokes respiration
  b. Ataxic breathing
  c. Central apnea
  d. Apneustic breathing

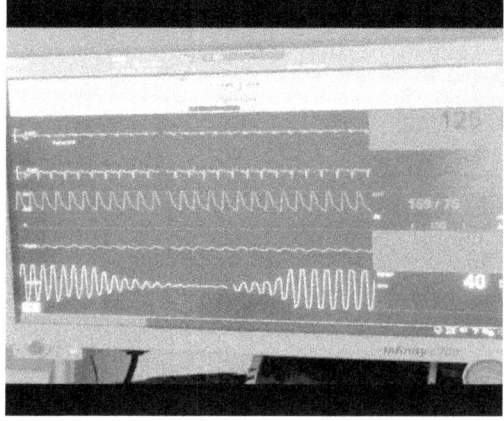

Ans. a

Explanation: Cheyne-Stokes respiration is a specific breathing pattern characterized by a cyclic sequence of increasing and decreasing tidal volumes, with periods of deep and rapid breaths (hyperpnea) followed by gradually decreasing tidal volumes leading to apnea (temporary cessation of breathing). This pattern is often associated with conditions that affect the central respiratory centers and the regulation of breathing. This patient may have hemorrhagic transformation immediate CT should be the next step after stabilizing airway.

Causes—cortical stroke, chronic heart failure (CHF), sleep apnea, and high altitude

Suggested Reading
1. Whited L, Graham DD. Abnormal Respirations. In: StatPearls [Internet]. Treasure Island (FL): StatPearls Publishing; 2023.

Q.24. A 55-year-old male patient presents with progressive shortness of breath, exercise intolerance, and chronic fatigue. He has a history of a pulmonary embolism that was treated 6 months ago. Despite anticoagulation therapy, his symptoms have worsened over time. On physical examination, he has elevated jugular venous pressure, a prominent pulmonic component of the second heart sound, and a systolic murmur over the pulmonary area as echocardiography and CT pulmonary angiogram (CTPA) shown. Which of the following conditions is the most likely the cause of this patient's symptoms?
a. Asthma
b. Chronic obstructive pulmonary disease (COPD)
c. Pulmonary arterial hypertension (PAH)
d. Chronic thromboembolic pulmonary hypertension (CTEPH)

Ans. d

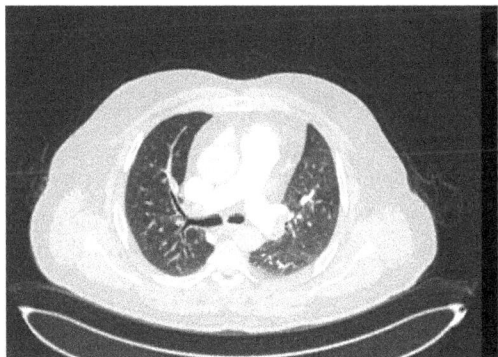
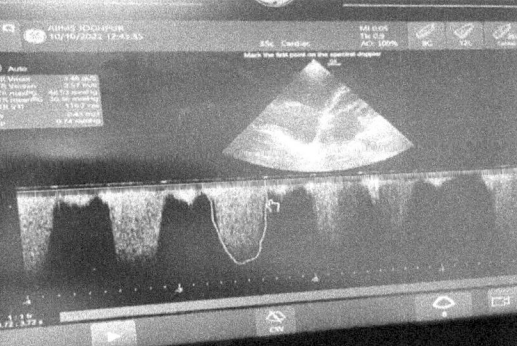

Explanation: The clinical presentation in the vignette, including a history of prior pulmonary embolism, progressive dyspnea, exercise intolerance, signs of right heart strain (elevated jugular venous pressure, prominent pulmonic component of the second heart sound), and echocardiographic evidence of right ventricular enlargement and pulmonary hypertension, is highly suggestive of chronic thromboembolic pulmonary hypertension (CTEPH). CTEPH occurs due to the incomplete resolution of acute pulmonary emboli, leading to the formation of organized fibrous thromboembolic material in the pulmonary vasculature. It is an important and potentially curable cause of pulmonary hypertension. Management is lifelong anticoagulant therapy.

Pulmonary endarterectomy (PEA) is the gold standard treatment for eligible CTEPH patients. It is a surgical procedure in which the organized thromboembolic material is removed from the pulmonary arteries. PEA is most effective in patients with accessible, surgically amenable lesions and is associated with significant improvements in symptoms and long-term survival.

Suggested Reading
1. Delcroix M, Torbicki A, Gopalan D, Sitbon O, Klok FA, Lang I, et al. ERS statement on chronic thromboembolic pulmonary hypertension. Eur Respir J. 2021;57(6):2002828.

Q.25. According to WHO classification of pulmonary hypertension, which category the abovementioned patient falls into?
a. Group 1
b. Group 2
c. Group 3
d. Group 4

Ans. d

Explanation: The World Health Organization (WHO) classification of pulmonary hypertension (PH) categorizes PH into five groups based on different etiologies and pathophysiological mechanisms. Here is an overview of the WHO classification:

Group 1: Pulmonary arterial hypertension (PAH)—it is characterized by elevated pulmonary arterial pressures due to increased resistance in the pulmonary vasculature. It includes idiopathic PAH, hereditary PAH, drug- and toxin-induced PAH, and PAH associated with other conditions such as connective tissue diseases, HIV infection, portal hypertension, congenital heart diseases, and others

Group 2: Pulmonary hypertension due to left heart disease—this group comprises pulmonary hypertension (PH) cases resulting from left-sided heart diseases, such as left ventricular systolic or diastolic dysfunction, valvular heart disease, and congenital/acquired left heart inflow/outflow tract obstructions.

Group 3: Pulmonary hypertension due to lung diseases and/or hypoxia—PH in this group is associated with chronic lung diseases, such as chronic obstructive pulmonary disease (COPD), interstitial lung disease (ILD), sleep-disordered breathing, and long-term exposure to high altitudes.

Group 4: Chronic thromboembolic pulmonary hypertension (CTEPH)—it occurs due to the incomplete resolution of acute pulmonary emboli, leading to the formation of organized fibrous thromboembolic material in the pulmonary vasculature. It is a unique form of PH that can be potentially cured with surgical intervention (pulmonary endarterectomy) or treated with balloon pulmonary angioplasty or medical therapy.

Group 5: Pulmonary hypertension with unclear multifactorial mechanisms—this group includes PH cases that cannot be classified under the other groups or have overlapping features from multiple groups. It comprises various conditions, such as blood disorders, systemic disorders, metabolic disorders, and others.

Suggested Reading
1. Rose-Jones LJ, Mclaughlin VV. Pulmonary hypertension: types and treatments. Curr Cardiol Rev. 2015;11(1):73-9.

Q.26. A 65-year-old male patient with a history of chronic smoking presents with a productive cough, fever, and right-sided chest pain. He is admitted in ICU on high-flow nasal oxygen (HFNO), due to progressive worsening of dyspnea over the past few weeks and severe hypoxemia. On examination, decreased breath sounds are noted on the right side of the chest, and chest X-ray reveals a right middle lobe opacity. A bronchoscopy is performed, which reveals a complete obstruction of the right middle lobe bronchus. Gram stain of bronchial secretions shows numerous neutrophils and no organisms. What is the most likely diagnosis, and what is the appropriate treatment for this condition?
   a. Lung cancer—surgical resection
   b. Pneumonia—broad-spectrum antibiotics
   c. Asthma exacerbation—bronchodilators and steroids
   d. Postobstructive pneumonia—bronchoscopic removal of the obstruction and antibiotics

Ans. d

Explanation: The clinical presentation in the vignette, including a history of chronic smoking, productive cough, fever, right-sided chest pain, decreased breath sounds on the affected side, and a chest X-ray showing a localized opacity, is highly suggestive of postobstructive pneumonia. In this condition, a bronchial obstruction, often caused by a mucous plug or a tumor, leads to distal lung infection and subsequent consolidation. The appropriate treatment for postobstructive pneumonia involves both removing the obstruction and administering antibiotics to treat the underlying infection. Bronchoscopy is performed to clear the obstructed bronchus and improve the airflow. Antibiotics should be selected based on the suspected pathogens and adjusted as necessary according to culture results. The other options listed in the Multiple Choice Questions (MCQs) can be ruled out based on the clinical findings and the presence of a bronchial obstruction. Lung cancer may cause obstruction but would typically require further evaluation and staging before considering surgical resection. Broad-spectrum antibiotics are suitable for treating pneumonia, but the underlying obstruction needs to be addressed. Asthma exacerbation may cause respiratory symptoms, but the presence of an obstruction and consolidation on imaging points toward a different diagnosis.

Suggested Reading
1. Rolston KVI, Nesher L. Post-obstructive pneumonia in patients with cancer: a review. Infect Dis Ther. 2018;7(1):29-38.

Q.27. When should be the adjunctive dose of steroids started in pneumocystis pneumonia (PCP) patients?
   a. Patient on face mask of 5 liters with PaO_2 <70 mm Hg
   b. Patient on room air with PaO_2 <70 mm Hg and with alveolar-arterial (A-a) gradient of >35 mm Hg

c. Patient on room air with SpO₂ <92% saturation
d. Patient already on co-trimoxazole (suphamethoxazole and trimethoprim) treatment with SpO₂ 98% on initiation and now has worsened hypoxemia.
e. Need to start steroids in all the above cases.

Ans. e

Explanation: Steroids have been given to HIV-positive patients with worsening hypoxemia; their use is not associated with any other opportunistic infection.
Criteria to start steroids are:
- PaO₂ <70 mm Hg on room air, or
- A-a gradient >35 mm Hg on room air, or
- Hypoxemia with SpO₂ of <92% on room air

And any patient who is already on PCP treatment with stable parameters initially and worsens later in the course of the disease needs to be put on steroids.
Regimen: Prednisone 40 mg orally twice daily for 5 days, followed by 40 mg orally once daily for 5 days, followed by 20 mg orally once daily for 11 days. However the use of steroids in HIV-negative patients with PCP with mild-to-moderate disease has not shown a good outcome benefits, but meta-analysis in severe PCP pneumonia cases without HIV, the use of steroids has been shown to reduce the ventilator free days and it needs to be given in severe cases.

Suggested Reading
1. Delclaux C, Zahar JR, Amraoui G, Leleu G, Lebargy F, Brochard L, et al. Corticosteroids as adjunctive therapy for severe pneumocystis carinii pneumonia in non-human immunodeficiency virus-infected patients: retrospective study of 31 patients. Clin Infect Dis. 1999;29(3):670-2.

Q.28. A 45-year-old female with a known diagnosis of systemic sclerosis presents to the emergency department with acute worsening of dyspnea and dry cough over the past week. She has a history of interstitial lung disease (ILD) associated with systemic sclerosis. On physical examination, her oxygen saturation on room air is 88%, respiratory rate is 28 breaths/min, and lung auscultation reveals bilateral inspiratory crackles. High-resolution CT scan of the chest shows worsening of bilateral interstitial opacities compared to previous imaging. What is the most appropriate initial treatment for this patient?
a. Intravenous cyclophosphamide
b. Noninvasive positive pressure ventilation (NPPV)
c. High-dose systemic corticosteroids
d. Empirical broad-spectrum antibiotics
e. Low-dose corticosteroid therapy

Ans. e

Explanation: There are no randomized studies for management of acute exacerbation of interstitial lung disease (AE-ILD), however according to the European Respiratory Society (ERS) guidelines idiopathic pulmonary fibrosis (IPF) treatment is mainly with supportive care, symptom palliation, and long-term oxygen therapy. Above the supportive care high dose corticosteroids are the main line of management with broad spectrum antibiotics to treat underlying cause of infection. Mechanical ventilation is weak evidence for AE-ILD and should not be the first line. HFNO/NIV should be given to reduce the hypoxemia symptoms. High-dose corticosteroids have benefit in idiopathic interstitial pneumonia, connective tissue-associated ILD, and in some cases of sarcoidosis and hypersensitive pneumonitis. However it should be taken into consideration that high-dose corticosteroids in case of systemic sclerosis-associated ILD (SSc-ILD) should be taken as a pinch of salt as it may lead into SRC scleroderma renal crisis (SRC).

Suggested Reading
1. Steen VD, Medsger TA Jr. Case-control study of corticosteroids and other drugs that either precipitate or protect from the development of scleroderma renal crisis. Arthritis Rheum. 1998;41:1613-19.

Q.29. A 25-year-old young patient comes with acute onset of shortness of breath, with tachycardia, sweating, and palpitation. Bedside echocardiogram in short axis at RVOT/aorta—shows a huge thrombus obstructing almost 80% of left main pulmonary artery, with RA and RV dilation. You decide and write the orders to give alteplase, 0.9 mg/kg 10% within 10 minutes and remaining infusion over next 1 hour. Half hour into infusion, patient suddenly collapses and has cardiac arrest. You start giving cardiopulmonary resuscitation (CPR). Next action should be:
   a. Continue CPR for next 30 minutes with infusion of alteplase to run as in written orders.
   b. Continue CPR for next 30 minutes with bolus push of remaining alteplase.
   c. Continue CPR for next 60–90 minutes with infusion of alteplase to run as in written orders.
   d. Continue CPR for next 60–90 minutes with bolus push of remaining alteplase.

Ans. d

Explanation: Post-thrombolysis in case of acute pulmonary embolism, CPR should be given for 60–90 minutes before calling off. And during cardiac arrest thrombolysis dose should be given as bolus push.

Suggested Reading
1. Konstantinides SV, Meyer G, Becattini C, Bueno H, Geersing GJ, Harjola VP, et al. 2019 ESC Guidelines for the diagnosis and management of acute pulmonary embolism developed in collaboration with the European Respiratory Society (ERS). Eur Heart J. 2020;41(4): 543-603.

Q.30. All of the following treatments can be used for PCP pneumonia, except:
   a. Dapsone 100 mg PO q24h + trimethoprim (TMP) 5 mg/kg PO q8h for 21 days
   b. Trimethoprim-sulfamethoxazole (TMP-SMX) 15–20 mg of TMP component/kg/day IV divided in q8h for 21 days
   c. Clindamycin 600 mg IV q8h + primaquine 15 mg PO q24h for 21 days

d. Pentamidine 4 mg /kg/day IV for 21 days
e. Pentamidine 300 mg in 6 mL sterile water by aerosol every 4 weeks

Ans. e

Explanation: Pentamidine aerosol is only used as prophylaxis in PCP pneumonia, not for the treatment. Above four options can be used for treatment of PCP pneumonia. Drugs used as prophylaxis are—aerosoled pentamidine, dapsone + pyrimethamine PO, atovaquone 1,500 mg PO with food.

Suggested Reading

1. Bozzette SA, Finkelstein DM, Spector SA, Frame P, Powderly WG, He W, et al. A randomized trial of three antipneumocystis agents in patients with advanced human immunodeficiency virus infection. NIAID AIDS Clinical Trials Group. N Engl J Med. 1995;332(11):693-9.

CHAPTER 6

Hemodynamic Monitoring

Harish Mallapura Maheshwarappa, Thilakchand KR, Ronak R Ankolekar

Q.1. A 56-year-old hypertensive male is shifted to the intensive care unit (ICU) postoperatively after robotic bilateral inguinal hernioplasty under general anesthesia. On arrival, patient has a blood pressure of 72/58 mm Hg and heart rate (HR) of 122 bpm. Arterial blood gas (ABG) shows lactates 2.3, hemoglobin on ABG is 8.9. Bedside ultrasonography reveals good LV contractility, inferior vena cava (IVC) distensibility index is 22%. Patient is on controlled ventilation. What is the best step to tackle hypotension?
   a. Crystalloid bolus
   b. Noradrenaline infusion
   c. Dobutamine infusion
   d. Blood transfusion

Ans. a

Explanation: As patient is on controlled ventilation, IVC distensibility index >18% is indicative of fluid responsiveness. Based on the information provided, volume resuscitation should be the ideal strategy.

Among the IVC indices, collapsibility index is performed in spontaneously breathing patients and distensibility and variability indices are calculated in patients on controlled mechanical ventilation.

$$CI\text{–}IVC \text{ (IVC collapsibility index): } [(IVC_{max} - IVC_{min})/IVC_{max}] \times 100$$
$$dIVC \text{ (IVC distensibility index): } [(IVC_{max} - IVC_{min})/IVC_{min}] \times 100$$
$$\Delta IVC: [(IVC_{max} - IVC_{min})/IVC_{median}] \times 100$$

The IVC index cut-off values for volume responsiveness are as follows:
1. CI–IVC of >50%
2. dIVC of >18%
3. ΔIVC of >12%

Suggested Reading
1. Sarıtaş A, Zincircioğlu Ç, Uzun Sarıtaş P, Uzun U, Köse I, Şenoğlu N. Comparison of inferior vena cava collapsibility, distensibility, and delta indices at different positive pressure supports and prediction values of indices for intravascular volume status. Turk J Med Sci. 2019;49(4):1170-8.

Q.2. A 65-year-old male, known case of hypertension, was admitted with anterior wall myocardial infarction (AWMI), underwent percutaneous coronary intervention (PCI) to left anterior descending artery, and is now shifted to the coronary care unit. He is hypotensive, his blood pressure (BP) is 76/50 mm Hg and HR is 124 bpm. On examination, he has cold, clammy peripheries. Bilateral basal crepitations are present on auscultation. ABG reveals lactates of 4.7. Transthoracic echocardiogram reveals a dP/dt of 760 mm Hg/s. What is the next best step in optimizing his hemodynamics? (dP/dt: rate of momentum transfer per unit time)

a. 1,000-mL fluid bolus
b. Noradrenaline infusion
c. IABP insertion
d. Dobutamine infusion

Ans. c

Explanation: dP/dt represents the ratio of pressure change in the ventricular cavity during the isovolemic contraction period. Normal value of dP/dt is >1,200 mm Hg/s. In this patient, dP/dt of 760 mm Hg/s is indicative of reduced cardiac contractility. As the patient is hypotensive and tachycardic, dobutamine infusion is more likely to worsen this predicament. Intra-aortic balloon pump (IABP) insertion would be the ideal strategy here to improve patient's hemodynamics.

Suggested Reading
1. Chengode S. Left ventricular global systolic function assessment by echocardiography. Ann Card Anaesth. 2016;19(Suppl 1):S26-34.

Q.3. An 82-year-old woman is admitted to the intensive treatment unit (ITU) after an elective triple vessel coronary artery bypass graft. Pulmonary artery catheter monitoring is initiated. After 6 hours postsurgery, she is found to have BP of 66/38 mm Hg and HR of 132 bpm. Her urine output is 15 mL/h over the past 2 hours. Pulmonary artery catheter data show: pulmonary artery pressure of 12/6 mm Hg, pulmonary artery occlusion pressure of 6 mm Hg, central venous pressure (CVP) of 5 cmH$_2$O, cardiac index of 1.5 L/min/m^2, and systemic vascular resistance of 2,800 dyne/s/cm^5. The most probable cause for his hemodynamic worsening is:

a. Cardiac tamponade
b. Sepsis
c. Hemorrhage
d. Pulmonary embolism

Ans. c

Explanation: Cardiac tamponade presents with high CVP and high values of pulmonary artery occluded pressure (PAOP) and pulmonary artery (PA) pressure. Sepsis presents with high-cardiac index due to hyperdynamic circulation and reduced systemic vascular resistance (SVR) as a result of vasodilatation. Pulmonary embolism is ruled out in this scenario with the presence of normal pulmonary artery pressure. Hemorrhagic shock is the most appropriate option here as the patient has low CVP, low PA pressures, and elevated SVR.

Suggested Reading
1. Saxena A, Garan AR, Kapur NK, O'Neill WW, Lindenfeld J, Pinney SP, et al. Value of hemodynamic monitoring in patients with cardiogenic shock undergoing mechanical circulatory support. Circulation. 2020;141(14):1184-97.

Q.4. A 74-year-old male, known case of diabetic nephropathy with end-stage renal disease (ESRD), has been shifted to the ICU postrenal transplant. On day 2 of ICU stay, nurse informs you of a drop in his urine output over the past 3 hours. ABG shows pH of 7.32, PCO_2 of 28, HCO_3 of 15, and BE of 11. Renal resistive index (RRI) was calculated, which was 1.1. Based on the parameters provided, which of the following can be ruled out?
   a. Graft rejection
   b. Septic shock
   c. Hypovolemia
   d. Renal artery stenosis

Ans. d

Explanation: The renal arterial resistive index (RI) is a sonographic index of intrarenal arteries defined as (peak systolic velocity – end-diastolic velocity)/peak systolic velocity. The normal range is 0.50–0.70.

Reasons for elevated values are:
- Ureteric obstruction
- Extreme hypotension
- Very young children
- Perinephric fluid collection
- Abdominal compartment syndrome

Reasons for decreased values are:
- Renal artery stenosis

Suggested Reading
1. Krumme B, Hollenbeck M. Doppler sonography in renal artery stenosis—does the Resistive Index predict the success of intervention? Nephrol Dial Transplant. 2007;22(3):692-6.
2. Weerakkody Y, Carroll D, Alsmair A; Radiopaedia.org. (2010). Renal arterial resistive index. [online] Available from https://radiopaedia.org/articles/renal-arterial-resistive-index?lang=us. [Last accessed June, 2023]

Q.5. A 58-year-old man underwent emergency laparotomy for suspected bowel perforation. Patient was hypotensive postinduction and esophageal Doppler monitoring showed the following values: cardiac output = 3.8 L/min, stroke volume = 44 mL, FTc (corrected flow time) = 260 ms, and peak velocity = 80 cm/s. Following a 250-mL bolus of colloid, there was improvement in stroke volume to 55 mL and FTc became 280 ms. What was the most possible cause of hypotension?
   a. Septic shock
   b. Cardiogenic shock
   c. Hypovolemic shock
   d. Obstructive shock

Ans. c

Explanation: Among esophageal Doppler measurements, FTc (corrected flow time) is a direct marker of preload. A low baseline FTc and increase in SV and FTc with fluid bolus are indicative of hypovolemic shock. Peak velocity is normal for patient's age ruling out cardiogenic shock. Septic shock presents with higher FTc as the afterload is reduced due to vasodilatation. Improvement in stroke volume with fluid administration rules out obstructive shock in this scenario.

Suggested Reading
1. Morris C. Oesophageal Doppler monitoring, doubt and equipoise: evidence based medicine means change. Anaesthesia. 2013;68(7):684-8.

Q.6. A 60-year-old female is admitted to the ICU with urinary tract infection. She has a background of coronary artery disease postpercutaneous coronary intervention. She is intubated in view of hemodynamic instability. ABG shows lactates of 3.2. Her esophageal Doppler values are as follows: Ftc (corrected flow time) = 390 ms, peak velocity = 100 cm/s, and cardiac index = 4.5. What is the most likely diagnosis?
   a. Septic shock
   b. Cardiogenic shock
   c. Obstructive shock
   d. Hypovolemic shock

Ans. a

Explanation: Cardiogenic shock would display a low CI with a high FTc as a result of increased afterload. Obstructive shock also displays a low CI with high FTc. Hypovolemic shock displays a low FTc as a result of reduced preload. Septic shock is the most appropriate answer here as the patient has a high FTc indicative of a reduced afterload due to vasodilatation and high cardiac index due to hyperdynamic circulation.

Suggested Reading
1. Morris C. Oesophageal Doppler monitoring, doubt and equipoise: evidence based medicine means change. Anaesthesia. 2013;68(7):684-8.

Q.7. A 48-year-old male was shifted to the ICU after on-pump coronary artery bypass graft (CABG) for triple vessel disease. On day 2, patient is hypotensive (BP – 80/50 mm Hg) and Tachycardic (HR – 122 bpm). ABG reveals lactates of 7.9. His peripheries appear cold and clammy. Patient is on esophageal Doppler monitoring, which shows: Ftc (corrected flow time) = 270 ms and peak velocity = 35 cm/s. Post-administration of 250 mL of crystalloid, FTc is 275 ms. Which is the most likely cause for the patient's deterioration?
   a. Cardiac tamponade
   b. Sepsis
   c. Hypovolemia
   d. Cardiac failure

Ans. d

Explanation: Esophageal Doppler monitoring enables several measured and derived parameters to be assessed. Three of the primary measurements are stroke distance, flow time, and peak velocity. Cardiac tamponade on esophageal Doppler reveals a high FTc and low peak velocity, hence ruled out in this scenario. Sepsis and hypovolemia are ruled out as peak velocity is normal in hypovolemia and sepsis presents with high FTc due to reduced afterload. This patient has cardiac failure as there is low FTc (not increasing with fluid administration) which is indicative of increased afterload, and reduced PV.

Suggested Reading
1. Morris C. Oesophageal Doppler monitoring, doubt and equipoise: evidence based medicine means change. Anaesthesia. 2013;68(7):684-8.

Q.8. A 64-year-old male was admitted with worsening respiratory distress, anasarca with tense ascites, and acute renal failure. He is a known case of ethanolic liver cirrhosis and severe congestive cardiac failure with ejection fraction (EF) of 15%. On admission, creatinine was 1.4 mg/dL which was increased to 3.2 mg/dL on day 3. On examination, patient was tachypneic with RR of 30 cpm, BP of 110/70 mm Hg, and HR of 82 bpm. His bedside ultrasonography examination revealed IVC of 2.1 cm, portal vein and hepatic vein Doppler revealed the following picture. Which of the following would not be an ideal treatment strategy?

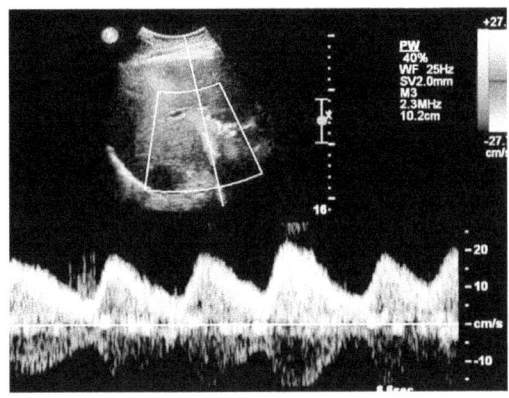

a. Frusemide infusion
b. Large-volume paracentesis
c. Crystalloid infusion
d. Dobutamine infusion

Ans. c

Explanation: The VEXUS examination is grade 3, indicating congestion in the portal vein producing pulsatility. Based on the available data, there is no role for crystalloid infusion in this patient. Patient could be having cardiorenal syndrome, hence dobutamine and furosemide infusion can help in improving the renal perfusion and improve urine output, respectively. As the patient has tense ascites, large volume paracentesis can relieve the intra-abdominal pressure and improve renal blood flow.

Suggested Reading
1. David J, Shaw AD. Utility of bedside ultrasound derived hepatic and renal parenchymal flow patterns to guide management of acute kidney injury. Curr Opin Crit Care. 2021;27(6):587-92.

Q.9. A 65-year-old male, known case of diabetes mellitus, was presented with right lower limb necrotizing fasciitis and underwent emergency fasciotomy and debridement of the necrotizing fasciitis under general anesthesia. Intraoperatively, FloTrac monitoring was initiated and stroke volume variation was 15% and then 2 L of crystalloids was transfused. Postprocedure, patient is shifted to ICU and is on controlled mechanical ventilation with tidal volume of 8 mL/kg. Patient remains hypotensive, with BP = 80/50 mm Hg, mean arterial pressure (MAP) = 62, and HR = 126. FloTrac monitoring values are as follows: cardiac output = 4, stroke volume variation = V9, systemic vascular resistance = 610 dyne/s/cm^5, stroke volume = 60 mL. What is the next best step?

a. Norepinephrine infusion
b. 250 mL of colloid
c. Blood transfusion
d. Administration of 500 mL isotonic crystalloid

Ans. a

Explanation: This patient does not appear to be fluid responsive anymore as suggested by the SVV. Hence, colloid administration, crystalloid bolus, and blood transfusion can be ruled out. The FloTrac readings of low SVR with normal stroke volume are suggestive of septic shock in this scenario. Hence, initiation of norepinephrine infusion is the next appropriate step in this patient. Controlled mechanical ventilation should be present to induce required changes in preload, it is inaccurate in spontaneously breathing patients. Tidal volume should be large enough to facilitate significant changes in preload (8 mL/kg). Regular heart rhythm should be present. Change in stroke volume is another dynamic parameter to assess for fluid responsiveness. This method is unique and it is shown to be highly predictive even in situations with arrhythmia and spontaneous breathing activity in contrast to systolic pressure variation (SPV) and pulse pressure variation (PPV).

Suggested Reading
1. Cherpanath TG, Geerts BF, Lagrand WK, Schultz MJ, Groeneveld AB. Basic concepts of fluid responsiveness. Neth Heart J. 2013;21(12):530-6.

Q.10. A 55-year-old male, known case of dilated cardiomyopathy with EF of 25% and AF with controlled ventricular rate on warfarin 2 mg OD, was presented with upper gastrointestinal (GI) bleed. On examination, patient was hypoxic on noninvasive ventilation (NIV) support and hypotensive with BP of 88/50 mm Hg. Arterial line was inserted and FloTrac monitoring initiated. Which of the parameters would help to guide fluid responsiveness in this patient?

a. SVV
b. PPV
c. SPV
d. ΔSV

Ans. d

Explanation: Several limitations are present in the use of dynamic parameters such as PPV, SPV, and SVV.
- Controlled mechanical ventilation with no spontaneous breaths
- No arrhythmias
- Tidal volume >8 mL/kg
- *Heart rate:* Respiratory rate >4
- Open abdomen can reduce the SVV/PPV by 40–50%

Suggested Reading
1. Deltexmedical. Stroke volume variation (SVV) and pulse pressure variation (PPV). [online] Available from https://www.deltexmedical.com/decision_tree/stroke-volume-variation-svv-and-pulse-pressure-variation-ppv/. [Last accessed June, 2023]
2. Suehiro K. Assessing fluid responsiveness during spontaneous breathing. J Anesth. 2022;36:579-82.

Q.11. A 45-year-old male, known case of coronary artery disease (CAD) on dual antiplatelets and ethanolic chronic liver disease, came with upper GI bleed. The patient got intubated in view of hemodynamic instability, patient is on controlled mechanical ventilation. Advanced hemodynamic monitoring is initiated, following values are noted: hypotension predictive index = 90, dP/dt = 750 mm Hg/s, and dynamic arterial elastance is 0.76. How do you manage the patient?
- a. Administer albumin
- b. Dobutamine infusion
- c. Noradrenaline infusion
- d. 500 mL fluid bolus

Ans. b

Explanation: Hypotension predictive index (HPI) is an algorithm based on detailed analysis of hemodynamic features from arterial pressure waveform as an input and occurrence of hypotension with MAP <65 mm Hg for at least 1 minute as output. The algorithm gives a unitless number ranging from 0 to 100, informing about likelihood that within 5–15 minutes, a hypotensive event will occur. Higher the value of HPI, greater the risk of hypotension. Dynamic arterial elastance (Eadyn) is a quotient of PPV and SVV. Optimal cut off value for Eadyn is 0.84. Lower values suggest poor response to fluid administration and advise use of vasopressors. Higher values suggest fluid responsiveness. In the given question, HPI is high indicating risk of hypotension. Eadyn is lower than the cutoff, supporting the initiation of vasopressors. As the dP/dt value is below normal (<1,200 dynes/s), which is an indicator of poor cardiac contractility, patient requires dobutamine infusion to prevent further hypoperfusion and hypotension.

Suggested Reading
1. Szrama J, Gradys A, Bartkowiak T, Woźniak A, Kusza K, Molnar Z. Intraoperative hypotension prediction: A proactive perioperative hemodynamic management—A Literature Review. Medicina (Kaunas). 2023;59(3):491.

Q.12. A 55-year-old gentleman, known case of hypertension and IHD post-percutaneous coronary intervention with EF of 50%, was presented with traumatic open left femur fracture, with extensive blood loss, and underwent emergency fixation of left femur under general anesthesia. Patient was resuscitated with 1,000 mL crystalloid and 2 unit PC intraoperatively. Patient was shifted to ICU after the procedure intubated on volume-controlled mode of ventilation. Arterial line was in situ and FloTrac monitoring was initiated. The parameters were as follows: systemic vascular resistance = 1450 dyne/s/cm^5, stroke volume variation = 22%, cardiac output = 3.2 L/min, and stroke volume = 65 mL. Postoperatively, hemoglobin was 9.6 g/dL. What is the next best step?
- a. Transfuse 1 unit of packed red blood cell (PRBC)
- b. Administration of 500 mL balanced crystalloid
- c. Noradrenaline infusion
- d. Dobutamine infusion

Ans. b

Explanation: Based on the values provided, this patient is still in hypovolemic shock, as the SVV is greater than 12% and SVR is elevated. The patient requires crystalloid infusion. The postoperative hemoglobin is >7 g% and does not warrant a blood transfusion. Patient has a normal SV, hence dobutamine is ruled out. As patient has elevated SVR, norepinephrine infusion can also be ruled out.

Suggested Reading
1. Suehiro K. Update on the assessment of fluid responsiveness. J Anesth. 2020;34:163-6.

Q.13. A 38-year-old male was admitted to the ICU after exploratory laparotomy for penetrating abdominal trauma with liver laceration. Intraoperatively, estimated blood loss was 1.2 L. 2 units of PRBCs and 2 units of fresh frozen plasma (FFPs) were transfused. He also received 3 L of crystalloids. He was also started on inotropes in view of hypotension. On day 2, patient continues to be on controlled ventilation, with 8 mL/kg TV, HR of 82 bpm, BP of 138/70 mm Hg, and MAP of 82 mm Hg with 0.2 µg/kg/min norepinephrine infusion. His SVV is 20%. ABG shows lactates of 0.8, hemoglobin of 9.8 g%, and urine output >0.5 mL/kg/h. How would you proceed further?
a. Fluid bolus of 250 mL RL
b. Taper norepinephrine
c. Furosemide infusion
d. Colloid bolus

Ans. b

Explanation: The presence of SVV >12% is indicative that the patient is fluid responsive, but we need to also take into account if the patient requires evaluation for fluid administration. This patient has minimal requirement of inotropic support, normal lactate levels, and producing >0.5 mL/kg/h urine output. Hence, the patient in this scenario does not require any fluid resuscitation. The noradrenaline requirement should be further tapered down as the MAP requirement is met as well.

Suggested Reading
1. Michard F. Volume management in critically ill patients. Eur Cardiol. 2008;4(1):99-100.

Q.14. A 75-year-old patient is admitted to the ICU postemergency laparotomy for colonic perforation. A Hartmann's procedure has been performed. Intraoperatively, she has received 3 L of Hartmann's solution and 500 mL of gelofusine. Advanced hemodynamic monitoring is initiated. She is now maintained intubated and ventilated with pressure support mode. Patient's abdomen is soft and intra-abdominal pressure is 7 mm Hg. Adequate analgesia is administered. She is becoming progressively more tachycardic and hypotensive. Which of the options would be the best indicator that a fluid bolus would be of benefit?
a. Central venous pressure of 6 mm Hg
b. Stroke volume variation of 14%
c. Pulmonary artery occlusion pressure of 10 mm Hg
d. Passive leg raise increment in stroke volume of 10%

Ans. d

Explanation: CVP and PAOP are static indices and do not give accurate information about fluid responsiveness. As the patient is spontaneously breathing and is on pressure support mode, the prerequisites for SVV estimation are not met and hence not reliable.

Passive leg raise (PLR) test can be performed in spontaneously breathing patients. An increase in ΔSV >10% with PLR is indicative of fluid responsiveness.

Suggested Reading
1. Suehiro K. Assessing fluid responsiveness during spontaneous breathing. J Anesth. 2022;36:579-82.

Q.15. A 62-year-old male, with ischemic heart disease and trple vessel disease has undergone coronary artery bypass surgery and is now admitted in the ICU under your care. Patient also suffers from diabetes mellitus for the past 15 years. The patient is under your care in ICU. On POD 2, drains are removed and on POD 3, patient is hypotensive with BP of 78/40 mm Hg and HR of 130 bpm. PA catheter shows right atrial pressure (RAP) of 24 mm Hg, right ventricle pressure (RVP) of 90/25 mm Hg, pulmonary artery pressure (PAP) of 80/24 mm Hg, and pulmonary artery occlusion pressure (PAOP) of 22 mm Hg. What could be the potential reason for worsening?
 a. Hemorrhagic shock
 b. Cardiac tamponade
 c. Right ventricular failure
 d. Pulmonary embolism

Ans. b

Explanation: Various hemodynamic parameters can be measured by PA catheter. Direct measurements obtained from PA catheter are CVP, right-sided intracardiac pressures (RA and RV), pulmonary artery pressure, PAOP, cardiac output, and mixed venous oxyhemoglobin saturation (SvO_2). Indirect measurements of PA catheter are SVR, PVR, CI, stroke volume index, oxygen delivery, and oxygen uptake. Normal RA pressure is 0–7 mm Hg, normal RV systolic pressure is 15–25 mm Hg, normal RV end-diastolic pressure is 3–12 mm Hg, normal systolic pulmonary artery pressure is 15–25 mm Hg, normal PA diastolic pressure is 8–15 mm Hg, and normal PAOP is 6–15 mm Hg. From the given values, there are increased RAP, RVP, PAP, and PAOP. In cardiac tamponade, RAP, RVP, PAP, and PAOP will be raised. In right ventricular failure, RAP, RVP, and PAP will be raised but PAOP will be low. In hemorrhagic shock, right-sided filling pressures will be low. So based on given values, cardiac tamponade is best possible answer.

Suggested Reading
1. Saxena A, Garan AR, Kapur NK, O'Neill WW, Lindenfeld J, Pinney SP, et al. Value of hemodynamic monitoring in patients with cardiogenic shock undergoing mechanical circulatory support. Circulation. 2020;141(14):1184-97.

Q.16. A 62-year-old male diabetic, bedridden with urinary catheter for 2 months, is admitted in the ICU with decreased responsiveness and diagnosed to have septic encephalopathy secondary to urosepsis. ECG rhythm shows atrial fibrillation. His vitals are as follows: MAP = 60 mm Hg and HR = 104 bpm. FloTrac monitoring is used and stroke volume is 55 mL. You perform a passive leg raise test and stroke volume increases to 59 mL. What is next best step?
 a. Crystalloid bolus of 500 mL
 b. Start noradrenaline infusion.
 c. Information not sufficient to decide
 d. Administration of 5% albumin

Ans. b

Explanation: Advantages of PLR over other dynamic methods of volume assessment are that it does not require sinus rhythm and it can also be performed in spontaneously ventilating patients. Change in stroke volume >10% after PLR implies that the patient is fluid responsive. In the given question, the stroke volume increases by 4 mL (<10% change), thus the patient is not fluid responsive. The best next step is to start inotropes.

Suggested Reading
1. Kulkarni AP, Kothekar AT, Divatia JV. Textbook of hemodynamic monitoring and therapy in critically ill. New Delhi: Jaypee Brothers Medical Publisher; 2020.

Q.17. A 56-year-old male, known case of diabetes, is admitted with urosepsis with septic shock. The patient is managed with IV antibiotics and IV fluids. Inotropes were gradually tapered and stopped. On day 4 in ICU, patient is off supports on room air. Which of the following does not help to assess readiness for deresuscitation?
a. B-lines on lung ultrasound
b. Absence of fluid responsiveness
c. Signs of hypoperfusion
d. Bioelectrical impedance analysis

Ans. c

Explanation:

Triggers to start fluid removal:	
• MAP/APP > 65/55 mm Hg	• PLR test negative
• GEDVI > 850 mL/m^2	• LVEDAI > 14 cm^2/m^2
• EVLWI > 10–12 mL/kg PBW	• High VEXUS score
• PVPI > 3	• IAP > 12–15 mm Hg
• PPV and SVV < 12%	• BIA: ECWI/ICW >1: V_E > 5%

(APP: abdominal perfusion pressure; EVLWI: extra-vascular lung water index; GEDVI: global end-diastolic volume index; LVEDAI: left ventricular end-diastolic area index; MAP: mean arterial pressure; PVPI: pulmonary vascular permeability index; PPV: pulse pressure variation; PLR: passive leg raising; SVV: stroke volume variation)

Deresuscitation should be started when there are signs of fluid accumulation. Signs of hypoperfusion imply that the patient is not adequately resuscitated to start deresuscitation.

Suggested Reading
1. Malbrain MLNG, Martin G, Ostermann M. Everything you need to know about deresuscitation. Intensive Care Med. 2022;48:1781-6.

Q.18. Which of the following is incorrect in a CVP trace?
a. Absent a wave—atrial fibrillation
b. Loss of y descent—cardiac tamponade
c. Junctional rhythm—cannon a wave
d. Tricuspid regurgitation—tall a wave

Ans. d

Explanation: Tricuspid regurgitation has giant v waves or ventricularization, because pressure generated during right ventricular contraction is transmitted. Absent a wave indicates atrial standstill as seen in atrial fibrillation. Cardiac tamponade: y descent is blunted due to decreased holodiastolic filling of the ventricle. Junctional rhythm: delayed atrial retrograde depolarization, which may cause to contract against closed tricuspid valve producing large waves called cannon a waves.

Suggested Reading
1. Reems MM, Aumann M. Central venous pressure: principles, measurement, and interpretation. Compend Contin Educ Vet. 2012;34(1):E1.

Q.19. A 58-year-old female is admitted in ICU with community-acquired pneumonia, intubated in view of worsening respiratory distress and severe metabolic acidosis. The patient develops anuric acute kidney injury (AKI) and is planned for dialysis. Which of the following parameters would most likely predict occurrence of intradialytic hypotension?

a. IVC distensibility index >18%
b. IVC collapsibility index <50%
c. IVC variability index <12%
d. IVC collapsibility index >50%

Ans. a

Explanation: Among the IVC indices, collapsibility index is performed in spontaneously breathing patients and distensibility and variability indices are calculated in patients on controlled mechanical ventilation.

$$CI\text{-}IVC \text{ (IVC collapsibility index)}: [(IVC_{max} - IVC_{min})/IVC_{max}] \times 100$$
$$dIVC \text{ (IVC distensibility index)}: [(IVC_{max} - IVC_{min})/IVC_{min}] \times 100$$
$$\Delta IVC: [(IVC_{max} - IVC_{min})/IVC_{median}] \times 100$$

The IVC index cut-off values for volume responsiveness are as follows:
a. CI–IVC of >50%
b. dIVC of >18%
c. ΔIVC of >12%.

Suggested Reading
1. Sarıtaş A, Zincircioğlu Ç, Uzun Sarıtaş P, Uzun U, Köse I, Şenoğlu N. Comparison of inferior vena cava collapsibility, distensibility, and delta indices at different positive pressure supports and prediction values of indices for intravascular volume status. Turk J Med Sci. 2019;49(4):1170-8.

Q.20. A 64-year-old female is admitted with no known comorbidities, she is known case of CA endometrium post total abdominal hysterectomy and bilateral salpingo-oophorectomy plus hyperthermic intraperitoneal chemotherapy. Patient is shifted to ICU after the procedure, intubated on controlled mechanical ventilation. Advanced hemodynamic monitoring was initiated, values of various parameters are as follows: hypotension predictive index = 94, cardiac index = 4.5, and dynamic arterial elastance = 0.92. How do you manage the patient?

a. 500 mL fluid bolus
b. Norepinephrine infusion
c. Dobutamine infusion
d. Wait and watch

Ans. a

Explanation: Hypotension predictive index is an algorithm based on detailed analysis of hemodynamic features from arterial pressure waveform as an input and occurrence of hypotension with MAP <65 mm Hg for at least 1 minute as output. The algorithm gives a unitless number ranging from 0 to 100, informing about likelihood that within 5–15 minutes, a hypotensive event will occur. Higher the value of HPI, greater the risk of hypotension. Dynamic arterial elastance (Eadyn) is a quotient of PPV and SVV. Optimal cut off value for Eadyn is 0.84. Lower values suggest poor response to fluid administration and advise use of vasopressors. Higher values suggest fluid responsiveness. In the given question, HPI is high indicating risk of hypotension. Eadyn value is more than cut off suggestive of fluid responsiveness. Thus, the next step would be to give fluid bolus.

Suggested Reading
1. Persona P, Tonetti T, Valeri I, Pivetta E, Zarantonello F, Pettenuzzo T, et al. Dynamic arterial elastance to predict mean arterial pressure decrease after reduction of vasopressor in septic shock patients. Life (Basel). 2022;13(1):28.
2. Szrama J, Gradys A, Bartkowiak T, Woźniak A, Kusza K, Molnar Z. Intraoperative hypotension prediction: A proactive perioperative hemodynamic management—A Literature Review. Medicina (Kaunas). 2023;59(3):491.

Q.21. A 40-year-old male, known case of CA pancreas, post two cycles of chemotherapy, was presented to cardiac emergency with sudden onset chest pain, got intubated in view of hemodynamic instability. His initial lactates was 4 mmol/L. PA catheter was inserted and it shows following values: right atrial pressure = 22 mm Hg, right ventricle pressure = 90/31 mm Hg, pulmonary artery pressure = 34/18 mm Hg, and pulmonary artery occlusion pressure = 4. Which of the following is most likely to be seen on bedside ultrasonography?
   a. Lung point
   b. RV apical hypokinesia
   c. Global hypokinesia
   d. RV diastolic collapse

Ans. b

Explanation: Based on measurements from PA catheter, normal RA pressure is 0–7 mm Hg, normal RV systolic pressure is 15–25 mm Hg, normal RV end-diastolic pressure is 3–12 mm Hg, normal systolic pulmonary artery pressure is 15–25 mm Hg, normal PA diastolic pressure is 8–15 mm Hg, and normal PAOP is 6–15 mm Hg. Based on the given values, there is increase in right-sided pressures and low PAOP. Findings are suggestive of pulmonary embolism. Of all the given options, RV apical hypokinesia is likely to be seen in pulmonary embolism. Lung point is seen in pneumothorax. RV diastolic collapse is seen in cardiac tamponade.

Suggested Reading
1. Saxena A, Garan AR, Kapur NK, O'Neill WW, Lindenfeld J, Pinney SP, et al. Value of hemodynamic monitoring in patients with cardiogenic shock undergoing mechanical circulatory support. Circulation. 2020;141(14):1184-97.

Q.22. A 58-year-old man is ventilated on the ICU following a Whipple's pancreatoduodenectomy. He is hypotensive (BP = 85/65 mm Hg) and tachycardic (HR = 120 bpm). Initial esophageal Doppler measurements include a flow time corrected

(FTc) of 290 ms, which changes to 320 ms following a 500 mL fluid challenge. Peak velocity is 90 cm/s. Which is the most likely cause for his hypotension?
a. Cardiogenic shock
b. Septic shock
c. Obstructive shock
d. Hypovolemic shock

Ans. d

Explanation: Based on Doppler-specific parameters, FTc (flow time corrected) is flow time duration of blood flow in the aorta normalized to 60 bpm. Typical values of normally hydrated resting individuals are 330–360 ms. FTc is inversely related to afterload. Low FTc is most commonly seen in low preload, hence generally should be given to fluid bolus in first instance. Peak velocity is indicator of contractility and typical values change with age. An approximate value of peak velocity appropriate for age is given by the formula: 140-age. From the given values, FTc was low initially, which increased after fluid challenge. Thus, it implies low preload as seen in hypovolemic shock. PV is normal, hence contractility is good.

Suggested Reading
1. Singer M. Oesophageal Doppler. Curr Opin Crit Care. 2009;15(3):244-8.

Q.23. Which of the following statements about SVC collapsibility index is incorrect:
a. It is obtained by TTE in midesophageal ascending aortic short-axis (ME–AA–SAX).
b. It is more sensitive than IVC collapsibility index in prediction of fluid responsiveness.
c. SVC collapsibility index >36% is indicative of fluid responsiveness.
d. It can be conducted in intubated and nonintubated patients.

Ans. a

Explanation: The SVC collapsibility index is measured in the midesophageal ascending aortic short-axis (ME–AA–SAX) via the transesophageal Doppler. It cannot be estimated in TTE. SVC collapsibility index >36% is indicative of fluid responsiveness.

Suggested Reading
1. Bubenek-Turconi ŞI, Hendy A, Băilă S, Drăgan A, Chioncel O, Văleanu L, et al. The value of a superior vena cava collapsibility index measured with a miniaturized transoesophageal monoplane continuous echocardiography probe to predict fluid responsiveness compared to stroke volume variations in open major vascular surgery: a prospective cohort study. J Clin Monit Comput. 2020;34(3):491-9.

Q.24. A 45-year-old female, known case of diabetes, is admitted in the ICU with community-acquired pneumonia with septic shock and managed initially with fluids and broad-spectrum antibiotics. On day 3, in ICU, patient is off inotropic supports and hemodynamically stable. Which of the following parameters does not help in assessing readiness for deresuscitation?
a. EVLWI
b. VEXUS
c. IAP
d. CI

Ans. d

Explanation: Deresuscitation is defined as active fluid removal in patients with fluid overload using drugs and/or ultrafiltration.

Triggers to start fluid removal:	
• MAP/APP >65/55 mm Hg	• PLR test negative
• GEDVI >850 mL/m^2	• LVEDAI >14 cm^2/m^2
• EVLWI >10–12 mL/kg PBW	• High VEXUS score
• PVPI >3	• IAP >12–15 mm Hg
• PPV and SVV <12%	

(APP: abdominal perfusion pressure; EVLWI: extra-vascular lung water index; GEDVI: global end-diastolic volume index; LVEDAI: left ventricular end-diastolic area index; MAP: mean arterial pressure; PVPI: pulmonary vascular permeability index; PPV: pulse pressure variation; PLR: passive leg raising; SVV: stroke volume variation)

Suggested Reading
1. Malbrain MLNG, Martin G, Ostermann M. Everything you need to know about deresuscitation. Intensive Care Med. 2022;48:1781-6.

Q.25. A 62-year-old male, with no known comorbidities, diagnosed with periampullary carcinoma, is posted for Whipple's procedure. In the intraoperative period, advanced hemodynamic monitoring is initiated. It shows the following values: hypotension prediction index = 90, cardiac index = 3.5, and dynamic arterial elastance = 0.78. What would be the next step to manage the patient?
 a. 500 mL fluid bolus
 b. Start noradrenaline infusion
 c. Start dobutamine infusion
 d. IABP insertion

Ans. b

Explanation: Hypotension predictive index is an algorithm based on detailed analysis of hemodynamic features from arterial pressure waveform as an input and occurrence of hypotension with MAP <65 mm Hg for at least 1 minute as output. The algorithm gives a unitless number ranging from 0 to 100, informing about likelihood that within 5–15 minutes a hypotensive event will occur. Higher the value of HPI, greater the risk of hypotension. Dynamic arterial elastance (Eadyn) is a quotient of PPV and SVV. Optimal cut off value for Eadyn is 0.84. Lower values suggest poor response to fluid administration and advise use of vasopressors. Higher values suggest fluid responsiveness. In the given question, HPI is high indicating risk of hypotension. Eadyn is lower than cutoff, supporting the initiation of vasopressors. Thus, starting noradrenaline is ideal step ahead. Cardiac index is normal.

Suggested Reading
1. Szrama J, Gradys A, Bartkowiak T, Woźniak A, Kusza K, Molnar Z. Intraoperative hypotension prediction: A proactive perioperative hemodynamic management—A Literature Review. Medicina (Kaunas). 2023;59(3):491.

Q.26. Which among the following statements about bioreactance is inaccurate?
 a. It requires four noninvasive sensor pads.
 b. The voltage is recorded between the inner pair of sensors.
 c. Flow of blood in the thorax induces a phase shift in the signal.
 d. It is inferior to bioimpedance in estimating cardiac output.

Ans. d

Explanation: Estimation of cardiac output by bioreactance requires four noninvasive sensor pads. The signal generation occurs between the outer pair of sensors and voltage is recorded between the inner pair of sensors. Blood flow in the thorax induces a phase shift in the signal. Bioreactance is based on the same principle but analyzes the signal of electrical reactance rather than the impedance. This considerably improves the signal-to-noise ratio.

Suggested Reading
1. Pavot A, Teboul J, Monnet X. Bioimpedance and Bioreactance. In: Kirov MY, Kuzkov VV, Saugel B (Eds). Advanced Hemodynamic Monitoring: Basics and New Horizons. Cham: Springer; 2021.

Q.27. Which of the following statements about renal resistive index (RRI) is accurate?
a. Performed at the level of interlobar or arcuate arteries
b. In patients with renal transplant, RRI of 0.9 is associated with lower risk of graft rejection.
c. RRI value is decreased in intra-abdominal hypertension.
d. Renal resistive index is a sonographic index of intrarenal arteries defined as (peak systolic velocity – end-diastolic velocity)/mean velocity.

Ans. a

Explanation: Renal arterial resistive index is a sonographic index of intrarenal arteries defined as (peak systolic velocity – end-diastolic velocity)/peak systolic velocity. Normal range is 0.5–0.7. Elevated values are associated with poorer prognosis in various renal disorders and renal transplant. RRI is measured using spectral Doppler at the arcuate arteries (at corticomedullary junction) or interlobar arteries (adjacent to medullary pyramids). Reasons for elevated values of RRI are abdominal compartment syndrome, perinephric fluid collection, extreme hypotension, and very young children.

Reason for decreased values of RRI is renal artery stenosis.

Suggested Reading
1. Weerakkody Y, Carroll D, Alsmair A; Radiopaedia.org. (2010). Renal arterial resistive index. Reference article. [online] Available from https://radiopaedia.org/articles/renal-arterial-resistive-index. [Last accessed June, 2023]

Q.28. Which of the following does not overestimate the cardiac output?
a. Left-to-right shunt
b. Low injectate
c. Extremely low-cardiac output
d. Severe tricuspid regurgitation

Ans. d

Explanation: PA catheter measures cardiac output by thermodilution technique. In cases with extremely low-cardiac output, blood is rewarmed by the walls of cardiac chamber and surrounding tissues resulting in overestimation of cardiac output. The back-and-forth flow across the tricuspid valve in severe TR can result in underestimation of cardiac output.

Suggested Reading
1. Chirinos JA. Textbook of Arterial Stiffness and Pulsatile Hemodynamics in Health and Disease. Cambridge: Academic Press; 2022.

Q.29. Which of the following arterial waveform patterns is incorrect for the clinical condition?
a. *Spike and dome pattern:* Hypertrophic cardiomyopathy
b. *Pulsus parvus et tardus:* Aortic stenosis
c. *Pulsus bisferiens:* Aortic regurgitation
d. *Pulsus alternans:* Mitral stenosis

Ans. d

Explanation: Pulsus alternans is characterized by the presence of large- and small-volume waveforms and is seen in severe left ventricular failure. Pulsus alternans occurs as a result of underlying cardiac distress and dysfunction. Pulsus alternans has been identified as left ventricular, right ventricular, or biventricular, and the etiology of pulsus alternans varies depending on the causative pathology. Left ventricular alternans occurs in the setting of severe left ventricular dysfunction. This includes cardiomyopathy, aortic stenosis, and coronary artery disease.

Suggested Reading
1. Henery D, Tummala R. (2022). Pulsus Alternans. [online] Available from https://www.ncbi.nlm.nih.gov/books/NBK557642/. [Last accessed June, 2023]

Q.30. Which of the following is not a limitation of PLR test?
a. It requires a real-time hemodynamic monitoring device for accurate assessment of volume responsiveness.
b. Patient should be in sinus rhythm and on controlled mechanical ventilation.
c. Contraindicated in patients with head trauma.
d. False negative values in intra-abdominal hypertension.

Ans. b

Explanation: Passive leg raise test does not require the patient to be in sinus rhythm and can also be performed in spontaneously breathing patients, unlike many other modalities of dynamic methods of volume assessment. Accurate measurements of hemodynamic changes require real-time monitoring which is able to distinguish the changes in cardiac output during 1 minute. It is contraindicated in patients with head trauma because of risk of raised ICP. In presence of intra-abdominal hypertension, the increased intra-abdominal volume results in squeezing of IVC, and hence generates false negatives.

Suggested Reading
1. Kulkarni AP, Kothekar AT, Divatia JV. Textbook of Hemodynamic Monitoring and Therapy in Critically Ill, 1st edition. New Delhi: Jaypee Brothers Medical Publisher;2020.

CHAPTER 7

Infection Control

Srinivas Samavedam

A newly established intensive care unit (ICU) is evaluating all options for handwash agents. The unit is also planning to screen all newly appointed healthcare professionals for transmissible infections.

Q.1. The choice is between iodophors, chlorhexidine, and alcohol-based handwash. The argument against chlorhexidine is:
   a. It has weak action against enveloped viruses.
   b. It has weak action against methicillin-resistant *Staphylococcus aureus* (MRSA).
   c. It has weak action against *Mycobacteria*.
   d. It has weak action against *enterococci*.

Ans. c

Explanation: *Mycobacteria* are killed less effectively by chlorhexidine in comparison to alcohol and iodophors.

Suggested Reading
1. Larson EL, Morton HE. Alcohols. In: Block SS (Ed). Disinfection, Sterilization and Preservation, 4th edition. Philadelphia, PA: Lea and Febiger; 1991. pp. 642-54;192-3.

Q.2. The unit decides to use consumption of handwash units as a measure of handwash compliance. Which of the following statements regarding this strategy is false?
   a. It is a recognized marker.
   b. Trends can be calculated over time period.
   c. It overcomes the problems associated with direct surveillance.
   d. It is a reliable indicator of actual compliance.

Ans. d

Explanation: Consumption of handwash products is a reliable and popular tool for surveillance but does not guarantee assessment of actual compliance.

Suggested Reading
1. Haas JP, Larson EL. Measurement of compliance with hand hygiene. J Hosp Infect. 2007;66(1):6-14.

Q.3. The senior administrators would like to screen all newly recruited nurses for nasal carriage of methicillin-resistant *Staphylococcus aureus* (MRSA). Which of the following statements regarding this strategy is false?
   a. Nasal carriage corresponds to hand carriage.
   b. It identifies those who are more likely to disseminate the infection.
   c. It is not proven to be cost-effective.
   d. Topical treatment is the first choice for those testing positive.

Ans. b

Explanation: Nasal carriage detection identifies asymptomatic carriers but does not identify those who are more likely to be transmitters. It has not been proven to be a cost-effective strategy to minimize transmission.

Suggested Reading
  1. Ouidri MA. Screening of nasal carriage of methicillin-resistant *Staphylococcus aureus* during admission of patients to Frantz Fanon Hospital, Blida, Algeria. New Microbes New Infect. 2018;23:52-60.

Q.4. The hospital plans to monitor all the patients admitted to the unit for infections during hospital stay and for a finite period after discharge. This form of surveillance is called:
   a. Prospective surveillance
   b. Retrospective surveillance
   c. Incidence surveillance
   d. Prevalence surveillance

Ans. a

Explanation: Retrospective surveillance is done by record review after discharge. Incidence surveillance measures new infections occurring in a definite period in hospital. Prevalence surveillance looks at active as well as previously documented infection rates.

Suggested Reading
  1. Mikulska M. Infection Control and Isolation Procedures. In: Carreras E, Dufour C, Mohty M, Krager N (Eds). The EBMT Handbook: Hematopoietic Stem Cell Transplantation and Cellular Therapies, 7th edition. Cham (CH): Springer; 2019. Chapter 27.

Q.5. The recommended method of isolation of patients with varicella infection is:
   a. Contact isolation
   b. Reverse isolation
   c. Droplet isolation
   d. Airborne isolation

Ans. d

Explanation: Contact isolation is advisable for *Clostridium difficile* and resistant bacterial infections. Droplet isolation is advisable for pathogens spread by droplets >5 µm.

Suggested Reading
  1. Kim SH, Park SH, Choi SM, Lee DG. Implementation of hospital policy for healthcare workers and patients exposed to varicella-zoster virus. J Korean Med Sci. 2018;33(36):e252.

Q.6. The most effective method of assessing adequacy of cleaning practices in an intensive care unit is:
   a. Visual inspection
   b. Fluorescent marker system
   c. Swab or contact plate culture
   d. ATP bioluminescence assay

Ans. c

Explanation: Swab or contact plate culture is the only method that gives specific measure of bacterial contamination.

Suggested Reading
1. World Health Organizations. Global Guidelines for the Prevention of Surgical Site Infection. Geneva: World Health Organization; 2018.

Q.7. According to Spaulding classification, items in contact with intact skin are classified as:
   a. Noncritical items
   b. Semicritical items
   c. Critical items
   d. Not included

Ans. a

Explanation: Instruments entering sterile body cavity are classified as critical and those in contact with intact mucous membrane are semicritical equipment.

Suggested Reading
1. Rowan NJ, Kremer T, McDonnell G. A review of Spaulding's classification system for effective cleaning, disinfection and sterilization of reusable medical devices: Viewed through a modern-day lens that will inform and enable future sustainability. Sci Total Environ. 2023;878:162976.

Q.8. Some recommendations were made for the standard policies for monitoring water and dialysis fluid in a hospital. Which of the following statements is false?
   a. Bacteriologic assays should be performed every month.
   b. Chemical analysis of water should be done before the system is installed.
   c. Samples should be collected as close to the source as possible.
   d. The maximum accepted concentration of microbial count is 100 CFU/mL.

Ans. c

Explanation: Samples for microbiological analysis of water and dialysate fluids should be collected as close to the point of entry into the dialysis unit.

Suggested Reading
1. Coulliette AD, Arduino MJ. Hemodialysis and water quality. Semin Dial. 2013;26(4):427-38.

Q.9. The recommended number of air exchanges for an operating room is:
   a. 8 exchanges per hour
   b. 10–12 exchanges per hour
   c. 14–16 exchanges per hour
   d. 20 exchanges per hour

Ans. d

Explanation: The recommended air exchanges inside an operating room is 20 per hour and outdoor air exchanges is 4 per hour.

Suggested Reading
1. Popp W, Alefelder C, Bauer S, Daeschlein G, Geistberger P, Gleich S, et al. Air quality in the operating room: Surgical site infections, HVAC systems and discipline—position paper of the German Society of Hospital Hygiene (DGKH). GMS Hyg Infect Control. 2019;14:Doc20.

Q.10. Which of the following steps is not a strategy for prevention of catheter-associated urinary tract infection?
a. Precatheterization antibiotics
b. Shorter duration of catheterization
c. Gravity drainage
d. Anti-infective catheters for special population

Ans. a

Explanation: Prior administration of antibiotics does not reduce the rate of catheter-associated urinary tract infection.

Suggested Reading
1. Chenoweth C, Saint S. Preventing catheter-associated urinary tract infections in the intensive care unit. Crit Care Clin. 2013;29(1):19-32.

Q.11. A 55-year-old patient was admitted to the ICU for management of acute intracerebral bleed. He was intubated for airway protection. He developed fever and leukocytosis with increase in endotracheal secretions on day 5. Chest X-ray did not show a new infiltrate. Oxygen requirements did not increase. Which of the following statements is false?
a. He is likely to have a ventilator-associated infective complication.
b. He is likely to have a ventilator-associated tracheobronchitis.
c. He needs escalation of antibiotics.
d. The diagnosis will be based on colony counts.

Ans. d

Explanation: The diagnosis of ventilator-associated pneumonia or tracheobronchitis is based on the effect of the infection on the gas exchange and radiological picture and not on the colony counts.

Suggested Reading
1. Koenig SM, Truwit JD. Ventilator-associated pneumonia: diagnosis, treatment, and prevention. Clin Microbiol Rev. 2006;19(4):637-57.

Q.12. Which of the following interventions is unlikely to help in reducing the incidence of ventilator-associated infective complications?
a. Sedation interruption
b. Tracheostomy in 1st week
c. Subglottic drainage
d. Head-end elevation

Ans. b

Explanation: Tracheostomy within the 1st week is not associated with a lesser incidence of ventilator-associated infective complication. Optimum timing seems to in the early 2nd week.

Suggested Reading
1. Terragni PP, Antonelli M, Fumagalli R, Faggiano C, Berardino M, Pallavicini FB, et al. Early vs late tracheotomy for prevention of pneumonia in mechanically ventilated adult ICU patients: a randomized controlled trial. JAMA. 2010;303(15):1483-9.

Q.13. A 26-year-old renal transplant recipient was admitted into the ICU with fever, abdominal pain, and watery diarrhea. He had leukocytosis with polymorphonuclear predominance. Abdomen was distended and plain radiograph showed features of colonic dilatation. Which of the following statements regarding *Clostridium difficile* infection is false?
   a. Toxin A is the main virulence factor.
   b. The disease spreads by transfer of spores by fecal–oral route.
   c. Humoral immunity plays a major role.
   d. Pseudomembranous colitis is commonly found.

Ans. a

Explanation: Both toxin A and B are independently associated with the pathogenesis and clinical manifestations of *Clostridium difficile* infection.

Suggested Reading
1. Kyne L, Warny M, Qamar A, Kelly CP. Association between antibody response to toxin A and protection against recurrent *Clostridium difficile* diarrhoea. Lancet. 2001;357(9251):189-93.

Q.14. The drug of choice for *Clostridium difficile* infection is:
   a. Intravenous metronidazole
   b. Oral metronidazole
   c. Intravenous vancomycin
   d. Oral vancomycin

Ans. d

Explanation: Drugs, which are locally active, are preferred. Oral route is preferred in *Clostridium difficile* infection. Vancomycin is probably more effective than metronidazole.

Suggested Reading
1. Rupnik M, Wilcox M, Gerding D. *Clostridium difficile* Infection: new developments in epidemiology and pathogenesis. Nat Rev Microbiol. 2009;7:526-36.

Q.15. A 43-year-old lady with rheumatoid arthritis underwent a total hip replacement for avascular necrosis of neck of femur. She presented with fever, pain on the operated site, and purulent discharge. Which of the following statements regarding a surgical site infection (SSI) is true?
   a. They are usually caused by exogenous bacteria.
   b. The organisms are same irrespective of the site of infection.
   c. Primary closures are not associated with SSI.
   d. The timelines for definition are different for implant-related surgeries.

Ans. d

Explanation: Surgical site infections are commonly caused by endogenous bacteria. Organisms differ based on the site of surgery. Infections caused after primary closure are classified as refined-clean infections. Infections occurring after implant surgery can be attributed up to 1 year while nonimplant surgeries have a cut off of 30 days.

Suggested Reading
1. Seidelman JL, Mantyh CR, Anderson DJ. Surgical site infection prevention: A review. JAMA. 2023;329(3):244-52.

Q.16. **Which of the following statements regarding preoperative antibiotic prophylaxis is true?**
a. Administration after incision is equally effective.
b. All biliary tract surgeries require prophylaxis.
c. Prophylactic dose should be repeated, if duration of surgery exceeds 3 hours.
d. The last dose should be given 48 hours after the first dose.

Ans. c

Explanation: Preoperative prophylaxis should ideally be given 30–60 minutes prior to incision. Biliary surgeries in high-risk patients and elderly need prophylaxis. The last dose should be given 12 hours after the first.

Suggested Reading
1. Centers for Disease Control and Prevention. (2020). Importing Patient Safety Procedure Data Using CSV. [online] Available from https://www.cdc.gov/nhsn/pdfs/ps-analysis-resources/ImportingProcedureData.pdf. [Last accessed June, 2023]

Q.17. **A 30-year-old lady was admitted for the management of 40% burns of varying thickness. She was resuscitated with fluids. She remained in the ICU for 2 weeks. During the 2nd week, she developed new-onset fever and shock. Which of the following infections is the most common infection among burn victims?**
a. Bacteremia followed by pneumonia and urinary tract infection
b. Wound infection followed by urinary tract infections
c. Pneumonia followed by bacteremia
d. Urinary tract infection followed by pneumonia

Ans. a

Explanation: The incidence of infections following burns is bacteremia (29%) followed by pneumonia (24%) and urinary tract infection (24%). Actual burn wound infections account for 3% of the infections.

Suggested Reading
1. Coban YK. Infection control in severely burned patients. World J Crit Care Med. 2012;1(4):94-101.

Q.18. **Which of the following statements regarding diagnosis of bloodstream infections is false?**
a. Samples should be drawn by separate punctures from different sites.
b. Timing of the blood drawn prior to next dose of antibiotic has no bearing on the yield.

c. The volume of blood drawn for culture has a bearing on the yield.
d. Catheter-drawn cultures have a high incidence of false positivity.

Ans. b

Explanation: If the patient is receiving antimicrobial therapy, blood cultures drawn immediately before the next dose may yield better results due to low levels of circulating antibiotics.

Suggested Reading
1. Mermel LA, Allon M, Bouza E, Craven DE, Flynn P, O'Grady NP, et al. Clinical practice guidelines for the diagnosis and management of intravascular catheter-related infection: 2009 Update by the Infectious Diseases Society of America. Clin Infect Dis. 2009;49(1):1-45.

Q.19. Which of the following statements is true regarding the definition of intravascular device-related bloodstream infection?
a. Catheter tip culture has no role.
b. Microbiologically proven exit-site infection is not relevant in the absence of a positive blood culture.
c. Infection evident >2 cm away from the exit site is considered a sign of infection of tunneled catheters.
d. Infusate culture has no role.

Ans. c

Explanation: The criteria for exit-site infection are different for tunneled versus nontunneled catheters. Evidence of infection >2 cm from the exit site of a tunneled catheter is evidence of device-related infection even in the absence of a positive blood culture.

Suggested Reading
1. Gahlot R, Nigam C, Kumar V, Yadav G, Anupurba S. Catheter-related bloodstream infections. Int J Crit Illn Inj Sci. 2014;4(2):162-7.

Q.20. A 21-year-old gentleman who had a prosthetic mitral valve implanted 1 year ago for severe mitral incompetence presents with fever rash and splenomegaly. Infective endocarditis is suspected. Which of the following statements is true?
a. Multiple valve implantations have a higher risk.
b. Longer bypass time has no bearing.
c. *Enterococcus* is the most common cause in the first 12 months.
d. HACEK group also is a common cause in the first 12 months.

Ans. a

Explanation: The risk factors for infective endocarditis include multiple implants and longer bypass times. HACEK (*Haemophilus* species, *Aggregatibacter* species, *Cardiobacterium hominis*, *Eikenella corrodens*, and *Kingella*) group and *enterococci* are more commonly implicated after the first 12 months.

Suggested Reading
1. Berisha B, Ragnarsson S, Olaison L, Rasmussen M. Microbiological etiology in prosthetic valve endocarditis: A nationwide registry study. J Intern Med. 2022;292:428-37.

Q.21. Which of the following statements regarding healthcare-related hepatitis B infection is true?
  a. Rural settings are at a higher risk.
  b. General incidence in the population has no impact.
  c. Professionals working in dialysis units are at a higher risk.
  d. Exposure to blood is the only risk factor.

Ans. c

Explanation: The general prevalence in the community and working in dialysis units are important risk factors in addition to exposure to blood. Incidence is higher in urban centers.

Suggested Reading
1. Berisha B, Ragnarsson S, Olaison L, Rasmussen M. Microbiological etiology in prosthetic valve endocarditis: A nationwide registry study. J Intern Med. 2022;292:428-37.

Q.22. Which of the following statements regarding the postexposure prophylaxis is true?
  a. For hepatitis B, prophylaxis is recommended irrespective of the worker's vaccination history if source is unknown.
  b. History of vaccination is enough to avoid further evaluation of an exposed worker.
  c. A worker who is hepatitis C negative and has been exposed to a positive patient should be initiated on treatment immediately.
  d. If the hepatitis C status of worker and source is unknown, watchful waiting with testing every 6–8 weeks is recommended.

Ans. d

Explanation: A worker whose vaccination history and titers are known may be managed without treatment if titers are high. For hepatitis C exposure if the source and worker's status is unknown, watchful observation is recommended with testing every 6–8 weeks.

Suggested Reading
1. Lewis JD, Enfield KB, Sifri CD. Hepatitis B in healthcare workers: Transmission events and guidance for management. World J Hepatol. 2015;7(3):488-97.

Q.23. The most common organism implicated in postliver transplant infections is:
  a. *Candida*
  b. Vancomycin-resistant *Enterococcus*
  c. *Klebsiella*
  d. Methicillin-resistant *Staphylococcus aureus*

Ans. d

Explanation: Methicillin-resistant *Staphylococcus aureus* is the most common organism isolated among patients with postliver transplant bloodstream and respiratory infections followed by vancomycin-resistant *enterococci*.

Suggested Reading
1. Hernandez Mdel P, Martin P, Simkins J. Infectious complications after liver transplantation. Gastroenterol Hepatol (N Y). 2015;11(11):741-53.

Infection Control

Q.24. Reverse isolation is indicated for:
   a. All patients with respiratory viral infections
   b. All patients with cutaneous lesions from exanthems
   c. Patients with low levels of immunity at high risk of infections
   d. All perioperative and postoperative patients

Ans. c

Explanation: Reverse isolation is the term used for the processes used to protect patients with low levels of immunity from infections transmitted from healthcare workers.

Suggested Reading
   1. Garner JS. Guideline for isolation precautions in hospitals. The Hospital Infection Control Practices Advisory Committee. Infect Control Hosp Epidemiol. 1996;17(1):53-80.

Q.25. The alternate name for reverse isolation is:
   a. Reverse nursing
   b. Protective nursing
   c. Barrier nursing
   d. All of the above

Ans. b

Explanation: Reverse isolation is also known as protective nursing or reverse barrier nursing.

Suggested Reading
   1. Garner JS. Guideline for isolation precautions in hospitals. The Hospital Infection Control Practices Advisory Committee. Infect Control Hosp Epidemiol. 1996;17(1):53-80.

Q.26. The recommended period of isolation for a patient with varicella-zoster infection is:
   a. 2 weeks
   b. 2 days prior to rash onset to crusting of lesions
   c. 2 weeks from rash onset
   d. Rash onset to 1 week after crusting of lesions

Ans. b

Explanation: The recommended period of isolation of a patient infected with chickenpox is 2 days prior to rash onset till all lesions have crusted.

Suggested Reading
   1. Gershon AA, Breuer J, Cohen JI, Cohrs RJ, Gershon MD, Gilden D, et al. Varicella zoster virus infection. Nat Rev Dis Primers. 2015;1:15016.

Q.27. Recommended mode of isolation of a patient with suspected or proven diphtheria is:
   a. Standard isolation
   b. Droplet isolation
   c. Contact isolation
   d. Combination of all three

Ans. d

Explanation: Transmission of *Corynebacterium diphtheriae* occurs from person to person through respiratory droplets (i.e., from coughing or sneezing) and close physical contact. Therefore, standard precautions, droplet, and contact precautions should be applied at all times.

Suggested Reading

1. Sharma NC, Efstratiou A, Mokrousov I, Mutreja A, Das B, Ramamurthy T. Diphtheria. Nat Rev Dis Primers. 2019;5:81.

Q.28. Which of the following statements regarding the disinfection of the expiratory cassette of a ventilator is true?
  a. Autoclave is recommended.
  b. Daily disinfection is recommended.
  c. Disinfection is not needed.
  d. ETO is recommended.

Ans. c

Explanation: Routine sterilization of the expiratory cassette is not recommended as it is not an invasive instrument. Autoclaving is not recommended.

Suggested Reading

1. World Health Organization. Infection Prevention and Control of Epidemic- and Pandemic-Prone Acute Respiratory Infections in Health Care. Geneva: World Health Organization; 2014. Annex I, Cleaning and disinfection of respiratory equipment. [online] Available from https://www.ncbi.nlm.nih.gov/books/NBK214361. [Last accessed June, 2023]

Q.29. Which of the following statements regarding the disinfection of oxygen flow meters is true?
  a. They should be disinfected daily.
  b. They should be disinfected after every patient discharge.
  c. ETO is recommended.
  d. They should be discarded after patient use.

Ans. a

Explanation: The oxygen flow meters should be cleaned and disinfected every day.

Suggested Reading

1. Mathur S. (2021). Cleaning, Disinfection and Proper Maintenance of Oxygen Concentrators. [online] Available from https://www.primedeq.com/blog/cleaning-disinfection-and-proper-maintenance-of-oxygen-concentrators. [Last accessed June, 2023]

Q.30. Which of the following is most effective against spores?
  a. Hydrogen peroxide
  b. Iodophor
  c. Glutaraldehyde
  d. Chlorhexidine

Ans. c

Explanation: The most effective agent against spores is glutaraldehyde, followed by peracetic acid.

Suggested Reading

1. Indian Council of Medical Research. Hospital Infection Control Guidelines. [online] Available from https://main.icmr.nic.in/sites/default/files/guidelines/Hospital_Infection_control_guidelines.pdf. [Last accessed June, 2023]

CHAPTER 8

Tropical Diseases

Dhruva Chaudhry, Jyothi Geetha Mohankumar, Vishal Raj

Q.1. A 42-year-old male presents to the emergency department with a 5-day history of fever, headache, muscle pain, and jaundice. He works as a farmer in a rural area and recalls being exposed to flooded fields during heavy rainfall 2 weeks ago. The patient reports feeling progressively worse over the past few days, with increasing fatigue and dark-colored urine. On examination, he appears severely ill with icteric sclera, hepatomegaly, and decreased urine output. Laboratory tests reveal elevated liver enzymes, acute kidney injury, thrombocytopenia, and hematuria. A chest X-ray shows bilateral interstitial infiltrates. Considering the clinical presentation, which of the following serological test is most appropriate for the diagnosis of leptospirosis?
   a. Polymerase chain reaction (PCR) for *Leptospira* DNA
   b. Microscopic agglutination test (MAT)
   c. Direct fluorescent antibody (DFA) test
   d. Enzyme-linked immunosorbent assay (ELISA) for Leptospira IgM antibodies
   e. Dark-field microscopy of blood smear

Ans. d

Explanation: Clinical presentation is consistent with leptospirosis, a zoonotic disease caused by spirochetes of the genus *Leptospira*. Leptospirosis is commonly associated with exposure to contaminated water, such as swimming or wading in freshwater or soil contaminated with the urine of infected animals.

Serological tests are the mainstay for the diagnosis of leptospirosis. The most appropriate initial serological test is the detection of *Leptospira*-specific immunoglobulin M (IgM) antibodies using an enzyme-linked immunosorbent assay (ELISA). IgM antibodies appear early in the course of the disease and are detectable within the first week of illness. A positive IgM result indicates recent infection with *Leptospira* and supports the diagnosis of leptospirosis.

Polymerase chain reaction (PCR) for *Leptospira* DNA (Option a) can be used to detect *Leptospira* DNA in blood or urine samples. However, it is most sensitive during the first week of illness and may not be as reliable in later stages of the disease. The microscopic agglutination test (MAT) (Option b) is considered the gold standard for the diagnosis of leptospirosis, but it requires specialized facilities and is time-consuming. Direct fluorescent antibody (DFA) test (Option c) and dark-field microscopy of blood smear (Option e) have limited sensitivity and specificity compared to serological tests.

Suggested Reading
1. Bharti AR, Nally JE, Ricaldi JN, Matthias MA, Diaz MM, Lovett MA, et al. Leptospirosis: a zoonotic disease of global importance. Lancet Infect Dis. 2003;3(12):757-71.

Q.2. Severe leptospirosis presents with multiorgan dysfunction. Which of the following clinicolaboratory findings is not consistent with it?
   a. Serum bilirubin levels may be high, whereas rises in aminotransferase and alkaline phosphatase levels are usually moderate.
   b. Amylase levels are often elevated.
   c. Nonoliguric hypokalemic renal failure is characteristic of late leptospirosis.
   d. A fourfold or greater rise in antibody titer is detected between acute- and convalescent-phase serum specimens.

Ans. c

Explanation: Nonhypokalemic oliguria is common in early leptospirosis. Serum bilirubin levels may be high, whereas rises in aminotransferase and alkaline phosphatase levels are usually moderate. Amylase levels are often elevated. A fourfold or greater rise in antibody titer is detected between acute- and convalescent-phase serum specimens.

Suggested Reading
1. Loscalzo. Harrison's Principles of Internal Medicine, 21st edition. Gautam Budh Nagar, Noida: McGraw Hill; 2022.

Q.3. Which among the following is most accurate regarding diagnostic tests of leptospirosis?
   a. Antibodies are usually detectable by day 6–10 of illness and peak within 3–4 weeks.
   b. Macroscopic agglutination tests are fast and easy serological method for diagnosis of leptospirosis.
   c. Blood culture requires samples in the second week of illness for isolation of organism.
   d. Dark-ground microscopy of body fluids has high sensitivity.

Ans. a

Explanation: While rapid diagnostic tests for leptospirosis can provide quick results, they are not always reliable. If the rapid diagnostic test is negative, perform a more specific test, such as the microscopic agglutination test (MAT). MAT is considered the gold standard for diagnosing leptospirosis and is based on the detection of antibodies against *Leptospira* in the patient's serum but it is very tedious and slow procedure.

Suggested Reading
1. Rajapakse S. Leptospirosis: Clinical aspects. Clin Med J R Coll Physicians London. 2022;22(1):14-7.

Q.4. The patient in the above question has severe leptospirosis. The treating consultant labels him as Weil's disease. Which of the following is not a feature of Weil's disease?
 a. Icterus
 b. Renal failure
 c. Hemorrhage
 d. Encephalitis

Ans. d

Explanation: Icteric leptospirosis occurs in approximately 5–10% of symptomatic leptospirosis cases and is a rapidly progressive multisystem illness associated with mortality rates of 5–15%. Usually, icteric leptospirosis is accompanied by fever, jaundice, and renal failure, a syndrome known as "Weil's disease". Pulmonary hemorrhage with acute respiratory distress syndrome (ARDS), myocarditis with electrocardiogram abnormalities, and rhabdomyolysis may also occur as part of this syndrome. Conjunctival suffusion is also common.

Suggested Reading
1. Pavli A, Maltezou HC. Travel-acquired leptospirosis. J Travel Med. 2008;15(6):447-53.

Q.5. What will be the appropriate treatment for the patient with severe leptospirosis?
 a. High-dose corticosteroids are recommended for severe leptospirosis requiring mechanical ventilation.
 b. Commence intravenous antibiotics either penicillin G or ceftriaxone.
 c. Plasmapheresis is recommended in all patients with multiorgan dysfunction and shock.
 d. Initiate intravenous (IV) ceftriaxone and doxycycline combination therapy.

Ans. b

Explanation: Patients who have clinical features of organ involvement, or those who have comorbidities, must be admitted for in-hospital care. Early initiation of antibiotic treatment is likely to improve outcome. Commence intravenous antibiotics—penicillin G 1.5 million units 6 hourly or ceftriaxone 1 g twice daily for 7 days. For those with penicillin or cephalosporin allergy, doxycycline or a macrolide (azithromycin or clarithromycin) may be used. Monitor fluid intake and urine output. The use of high-dose corticosteroids for treatment of leptospirosis is not supported by high-quality evidence, and routine use is not recommended. There are reports of potential adjunctive benefit with high-dose corticosteroids in severely ill patients. Plasmapheresis has been used in severe leptospirosis, with some nonrandomized trials showing benefit, but the evidence is of low quality.

Suggested Reading
1. Rajapakse S. Leptospirosis: Clinical aspects. Clin Med (Lond). 2022;22(1):14-7.

Q.6. Relatives of the patient are anxious and asks about the prognosis and morbidities if the disease. which among the following will help in you in counseling the relatives?
 a. The involvement of liver and kidney will cause scarring and leads to long-term sequalae.
 b. Pulmonary involvement is common in severe disease and has high case fatality rate.

c. Neurological involvement is mild and generally not manifested as symptoms.
d. Cholecystitis and pancreatitis though reported in this disease have mild prognostic value.

Ans. b

Explanation: The infection may progress to severe systemic inflammatory syndrome with hemorrhagic features. Findings of disseminated intravascular coagulation may occur with bleeding. The onset of mental status alterations indicates progression to parenchymal involvement of the cerebral cortex with meningoencephalitis, heralding a high mortality risk. Severe and diffuse alveolar hemorrhage with massive hemoptysis can occur in the absence of typical Weil disease. Myocarditis may occur in severe disease. All the physical findings of biventricular heart failure can be found, including elevated jugular venous pulsations; a new S3 gallop; and dysrhythmia, including atrial fibrillation, heart blocks of varying severity, and ventricular ectopy. Acalculous cholecystitis is a finding of profound systemic illness. Pancreatitis has also been described in severe cases. The incidence of pulmonary involvement has increased over the past few years, affecting up to 70% of patients. Pulmonary involvement has emerged as a serious cause of mortality, becoming the main cause of leptospirosis-associated death in some countries. Uveitis, iridocyclitis, and chorioretinitis may occur late into illness and may persist for years.

Suggested Reading
1. Dall'Antonia M, Sluga G, Whitfield S, Teall A, Wilson P, Krahé D. Leptospirosis pulmonary haemorrhage: a diagnostic challenge. Emerg Med J. 2008;25(1):51-2.
2. Gulati S, Gulati A. Pulmonary manifestations of leptospirosis. Lung India. 2012;29(4):347-53.

Q.7. **A 35-year-old male farmer presented with complaints of fever, myalgia, jaundice, and rashes of 8-day duration. At admission, he had tachypnea and tachycardia and febrile. Urine output was reduced, laboratory investigations came positive for IgM *Leptospira*. He was admitted and required oxygen supplementation via face mask at 4 L/min. He was started on IV ceftriaxone. He developed fever spikes, increased oxygen requirement and hypotension after 8 hours of antibiotic infusion. Which among the following is not a feature/association of Jarisch–Herxheimer reaction?**
a. It is known to be associated with beta-lactam antibiotic administration in patients with spirochetes infection.
b. One of the risk factors includes short duration between antibiotic and symptom onset interval.
c. It is acute inflammatory response to clearance of spirochetes from circulation.
d. It was originally reported in Lyme's disease.

Ans. d

Explanation: Initiation of chemotherapy in spirochetal diseases may precipitate a febrile inflammatory reaction, known as the Jarisch–Herxheimer reaction (JHR), originally described in patients with syphilis receiving mercury treatment. This reaction is characterized by an acute inflammatory response associated with the release of large amounts of cytokines, resulting from clearance of spirochetes from the circulation. Prevalence, clinical manifestations, and outcome of JHR have been well studied in syphilis, Lyme disease, tick-borne relapsing fever, and louse-borne relapsing fever. Though reported predominantly in syphilis, importance of JHR in leptospirosis is evolving.

Suggested Reading
1. Guerrier G, D'Ortenzio E. The Jarisch-Herxheimer reaction in leptospirosis: a systematic review. PLoS One. 2013;8(3):e59266.

Q.8. A 36-year-old hiker, who recently explored some rural, tropical terrains in India, is admitted to ICU with high-grade fever, intense headaches, diffuse arthralgia, and a widespread maculopapular rash. His complete blood count reveals leukopenia and thrombocytopenia. Serological tests came back positive for IgM against *Orientia tsutsugamushi*, leading to a diagnosis of scrub typhus. Given the clinical presentation and test results, which of the following statements is the most accurate in regard to scrub typhus in an ICU scenario?
   a. Central nervous system involvement, presenting as meningitis or encephalitis, is extremely rare in scrub typhus.
   b. Renal involvement is usually not a concern in scrub typhus, even in severe cases.
   c. Scrub typhus patients rarely develop pneumonitis, making respiratory support unnecessary in the ICU setting.
   d. The management of scrub typhus involves a course of doxycycline, even in severe cases.

Ans. d

Explanation: Despite the severity of symptoms and the requirement for ICU admission, the treatment of scrub typhus includes a course of doxycycline. Other options can also involve macrolides or chloramphenicol. However, complications involving central nervous system, kidneys, and the development of pneumonitis are not uncommon, thus contradicting options a, b, and c.

Suggested Reading
1. Taylor AJ, Paris DH, Newton PN. A systematic review of mortality from untreated scrub typhus (Orientia tsutsugamushi). PLoS Negl Trop Dis. 2015;9(8):e0003971.
2. Weitzel T, Dittrich S, López J, Phuklia W, Martinez-Valdebenito C, Velásquez K, et al. Endemic Scrub Typhus in South America. N Engl J Med. 2016;375(10):954-61.

Q.9. A 38-year-old patient working in agricultural fields in a rural part of India is admitted to your ICU. He has been experiencing high-grade fever, severe headaches, diffuse arthralgia, and a disseminated maculopapular rash for a week. Blood investigations reveal leukocytosis, thrombocytopenia, and elevated liver enzymes. Serological tests confirm the presence of IgM antibodies against *Orientia tsutsugamushi*, indicative of scrub typhus. Which of the following statements is the most accurate regarding scrub typhus, especially in an ICU setting?
   a. Classic eschars, indicative of scrub typhus, are seen in <20% of ICU patients diagnosed with the condition.

b. Unlike other rickettsial diseases, repeated infections with scrub typhus can occur as immunity does not provide protection against heterologous strains.
c. The Weil–Felix test, which detects antigens, is the most reliable diagnostic test for scrub typhus due to its high specificity and sensitivity.
d. The case fatality rate of scrub typhus is <5–7% in ICU settings.

Ans. b

Explanation: Unlike other rickettsial diseases, repeated infections can occur in scrub typhus as immunity does not protect against heterologous strains. The case fatality rate of scrub typhus is indeed higher than 5–7% in ICU settings (refuting statement d). Classic eschars are found in about 30–50% of the cases (refuting statement a). Lastly, the Weil–Felix test lacks specificity and sensitivity compared to more specific assays (refuting statement c).

Suggested Reading
1. Devasagayam E, Dayanand D, Kundu D, Kamath MS, Kirubakaran R, Varghese GM. The burden of scrub typhus in India: A systematic review. PLoS Negl Trop Dis. 2021;15(7):e0009619.
2. Loscalzo. Harrison's Principles of Internal Medicine, 21st edition. India: McGraw Hill; 2022.

Q.10. A 45-year-old farmer is admitted to the ICU after presenting with a high-grade fever, intense headaches, joint pain, and generalized muscle soreness persisting for 1 week. The patient, residing in a rural area, has also observed a nontender eschar on his lower leg. His physical examination reveals a weary and feverish appearance with a body temperature of 39.2°C (102.5°F). Vital signs include a rapid heart rate of 110 beats/min and a low blood pressure of 90/60 mm Hg. Furthermore, he exhibits signs of conjunctival injection and a generalized erythematous maculopapular rash on his torso and extremities. Laboratory investigations reveal low platelet count, high liver enzymes, and leukopenia. The collective clinical presentation of a rural dwelling patient with high fever, headache, myalgia, eschar, conjunctival injection, and rash accompanied by specific laboratory findings arouses suspicion for scrub typhus. Considering this patient's constellation of symptoms, signs, and laboratory findings, which of the following would be the most definitive diagnostic test to confirm a suspected diagnosis of scrub typhus?
a. Polymerase chain reaction (PCR) for *Orientia tsutsugamushi* DNA
b. Weil–Felix test
c. Indirect immunofluorescence assay (IFA) for scrub typhus-specific IgM antibodies
d. Wright's agglutination test
e. Microscopic examination of peripheral blood smear to reveal morulae within monocytes

Ans. c

Explanation: In suspected cases of scrub typhus, characterized by the patient's symptoms, signs, and laboratory findings, the most definitive diagnostic test is the detection of scrub typhus-specific IgM antibodies using an indirect immunofluorescence assay (IFA). These IgM antibodies typically become detectable around 7–10 days after symptom onset. While PCR for *Orientia tsutsugamushi* DNA can be used, it has limited availability and potential sensitivity issues. The Weil–Felix test, an older serological test, lacks both specificity and sensitivity for scrub typhus. Wright's agglutination test is not specific for scrub typhus, and although microscopic examination of a peripheral blood smear may be helpful, it is less sensitive and specific than serological tests.

Suggested Reading
1. Chrispal A, Boorugu H, Gopinath KG, Prakash JAJ, Chandy S, Abraham OC, et al. Scrub typhus: an unrecognized threat in South India—clinical profile and predictors of mortality. Trop Doct. 2010;40(3):129-33.
2. Paris DH, Dumler JS. State of the art of diagnosis of rickettsial diseases: the use of blood specimens for diagnosis of scrub typhus, spotted fever group rickettsiosis, and murine typhus. Curr Opin Infect Dis. 2016;29(5):433-9.

Q.11. A 50-year-old farmer, who has spent considerable time working in dense vegetation areas, is admitted to the ICU. He presents with symptoms including a high-grade fever, headache, myalgia, and a maculopapular rash that has persisted for a week. Laboratory investigations confirm positive IgM scrub typhus, suggesting a probable infection with the bacteria. In addition to these symptoms, he shows signs of respiratory distress, and his chest X-ray indicates bilateral alveolar infiltrates. Laboratory parameters also note nonoliguric acute kidney injury and a mild increase in liver enzymes. Given this clinical picture, a diagnosis of severe scrub typhus is made, prompting immediate treatment. In the context of his clinical scenario and considering the INTEREST trial findings on the treatment of severe scrub typhus, which of the following statements is most accurate?
  a. Treatment with a combination of intravenous (IV) doxycycline and azithromycin is more effective in managing severe scrub typhus than either of the drugs used alone.
  b. IV azithromycin is preferred over IV doxycycline in the treatment of severe scrub typhus.
  c. IV penicillin combined with azithromycin is a more effective strategy for treating severe scrub typhus.
  d. The INTEREST trial found no significant differences in treatment outcomes between severe and mild forms of scrub typhus.

Ans. a

Explanation: The recent INTEREST trial, a multicenter randomized controlled study, explored the efficacy of different treatment strategies for severe scrub typhus. It compared the use of IV doxycycline, IV azithromycin, and a combination of both. Among the 794 patients included in the study, the combination treatment led to a significantly lower mortality rate at 28 days compared to either doxycycline or azithromycin alone.

Suggested Reading
1. Varghese GM, Dayanand D, Gunasekaran K, Kundu D, Wyawahare M, Sharma N, et al. Intravenous doxycycline, azithromycin, or both for severe scrub typhus. N Engl J Med. 2023;388(9):792-803.

Q.12. A 32-year-old female is brought to the emergency department (ED) with a history of high-grade fever, severe headache, and retro-orbital pain that has been ongoing for the past few days. She recently returned from Singapore but denies any specific insect bite or contact with sick individuals. Laboratory investigations reveal thrombocytopenia and PCV of 52. Her platelet count was found to be 15,000 cells/mm^3 on the 4th day of her illness, with absence of clinically significant bleeding or petechiae. Given this clinical scenario, which of the following statements is incorrect in a suspected case of dengue fever?
   a. Prophylactic platelet transfusions are generally not recommended in patients who do not have clinically significant bleeding, even in the presence of severe thrombocytopenia.
   b. To mitigate the risk of fluid overload, the amount of parenteral fluid therapy should be the minimum required to maintain cardiovascular stability until normal permeability returns.
   c. Initial fluid therapy should preferentially employ isotonic crystalloid solutions, with isotonic colloid solutions reserved for patients in profound shock or those who do not respond to initial crystalloid therapy.
   d. The thrombocytopenia seen in this patient is predominantly due to bone marrow suppression.

Ans. d

Explanation: Thrombocytopenia in dengue fever is less likely to be due to bone marrow suppression and is more often attributed to a combination of peripheral platelet destruction and deregulated platelet production. The other options correctly reflect the evidence-based approach to managing patients presenting with similar symptoms and laboratory findings.

Suggested Reading
   1. Quirino-Teixeira AC, Andrade FB, Pinheiro MBM, Rozini SV, Bottz ED. Platelets in dengue infection: more than a numbers game. Platelets. 2022;33(2):176-83.
   2. Simmons CP, Farrar JJ, van Vinh Chau N, Wills B. Dengue. N Engl J Med. 2012;366(15): 1423-32.

Q.13. A 34-year-old male is rushed to the emergency department, complaining of a high-grade fever, intense headache particularly behind the eyes, severe muscle pain, and increasingly shortness of breath for the past 5 days. He looks severely ill with a temperature of 39.7°C (103.4°F), a diffuse nonblanching maculopapular rash on his trunk and extremities, and signs of respiratory distress. Laboratory reports indicate thrombocytopenia with a platelet count of 50,000/mm^3 and increased liver enzymes. His arterial blood gas measurement reveals a PaO$_2$ of 70 mm Hg. With respect to the management of this patient, which statement would be accurate?
   a. Acute respiratory distress should be addressed with immediate intubation and mechanical ventilation.
   b. A platelet transfusion should be immediately administered due to the significantly low platelet count.

    c. NSAIDs are the first choice for managing the patient's fever and pain.
    d. Intravenous fluid therapy should be judiciously used to prevent the risk of fluid overload.

Ans. d

Explanation: The patient's clinical presentation suggests a severe systemic infection that has led to a critical state, possibly complicated by plasma leakage, a hallmark of severe dengue infection. Fluid management is crucial in these patients. In the critical phase of dengue, plasma leakage can lead to hypovolemic shock. Hence, intravenous fluid replacement is required. However, during the recovery phase, reabsorption of the extravasated fluid can lead to fluid overload if excessive fluid is given, especially in the presence of concurrent organ impairment. Thus, fluid therapy should be meticulously managed to prevent fluid overload.

Suggested Reading
1. Rajapakse S, Rodrigo C, Rajapakse A. Management of dengue fever in the ICU. Curr Opin Crit Care. 2020;26(2):149-54.
2. World Health Organization. Dengue: Guidelines for Diagnosis, Treatment, Prevention and Control. Geneva, Switzerland: World Health Organization; 2009.

Q.14. A 36-year-old male is admitted to an intensive care unit in a rural region of India. His wife reports a history of fever and headaches for the past week, with increasing disorientation and confusion over the past 48 hours. Upon admission, the patient presents with tachypnea, decreased oxygen saturation (SpO$_2$ 85% on room air), and diffuse bilateral crackles on auscultation. Laboratory investigations reveal significant thrombocytopenia, and a peripheral blood smear confirms the presence of *Plasmodium falciparum*. A chest X-ray shows bilateral infiltrates indicative of potential acute respiratory distress syndrome (ARDS).

Based on this information, what would be the most appropriate immediate management?
   a. Commence intravenous ceftriaxone and apply high-flow oxygen therapy
   b. Initiate noninvasive ventilation and intravenous quinine
   c. Administer intravenous artesunate and provide oxygen via a Venturi mask
   d. Start intravenous artesunate and mechanical ventilation
   e. Administer intravenous dexamethasone and commence bilevel positive airway pressure (BiPAP) ventilation

Ans. d

Explanation: The patient appears to be suffering from severe malaria complicated by cerebral symptoms and ARDS, which can be fatal if not managed promptly. The World Health Organization currently recommends intravenous artesunate as the first-line treatment for severe malaria. This is supported by strong evidence indicating a lower mortality rate with artesunate than with quinine. Furthermore, the patient's respiratory distress and decreased oxygen saturation strongly suggest the need for mechanical ventilation. Other treatments such as antibiotics, noninvasive ventilation, corticosteroids, or less aggressive oxygen support methods might not be adequate given the severity and specifics of the situation.

Suggested Reading
1. ARDS Definition Task Force; Ranieri VM, Rubenfeld GD, Thompson BT, Ferguson ND, Caldwell, Fan E, et al. Acute respiratory distress syndrome: The Berlin Definition. JAMA. 2012;307(23):2526-33.
2. Hanson J, Lee SJ, Hossain MA, Anstey NM, Charunwatthana P, Maude RJ, et al. Microvascular obstruction and endothelial activation are independently associated with the clinical manifestations of severe falciparum malaria in adults: an observational study. BMC Med. 2015;13:122.
3. World Health Organization. Guidelines for the treatment of malaria, 3rd edition. Geneva: World Health Organization; 2015.

Q.15. A 35-year-old woman is brought to the emergency department in a semiconscious state. She has had a fever and headache for the past week, and she had a seizure shortly before arrival. On admission, her blood glucose levels are found to be abnormally low, and brain imaging reveals signs of cerebral edema. The patient resides in a region of India where malaria is endemic. Considering her clinical presentation and background, what is the most appropriate next step in managing this patient?
a. Start empirical antimalarial therapy
b. Administer intravenous glucose to correct the hypoglycemia
c. Start empirical antibiotics for suspected bacterial meningitis
d. Start antiepileptic drugs to manage the seizure
e. Start antiviral therapy for a potential case of encephalitis

Ans. a

Explanation: This patient's symptoms of fever, headache, seizure, and the development of neurological deficits suggest a severe case of cerebral malaria, especially given her residence in a malaria-endemic region. Hypoglycemia is a known complication of severe malaria, and it arises due to a combination of decreased glucose production (from hepatic dysfunction) and increased glucose consumption (high metabolic demand from parasitized erythrocytes). While managing hypoglycemia and seizures is necessary, the priority in this case should be initiating empirical antimalarial therapy, given the strong suspicion of cerebral malaria.

Suggested Reading
1. Mishra SK, Newton CR. Diagnosis and management of the neurological complications of falciparum malaria. Nat Rev Neurol. 2009;5(4):189-98.
2. White NJ, Pukrittayakamee S, Hien TT, Faiz MA, Mokuolu OA, Dondorp AM. Malaria. Lancet. 2014;383(9918):723-35.

Q.16. As you are attending the patient, the emergency department resident calls you to inform the details and action he took, while receiving the patient. Which among the following was correctly reported by the resident?
a. The patient belonged to group 2 of the WHO classification of severe malaria subgroup.
b. Exchange transfusion option was discussed with the family.

c. The infection could be due to *Plasmodium malariae* because of the severity.
d. He had sent the patient's blood samples to rule out other viral hemorrhagic fever also.

Ans. d

Explanation: *P. malariae* infection is generally more benign, whereas *P. falciparum* and *P. knowlesi* are more likely to cause severe malaria and latter can be confused with *P. falciparum* or *P. malariae*. It should be noted that *P. vivax* is more common globally and that it may also cause severe malaria. Risk assessment and testing for *Plasmodium* and viral hemorrhagic fever, as the two may overlap in presentation and may coexist in a single patient, should preferably be done.

If parasitemia is known to be >10% or if the patient is experiencing life-threatening complications (i.e., coma, respiratory failure, coagulopathy, and fulminant kidney failure), exchange transfusion may be investigated as a treatment option. The CDC no longer recommends the use of exchange transfusion for the treatment of severe malaria.

The WHO updated the classification of severe malaria in 2014 and recommended dividing patients into three subgroups.

1. In group 1, the most critical patients are generally treated with parenteral antimalarial medication and require intensive supportive care and resuscitation. Group 1 includes all patients who present with prostration or altered mental status (i.e., confusion, agitation, or coma). Furthermore, any patient who presents with extreme acidotic breathing (rapid, deep breathing with retractions), hypotension, anuria, or significant GI bleeding belongs in this group.
2. Group 2 can usually be treated with oral artemisinin-based combination therapy (ACT) but requires close medical observation owing to an increased risk for clinical decompensation. Group 2 consists of patients who do not possess any characteristics of those in group 1 but who present with anemia (hemoglobin <7 g/dL or hematocrit <20%), hemoglobinuria, jaundice, or one or more convulsions during the preceding 24-hour period.
3. Group 3 is the designation reserved for patients who require parenteral antimalarials due to continuing intractable vomiting but do not exhibit any of the features of group 1 or 2.

Suggested Reading
1. CDC. (2013). Exchange Transfusion for Treatment of Severe Malaria No Longer Recommended. [online] Available from: http://www.cdc.gov/malaria/new_info/2013/exchange_transfusion.html [Last accessed June, 2023].
2. Severe malaria. Tropical medicine and international health. Trop Med Int Health. 2014;19:7-137.

Q.17. A 26-year-old pregnant female at 30 weeks gestation presents to the emergency department with a 5-day history of fever, headache, and myalgia. She recently traveled to a malaria-endemic region in sub-Saharan Africa. On examination, she appears pale and febrile. Laboratory tests reveal thrombocytopenia, anemia, and

elevated lactate levels. A peripheral blood smear confirms the diagnosis of severe malaria due to *Plasmodium falciparum*. The patient's condition deteriorates rapidly with the development of respiratory distress and altered mental status. She is promptly admitted to the intensive care unit (ICU). What is the most appropriate management for this patient?
a. Initiate intravenous (IV) artesunate
b. Administer IV quinine
c. Administer mefloquine + clindamycin
d. Begin IV doxycycline

Ans. a

Explanation: In pregnant women, severe malaria poses additional risks to both the mother and fetus. Gravid women who contract malaria have a greater tendency to develop severe malaria. Unlike malarial infection in nongravid individuals, pregnant individuals with *P. vivax* are at high risk for severe malaria, and those with *P. falciparum* have a greatly increased predisposition for severe malaria as well.

The most appropriate management for severe malaria in a pregnant female in the ICU is the initiation of intravenous (IV) artesunate. Artesunate is the recommended first-line treatment for severe malaria due to *P. falciparum*, including in pregnant women. It has shown superior efficacy and safety compared to intravenous quinine, which was previously used as the standard treatment. Artesunate rapidly reduces parasite burden, decreases mortality rates, and improves clinical outcomes. Treatment options for uncomplicated chloroquine-resistant *P. falciparum* and *P. vivax* malaria in pregnant individuals were limited to mefloquine or quinine plus clindamycin. Although the limited availability of quinine and increasing resistance to mefloquine limits these options, strong evidence demonstrates that artemether-lumefantrine (Coartem) is effective and safe in the treatment of malaria in pregnancy. These data are supported by the World Health Organization.

Mechanical ventilation and IV fluids are supportive measures that may be necessary in the management of severe malaria, especially if the patient develops respiratory distress or signs of hypovolemia. However, the priority is to start specific antimalarial therapy with IV artesunate.

Doxycycline is contraindicated in pregnancy due to potential adverse effects on the fetus and should not be used for the treatment of malaria in pregnant women.

Suggested Reading
1. Centers for Disease Control and Prevention. (2020). Treatment of Malaria: Guidelines for Clinicians (United States). Available from: https://www.cdc.gov/malaria/resources/pdf/treatmenttable.pdf [Last accessed June, 2023].
2. Rijken MJ, McGready R, Boel ME, Poespoprodjo R, Singh N, Syafruddin D, et al. Malaria in Pregnancy in the Asia-Pacific Region. Lancet Infect Dis. 2012;12(1):75-88.
3. World Health Organization. Guidelines for the Treatment of Malaria, 3rd edition. Geneva: World Health Organization; 2015.

Q.18. Which of the following statements regarding tafenoquine in the treatment of malaria is true?

a. Tafenoquine is effective against all species of *Plasmodium*.
b. Tafenoquine is primarily used for the treatment of uncomplicated malaria.
c. Tafenoquine is contraindicated in patients with glucose-6-phosphate dehydrogenase (G6PD) deficiency.
d. Tafenoquine has a short half-life and requires daily dosing.

Ans. c

Explanation: Tafenoquine is an antimalarial medication that is used for the radical cure of *Plasmodium vivax* malaria, targeting both the blood and liver stages of the parasite. It was approved by FDA in 2018 in aged 16 years. And older, also for prophylaxis in adults travelling to malaria's endemic areas. While tafenoquine is used for the treatment of malaria, its primary indication is for the radical cure of *P. vivax* malaria to prevent relapse. One of the most important considerations when using tafenoquine is the risk of hemolytic anemia in patients with glucose-6-phosphate dehydrogenase (G6PD) deficiency. G6PD deficiency is an inherited condition that can lead to the breakdown of red blood cells upon exposure to certain medications, including tafenoquine. Therefore, tafenoquine is contraindicated in patients with G6PD deficiency due to the risk of severe hemolysis. Tafenoquine has a long half-life, which allows for a single-dose treatment regimen. It is administered as a single oral dose after an initial loading dose of chloroquine or an artemisinin-based combination therapy.

Suggested Reading
1. Llanos-Cuentas A, Lacerda MV, Rueangweerayut R, Vélez ID, Namaik-Larp C, Chu CS, et al. Tafenoquine versus Primaquine to Prevent Relapse of Plasmodium vivax Malaria. N Engl J Med. 2019;380(25):229-41.
2. Tafenoquine [package insert]. Research Triangle Park, NC: GlaxoSmithKline; 2018.
3. White NJ, Duong TT, Uthaisin C, Nosten F, Phyo AP, Hanboonkunupakarn B. Antimalarial activity of tafenoquine in a human challenge model. Trans R Soc Trop Med Hyg. 2014;108(1):13-7.

Q.19. Which of the following are not seen in cerebral malaria?

a. Granulomas of Durck
b. Orange and white hemorrhagic streaks on retina on ophthalmoscopy
c. Vessel blockage due to hyperparasites and RBC adhesion
d. All can be seen

Ans. d

Explanation: The World Health Organization defines cerebral malaria as a clinical syndrome characterized by coma at least 1 hour after termination of a seizure or correction of hypoglycemia, asexual forms of *Plasmodium falciparum* parasites on peripheral blood smears and no other cause to explain the coma. Durck's granuloma is an area of rarefied brain containing activated microglial/macrophages appearing at the site of a prior ring hemorrhage. Coma is due to parasitized red blood cells (pRBCs) sequestered in cerebral microcirculation. In the eye, multiple discrete areas of retinal whitening are observed in most children with cerebral malaria. These areas have impaired capillary perfusion on fluorescein angiography.

Suggested Reading
1. Idro R, Marsh K, John CC, Newton CR. Cerebral malaria: Mechanisms of brain injury and strategies for improved neurocognitive outcome. Pediatr Res. 2010;68(4):267-74.

Q.20. **A 30-year-old female presents with continuous fever, headache, and malaise of 5 days duration with constipation. She reports a history of recent travel. On examination, there is mild hepatomegaly and splenomegaly. Laboratory investigations reveal leukopenia and elevated transaminases. Which of the following tests would be most helpful in confirming the diagnosis of typhoid fever in this patient?**
   a. Blood culture
   b. Stool culture
   c. Serological testing for *Salmonella* antibodies
   d. Polymerase chain reaction (PCR) for *Salmonella* DNA

Ans. a

Explanation: Blood culture is often used in definitive diagnosis of typhoid fever while, bone marrow culture has a greater sensitivity and considered reference standard. Maximum blood culture yield will be achieved when bacteremia is at peak such as in the first to third week from the onset of the illness. Culturing the bacteria from body fluids is the definitive test for the diagnosis of typhoid fever although inconclusive serological methods such as Widal test are commonly employed in many healthcare settings. A previous literature review on the sensitivity of blood culture suggested 40-60%

Suggested Reading
1. Mogasale V, Ramani E, Mogasale VV, Park J. What proportion of *Salmonella typhi* cases are detected by blood culture? A systematic literature review. Ann Clin Microbiol Antimicrob. 2016;15(1):32.

Q.21. **Which of the following is accurate regarding culture for typhoid fever?**
   a. Stool culture alone may be used to diagnose typhoid fever.
   b. Blood, intestinal secretions, and stool culture results are only positive in 20-30% of patients who present in the first week of onset.
   c. Culture of bone marrow aspirate is 90% sensitive until at least 5 days after antibiotics are initiated.
   d. A urine culture is the criterion standard diagnostic tool for typhoid fever.

Ans. c

Explanation: The criterion standard for diagnosis of typhoid fever has long been culture isolation of the organism. Cultures are widely considered 100% specific. Culture of bone marrow aspirate is 90% sensitive until at least 5 days after commencement of antibiotics. Blood, intestinal secretions (vomitus or duodenal aspirate), and stool culture results are positive for *S. typhi* in approximately 85-90% of patients with typhoid fever who present within the first week of onset. They decline to 20-30% later in the disease course. Stool culture may be positive for *S. typhi* several days after ingestion of the bacteria secondary to inflammation of the intraluminal dendritic cells. Later in the illness, stool culture results are positive because of bacteria are shed through the gallbladder. Multiple blood cultures (three or more) yield a sensitivity of 73-97%. Large-volume (10-30 mL) blood culture and clot culture may increase the likelihood of detection. Stool culture alone yields a sensitivity of <50%, and urine culture alone is even less sensitive.

Suggested Reading
1. Mogasale V, Ramani E, Mogasale VV, Park J. What proportion of *Salmonella typhi* cases are detected by blood culture? A systematic literature review. Ann Clin Microbiol Antimicrob. 2016;15(1):32.

Q.22. **A 45-year-old man presented with fever, chills, headache, and muscle aches. Laboratory tests show hemolytic anemia, thrombocytopenia, and the presence of intraerythrocytic parasites. Which of the following is the most likely diagnosis?**
   a. Babesiosis
   b. Malaria
   c. Lyme disease
   d. Rocky Mountain spotted fever

Ans. a

Explanation: The clinical presentation of fever, chills, headache, muscle aches, along with laboratory findings of hemolytic anemia, thrombocytopenia, and intraerythrocytic parasites, is consistent with babesiosis. Babesiosis is a tick-borne disease caused by the protozoan parasite *Babesia*, which infects and destroys red blood cells, leading to the characteristic findings. Polymerase chain reaction (PCR) is the most sensitive and specific diagnostic test for confirming the presence of *Babesia* DNA in the blood. The most effective treatment for babesiosis is a combination therapy of atovaquone and azithromycin. Atovaquone targets the parasite within the red blood cells, while azithromycin helps to control the infection and reduce the parasitic load.

Suggested Reading
1. Vannier E, Krause PJ. Human babesiosis. N Engl J Med. 2012;366(25):2397-407.

Q.23. **During a recent outbreak in Kerala, India, a 32 year-old male presents to the emergency department with acute respiratory distress. He reports a sudden onset of fever, headache, and myalgia 2 days ago. He had history of contact with suspected case of the viral infection. He also complains of dizziness, confusion, and nausea. On examination, the patient is febrile and tachypneic. Neurological examination reveals signs of meningeal irritation. Chest X-ray shows bilateral infiltrates. Laboratory investigations show lymphocytic leukocytosis and elevated liver enzymes. Considering the recent outbreak in Kerala, which of the following is the most likely diagnosis?**
   a. Influenza pneumonia
   b. Tuberculosis meningitis
   c. Nipah virus infection
   d. Dengue fever
   e. Malaria

Ans. c

Explanation: This patient's clinical presentation is highly suggestive of Nipah virus infection, particularly during the context of the recent outbreak in Kerala, India. Nipah virus is a zoonotic paramyxovirus that causes severe respiratory and neurological symptoms in humans. The infection is associated with a high mortality rate. The clinical features of Nipah virus infection include the sudden onset of fever, headache, myalgia, and respiratory distress. Neurological symptoms such as dizziness, confusion, and meningeal signs can also be present. The disease often progresses rapidly and can lead to encephalitis and acute respiratory distress syndrome (ARDS). Bilateral infiltrates on chest X-ray are commonly observed. Laboratory findings may include lymphocytic leukocytosis and elevated liver enzymes.

Influenza pneumonia (Option a) typically presents with a more gradual onset of symptoms, such as cough, sore throat, and malaise, and is less likely to cause neurological manifestations. Tuberculosis meningitis (Option b) typically has a subacute presentation with gradually worsening symptoms, including fever, headache, and altered mental status. Dengue fever (Option d) and malaria (Option e) present with fever and systemic symptoms but do not typically cause respiratory distress or meningeal signs seen in Nipah virus infection.

Suggested Reading
1. Arunkumar G, Chandni R, Mourya DT, Singh SK, Sadanandan R, Sudan P, et al. Outbreak investigation of Nipah virus disease in Kerala, India, 2018. J Infect Dis. 2019;219(12):1867-78.
2. Chadha MS, Comer JA, Lowe L, Rota PA, Rollin PE, Bellini WJ, et al. Nipah virus-associated encephalitis outbreak, Siliguri, India. Emerg Infect Dis. 2006;12(2):235-40.

Q.24. **A 56-year-old farmer with history of diabetes on insulin presented with history of cough, shortness of breath, left abdominal pain, and malaise, reduced appetite for last 2 weeks. He resented to the emergency with respiratory distress and examination revealed bilateral crackles over chest and tender left hypochondrium. Chest X-ray suggested multilobar consolidation USG abdomen revealed left splenic abscess. Sputum culture yielded gram-negative oxidase positive organism. Which of the following is the most appropriate initial management step for this patient?**
   a. Initiate empirical treatment with amoxicillin-clavulanate.
   b. Start azithromycin therapy.
   c. Obtain blood cultures and start intravenous ceftazidime.
   d. Administer oral trimethoprim-sulfamethoxazole.
   e. Order a sputum culture and start doxycycline therapy.

Ans. c

Explanation: This patient's clinical presentation is highly suggestive of melioidosis, an infectious disease caused by the bacterium *Burkholderia pseudomallei*. Melioidosis is commonly seen in individuals with underlying risk factors such as diabetes, chronic kidney disease, or immunosuppression. The clinical manifestations vary widely and can involve multiple organ systems, including the lungs, liver, spleen, and skin. The initial management of suspected melioidosis includes obtaining blood cultures to identify the causative organism and initiating empirical antibiotic therapy. Ceftazidime is the drug of choice for severe melioidosis and should be started intravenously. It provides broad-spectrum coverage against *Burkholderia pseudomallei* and is usually given for a minimum of 10–14 days, followed by oral eradication therapy with a combination of trimethoprim-sulfamethoxazole (TMP-SMX) or doxycycline for 3–6 months to prevent relapse. Amoxicillin-clavulanate (Option a) is not effective against *Burkholderia pseudomallei* and should not be used as empirical therapy for melioidosis. Azithromycin (Option b) and doxycycline (Option e) have limited efficacy against *Burkholderia pseudomallei* and are not the preferred initial treatment choices. While TMP-SMX (Option d) is used for eradication therapy, intravenous ceftazidime is the appropriate initial step to cover the severe infection.

Suggested Reading
1. Wiersinga WJ, Currie BJ, Peacock SJ. Melioidosis. N Engl J Med. 2012;367(11):1035-44.

Q.25. **A 15-year-old boy presents to the emergency department with a 2-day history of fever, headache, and altered mental status. On examination, the patient is drowsy and confused. Neck stiffness and positive Kernig's sign are noted. Neurological examination reveals tremors and generalized hyperreflexia. Laboratory investigations show leukocytosis with a shift to the left, thrombocytopenia, and elevated liver enzymes. A lumbar puncture is performed, and cerebrospinal fluid (CSF) analysis reveals lymphocytic pleocytosis and increased protein levels. Which of the following is the most likely diagnosis?**
   a. Meningococcal meningitis
   b. Tuberculous meningitis
   c. Japanese encephalitis
   d. Herpes simplex encephalitis
   e. West Nile encephalitis

Ans. c

Explanation: This patient's clinical presentation is highly suggestive of Japanese encephalitis. Japanese encephalitis is caused by the Japanese encephalitis virus, a mosquito-borne flavivirus. The disease typically presents with fever, headache, and altered mental status, which may progress to seizures, tremors, and focal neurological deficits. Laboratory findings often include leukocytosis with a left shift, thrombocytopenia, and elevated liver enzymes. Lumbar puncture is performed to evaluate CSF, which typically shows lymphocytic pleocytosis and increased protein levels.

Meningococcal meningitis (Option a) is characterized by sudden onset of fever, headache, neck stiffness, and a petechial rash. Tuberculous meningitis (Option b) typically presents with subacute symptoms, such as fever, headache, altered mental status, and focal neurological deficits. Herpes simplex encephalitis (Option d) usually presents with a prodrome of fever, headache, and behavioral changes followed by the development of seizures, focal neurological deficits, and altered mental status. West Nile encephalitis (Option e) presents with fever, headache, and meningeal signs, but focal neurological deficits are less common compared to Japanese encephalitis.

Suggested Reading
1. Kulkarni R, Sapkal GN, Kaushal H, Mourya DT. Japanese Encephalitis: A Brief Review on Indian Perspectives. Open Virol J. 2018;12:121-30.
2. Van K, Korman TM, Nicholson S, Troutbeck R, Lister DM, Woolley I. Case report: Japanese encephalitis associated with chorioretinitis after short-term travel to Bali, Indonesia. Am J Trop Med Hyg. 2020;103(4):1691–3.

Q.26. A 62-years-old Indian woman, housewife by occupation living in crowded settings, presented to emergency with complaints of recurrent vomiting for last 7 months. Her general hygiene was very poor. On blood investigations, her counts were within normal limits, but there was eosinophilia. Ultrasonography (USG) abdomen revealed ill-defined circumferential hypoechoic wall thickening of pylorus causing luminal narrowing with dilated proximal stomach. Strongyloidiasis was suspected. Which is most accurate?
a. *Strongyloides* travels from the skin to the gastrointestinal (GI) tract of its host and then invades pleura and reaches the lung.
b. There are stages of hyperinfection and disseminated stage of the disease in humans.
c. Sensitivity of a single direct fecal microscopic examination is said to be <10% and it increases to 40% if three fecal specimens are screened.
d. Albendazole is the treatment of choice for the condition with a cure rate of 97%.

Ans. b

Explanation: Strongyloidiasis travels from the skin to the lung and then reaches the GI tract. Ivermectin is the treatment of choice with a cure rate of 97%. Stool microscopy is the simplest method to diagnose the disease with sensitivity going up to 70% with 3 stool specimen.

Suggested Reading
1. Paul M, Meena S, Gupta P, Jha S, Rekha US, Kumar P. Clinico-epidemiological spectrum of strongyloidiasis in India: Review of 166 cases. J Fam Med Prim Care. 2020;9:485.

Q.27. A 24-year-old female with fever, myalgia of 1 week duration presented to the emergency. She had thrombocytopenia rising hematocrit. Her serology was positive for IgM dengue. She was admitted for observation and monitoring. She was given supportive treatment with fluids and was responding with resolution of fever. However, developed new onset fever, bicytopenia, hepatosplenomegaly after a brief resolution of her initial symptoms. The treating physician suspected hemophagocytic lymphohistiocytosis (HLH). Which among the following is most accurate regarding secondary HLH?
a. In India, tuberculosis is the main cause for infection-related hemophagocytes syndrome.
b. HLH-2004 protocol is necessary in all cases of secondary HLH.
c. Bone marrow is needed to fulfil the criteria for HLH.
d. 60–70% of infection-related HLH responds to appropriate treatment and control of the underlying disease.

Ans. d

Explanation: Hemophagocytic lymphohistiocytosis (HLH) is a potentially fatal hyperinflammatory condition, if not recognized and treated in time. A high index of suspicion can help identify the condition early. This condition can occur in the primary or secondary form. Secondary HLH or hemophagocytic syndrome (HPS) secondary to infections is an important clinical entity especially in tropical world. Srinivas et al. in a systematic review found that infectious cause in 51% of HLH. Dengue and malaria accounted for most of the cases of HLH. Most of the times patient responded to less aggressive immunosuppression than the HLH-2004 regimens like steroids.

Suggested Reading
1. Kodan P, Chakrapani M, Shetty M, Pavan R, Bhat P. Hemophagocytic lymphohistiocytosis secondary to infections: A tropical experience! J Postgrad Med. 2015;61(2):112-5.

Q.28. **A 20-year-old male livestock owner came with fever, photophobia, and confusion. On clinical examination, there was tachycardia, lymphadenopathy, petechiae, and ecchymosis. He gives a history of unknown bite from the farm while taking care of animals 10 days back. His RT-PCR assay was positive for Congo hemorrhagic fever. Which of the following is inaccurate regarding Congo hemorrhagic fever, CCHF?**
  a. The virus causing the disease requires biosafety level 4 for handling the specimen.
  b. It belongs to the family of Bunyaviridae, transmitted by ixodid ticks.
  c. In India, the disease has been mostly reported from Gujarat and Rajasthan.
  d. The antiviral ribavirin has been approved by the FDA for the treatment of CCHF.

Ans. d

Explanation: Crimean-Congo hemorrhagic fever (CCHF) is a high priority disease because of possibility of outbreaks and high case fatality rate of around 50%. Tests on patient samples present an extreme biohazard risk and should only be conducted under maximum biological containment conditions. The antiviral drug ribavirin has been used to treat CCHF infection only with apparent benefit and not approved by FDA. It belongs to the family of Bunyaviridae, transmitted by ixodid ticks. In India, the disease have been mostly reported from Gujarat and Rajasthan.

Suggested Reading
1. Spengler JR, Bente DA, Bray M, Burt F, Hewson R, Korukluoglu G, et al. Second International Conference on Crimean-Congo Hemorrhagic Fever. Antiviral Res. 2018;150:137-47.

Q.29. **A 40-year-old male travelled in slums for camp activity and had food and water from the place. He developed multiple episodes of watery loose stools along with vomiting after 1 day. Similar symptoms were reported among his colleagues. He was brought to emergency department and had dehydration and hypotension. As the attending physician your first suspicion is cholera. What is not true about cholera and its treatment?**
  a. Watery diarrhea, which may be profuse, and vomiting are usually the initial symptoms.
  b. Although along with loss of water and electrolytes, hypokalemia occurs but not hyponatremia.

c. If ORS packets are not available, other substitutes must not be tried.
d. The mainstay of the management is IV fluids and IV antibiotics.

Ans. b

Explanation: Cholera is an acute gastrointestinal infection caused by ingestion of food or water contaminated with the bacterium *Vibrio cholerae*. Usually has an incubation period of 1–2 days. Symptoms classically described as abrupt onset of painless, rice water stools. Most of those infected can be successfully treated with oral rehydration solution. Cholera is most often associated with isonatremic hyponantremia. Only severe cases require IV antibiotics and fluids.

Suggested Reading
1. Version P. MSD manual: Professional version. JAC Antimicrob Resist. 2020;2(3):1-5.

Q.30. A 35-year-old male working in veterinary college presented with complaints of intermittent fever, malaise, and anorexia of 1 month duration. On detailed history, he was part of the team which evaluated pregnant cattle's having abortions. Clinical evaluation revealed anemia, hepatosplenomegaly. Rose Bengal test was positive. Which among the following is accurate regarding brucellosis?
a. It is a focal disease with a particular affinity for the musculoskeletal system.
b. Ageusia is a common manifestation in neurobrucellosis.
c. Longer duration of combination of antibiotics active in acidic environment is required for the treatment.
d. The WHO suggests use of clarithromycin and rifampicin combination for 6 weeks.

Ans. c

Explanation: Brucellosis called Malta fever or Mediterranean fever is an acute infection which can become chronic with complications. It is an infection causing systemic manifestations with cytopenia's, vasculitis lymphadenopathy, organomegaly, and infective endocarditis. Sensorineural hearing loss is a feature in neuroborreliosis. General principles of brucellosis treatment include use of antibiotics with activity in acidic intracellular environments (such as doxycycline and rifampin), use of combination therapy (given high relapse rates with monotherapy), and prolonged duration of treatment. WHO recommends doxycycline 100 mg twice a day for 45 days, plus streptomycin 1 g daily for 15 days. The main alternative therapy is doxycycline at 100 mg, twice a day for 45 days, plus rifampicin at 15 mg/kg/day (600–900 mg) for 45 days.

Suggested Reading
1. O'Callaghan D. Human brucellosis: Recent advances and future challenges. Infect Dis Poverty. 2020;9(1):101.
2. Solera J, Solís García Del Pozo J. Treatment of pulmonary brucellosis: A systematic review. Expert Rev Anti Infect Ther. 2017;15(1):33-42.

CHAPTER 9

Gastrointestinal System

Sushil Kumar Yadav, Priyanka Akshay Metgud

Q.1. Which of the following best describes severe acute pancreatitis based on the revised Atlanta classification?
 a. Acute necrotic collections
 b. Local or systemic complications without persistent organ failure
 c. Acute inflammation of the pancreatic parenchyma and peripancreatic tissues, but without recognizable tissue necrosis
 d. Persistent organ failure >48 hours
 e. Organ failure that resolves within 48 hours

Ans. d

Explanation: Severe acute pancreatitis should be diagnosed if a patient exhibits signs of persistent organ failure for >48 hours despite adequate intravenous fluid resuscitation. Definitions of key terms [*based on the 2012 Atlanta Classification of Acute Pancreatitis-Diagnosis of acute pancreatitis (two of the following)*]:

- Abdominal pain (acute onset of a persistent, severe, epigastric pain often radiating to the back)
- Serum lipase activity (or amylase) at least three times greater than the upper limit of normal
- Characteristic findings of acute pancreatitis on computed tomography or magnetic resonance imaging

Mild acute pancreatitis: No organ failure, local or systemic complications

Moderately severe acute pancreatitis:
- Organ failure that resolves within 48 hours
- Local or systemic complications without persistent organ failure

Severe acute pancreatitis: Persistent organ failure >48 hours

Interstitial edematous acute pancreatitis: Acute inflammation of the pancreatic parenchyma and peripancreatic tissues, but without recognizable tissue necrosis

Necrotizing acute pancreatitis: Inflammation associated with pancreatic parenchymal necrosis and/or peripancreatic necrosis

Organ failure and systemic complications of acute pancreatitis:
- *Respiratory:* Partial pressure of oxygen (PaO_2)/fraction of inspired oxygen (FiO_2) ≤ 300
- *Cardiovascular:* Systolic blood pressure <90 mm Hg (off inotropic support), not fluid responsive, or pH <7.3
- *Renal:* Serum creatinine ≥170 mmol/L

Localized complications:
- Walled-off necrosis
- Peripancreatic fluid collections
- Necrotic fluid collections
- Pseudocysts of pancreas

Suggested Reading
1. Greenberg JA, Hsu J, Bawazeer M, Marshall J, Friedrich JO, Nathens A, et al. Clinical practice guideline: management of acute pancreatitis. Can J Surg. 2016;59(2):128-40.

Q.2. A 28-year-old man came to the hospital 4 days after being involved in road traffic accident (RTA). He was the restrained driver in the vehicle during a front-on collision at 80 miles/h. He was discharged home as he had no complaints and signs of trauma. After 3 days, he started complaints of abdominal pain with nausea. His laboratory workup reveals a hemoglobin of 10.8 g/dL and lipase level of 1,350 IU/L. A CT abdomen showed acute pancreatitis. Which is the most vulnerable part of pancreas that gets injured in the setting of restrained motor vehicle accident?
a. Body of the pancreas
b. Tail of the pancreas
c. Head of the pancreas
d. Uncinate process

Ans. a

Explanation: The pancreas is a long J-shaped, soft, and lobulated retroperitoneal organ. It is situated transversely across the posterior abdominal wall, at the back of the epigastric and left hypochondriac regions at level of lumbar (L1-2) spine. Blunt trauma to the pancreas is, in most instances, caused by a sudden localized force to the upper abdomen that compresses the pancreas against the vertebral column (e.g., steering-wheel injury in a motor vehicle accident in adults and from bicycle handlebar injury or direct blow from a kick or fall in children). In order of frequency, injuries to the pancreas involve the body, head, and tail. Midline of part of the pancreatic body overlies the lumber spine, making this area most susceptible to abdomen trauma.

Suggested Reading
1. Debi U, Kaur R, Prasad KK, Sinha SK, Sinha A, Singh K. Pancreatic trauma: A concise review. World J Gastroenterol. 2013;19(47):9003-11.

Q.3. A 38-year-old man presented to emergency department with epigastric pain for the last 24 hours. His abdomen is tender to palpation in the epigastrium region. Investigation reveals elevated amylase and lipase, and a diagnosis of acute pancreatitis is made. The patient admitted is started on intravenous (IV) fluids, IV

analgesia, and kept nil per os (NPO). **Which of the following scoring systems can be used within 12 hours of admission for early mortality risk stratification?**
a. Rockall score
b. Bedside Index for Severity in Acute Pancreatitis (BISAP) score
c. Acute Physiology and Chronic Health Evaluation (APACHE II) score
d. CT severity index

Ans. b

Explanation: BISAP score is a simple scoring system for acute pancreatitis that can be used within the first 12 hours to predict severity and identify patients at risk for complications and mortality. This score gives one point for each of the following: blood urea nitrogen (BUN) >25 mg/dL, impaired mental status, systemic inflammatory response syndrome, age older than 60 years, and pleural effusion. A score of 4 or 5 indicates a 7–12-fold increased risk of organ failure.

The Rockall score is used to assess severity in acute upper gastrointestinal (GI) bleeding.

Suggested Reading
1. Hagjer S, Kumar N. Evaluation of the BISAP scoring system in prognostication of acute pancreatitis—A prospective observational study. Int J Surg. 2018;54(Pt A):76-81.

Q.4. Which of the following are the most common causes of acute pancreatitis?
a. Autoimmune
b. Gallstones
c. Drugs and toxins
d. Postendoscopic retrograde cholangiopancreatography (ERCP)
e. Binge alcohol consumption

Ans. b

Explanation: Gallstones and increased alcohol consumption are the most common causes of pancreatitis.

Suggested Reading
1. Banks PA. Epidemiology, natural history, and predictors of disease outcome in acute and chronic pancreatitis. Gastrointest Endosc. 2002;56(Suppl):S226-30.

Q.5. A 45-year-old acute pancreatitis patient admitted with heart rate (HR) of 122 bpm, oxygen saturation (SpO$_2$) of 96%, and blood pressure (BP) of 90/62 mm Hg. What would be the imaging to be done now in this patient?
a. Contrast-enhanced computed tomography abdomen
b. Ultrasonography abdomen
c. Computed tomography abdomen plain
d. MRCP

Ans. b

Explanation: Baseline ultrasonography should be done in all patients of acute pancreatitis.

Magnetic resonance cholangiopancreatography (MRCP) is recommended when ultrasonography was not conclusive and liver enzymes are elevated.

Selected patients need CT evolution:
- A patient with broad differential diagnosis that includes acute pancreatitis.
- Acute pancreatitis with suspected local complication.

Suggested Reading
1. Greenberg JA, Hsu J, Bawazeer M, Marshall J, Friedrich JO, Nathens A, et al. Clinical practice guideline: management of acute pancreatitis. Can J Surg. 2016;59(2):128-40.

Q.6. A most appropriate nutrition support in a 40-year-old pancreatitis patient is:
a. Early total parenteral nutrition
b. Total parenteral nutrition (TPN) preferred over enteral nutrition
c. Enteral nutrition initiation as early as possible
d. Initiation of nutrition after resolution of pancreatitis

Ans. c

Explanation: Patients with mild acute pancreatitis should be initiated on oral feeds as tolerated on admission. Patients of severe acute pancreatitis should be commenced on enteral feeds as soon as possible preferably within 48 hours of admission. Enteral feeding is recommended over parenteral nutrition.

Suggested Reading
1. Greenberg JA, Hsu J, Bawazeer M, Marshall J, Friedrich JO, Nathens A, et al. Clinical practice guideline: management of acute pancreatitis. Can J Surg. 2016;59(2):128-40.

Q.7. A 48-year-old male patient was admitted to the hospital and diagnosed with gallstone pancreatitis. After initial stabilization with intravenous fluid and analgesia, on day 4, patient developed severe abdominal pain and distension. CT abdomen reveals pancreatic necrosis with CT severity score of 6/10. What is next for management?
a. Surgical intervention
b. Percutaneous drainage of necrosis
c. Broad-spectrum antibiotics
d. Continue supportive care

Ans. d

Explanation: Pancreatic necrosis may occur after 4th day of onset of pancreatitis. Acute noninfected pancreatic necrosis is best managed conservatively with early introduction of nutritional support, preferably enteral route. Early surgical intervention in sterile necrosis has worse outcomes than conservative management. Antibiotic prophylaxis is no longer recommended for sterile necrosis because it has no survival advantage and may lead to development of antibiotic resistance or fungal infection.

Suggested Reading
1. Greenberg JA, Hsu J, Bawazeer M, Marshall J, Friedrich JO, Nathens A, et al. Clinical practice guideline: management of acute pancreatitis. Can J Surg. 2016;59(2):128-40.

Q.8. A 25-year-old male patient presented with abdominal pain in epigastric region, and provisional diagnosis was made as acute pancreatitis. Which of the following are initial lines of management, except?
   a. Hydration guided by hematocrit and BUN
   b. Pain management
   c. Prophylactic antibiotics
   d. Early enteral nutrition

Ans. c

Explanation:
Initial management of acute pancreatitis includes:
- Resuscitation with intravenous crystalloids
- Analgesia
- Early enteral nutrition

Prophylactic antibiotics are not recommended in patients with mild or severe acute pancreatitis. Antibiotics should be given for an extrapancreatic infection, such as cholangitis, catheter-acquired infections, bacteremia, urinary tract infections, and pneumonia.

Suggested Reading
1. Tenner S, Baillie J, DeWitt J, Vege SS; American College of Gastroenterology. American College of Gastroenterology Guideline: Management of Acute Pancreatitis. Am J Gastroenterol. 2013;108:1400-15.

Q.9. What is the most common cause for acute liver failure in developed countries?
   a. Alcoholic hepatitis   b. Hepatitis B infection
   c. Acetaminophen toxicity   d. Hepatitis E virus

Ans. c

Explanation: In developed countries, drug-induced liver injury (DILI) is most common cause for acute liver failure. Paracetamol (acetaminophen) is most common overdose seen, while viral hepatitis is most common cause of acute liver failure in developing countries.

Suggested Reading
1. European Association for the Study of the Liver. EASL Clinical Practical Guidelines on the management of acute (fulminant) liver failure. J Hepatol. 2017;66(5):1047-81.

Q.10. Criteria to fulfill diagnosis of acute liver failure include all, except:
   a. Jaundice
   b. Coagulopathy with international normalized ratio (INR) >1.5
   c. Encephalopathy
   d. Duration of illness >28 days

Ans. d

Explanation: Based on the duration between development of encephalopathy and jaundice, acute liver failure is classified as:
- *Hyperacute liver failure:* Encephalopathy occurring within 7 days of jaundice onset.

- *Acute liver failure:* Encephalopathy occurring within 8–28 days of jaundice onset.
- *Subacute liver failure:* Encephalopathy occurring within 5–12 weeks of jaundice onset.

  If duration is >28 weeks before the onset of encephalopathy, it is categorized as chronic liver disease.

Suggested Reading
1. European Association for the Study of the Liver. EASL Clinical Practical Guidelines on the management of acute (fulminant) liver failure. J Hepatol. 2017;66(5):1047-81.

Q.11. All are included in King's College criteria for nonparacetamol-related acute liver failure, except:
a. Age <10 years and >40 years
b. INR > 3.5
c. Bilirubin > 17 mg/dL
d. Serum creatinine

Ans. d

Explanation:
King's College criteria:
Acute liver failure due to paracetamol:
- *Paracetamol-related acute liver failure single criteria:*
  - Arterial pH < 7.3 after resuscitation and >24 hours since ingestion
  - Lactate > 3 mmol/L
- *Three of following criteria:*
  1. >grade-3 hepatic encephalopathy
  2. Serum creatinine >3.4 mg/dL
  3. INR > 6.5

Acute liver failure due to nonparacetamol:
- *Nonparacetamol-related acute liver failure single criteria:*
  - INR > 6.5
- *Three out of five following criteria:*
  - *Etiology:* Indeterminate etiology—hepatitis and drug-induced hepatitis
  - Age <10 years or >40 years
  - Interval jaundice—encephalopathy >7 days
  - Bilirubin > 17 mg/dL
  - INR > 3.5

Suggested Reading
1. European Association for the Study of the Liver. EASL Clinical Practical Guidelines on the management of acute (fulminant) liver failure. J Hepatol. 2017;66:1047-81.

Q.12. All are the prognostic criteria for acute liver failure (ALF), except:
a. APACHE score
b. Acute Liver Failure Study Groups (ALFSG)
c. Model for end-stage liver disease
d. ALF early dynamic model
e. Child–Pugh criteria

Ans. e

Explanation:
Following prognostic criteria have been studied to evaluate acute liver failure:
- King's College criteria
- Model for end-stage liver disease (MELD)
- Acute Physiology and Chronic Health Evaluation-2 (APACHE 2)
- Sequential organ failure assessment (SOFA)
- ALF study group (ALFSG)
- ALF early dynamic model (ALFD)
- Clichy criteria

Suggested Reading
1. Carmi S. Acute liver failure: Diagnosis and management. J Intensive Care Med. 2016;31(10):642-53.

Q.13. A 20-year-old female admitted to the casualty after ingestion of 80 tablets of acetaminophen 500 mg, approximately 21 hours before. On admission, patient was alert with HR = 102 bpm, BP = 110/60 mm Hg, respiratory rate (RR) = 22 breaths/min, with laboratory values: aspartate transaminase (AST) = 7,020, alanine transaminase (ALT) = 5,200, total bilirubin = 4 mg/dL, INR = 3, platelets = 1.52 lakh, white blood cell (WBC) = 7,000. Which of the following statement is incorrect for the role of N-acetyl cysteine in management of this patient?
 a. N-acetyl cysteine is standard of care.
 b. Efficacy of N-acetyl cysteine is best when given within 8 hours.
 c. N-acetyl cysteine is recommended for up to 72 hours.
 d. N-acetyl cysteine should not be administered to at-risk patients if levels are nontoxic.

Ans. d

Explanation: N-acetyl cysteine (NAC) is standard of care for acetaminophen overdose. Acetaminophen (APAP) levels do not necessarily rule out overdose. Efficacy of NAC is best when used within 8 hours, but it can be used even up to 72 hours of ingestion.

Oral preparation of NAC may be used in grade-1 hepatic encephalopathy and intravenous NAC in severe cases. NAC is continued until hepatic function improves and may be continued for several days.

Suggested Reading
1. Carmi S. Acute liver failure: Diagnosis and management. J Intensive Care Med. 2016;31(10):642-53.

Q.14. What is the most appropriate line of management for 35 weeks' gestation of pregnancy with fatty liver of pregnancy with altered mental status?
 a. Use of corticosteroids
 b. Ursodeoxycholic acid
 c. Delivery of fetus
 d. N-acetyl cysteine is standard of care

Ans. c

Explanation: Hepatic emergencies commonly encountered in third trimester of pregnancy are:
- HELLP (hemolysis, elevated liver enzymes, and low platelets) syndrome
- AFLP (acute fatty liver of pregnancy)

The AFLP is present with abdominal pain, malaise, and findings of hepatic steatosis. HELLP syndrome should be differentiated from atypical hemolytic uremic syndrome and thrombotic thrombocytopenic purpura. Maternal mortality is around 20% in above hepatic emergencies of pregnancy. Prompt delivery of the baby in both these conditions offers a good outcome.

Suggested Reading
1. European Association for the Study of the Liver. EASL Clinical Practical Guidelines on the management of acute (fulminant) liver failure. J Hepatol. 2017;66:1047-81.

Q.15. **Which of the following is the most common leading cause of death in acute liver failure patient?**
a. Cerebral edema
b. Infections
c. Bleeding due to coagulopathy
d. Acute kidney injury

Ans. b

Explanation: Infections are associated with leading cause of death in acute liver failure; in that, majority (70%) are respiratory and urinary tract infections. Infection control to prevent nosocomial infection is strongly recommended. 80% of acute liver failure patients have bacteriologically proven infection, while 32% have concomitant fungal infection. The lung is the most common site of infection followed by urinary tract.

Suggested Reading
1. Carmi S. Acute liver failure, diagnosis and management. J Intensive Care Med. 2016;31(10):642-53.

Q.16. **A 40-year-old male intravenous drug abuser presented with lethargy and pruritus. He is drowsy but arousable, incoherent, and extremely confused. Laboratories confirmed hepatitis B infection and deranged prothrombin time (PT)/INR with PT = 74 seconds. Which of the following statements is incorrect?**
a. The patient is in grade-3 hepatic encephalopathy.
b. Prognosis of HBV-related hepatic failure is worse in elderly.
c. Cerebral edema can likely cause confusion state.
d. Coagulopathy should be corrected with fresh frozen plasma (FFP)/cryoprecipitate.

Ans. d

Explanation: Infection with HBV is commonly seen viral cause of severe acute liver injury or acute liver failure either due to de novo infection, delta superinfection, or reactivation of previous HBV infection. The outcome of HBV-related acute liver failure is worse in the elderly patients and in those with multiple comorbidities. Rapid changes in the PT or INR have significant prognostic value. The routine correction of coagulopathy in acute liver failure is not recommended and should be limited to specific situations, such as active bleeding or insertion of intracranial pressure (ICP) monitors.

Suggested Reading
1. European Association for the Study of the Liver. EASL Clinical Practical Guidelines on the management of acute (fulminant) liver failure. J Hepatol. 2017;66:1047-81.

Q.17. Cerebral edema in acute liver failure is a complex interplay between inflammation of brain parenchyma, ammonia level, altered neurotransmission pathways, and cerebral dysautoregulation. Which of following is not a rescue therapeutic option for raised intracranial pressure secondary to cerebral edema in acute liver failure?
   a. Early initiation of continuous renal replacement therapy (CRRT)
   b. Elective intubation and keep sedated
   c. Maximize osmotherapy
   d. Continuous neuromuscular blockage for sustained refractory ICP
   e. Noninvasive ventilation

Ans. e

Explanation: High ammonia level contributes a significant role in pathogenesis of hepatic encephalopathy in acute liver failure. Severe cerebral edema results in increased intracranial pressure and brain herniation.

Management of acute liver failure with advanced hepatic encephalopathy and intracranial hypertension:
- Treat the cause of acute liver failure.
- Identify risk factors for intracranial hypertension, mortality, and start preparation for liver transplant in high-risk patients.
- *Neuromonitoring strategies in acute liver failure:* Glasgow coma scale assessment, optic nerve sonography, transcranial Doppler (TCD), jugular bulb oxygen saturation, brain imaging, and invasive intracranial monitoring
- *Neuroprotective strategies to decrease intracranial hypertension:*
    - Keep head elevation of bed and neck in midline position.
    - Use of hyperosmolar therapy.
    - Early use of CRRT.
- *Rescue strategies for increased intracranial pressure or refractory intracranial hypertension:*
    - Maximize osmotherapy with hypertonic saline or mannitol.
    - Try to maintain adequate cerebral perfusion pressure.
    - Increased sedation for metabolic suppression.
    - Targeted temperature management (TTM)
    - Continuous neuromuscular blockade infusion
- *Stepwise and slow de-escalation of neuroprotective therapies in post-transplant or transplant-free recovery:*
    - Slow normalization of serum sodium levels.
    - Slow rewarming if induced hypothermia initiated.
    - Watch for rebound edema or dialysis disequilibrium syndrome.

Suggested Reading

1. Kandiaha PA, Olson JC, Subramanian RM. Emerging strategies for the treatment of patients with acute hepatic failure. Curr Opin Crit Care. 2016;22(2):142-51.

Q.18. Which of the following strategies are used in management of ascites in a patient of liver cirrhosis, except:
   a. Salt restriction (intake of sodium 80–120 mmol/day)
   b. Spironolactone initiation if salt restriction fails.
   c. Use of furosemide and spironolactone combination
   d. Fluid restriction to <1 L/day

Ans. d

Explanation: European Association for the Study of the Liver (EASL) clinical practice guidelines on the management of ascites are:
- Restriction of salt intake is an important component of the management of ascites (intake of sodium of 80–120 mmol/day, which corresponds to 4.6–6.9 g of salt/day) in liver cirrhosis patients.
- Bed rest is not recommended for treatment for ascites.
- Fluid restriction is also not recommended in patients who have ascites with normal serum sodium level.
- Patients with the first episode of grade-2 (moderate) ascites should receive an aldosterone antagonist such as spironolactone, starting at dose of 100 mg/day and stepwise increased to a maximum of 400 mg/day. In patients who do not respond to aldosterone antagonists, furosemide should be added at dose from 40 mg/day to a maximum of 160 mg/day. Patients should undergo frequent clinical and biochemical monitoring for responsiveness and complication of diuretics.

Suggested Reading

1. European Association for the Study of the Liver. EASL clinical practice guidelines on the management of ascites, spontaneous bacterial peritonitis, and hepatorenal syndrome in cirrhosis. J Hepatol. 2010;53:397-417.

Q.19. A 62-year-old male patient presented to casualty with breathing difficulty due abdominal distension. He had history of decompensated liver disease due to chronic hepatitis B and repeated hospitalization for ascitic tapping. On examination, there was a tense ascites with pitting edema on lower limbs. Which of the following are criteria to diagnose refractory ascites in cirrhosis?
   a. Reappearance of grade-2 or -3 ascites within 4 weeks of initial mobilization
   b. Mean weight loss of <0.8 kg over 4 days
   c. No response on intensive diuretic therapy (spironolactone 400 mg/day and furosemide 160 mg/day) for at least 1 week
   d. Diuretic-induced hepatic encephalopathy
   e. All of the above

Ans. e

Explanation: According to International Ascites Club, refractory ascites is defined as "ascites that cannot be mobilized or the early recurrence of which (i.e., after LVP) cannot be satisfactorily prevented by medical therapy". Once ascites becomes refractory to medical treatment, the median survival of patients is approximately 6 months.
- *Diuretic-resistant ascites:* Ascites that cannot be mobilized or the early recurrence of which cannot be prevented because of a lack of response to sodium restriction and diuretic treatment.
- *Diuretic-intractable ascites:* Ascites that cannot be mobilized or the early recurrence of which cannot be prevented because of the development of diuretic-induced complications that preclude the use of an effective diuretic dosage.

Diagnosis of refractory ascites liver cirrhosis:
- *Treatment duration:* Patients must be on intensive diuretic therapy (spironolactone 400 mg/day and furosemide 160 mg/day) for at least 1 week and on a salt-restricted diet of <90 mmol/day.
- *Lack of response:* Mean weight loss <0.8 kg over 4 days and urinary sodium output less than the sodium intake
- *Early ascites recurrence:* Reappearance of grade-2 or -3 ascites within 4 weeks of initial mobilization.
- *Diuretic-induced complications:* These are diuretic-induced hepatic encephalopathy, diuretic-induced acute kidney injury, and diuretic-induced electrolyte imbalance (hyponatremia, hypokalemia/hyperkalemia).

Suggested Reading
1. European Association for the Study of the Liver. EASL clinical practice guidelines on the management of ascites, spontaneous bacterial peritonitis, and hepatorenal syndrome in cirrhosis. J Hepatol. 2010;53:397-417.

Q.20. **Which of following is not a feature of acute liver injury?**
   a. Coagulopathy
   b. Altered level of consciousness
   c. Increased serum transaminase
   d. Abnormal bilirubin

Ans. b

Explanation: In acute liver injury (ALI), patients develop coagulopathy, but do not have any alteration to their level of consciousness; and in acute liver failure (ALF), patients develop both coagulopathy and altered mentation.

The clinical features of coagulopathy, increased serum transaminases, abnormal bilirubin, and altered mentation may be seen in variety of systemic diseases. Therefore, if there is no primary liver insult, these patients should be considered to have a secondary liver injury and management should focus on the treatment of any underlying disease.

Suggested Reading
1. European Association for the Study of the Liver. EASL Clinical Practical Guidelines on the management of acute (fulminant) liver failure. J Hepatol. 2017;66:1047-81.

Q.21. All of the following are part of management for hepatic encephalopathy in liver cirrhosis, except?
   a. Rifaximin
   b. Oral branched-chain amino acids (BCAAs)
   c. Decrease dietary protein to reduce ammonia production
   d. Correct precipitating factors

Ans. c

Explanation: Hepatic encephalopathy (HE) is a frequent complication and one of the most debilitating manifestations of liver disease, severely affecting the lives of patients and their caregivers. The agents used for hepatic encephalopathy in cirrhosis include nonabsorbable disaccharides, such as lactulose, and antibiotics, such as rifaximin. Other therapies, such as oral branched-chain amino acids (BCAAs), intravenous (IV) L-ornithine L-aspartate (LOLA), probiotics, and other antibiotics, have also been used. In the hospital, a nasogastric tube can be used to administer oral therapies in patients who are unable to swallow or have an aspiration risk.

According to ASPEN guidelines, nutrition regimens should avoid restriction of protein in patients with liver disease, and similar amount of calorie and protein should be provided as recommended for other critically ill patients.

Suggested Reading
1. McClave SA, Taylor BE, Martindale RG, Warren MM, Johnson DR, Braunschweig C, et al. Guidelines for the provision and assessment of nutrition support therapy in the adult critically ill patient: Society of Critical Care Medicine (SCCM) and American Society for Parenteral and Enteral Nutrition (A.S.P.E.N.). JPEN J Parenteral Enteral Nutr. 2016;40(2):159-211.
2. Vilstrup H, Amodio P, Bajaj J, Cordoba J, Ferenci P, Mullen KD, et al. Hepatic encephalopathy in chronic liver disease: 2014 Practice Guideline by the American Association for the Study of Liver Diseases and the European Association for the Study of the Liver. Hepatology. 2014;60(2):715-35.

Q.22. A 40-year-old female with esophageal varices presented with massive GI bleed. Despite pharmacological treatment, bleeding persisted. Balloon tamponade with Sengstaken–Blakemore tube was decided. Which is false for Sengstaken–Blakemore tube usage?
   a. Acute bleeding is likely to be controlled in 80% of the cases.
   b. The tube has three lumen and two balloons.
   c. The tube should be inserted 30 cm before inflation of the gastric balloon.
   d. Traction of approximately a bag of 500 mL IVF to be applied.
   e. Chances of bleeding are common following balloon deflation.

Ans. c

Explanation: Despite urgent endoscopic and/or pharmacological therapy, variceal bleeding cannot be controlled or recurs early in about 10–20% of patients. Shunt therapy, either shunt surgery or transjugular intrahepatic portosystemic shunt (TIPS), has proven clinical efficacy as salvage therapy for patients who fail to respond to endoscopic or pharmacological therapy.

Balloon tamponade (Sengstaken–Blackemore tube) is very effective in controlling bleeding temporarily with immediate control of hemorrhage in over 80% of patients. However, its use is associated with potentially lethal complications such as aspiration, migration, and necrosis/perforation of the esophagus with mortality rates as high as 20%. Therefore, it should be restricted to patients with uncontrollable bleeding for whom a more definitive therapy (e.g., TIPS) is planned within 24 hours of placement. Airway protection is strongly recommended when balloon tamponade is used.

Sengstaken–Blakemore tube is a three-lumen tube—one lumen to inflate gastric balloon, second lumen to inflate esophageal balloon, and third lumen to aspirate gastric contents. There is no esophageal suction port. While tube insertion, once it has gone up to 45 cm mark, its tip is expected to lie in the gastric lumen—confirm by aspirating stomach content and checking pH—position to be checked later by portable chest X-ray (CXR). Once you are sure that the tip is in the stomach, inflate the gastric balloon by inflating it with 200 mL of air. Gentle traction is applied to the tube approximately 1 pound of weight attached to tube with balance suspension traction or alternative traction, use a bag with 500 mL of NS solution.

Suggested Reading
1. Garcia-Tsao G, Sanyal AJ, Grace ND, Carey W; Practice Guidelines Committee of American Association for Study of Liver Diseases; Practice Parameters Committee of American College of Gastroenterology. Prevention and management of gastroesophageal varices and variceal hemorrhage in cirrhosis. Hepatology. 2007;46(3):922-38.
2. Lee R. Esophagogastric Tamponade Tube, Special Gastrointestinal Procedures. AACN Procedure Manual for High Acuity, Progressive, and Critical Care, 7th edition. Amsterdam: Elsevier; 2017. pp. 958-69.e1.

Q.23. Which of following is not a management for refractory ascites?
   a. Large-volume paracentesis.
   b. Transjugular intrahepatic portosystemic shunt.
   c. Fluid restriction
   d. Liver transplantation

Ans. c

Explanation: Management of refractory ascites in liver cirrhosis includes large-volume paracentesis (LVP) with albumin, diuretic therapy, insertion of transjugular intrahepatic portosystemic shunt (TIPS), and liver transplantation.

Suggested Reading
1. European Association for the Study of the Liver. EASL clinical practice guidelines on the management of ascites, spontaneous bacterial peritonitis, and hepatorenal syndrome in cirrhosis. J Hepatol. 2010;53:397-417.

Q.24. All of the following are correct about classification of hepatic encephalopathy (HE) according to underlying disease, except:
   a. Type A resulting from ALF
   b. Type B resulting predominantly from portosystemic bypass or shunting

c. Type C resulting from hepatitis C
d. Type C resulting from cirrhosis

Ans. c

Explanation: Hepatic encephalopathy should be classified according to all of the following four factors:
1. According to the underlying disease, HE is subdivided into:
   - Type A resulting from ALF
   - Type B resulting predominantly from portosystemic bypass or shunting
   - Type C resulting from cirrhosis
2. According to the severity of manifestations
3. According to its time course, HE is subdivided into:
   - Episodic HE
   - Recurrent HE denotes bouts of HE that occur with a time interval of 6 months or less.
   - Persistent HE denotes a pattern of behavioral alterations that are always present and interspersed with relapses of overt HE.
4. According to the existence of precipitating factors, HE is subdivided into:
   - No precipitated
   - Precipitated, and the precipitating factors should be specified.

Suggested Reading
1. Vilstrup H, Amodio P, Bajaj J, Cordoba J, Ferenci P, Mullen KD, et al. Hepatic Encephalopathy in Chronic Liver Disease: 2014 Practice Guideline by the American Association for the Study of Liver Diseases and the European Association for the Study of the Liver. Hepatology. 2014;60(2):715-35.

Q.25. A 43-year-old male, known case of cirrhosis, presented to the hospital with worsening of ascites and on investigation, he was found to be in acute kidney injury. All are included in diagnostic criteria of hepatorenal syndrome, except:
a. Cirrhosis without ascites
b. Cirrhosis with ascites
c. Absence of shock
d. Absence of renal parenchymal disease

Ans. a

Explanation: Hepatorenal syndrome (HRS) is defined as the occurrence of renal failure in a patient with advanced liver disease in the absence of an identifiable cause of renal failure. Thus, the diagnosis is essentially one of exclusions of other causes of renal failure.

Criteria for diagnosis of hepatorenal syndrome in cirrhosis:
- Cirrhosis with ascites
- Serum creatinine >1.5 mg/dL
- Absence of shock

- Absence of hypovolemia as defined by no sustained improvement of renal function (creatinine decreasing to <133 μmol/L) following at least 2 days of diuretic withdrawal (if on diuretics) and volume expansion with albumin at 1 g/kg/day up to maximum of 100 g/day.
- No current or recent treatment with nephrotoxic drugs
- Absence of parenchymal renal disease as defined by proteinuria <0.5 g/day, no microhematuria (<50 red cell/high-powered field) and normal renal ultrasonography.

Suggested Reading
1. European Association for the Study of the Liver. EASL clinical practice guidelines on the management of ascites, spontaneous bacterial peritonitis, and hepatorenal syndrome in cirrhosis. J Hepatol. 2010;53:397-417.

Q.26. A 52-year-old male with a history of chronic alcoholism presented to emergency department with complaint of hematemesis. Which of the following risk stratification score uses preendoscopic findings to predict rebleeding and mortality?
 a. Glasgow–Blatchford score
 b. Cedars–Sinai medical center predictive index
 c. Forrest classification
 d. Complete Rockall score

Ans. a

Explanation: Glasgow–Blatchford score relies solely on preendoscopic parameters to predict the need for interventions, rebleeding, and death; whereas, the complete Rockall score and Cedars–Sinai medical center predictive score both of have additional endoscopic criteria.

Suggested Reading
1. Klein A, Gralnek IM. Acute, nonvariceal upper gastrointestinal bleeding. Curr Opin Crit Care. 2015;21(2):154-62.

Q.27. A 32-year-old female presented with pain in abdomen and vomiting. No significant past history except deep vein thrombosis (DVT) in pregnancy. She is on no medication, except oral contraceptive pill (OCP). There is no history of any habits. Clinical examination reveals hepatomegaly, ascites, and peripheral edema. Ascitic fluid analysis shows neutrophil count = <20/mm^3 and serum-ascites albumin gradient (SAAG) of 1.4. What is likely diagnosis?
 a. Spontaneous bacterial peritonitis b. Alcoholic hepatitis
 c. Budd–Chiari syndrome d. Metastatic disease.

Ans. c

Explanation: Budd–Chiari syndrome is a congestive hepatopathy caused by blockage of hepatic veins. This syndrome occurs in 1/100,000 in the general population. Hypercoagulable state could be identified in 75% of the patients; more than one etiologic factor may play a role in 25% of the patients. Primary myeloproliferative diseases are the leading cause of the disease. Two of the hepatic veins must be blocked for clinically evident disease. Liver congestion and hypoxic damage of hepatocytes eventually result in predominantly centrilobular fibrosis. OCP is risk factor for hypercoagulable state.

Suggested Reading
1. Aydinli M, Bayraktar Y. Budd–Chiari syndrome: Etiology, pathogenesis, and diagnosis. World J Gastroenterol. 2007;13(19):2693-6.

Q.28. **A patient with liver cirrhosis presented with upper GI bleed. All are effective for acute management, except:**
   a. Terlipressin
   b. Coagulation correction
   c. Propranolol
   d. Endoscopic intervention

Ans. c

Explanation:
- Endoscopic management is recommended as preferred treatment to unstable patients with severe acute upper GI bleed immediately after resuscitation and within 24 hours of admission to stable patients.
- Vasoconstrictors like Terlipressin are recommended and should be started immediately and continued for 5 days.
- Nonselective β-blocker (NSBB) is recommended as secondary prophylaxis.
- Base decisions on blood transfusion on the full clinical picture, recognizing that overtransfusion may be as damaging as undertransfusion. A restrictive transfusion policy aiming for a hemoglobin of 70–80 g/L is suggested in hemodynamically stable patients.
- Offer platelet transfusion to patients who are actively bleeding and have a platelet count of <50 × 109/L.
- Offer fresh frozen plasma to patients who have either:
  - A fibrinogen level of 1.5 times normal
  - A prothrombin time (international normalized ratio) or activated partial thromboplastin time >1.5 times normal

Suggested Reading
1. Tripathi D, Stanley AJ, Hayes PC, Patch D, Millson C, Mehrzad H, et al. U.K. guidelines on management of variceal haemorrhage in cirrhotic patients. Gut. 2015;64(11):1680-704.

Q.29. **A 56-year-old gentleman, a case of decompensated chronic liver diseases, had multiple episodes of hepatorenal syndrome (HRS). His last creatinine at the time of hospital admission was 2.5 mg. Which of the following factors are involved in pathophysiology of hepatorenal syndrome in cirrhosis?**
   a. Splanchnic vasodilatation
   b. Increased synthesis of several vasoactive mediators
   c. Cirrhotic cardiomyopathy
   d. All of above

Ans. d

Explanation:
There are four factors involved in the pathogenesis of HRS:
1. Development of splanchnic vasodilatation, which causes a reduction in effective arterial blood volume and a decrease in mean arterial pressure.
2. Activation of the sympathetic nervous system and the renin–angiotensin–aldosterone system, which causes renal vasoconstriction and a shift in the renal autoregulatory curve, which makes renal blood flow much more sensitive to changes in mean arterial pressure.
3. Impairment of cardiac function due to the development of cirrhotic cardiomyopathy, which leads to a relative impairment of the compensatory increase in cardiac output secondary to vasodilatation.
4. Increased synthesis of several vasoactive mediators, which may affect renal blood flow or glomerular microcirculatory hemodynamics, such as cysteinyl leukotrienes, thromboxane A2, F2-isoprostanes, and endothelin-1; yet the role of these factors in the pathogenesis of HRS remains unknown.

Suggested Reading
1. European Association for the Study of the Liver. EASL clinical practice guidelines on the management of ascites, spontaneous bacterial peritonitis, and hepatorenal syndrome in cirrhosis. J Hepatol. 2010;53:397-17.

Q.30. Which of the following are mechanisms of impaired gas exchange in hepatopulmonary syndrome in cirrhosis?
   a. Presence of direct AV communication
   b. Diffusion limitation
   c. V/Q mismatch
   d. All the above

Ans. d

Explanation: Hepatopulmonary syndrome (HPS) is a pulmonary vascular complication of liver disease, which adversely affects prognosis. The disease is characterized by intrapulmonary vascular dilatations and shunts, resulting in impaired gas exchange. A complex interaction between the liver, the gut, and the lungs, predominately impacting pulmonary endothelial cells, immune cells, and respiratory epithelial cells, is responsible for the development of typical pulmonary alterations seen in HPS.

The development of impaired gas exchange in HPS has been attributed to three mechanisms resulting from alterations in the alveolar microcirculation: V/Q mismatch, diffusion limitation, and the presence of direct AV communications. V/Q mismatch results from increased pulmonary blood flow due to microvascular alterations, while ventilation remains unchanged. Diffusion limitation occurs because oxygen must travel a greater distance to bind hemoglobin due to vascular dilation. Direct AV communications bypass the alveolar microcirculation, resulting in direct mixing of venous and arterial blood.

Suggested Reading
1. Raevens S, Boret M, Fallon MB. Hepatopulmonary syndrome. JHEP Rep. 2022;4:100527.

Q.31. Which of the following is not a component of Milan criteria used for liver transplantation in hepatocellular carcinoma?
   a. Single tumor not >5 cm or three tumors none >3 cm
   b. Absence of macrovascular invasion
   c. Tumor >6 cm
   d. Absence of extrahepatic spread

Ans. c

Explanation: Liver transplantation is best treatment modality for patients with liver cirrhosis and hepatocellular carcinoma. Milan criteria include following:
- *Tumor size/number:* <5 cm single tumor or three tumors none >3 cm
- Absence of macrovascular invasion
- No extrahepatic diseases
- Recurrence rate <15% over 5 years

Suggested Reading
1. Mazzaferro V, Regalia E, Doci R, Andreola S, Pulvirenti A, Bozzetti F, et al. Liver transplantation for treatment of small hepatocellular carcinoma in patients with cirrhosis. N Engl J Med. 1996;334(11):693-9.

Q.32. Which of following is incorrect about acute acalculous cholecystitis?
   a. Mortality rate is high.
   b. Common in older men
   c. Predominance among younger and middle-aged
   d. Prognosis is better in acute calculous cholecystitis than acute acalculous cholecystitis.

Ans. c

Explanation: Acalculous cholecystitis is most common in older men. The mortality rate is high, ranging from 10 to 50% compared with a 1% mortality rate in patients with calculous cholecystitis. Patients with a history of trauma, burn, surgery, hemodynamic instability, prolonged immobility, and fasting are at highest risks for acalculous cholecystitis.

Suggested Reading
1. Gallaher JR, Charles A. Acute cholecystitis: A review. JAMA. 2022;327(10):965-75.

CHAPTER

Critical Care Nutrition

Sanjith Saseedharan

Q.1. All patients who get admitted to the intensive care unit need a nutritional risk screening. When it comes to nutritional screening, the preferable way to do it is:
a. Take the weight loss and albumin level of the patient.
b. Look at triceps skinfold thickness and calf circumference
c. The NUTRIC score and the NRS 2002 remain the gold standard in screening of critically ill patient.
d. There is no gold standard to screen malnutrition in patient who is critically ill.

Ans. d

Explanation: Patients entering to the intensive care unit (ICU) have a higher risk of malnutrition as compared to admissions at various other wards and it is clear that nutritional screening should be performed within 24 hours of admission to the ICU. Anthropometric data and laboratory values such as albumin and weight loss cannot be taken individually or as a group to assess nutrition. The Nutrition Risk Screening (NRS) 2002 factored recent dietary intake, disease severity, and weight loss, and a high NRS 2002 score (>3) was able to predict poor outcomes in noncritically ill patients, but not in critically ill patients. As per this tool, any patient with APACHE score >10 will fall into the high-risk category. The NUTRTIC score was developed for critically ill patients; however, this score did not include nutritional parameters and has not been tested in a randomized clinical trial. However, major nutritional societies such as the ASPEN and the Society of Critical Care Medicine guidelines suggest using either NRS 2002 or NUTRIC/m NUTRIC for nutritional screening in critically ill patients. However, at this present juncture there is no gold standard in the screening of malnutrition in critically ill patients.

Suggested Reading
1. McClave SA, Taylor BE, Martindale RG, Warren MM, Johnson DR, Braunschweig C, et al. Guidelines for the provision and assessment of nutrition support therapy in the adult critically ill patient: Society of critical care medicine (SCCM) and American Society for Parenteral and Enteral Nutrition (A.S.P.E.N.). J Parenter Enteral Nutr. 2016;40(2): 159-211.
2. Narayan SK, Gudivada KK, Krishna B. Assessment of nutritional status in the critically ill. Indian J Crit Care Med. 2020;24(Suppl 4):S152-6.

Q.2. The diagnosis of malnutrition is essential in the ICU for directing goal-directed nutritional interventions and monitoring. The Global Leadership Initiative on Malnutrition (GLIM) criteria have potential benefits in this area. The GLIM criteria would include:
  a. GLIM criteria consist of weight loss and low BMI.
  b. A weight loss of >5% in last month along with a closed head injury would qualify for the diagnosis of malnutrition.
  c. Consuming <50% of the energy requirements for >1 week qualifies as malnourishment.
  d. BMI of 21 with diarrheal illness for 4 days qualifies for diagnosis of malnutrition.

Ans. b

Explanation: To form a common malnutrition language and thus develop global standards, the Global Leadership Initiative on Malnutrition (GLIM) was convened by several of the major global clinical nutrition societies. Diagnosis of malnutrition needs a two-step process which includes screening (using any of the validated screening tools like NRS 2002 NUTRIC/mNUTRIC, etc.) followed by diagnosis assessment (using the GLIM criteria). The diagnosis of malnutrition would require one etiologic criterion and one phenotypic criterion. The etiologic criteria would include criteria for weight loss (>5% within past 6 months, or >10% beyond 6 months) or low body mass index (<18.5 if <70 or <20 if >70 years) or reduced muscle mass (reduced by validated body composition measuring technique). The phenotypic criteria would involve reduced food intake [≤50% of ER >1 week, or any reduction for >2 weeks, or any chronic gastrointestinal (GI) condition that adversely impacts food assimilation or absorption] or assimilation and inflammation (acute disease/injury or chronic disease related). Here, it is important to note the GLIM criteria needs still be vigorously studied in critically ill patients. Some studies have also demonstrated the potential in critically ill patients and there seems no reason to believe that it may not do so.

Suggested Reading
  1. Cederholm T, Jensen GL, Correia MITD, Gonzalez MC, Fukushima R, Higashiguchi T, et al.; GLIM Core Leadership Committee; GLIM Working Group. GLIM criteria for the diagnosis of malnutrition—A consensus report from the global clinical nutrition community. Clin Nutr. 2019;38(1):1-9.
  2. Díaz G, T D Correia MI, Gonzalez MC, Reyes M. The global leadership initiative on malnutrition criteria for the diagnosis of malnutrition in patients admitted to the intensive care unit: A systematic review and meta-analysis. Clin Nutr. 2023;42(2):182-9.

Q.3. In critically ill patients, it is advisable to start medical nutrition therapy and for the conduct of this:
  a. It is important to pass nasogastric tube routinely to feed these patients well.
  b. Immediate commencement of parenteral nutrition is found to be beneficial.
  c. An oral diet is the preferred form of nutrition.
  d. A combination of oral and parenteral nutrition is optimum.

Ans. c

Explanation: There is strong consensus among major guidelines groups and societies that the oral route is the preferred route of nutrition in critically ill patients who are able to eat with a gradual progression to full feeds which is defined as approximately 70% of the energy expenditure. It is not advisable to feed to 100% of the energy goals. A routine use of nasogastric tube is not indicated in order to feed the patient. If the patient is unable to take oral nutritional therapy then it is important to start enteral nutrition (EN) and progressively increase the rate as per local protocols. It is advisable to avoid commencement of parenteral nutrition till all attempts at using the gut have been exhausted. A combination of oral and parenteral nutrition is not recommended to be routinely used. However, a combination of parenteral nutrition (supplemental) can be considered at 5-7 days if oral nutrition cannot reach at least 70% of the energy requirements. However, if a patient has been classified as high-nutrition risk by any criteria and EN is not feasible at all (for example, has mesenteric ischemia with gangrene bowel), we should consider the use of parenteral nutrition at a lower dose. At this point, it is important to remember that there is a risk of refeeding which needs to be kept in mind.

Suggested Reading
1. Dhaliwal R, Cahill N, Lemieux M, Heyland DK. The Canadian Critical Care Nutrition guidelines in 2013: an update on current recommendations and implementation strategies. Nutr Clin Pract. 2014;29:29-43.
2. Singer P, Blaser AR, Berger MM, Alhazzani W, Calder PC, Casaer MP, et al. ESPEN guideline on clinical nutrition in the intensive care unit. Clin Nutr. 2019;38(1):48-79.
3. Taylor BE, McClave SA, Martindale RG, Warren MM, Johnson DR, Braunschweig C, et al. Guidelines for the provision and assessment of nutrition support therapy in the adult critically ill patient: Society of Critical Care Medicine (SCCM) and American Society for Parenteral and Enteral Nutrition (A.S.P.E.N.). Crit Care Med. 2016;44:390-438.

Q.4. In the event that the patient needs enteral nutrition:
   a. It is advisable to secure postpyloric access as the incidence of aspiration would reduce.
   b. There is clear data that bolus nutrition is better than continuous nutrition.
   c. A nasogastric access is the recommended route during the initiation of enteral nutrition if oral nutrition is insufficient.
   d. There is no indication of postpyloric feeding in critically ill patients.

Ans. c

Explanation: In patients where there is insufficient oral intake, which means <70% of energy requirements, there should be consideration for the use for a nasogastric tube and feeding via this route. This route can be easily secured by passing a nasogastric tube in comparison to a postpyloric tube, which entails the requirement of specialized team, specialized care, specialized feeding, specialized tube, and an extra cost. Postpyloric route should not be considered as a routine in critically ill patient. However, there are certain indications for postpyloric feeding. Consideration should be given for postpyloric route in the event that the patient has a high chance of aspiration. Postpyloric

EN has been associated with a decrease in ventilator-acquired pneumonia but has not shown any superiority when it comes to length of ventilation, ICU or hospital stay, or mortality. When it comes to method of feeding, there is no clear data to confirm that bolus feeding is superior to continuous form of nutrition. Bolus feeding is known to stimulate protein production. Continuous nutrition was associated with a lower risk of diarrhea as compared to bolus nutrition. Both the feeding types appear to achieve the same gastric volume, caloric delivery, time to goal therapy, and insulin requirement. Studies have not demonstrated a discernible clinical advantage of one form of therapy as compared to the other.

Suggested Reading
1. Mahadeva S, Malik A, Hilmi I, Qua CS, Wong CH, Goh KL. Difference in reflux between duodenal and jejunal transnasal endoscopic placement of nasoenteric feeding tubes: outcomes and limitations in non-critically ill patients. Nutr Clin Pract. 2008;23:176-81.
2. Patel JJ, Rosenthal MD, Heyland DK. Intermittent versus continuous feeding in critically ill adults. Curr Opin Clin Nutr Metab Care. 2018;21:116-20.

Q.5. When feeding the patient via nasogastric tube:
 a. Gastric residuals >200 mL are considered significant and should involve automatic cessation of feeding.
 b. In the event that there is increased gastric residual volume (GRV) then immediate conversion to nasojejunal route should be done.
 c. The use of prokinetic agents should be considered when there are increased gastric residual volumes.
 d. Parenteral nutrition should be started when there are increased gastric residual volumes for fear of aspiration.

Ans. c

Explanation: Major societies like the ASPEN have suggested to avoid checking the gastric residual volumes routinely for patients receiving enteral nutrition. The ESPEN suggests withholding feeds in the event that the gastric residual volume exceeds >500 mL/6 hours. However, it is important to note that there is no association of high-gastric residuals and infection. In spite of these recommendations, it is a common practice in many ICUs to monitor gastric residuals. Gastric residual volume measurement is not well standardized; they are operator, patient, and tube dependent. In the event there is an increase in gastric residual volume of >500 mL in 6 hours, it is prudent to initiate measures to tackle this. After ensuring that this is not an acute abdominal problem (e.g., perforation), it is very important to consider the use of prokinetics as there is clear evidence to suggest improved enteral feed tolerance. Here, there is a definite role of erythromycin and, if required, metoclopramide for a period of 48 hours. In the event that even after 48 hours the problem of the GRV is not solved, then this would need securing a nasojejunal tube. Commencement of parenteral nutrition should be delayed till all attempts to feed the patient enterally have failed.

Suggested Reading
1. Lewis K, Alqahtani Z, McIntyre L, Almenawer S, Alshamsi F, Rhodes A, et al. The efficacy and safety of prokinetic agents in critically ill patients receiving enteral nutrition: a systematic review and meta-analysis of randomized trials. Crit Care. 2016;20:259.
2. Rhodes A, Evans LE, Alhazzani W, Levy MM, Antonelli M, Ferrer R, et al. Surviving sepsis initiative. Intensive Care Med. 2017;43:304-77.

Q.6. When determining the right amount of kcal to be delivered to a critically ill mechanically ventilated patient, the optimal method/equation to use is:
   a. Harris–Benedict formula
   b. Penn State equation
   c. Simple predictive equations
   d. Indirect calorimetry

Ans. d

Explanation: Worldwide, it is a practice to use predictive equations. However, the predictive equations do not have agreement among themselves too. Many predictive equations like the Harris–Benedict equations also have the multiplication of a stress factor to factor the illness severity. However, what we know is that the predictive equations are not optimal and may lead to overfeeding and underfeeding of our critically ill patient. Simple weight-based predictive equations also have an inherent disability to monitor weight as it is difficult to do so in bedridden mechanically ventilated patients, and beds available to do so are very costly. Also, it is important to understand that patients go from various states from admission to discharge and hence will have different energy expenditures at different time periods and the same equation cannot be used in such different periods. The gold standard in the determination of energy expenditure in the intensive care unit is to use indirect calorimetry. In the absence of indirect calorimetry, one can determine VO_2 from the pulmonary catheter or VCO_2 from the ventilator, which will give more accurate values (however not as accurate as the indirect calorimeter) than predictive equations.

Suggested Reading
1. Frankenfield DC, Coleman A, Alam S, Cooney RN. Analysis of estimation methods for resting metabolic rate in critically ill adults. J Parenter Enteral Nutr. 2009;33:27-36.
2. Oshima T, Graf S, Heiddeger CP, Genton L, Pugin J, Pichard C. Can calculation of energy expenditure based on CO_2 measurements replace indirect calorimetry? Crit Care. 2017;21:13.

Q.7. When it comes to energy expenditure as monitored by indirect calorimetry:
   a. Indirect calorimetry can be done in spontaneously breathing patients.
   b. In mechanically ventilated polytrauma patient with intercostal drainage, the indirect calorimetry can easily be performed.
   c. There is data to show mortality benefit with the use of indirect calorimetry.
   d. Indirect calorimetry can also give protein requirements.

Ans. a

Explanation: Indirect calorimetry (IC) is used for the measurement of energy expenditure (REE or kcal). IC does not give the protein requirements. Accurate measurement of energy expenditure can be performed in mechanically ventilated as well as spontaneously breathing patients. In fact, the Q-NRG® is the only commercially available IC tested against mass spectrometry to ensure gas accuracy, while being very easy-to-use. However, there are few caveats in the performance of IC, which include the following. The ventilator system and connections should be leak free. In the presence of leak, there would be an underestimation of resting energy expenditure (REE). The measurement cannot be performed when there is active resuscitation or changes being done on the ventilator (for example, a hyperventilation). The measurement should also be avoided during hemodialysis and peritoneal dialysis. The presence of high levels of PEEP and use of anesthetic gases may also interfere with the IC readings and invalidate the same. There is no data to demonstrate a mortality benefit when it comes to IC. There is also an error in measurement when the fraction of inspired oxygen (FiO_2) approaches 80% and hence IC cannot be performed at these FiO_2.

Suggested Reading
1. Bishop M, Benson MS, Pierson DJ. Carbon dioxide excretion via bronchopleural fistulas in adult respiratory distress syndrome. Chest. 1987;91:400-4.
2. Henneberg S, Soderberg D, Groth T, Stjernsrom H, Wiklund L. Carbon dioxide production during mechanical ventilation. Crit Care Med. 1987;15:8-12.
3. Norton AC. Accuracy in pulmonary measurement. Respir Care. 1979;24:131-7.
4. Oshima T, Delsoglio M, Dupertuis YM, Singer P, De Waele E, Veraar C, et al. The clinical evaluation of the new indirect calorimeter developed by the ICALIC project. Clin Nutr. 2020;39(10):3105-11.

Q.8. Energy provision for chronic kidney disease (CKD) patients is very important for the overall health of these patients. In this aspect, the true statement here is:
a. The average energy requirement for a patient on renal replacement therapy is 40 kcal/kg/day.
b. Weight-based simple predictive equations are the most accurate method to judge the energy requirements in these patients on continuous veno-venous hemofiltration (CVVH).
c. Indirect calorimetry can be done while the patient is on intermittent hemodialysis.
d. Indirect calorimetry can be done while the patient is on continuous renal replacement therapy (CRRT).

Ans. d

Explanation: It is important to note that when energy provision was increased to 40 kcal/kg/day, there was no improvement in the nitrogen balance; however, there was an increased incidence of hyperglycemia and hypertriglyceridemia. Hence, to provide the right amount of energy for these patients is extremely difficult as weight is not only difficult to measure, but also the fluid shifts in these patients makes it impossible to judge the right reference weight and hence the right amount of energy requirements making this a fallacy of the simple weight-based predictive equations. Hence, indirect calorimetry is the only way to figure out the real energy requirements in these patients. However, there are some caveats in the performance of indirect calorimetry. Indirect calorimetry needs to be performed 2 hours after a session on intermittent hemodialysis to improve the precision of the measurement. Theoretically during CRRT, it is known that a good amount of effluent is removed via the effluent and hence the VCO_2 estimates might not be OK, which may thus make the REE not very accurate. However, what has been seen in a study is that the influence of CO_2 is actually minimal and thus the measurement is reasonably better than predictive equations.

Suggested Reading
1. Fiaccadori E, Maggiore U, Rotelli C, Giacosa R, Picetti E, Parenti E, et al. Effects of different energy intakes on nitrogen balance in patients with acute renal failure: a pilot study. Nephrol Dial Transplant. 2005;20:1976-80.
2. Jonckheer J, Demol J, Lanckmans K, Malbrain M, Spapen H, De Waele E. MECCIAS trial: metabolic consequences of continuous veno-venous hemofiltration on indirect calorimetry. Clin Nutr. 2020;39(12):3797-803.
3. Jonckheer J, Spapen H, Debain A, Demol J, Diltoer M, Costa O, et al. CO_2 and O_2 removal during continuous veno-venous hemofiltration: a pilot study. BMC Nephrol. 2019;20:222.

Q.9. With regards to energy provision in acute liver failure, all are true, except:
a. The energy requirement in acute liver failure is usually increased.
b. The intake of energy has a clear relation to muscle mass.
c. A minimum of 1.5–2 g/kg of carbohydrate per day is required in these patients.
d. A disease-specific (liver-specific formula feed) feed is known to improve outcomes in these patients.

Ans. d

Explanation: Energy requirement in acute liver failure is generally increased by 15–30% and it is important to note that the optimal intake of energy, protein, and essential amino acids is necessary in maintaining muscle mass and avoiding sarcopenia, which portends a poor prognosis in these patients. Hence, the gold standard in estimating energy requirements in this group of patients remains the use of indirect calorimetry. These patients are also known to develop hepatic glycolysis and impaired gluconeogenesis, which predispose these patients to recurrent hypoglycemia and hence require accurate glycemia monitoring. Disease-specific formulae do not make any difference in acute liver failure patients. There is no data to show that branched-chain amino acid (BCAA)-enriched formula makes any difference in outcomes in acute liver failure patients. However, it is important to note that there are a very few studies in this regards.

Suggested Reading
1. Abenavoli L, Maurizi V, Boccuto L, Di Berardino A, Giostra N, Santori P, et al. Nutritional support in acute liver failure. Diseases. 2022;10(4):108.

Q.10. A 66-year-old female gets admitted to the intensive care unit with an acute exacerbation of chronic obstructive pulmonary disease (COPD) along with diarrhea. She was also given a fluid resuscitation on arrival to the emergency room (ER) in view of a low blood pressure. An X-ray revealed a pneumothorax too and an implantable cardioverter-defibrillator (ICD) was promptly placed. The energy

requirements were measured by using indirect calorimetry. However, with regards to the assessment of the protein, the right statement is:
a. This can be easily done by assessing nitrogen balance in such acutely ill individuals.
b. Albumin is a good judge of protein status during enteral nutrition.
c. A bioelectrical impedance analysis is a good option in this patient to assess lean body mass and skeletal muscle mass status, and thus protein status.
d. Computed tomography (CT) has emerged as very well-validated tool in the assessment of sarcopenia and thus assessment of protein malnutrition.

Ans. d

Explanation: Nitrogen balance needs a 24-hour urinary collection, which is a cumbersome procedure in ICU patients. There are simplified equations for the same. However, these equations usually are not right as they do not take into consideration losses from wounds, drainage tubes, pulmonary and gastrointestinal output. Moreover, patients requiring ICU due to critical illness and patients with renal insufficiency need corrections for elevations in blood urea, which again is an estimation. Hence, it is definitely not an easy task to find the nitrogen balance in critically ill individuals. Albumin has a half-life of around 20 days and hence will not be a great judge to monitor trends in short intervals. In fact, all the capillary leakage that is associated with critical illness will make the serum albumin appear to be falsely low. Hence, serum albumin is not a good judge for protein status. Bioelectrical impedance analysis (BIA) has been proven to be a good tool in the assessment of healthy individuals and the patients in whom there are no major shifts in fluids. Hence, this may not be a great tool in our patient who has just had a major fluid resuscitation.

Suggested Reading
1. Serón-Arbeloa C, Labarta-Monzón L, Puzo-Foncillas J, Mallor-Bonet T, Lafita-López A, Bueno-Vidales N, et al. Malnutrition screening and assessment. Nutrients. 2022;14(12):2392. doi: 10.3390/nu14122392.

Q.11. Proteins are an essential requirement of critically ill patient. In this aspect, which among the following is the right answer?
a. The protein requirement of a hospitalized chronic kidney patient should be 0.8 g/kg.
b. The protein requirement for critically ill patient is 1.5–2.5 g/kg per day.
c. Protein intake should be deferred in case of high ammonia with acute hepatic failure and cerebral edema.
d. High-protein intake could contribute to higher serum creatinine.

Ans. a

Explanation: All normal healthy individuals require >0.8 g/kg of proteins. Critical illness is a catabolic state and hence these patients may lose protein signified and shown as a drop in muscle mass daily while being admitted to the ICU. Hence, there is a clear role in the provision of adequate proteins. Studies have demonstrated survival benefits when >80% of the protein goals are met clearly showing a dose-dependent mortality advantage. Patient admitted to the intensive care unit will require 1.3-1.5 g/kg of proteins daily. Patient who has chronic kidney disease and is hospitalized for any other issue should receive 0.6-0.8 g/kg/day of proteins. These are patients who have noncatabolic conditions where they could be metabolically stable and thus do not require increased protein regimens. However, in the presence of high ammonia (especially >150 mmol/L), it may be wise to defer the delivery of proteins for 24-48 hours till the ammonia is corrected and the encephalopathy improves. This is because this may be a short-lived entity, and risks of cerebral edema as a result of ammonia from the protein delivery may be much higher than the benefits of delivering a protein load. Importantly, it is logical to repeat ammonia when commencing to deliver proteins.

Suggested Reading
1. Fiaccadori E, Sabatino A, Barazzoni R, Carrero JJ, Cupisti A, De Waele E, et al. ESPEN guideline on clinical nutrition in hospitalized patients with acute or chronic kidney disease. Clin Nutr. 2021;40(4):1644-68.
2. Plauth M, Bernal W, Dasarathy S, Merli M, Plank LD, Schütz T, et al. ESPEN guideline on clinical nutrition in liver disease. Clin Nutr. 2019;38(2):485-521.
3. Scheinkestel CD, Adams F, Mahony L, Bailey M, Davies AR, Nyulasi I, et al. Impact of increasing parenteral protein loads on amino acid levels and balance in critically ill anuric patients on continuous renal replacement therapy. Nutrition. 2003;19:733-40.

Q.12. When it comes to protein delivery in patients undergoing renal replacement therapy, all of the following are true, except:
  a. Patients with acute kidney injury (AKI) on intermittent hemodialysis should be provided with 1.3-1.5 g/kg/day of proteins.
  b. Patients with AKI on prolonged CRRT should be provided with 1.5-2 g/kg/day of proteins.
  c. In patients with AKI, proteins should be reduced or delayed to prevent hemodialysis.
  d. Total nitrogen loss in a patient on CRRT is about 25 g/day.

Ans. b

Explanation: Medical nutrition therapy with proteins supplementation is required during any form of renal replacement therapy or in any stage of AKI or CKD. The protein catabolic rate is not influenced by the provision or delivery of nutrition and hence proteins should be reduced to avoid or delay renal replacement therapy. In CRRT, apart from uremic toxins and macronutrients including small proteins and peptides, micronutrients, such as amino acids, glucose, trace elements, and water-soluble vitamins, are cleared from the patient's blood into the effluent. Small studies have demonstrated a high-protein catabolic rate (1.2-2.1 g/kg/d) among patients who are on CRRT and intermittent hemodialysis with a typical nitrogen loss of around 25 g/day. What is also known is that patients who received a higher dose of proteins, >1.5-2 g/kg/day, achieved a positive nitrogen balance. A positive nitrogen balance in these cases is known to impact survival and morbidity in these groups of patients. Major societies like the ESPEN have recommended a total protein intake of up to 1.7 g/kg/day on CRRT, and the ASPEN has recommended 2-2.5 g/kg/day for such group of patients. What is also known is that >2–2.5 g/kg/day will not cause an increase in blood urea nitrogen (BUN) necessitating an increase in the CRRT dose or increase in the amino acid loss.

Suggested Reading
1. Fishman G, Pierre S. Metabolic and nutritional aspects in continuous renal replacement therapy. J Intens Med. 2023. Article in press.
2. Ganesan MV, Annigeri RA, Shankar B, Rao BS, Prakash KC, Seshadri R, et al. The protein equivalent of nitrogen appearance in critically ill acute renal failure patients undergoing continuous renal replacement therapy. J Ren Nutr. 2009;19:161-6.

Q.13. A 60-year-old male was admitted to the hospital with very low blood pressure and pain in the abdomen. He needed large-volume resuscitation. The resuscitation continued to the next day and he needed additional vasopressor support. Over a period of the day, his vasopressor requirement increased and he did require high doses of noradrenaline, adrenaline, and vasopressin. In such a scenario, what among the following is correct?
a. Even trickle feeding should not be attempted.
b. There is an increased incidence of adverse outcomes or effects when full enteral nutrition is initiated in patients with unstable hemodynamics.
c. Even with controlled shock, it is wise to withhold enteral nutrition.
d. It is impossible to identify intestinal ischemia and hence it is important not to feed such patients.

Ans. b

Explanation: Patients on vasopressors with hemodynamic instability are a specific group where the benefits of feeding the patient should be weighed against the risks of doing so. There is data to suggest that absorption is not completely hampered but it is only delayed owing to hypomotility. Hence, administration of trickle feeds can be attempted without side effects. However, when full enteral nutrition is attempted in such patients with hemodynamic instability, there is an increased incidence of bowel ischemia and acute colonic pseudo-obstruction. In the presence of controlled shock, however, enteral nutrition should be started slowly and progressed over the next 3–5 days to full feeding. Here, it is also wise to note that studies have documented that around 3–10 μg/kg/min of dopamine, 12 μg/kg/min of dobutamine, and 6–25 μg/min of norepinephrine are safe for EN tolerance. At this time, it is important to monitor for feed intolerance and worsening of hemodynamic status. The usual signs seen include vomiting, diarrhea, and abdominal pain, which signify feed intolerance. Problems of ischemia can be identified by the presence of abdominal distension; pain disproportionate to physical examination of the abdomen, high nasogastric output, metabolic acidosis without obvious cause, and digestive hemorrhage may be indicative of this complication, although there are no specific clinical signs or markers for early diagnosis. There are also radiological signs such as thickened loops of bowel with thumbprinting, air in the wall of gastrointestinal tract, portal venous gas, and air in the peritoneal space, which can help in the identification of this side effect.

Suggested Reading
1. Berger MM, Berger-Gryllaki M, Wiesel PH, Revelly JP, Hurni M, Cayeux C, et al. Intestinal absorption in patients after cardiac surgery. Crit Care Med. 2000;28(7):2217-23.
2. Reignier J, Boisramé-Helms J, Brisard L, Lascarrou JB, Ait Hssain A, Anguel N, et al. NUTRIREA-2 trial investigators; clinical research in intensive care and sepsis (CRICS) group. Enteral versus parenteral early nutrition in ventilated adults with shock: a randomised, controlled, multicentre, open-label, parallel-group study (NUTRIREA-2). Lancet. 2018;391:133-43.

Q.14. When all attempts made to establish enteral nutrition have been failed then it is advisable to start parenteral nutrition. All of the following are metabolic complications of parenteral nutrition, except:
a. Fluid overload
b. Hypoglycemia
c. Fat overload syndrome
d. Hypersensitivity reactions

Ans. b

Explanation: Parenteral nutrition would require the administration of a large volume to meet the energy and protein requirements. Needless to say that this can lead to fluid overload in the critically ill patients which may cause complications that include pulmonary edema, generalized edema, and related issues. Hence, it becomes imperative to watch the fluid balance in such situations. Because of the high amount of glucose load in parenteral nutrition, there are always a chance of hyperglycemia and its related complications including increased chances of infections, etc. A limited ability to metabolize fat and a prolonged clearance time sometimes seen in critically ill patient may rarely lead to fat overload syndrome in patients on intravenous lipid emulsion containing total parenteral nutrition. This can be noticed by sudden anemia, leukopenia, thrombocytopenia, fatty infiltration of liver, hepatomegaly, and central nervous system manifestation. An allergic reaction characterized by tachypnea, tachycardia, fever, hypotension, nausea, vomiting, headache, and dizziness may develop in any patient being infused with parenteral nutrition as a result of a hypersensitivity reaction to any of the products being transfused.

Suggested Reading
1. Cotogni P. Management of parenteral nutrition in critically ill patients. World J Crit Care Med. 2017;6(1):13-20.

Q.15. A 55-year-old patient presented to the hospital with intractable vomiting, abdominal pain, and dehydration for 5 days. For the last 5 days, patient has had nothing by mouth due to these symptoms. He was admitted and diagnosed to have intestinal obstruction. He underwent surgery and was found to have gangrenous bowel with adhesion. An adhesiolysis and end-to-end anastomosis of bowel with removal of gangrenous segment were done. Post this, the patient was shifted to the ICU (almost 7 days after the event). It was decided to start this patient on parenteral nutrition. 16 hours later, this patient developed hypotension, cardiac arrhythmias, and metabolic acidosis. Considering refeeding syndrome, the correct statement is:
a. This usually occurs due to sudden drop in the insulin levels.
b. Refeeding syndrome could precipitate acute respiratory failure.

c. The diagnosis of refeeding would require a decrease in phosphorous, potassium, and magnesium.
d. Individuals with a BMI of <21 have a high chance of refeeding syndrome.

Ans. b

Explanation: Refeeding syndrome is postulated to occur due to a rise in insulin as a result of reintroduction of glucose. This would then cause hypokalemia and hypophosphatemia due to phosphorylation of glucose and stimulation of Na^+-K^+-ATPase pump. Apart from reduction in cardiac contractility and cardiac arrhythmia, the severe hypophosphatemia could cause respiratory muscle dysfunction and thus acute respiratory failure. The diagnosis of refeeding syndrome would require a decrease in any 1, 2, or 3 of serum phosphorus, potassium, and/or magnesium levels by 10–20% (mild RS), 20–30% (moderate RS), or >30% and/or organ dysfunction resulting from a decrease in any of these and/or due to thiamin deficiency (severe RS). Along with this, it is also required that these above features occur with a span of 5 days after starting feeds or substantially increasing the feeds. Patients deemed to be having a significant risk for refeeding syndrome are those whose BMI is <16 kg/m^2, with a weight loss of >7.5% in 3 month or >10% in 6 months, taking <50% of EE in the 5 days of admission in ICU, having low levels of potassium, phosphorous, and magnesium, requiring multiple doses of supplementation with evidence of severe loss of muscle and subcutaneous fat.

Suggested Reading

1. Boateng AA, Sriram K, Meguid MM, Crook M. Refeeding syndrome: treatment considerations based on collective analysis of literature case reports. Nutrition. 2010;26(2):156-67.
2. da Silva JSV, Seres DS, Sabino K, Adams SC, Berdahl GJ, Citty SW, et al.; Parenteral Nutrition Safety and Clinical Practice Committees, American Society for Parenteral and Enteral Nutrition. ASPEN Consensus Recommendations for Refeeding Syndrome. Nutr Clin Pract. 2020;35(2):178-95.

Q.16. The above patient was deemed as a high risk for refeeding syndrome due to low BMI, no feeding for >5 days, and also had repeated requirement potassium and phosphate replacement. Keeping the high chances of refeeding in mind, all except one are correct:
a. Do not initiate glucose first. First start with proteins alone with close watch on hemodynamics.
b. There is no need to restrict fluids.
c. It is important to monitor electrolytes 12 hourly.
d. Supplementing thiamine (100 mg) is a good practice in the prevention of this syndrome.

Ans. a

Explanation: The ASPEN consensus recommendations for avoidance and treatment of refeeding syndrome in at-risk individuals are that—in such a case, one should be starting with 100–150 g of glucose for the first 24 hours and gradually (by around 33%) rise every 1–2 days. However, this needs to be done when all the electrolyte abnormalities are corrected. The dextrose should be calculated from all sources, which include drug dilutions, etc. There is no need for restriction of fluids, proteins, or sodium. Potassium, calcium, and magnesium need to be monitored 12 hourly and, at times, even more frequently as sometimes there is a precipitous drop in these, which may then cause cardiac arrhythmia and death if not attended and corrected urgently. In the event that there is a drop in any of these electrolytes then it is essential to halve the dextrose or glucose load by half and reinitiate again slowly with close watch on the electrolytes and vitals. All glucose-dependent metabolic pathways will require thiamine and hence deficiency will manifest during refeeding syndrome which may lead to confusion, encephalopathy (Wernicke's syndrome and Korsakoff psychosis), oculomotor abnormalities (mainly horizontal ophthalmoplegia), hypothermia, and even coma. Inadequate ATP generation as a result of this may also cause decreased cardiac contractility and heart failure.

Suggested Reading
1. Coelho LS, Hueb JC, Minicucci MF, Azevedo PS, Paiva SA, Zornoff LA. Thiamin deficiency as a cause of reversible cor pulmonale. Arq Bras Cardiol. 2008;91(1):e7-9.
2. White JV, Guenter P, Jensen G, Malone A, Schofield M. Consensus statement: Academy of Nutrition and Dietetics and American Society for Parenteral and Enteral Nutrition: characteristics recommended for the identification and documentation of adult malnutrition (undernutrition). J Parenter Enteral Nutr. 2012;36(3):275-83.

Q.17. **A 70-year-old male presented to the hospital with a boring central pain for the last 4 days. The lipase levels were found to be elevated with leukocytosis. A CT scan revealed a picture of pancreatitis. In this situation:**
   a. It is important to start parenteral nutrition immediately.
   b. Oral feeding should be started only when the enzymes and the pain improve.
   c. Oral feeds can be attempted.
   d. Insert a nasojejunal tube immediately and start feeding.

Ans. c

Explanation: All patients of pancreatitis should be started on EN within 24-48 hours of admission. All patients for pancreatitis should be started on oral feeding if there is no gross hemodynamic embarrassment. There should not be any form of delay for improvement of pain, bowel sounds, or reduction in enzymes. Importantly, a soft diet is usually well tolerated and gives more calories and proteins when compared to a liquid diet. Some patients, who have a higher grade of severity of pancreatitis, will have intolerance and hence this has to be monitored well. Such a policy is known to be beneficial as it is associated with a shorter length of stay and a general feeling of wellbeing. Parenteral nutrition should not be attempted until all attempts of securing enteral nutrition have failed. In the event that there is intolerance to enteral nutrition via the oral route, it is advisable to first pass a nasogastric tube; in case the nasogastric tube is intolerant, then it is advisable to pass a nasojejunal tube. At this point, it is important to note that studies have demonstrated no difference when it comes to tolerance, complications rates, and mortality. Nevertheless, a small proportion of patients do develop a delayed gastric emptying and gastric outlet syndrome and may thus require nasojejunal feeding. However, a nasojejunal feed should not be placed routinely in all cases of pancreatitis.

Suggested Reading
1. Arvanitakis M, Ockenga J, Bezmarevic M, Gianotti L, Krznarić Ž, Lobo DN, et al. ESPEN guideline on clinical nutrition in acute and chronic pancreatitis. Clin Nutr. 2020;39(3):612-31.

Q.18. A 50-year-old patient presented to the ICU with the features of severe pancreatitis with >50% necrosis of the pancreas. He required large volume resuscitation. Subsequently, his intra-abdominal pressure (IAP) was measured and found to be 12 mm Hg. His pain by now had reduced:
a. As this patient has IAP of 12 mm Hg, it is not advisable to start enteral nutrition.
b. This is an optimal candidate for parenteral nutrition.
c. There is no reason to stop enteral feeding even if the IAP is >20 mm Hg.
d. It is recommended to start nasojejunal feeding if the IAP is >15 mm Hg.

Ans. d

Explanation: One of the after effects of large-volume resuscitation is raised intra-abdominal pressure and abdominal compartment syndrome. This is defined as sustained pressure of >12 mm Hg, whereas abdominal compartment syndrome is defined as a sustained increase in intra-abdominal pressure of >20 mm Hg associated with a new organ dysfunction or failure. Patients of severe acute pancreatitis have raised resting energy expenditure and excessive nitrogen losses. It has been clearly demonstrated that EN in patients with severe AP reduces mortality and infectious complications, decreases organ failure and surgical intervention rate, has a trend toward reduction of hospital stay, and is safer and more effective than PN. In the presence of severe pancreatitis and intra-abdominal hypertension of <15, a nasogastric feeding could be attempted; however, the preferred route remains to be nasojejunal feed. Patients with intra-abdominal pressure of >15 mm Hg and acute pancreatitis are known to have increased gastrointestinal symptoms and signs (absence of bowel movements, abdominal distension, high gastric residual volume, etc.), and it is advisable to use the nasojejunal route for initiation of enteral nutrition.

Suggested Reading
1. McClave SA, Taylor BE, Martindale RG, Warren MM, Johnson DR, Braunschweig C, et al. Guidelines for the provision and assessment of nutrition support therapy in the adult critically ill patient: Society of Critical Care Medicine (SCCM) and American Society for Parenteral and Enteral Nutrition (A.S.P.E.N.). J Parenter Enter Nutr. 2016;40:159-211.
2. Reintam Blaser A, Malbrain M, Regli A. Abdominal pressure and gastrointestinal function: an inseparable couple? Anaesthesiol Intensive Ther. 2017;49:146-58.

Q.19. A 50-year-old gentleman was admitted to the surgical ICU after a Whipple surgery for CA pancreas. Patient is hemodynamically stable on admission. This patient was otherwise healthy and did not have any feature of malnutrition prior to surgery. Considering the nutrition care plan in this case, all of the following are false, except:
a. This patient will be not benefitted with nutrition enriched with omega-3 fatty acids and arginine.

b. Oral glutamine supplementation is very important during these stressful conditions.
c. It would have been beneficial to provide nutrition therapy for a period of 7-14 days.
d. This patient should be started on early tube feeding.

Ans. c

Explanation: Cancer itself is a cachectic and catabolic state. However, this is not the norm. All cancer patients may not be malnourished. Immune-enhancing formulae (enriched with arginine, nucleotides, and omega-3 fatty acids), however, should be given perioperatively. Studies have shown that this practice decreased rate of postoperative complications and consequently to a decreased length of stay in the hospital. In fact, there are studies to show that at least 5-6 days of immune-enriched supplements preoperatively have improved outcomes for surgeries involving the upper GI malignancy. It is only in patients who have very severe malnourishment indicated by any one of the following: weight loss >10-15% within 6 months, BMI <18.5 kg/m^2, serum albumin <30 g/dL, and NRS >5 that it is advisable to postpone surgery if required in order to provide nutritional therapy for a period of 7-14 days. There is no evidence to recommend the use of oral glutamine for such patients. However, in the event that patient is on exclusive parenteral nutrition then it may be beneficial to supplement with IV glutamine at a dose of 0.5 g/kg/d because this practice is not only safe but also has shown to reduce the rate of infections. All patients after Whipple surgery should be started on oral diet within 24-48 hours after surgery. Early tube feeding (within 24 hours) shall be initiated in patients in whom early oral nutrition cannot be started, and in whom oral intake will be inadequate.

Suggested Reading
1. Braga M, Gianotti L, Radaelli G, Vignali A, Mari G, Gentilini O, et al. Perioperative immunonutrition in patients undergoing cancer surgery: results of a randomized double-blind phase 3 trial. Arch Surg. 1999;134:428-33.
2. Braga M, Gianotti L, Vignali A, Carlo VD. Preoperative oral arginine and n-3 fatty acid supplementation improves the immunometabolic host response and outcome after colorectal resection for cancer. Surgery. 2002;132:805-14.

Q.20. Postpancreatic surgery, patient was tolerating an oral diet and all tubes and lines were removed. On day 5, the patient did develop fever which was unrelenting. On the next day, the blood pressure dropped. Antibiotics were escalated. However, the condition worsened on the next day. Patient developed thrombocytopenia and coagulopathy. A repeat CT scan revealed a leak in the abdomen with clinical features of peritonitis. Patient also had a bout of hematemesis. All of the following are relative contraindications to secure a percutaneous enteral access, except:
a. Recent surgery
b. Profound thrombocytopenia
c. Hematemesis
d. Uncontrolled peritonitis

Ans. a

Explanation: As in any invasive procedure, securing a percutaneous access for feeding [for example, percutaneous endoscopic gastrostomy (PEG)] the patient should not be having any coagulopathy, hence deranged INR, PTT, and thrombocytopenia (with platelets counts <80,000) would serve as contraindications for securing peripheral access. EN is in itself contraindicated when there are prolonged ileus, upper GI bleeding, extreme hemodynamic instability, high-output fistula, and gastrointestinal ischemia. Similarly in the presence of uncontrolled peritonitis, an elective surgery to secure a percutaneous feeding route should be avoided as the outcomes are poor along with a possibility of flare up of sepsis and septic shock.

Suggested Reading
1. Rahnemai-Azar AA, Rahnemaiazar AA, Naghshizadian R, Kurtz A, Farkas DT. Percutaneous endoscopic gastrostomy: indications, technique, complications and management. World J Gastroenterol. 2014;20(24):7739-51.

Q.21. A 35-year-old male presented with a history of weight loss of >10% in the last 3 months with septic shock from urinary origin. He was resuscitated with IV fluids and required escalating doses of vasopressors. After the first 2 days, the inotropes stabilized to a much lower dose. It was decided to initiate nutrition. However on starting oral diet, then nasogastric and further nasojejunal feeding in the next 3 days, the patient still had features of intolerance. With respect to starting PN in such a case, which among the following is optimal?
  a. Since this patient is malnourished, it is important to wait for at least 7 days before starting parenteral nutrition.
  b. Parenteral nutrition should have started earlier itself (at day 3) when it was found that enteral nutrition was not sufficient.
  c. Since the patient has just recovered from severe septic shock, it is important to wait for few days more before starting nutrition.
  d. Parenteral nutrition should have started at the time of admission.

Ans. b

Explanation: In a well-nourished individual who is not able to take sufficient oral or enteral nutrition, it is advisable to wait for 7 days before commencing parenteral nutrition. However, this is not true in cases like the one presented. In patients who are severely malnourished, parenteral nutrition should be initiated by day 3 (as per the ESPEN recommendations). In this case, it is right to delay the initiation of parenteral nutrition as higher adverse effects are noticed when parenteral nutrition is initiated in the presence of hemodynamic instability, hypovolemia, and tissue hypoxia. This phase is characterized with more intolerance to feeds and associated complications. The presence of hemodynamic instability also leads to gross metabolic derangements and electrolyte abnormalities, which may be even worsened with addition of parenteral nutrition. Hence, it is wise to defer provision of PN till resuscitation is complete and baseline hemodynamic status has stabilized.

Suggested Reading
1. Worthington P, Balint J, Bechtold M, Bingham A, Chan LN, Durfee S, et al. When is parenteral nutrition appropriate? J Parenter Enteral Nutr. 2017;41:324-77.

Critical Care Nutrition

Q.22. **All attempts to start enteral nutrition failed in a 60-year-old patient with pancreatitis and it was decided to initiate total parenteral nutrition (TPN). All among the following are right, except:**
   a. Delivery of total parenteral nutrition would require a central line.
   b. It is important to correct all electrolyte abnormalities before staring TPN.
   c. There is a high chance of refeeding when TPN is started on the background of severe malnourishment.
   d. It is not important to provide trace elements with every dose of TPN.

Ans. d

Explanation: There is high chance of refeeding syndrome especially in patients who are deemed at high risk, which includes those patients with severe malnourishment and electrolytes abnormalities such as hypokalemia and hypophosphatemia. This would generally occur if TPN is started at a high rate as there is an immediate provision of high dose of dextrose into the circulation leading to hyperinsulinemia and its related consequences. Hence, it is imperative to correct electrolyte abnormalities and administer a dose of thiamine to at-risk individuals. PN is usually provided when enteral nutrition is not provided and not safe. Almost all micronutrients are absorbed in the gut and help in the metabolism and utilization of macronutrients and other homeostatic mechanisms. Hence, it is imperative that micronutrients and trace elements should be supplemented when parenteral nutrition is in the form of nutritional therapy as usual TPN mixture does not contain them.

Suggested Reading
1. Blaauw R, Osland E, Sriram K, Ali A, Allard JP, Ball P, et al. Parenteral provision of micronutrients to adult patients: An Expert Consensus Paper. J Parenter Enteral Nutr. 2019;43:S5-S23.

Q.23. **When total parenteral nutrition is prescribed to the patient, a frequent complication is hyperglycemia.**
   Which statement is correct among the following?
   a. This complication can be managed by using oral hypoglycemic agents promptly.
   b. Adding insulin to the TPN is better than adding insulin through a separate infusion.
   c. Adding glargine to the TPN may help in controlling the blood glucose better.
   d. Parenteral nutrition usually causes hypoglycemia and not hyperglycemia.

Ans. b

Explanation: The hyperglycemia as a result of parenteral nutrition should be managed using intravenous insulin as in such situation, oral hypoglycemic agents are found to be inferior. What is also known is that combining oral nutrition in small amounts, in addition to parenteral nutrition, will cause the release of insulin and help in the control of sugar. An olive oil-based parenteral nutrition along with an addition of glutamine is also said to be beneficial possibly due to the effect on insulin resistance and glucose oxidation. Adding insulin to the bag seems more practical as in the event that TPN is stopped for any reason, the insulin would thus stop automatically; however, if insulin is given in a separate infusion then in the event that the TPN is stopped, there is a chance for insulin to go on and create hypoglycemia. The amount of insulin could be calculated as 15 U per 150 g of glucose/L of PN if patient is euglycemic or 15 U per 100 g of glucose/L of PN if patient's sugar is more than 200 most of the time. Neutral protamine Hagedorn (NPH), lispro, aspart, or glargine should not be added to PN admixtures as studies regarding the compatibility are awaited in this regards. Reasonable amount of stability of PN is only seen with regular/short-acting insulin.

Suggested Reading
1. McCulloch A, Bansiya V, Woodward JM. Addition of insulin to parenteral nutrition for control of hyperglycemia. J Parenteral Enteral Nutr. 2018;42(5):846-54.
2. Schönenberger KA, Reber E, Dürig C, Baumgartner A, Efthymiou A, Huwiler VV, et al. Management of hyperglycemia in hospitalized patients receiving parenteral nutrition. Front Clin Diabetes Healthc. 2022;3:829412.

Q.24. The nurse was given the order to start parenteral nutrition on our patient who already had a central line in place. At this stage, what among the following is false?
a. There is no particulate matter in total nutrient admixtures.
b. A 0.22-µ filter should be used during the administration of total parenteral nutrition.
c. Addition of other fluids/drugs that are incompatible may increase the particulate matter.
d. Respiratory compromise is the predominant side effect of infusing particulate matter in the parenteral nutrition infusion.

Ans. b

Explanation: There are particulate matters nearing 2 µ in size in total nutrient admixtures which might cause adverse outcomes. This particulate matter can be any of the following which includes dust, glass, rubber, plastic, silicone, fibers, metal, and precipitates resulting from drug incompatibility. In fact, additives that are commonly added into the TPN may cause alteration in the pH and concentration of the nutrients, which may lead to drug and mineral precipitation. Infusion of this particulate matter may cause respiratory compromise and may include symptoms such as fever, dyspnea, cough, respiratory failure, and sudden unexpected death from cardiopulmonary arrest. A filter size as small as 0.22 µ is designed to retain microorganisms; however, this may not be suitable for lipid-containing emulsions as this may cause the compression of the lipid droplets, which may cause the emulsion to destabilize. Hence, a 1.2-µ filter is recommended with a change of the filter every 24 hours, which will help to trap the particulate matter of nearly 2 µ, which may cause a serious threat.

Suggested Reading
1. Worthington P, Gura KM, Kraft MD, Nishikawa R, Guenter P, Sacks GS. Update on the use of filters for parenteral nutrition: An ASPEN Position Paper. Nutr Clin Pract. 2021;36:29-39.

Q.25. A patient of high-output bowel fistula was admitted to the ICU. On the 1st day, the patient was resuscitated with intravenous fluids. His electrolytes were repleted and a decision was taken to initiate the patient on total parenteral nutrition gradually.

With regards to the supplementation of trace elements, only one among the following is right:
a. Any deficiency of any trace elements indicates deficiency in acute illness.
b. Any micronutrient deficiency in acute care needs to be corrected.
c. It is not necessary to supplement multivitamins and trace elements during the provision of parenteral nutrition.
d. Apart from the coadministration with PN, there are no other indications for trace elements.

Ans. a

Explanation: It is not necessary that low levels of trace elements on testing may not mean that there is a total body deficiency as this might just a redistribution out of the vascular compartment from which blood is taken for testing. The context of the testing thus becomes important and hence markers of inflammation like C-reactive protein (CRP) may help in guiding the diagnosis of deficiency (e.g., normal CRP with a low level). In the event that there is a deficiency then it is important to correct the deficiency as it plays a very important role in antioxidant defense mechanisms, metabolic pathways, and general immune pathways. Importantly, it is important to routinely supplement with trace elements and multivitamins when the patient is being given parenteral nutrition. Apart from PN, there are multiple reasons to provide parenteral trace elements and multivitamins, which include oxidative stress states such as sepsis and septic shock, insufficient enteral intakes, hemodialysis, CRRT, high-output fistula, and major burns.

Suggested Reading
1. Blaauw R, Osland E, Sriram K, Ali A, Allard JP, Ball P, et al. Parenteral provision of micronutrients to adult patients: An Expert Consensus Paper. J Parenter Enteral Nutr. 2019;43 (Suppl 1):S5-S23.

Q.26. A patient was rescued from a burning car, had suffered 40% burns, and was admitted to the ICU. This patient required large-volume resuscitation and stabilized after 2 days. It was decided to start enteral nutrition in this patient. With regards to enteral nutrition, which among the following is the wrong statement?
a. Indirect calorimetry is the gold standard for energy estimation in this patient.
b. Simple weight-based predictive equations may not be the optimal formula for energy estimation.
c. Enteral nutrition via the GI tract in burns patient is comparable to other pathological states.
d. Burn is one of the few indications where supplementation of glutamine is found to be beneficial.

Ans. c

Explanation: The use of simple predictive equations, Harris–Benedict formula, has been known to result in underfeeding and overfeeding both, both of which have resulted in poor outcomes in this class of patients. What is also known is that there is moderate increase in the feeding targets due to an increased hypermetabolic state. Hence, the only way to accurately determine the energy expenditure would be the measurement using the indirect calorimeter. In the absence of indirect calorimeter, the "Toronto" $(-4343 ƥ (10.5 \times \% \ TBSA) ƥ (0.23 \times caloric\ intake) + (0.84 \times REE\ by\ Harris-Benedict «crude») + (114 \times t^o) - (4.5 \times days\ after\ injury)$ equation may be a better alternative. Enteral nutrition is complicated in burns patients as it is difficult to secure a safe enteral access, also these patients are generally subjected to large-volume resuscitation. The leaky capillaries contribute to the excess edema in the GI tract which might cause an increased incidence of GI intolerance. Hence, EN in burns cannot be compared to EN in other intensive care unit patient. Trials looking at glutamine in burns do demonstrate significant reductions of gram-negative bacteremia in burn injury. This might be occurring due to maintenance of the gut barrier or gut immune function. Among all intensive care unit patients, burn patients seem to have better outcomes when supplemented with glutamine. Current societal recommendations continue to suggest the use of glutamine in burn injury.

Suggested Reading
1. Rousseau AF, Losser MR, Ichai C, Berger MM. ESPEN endorsed recommendations: nutritional therapy in major burns. Clin Nutr. 2013;32(4):497-502.

Q.27. **An 82-year-old gentleman with diabetes as his comorbidity was admitted to the ICU with a diagnosis of respiratory tract infection. He was diagnosed to have acute respiratory distress syndrome (ARDS). He needed mechanical ventilation and was still on vasopressors in view of septic shock. It was decided to start this patient on feeds and was provided 200 kcal for the first 3 days with regards to feeding what among the following is correct?**
a. This is a trophic feed.
b. Trophic feed is generally 25–50% of the actual energy requirement.
c. This is adequate feeding.
d. Trophic feeding is purely dependent on the volume of feeds.

Ans. a

Explanation: This is broadly defined as a feeding rate of <500 kcal/day and not >25% of the total calorie requirement, which works to around 7 kcal/day. This will definitely not meet nutritional needs; however, this may potentially preserve the intestinal epithelium, stimulate secretion of brush border enzymes, maintain the immune function, preserve epithelial tight cell junctions, and may also prevent bacterial translocation. What is known is that it is beneficial to provide trophic feeding than keeping the patient without any enteral nutrition at all. Trophic feeding will definitely preserve the autophagy (the mechanism proposed to clear damaged cellular substances like organelles). These patients at this stage also are known to have endogenous energy consumption, which can help them to subsist. Potentially feeding this patient the full feeds may lead to overfeeding.

Suggested Reading
1. Rice TW, Wheeler AP, Thompson BT, Steingrub J, Hite RD, Moss M, et al. Initial Trophic vs Full Enteral Feeding in Patients with Acute Lung Injury: The EDEN Randomized Trial. JAMA. 2012;307(8):795-803.

Q.28. A 60-year-old gentleman with diabetes and hypertension as his comorbidities was admitted to the ICU with a diagnosis of urosepsis. Postresuscitation, he was stabilized in the first day. Decision was taken to start enteral nutrition as his appetite and intake were very low for the last 5 days. In this aspect, the right answer would be:
a. We should provide 30–35 kcal/kg of energy per day as this patient is found to be catabolic.
b. Excess energy provision is not a problem.
c. It is optimal to provide 70% or two-thirds of the measured energy expenditure.
d. We should provide 100% of the energy expenditure.

Ans. c

Explanation: When it comes to energy, the gold standard to measure energy expenditure is indirect calorimetry. It is not advisable to give more than or even 100% of the measured energy expenditure as there are problems that arise with overfeeding. Autophagy is considered as "housekeeping process" that washes out intracellular organism and clears macromolecular damaged protein/organelles thus having roles in immune regulation, response to stress, infection, malignancy, aging, pulmonary disease, metabolic disease, and neurodegenerative disorders. There is a possibility of switching off of this process which has been the potential reason as suggested by the EPaNIC investigators where those patients who were overfed had worse outcomes. An excess amount of energy provision may need more volume, which can come with its own set of challenges such as fluid overload, increased edema, and intolerance. Moreover, this may also cause high degree of hyperglycemia as a result of excess provision of carbohydrates. Moreover, many of these patients may be acutely ill with low intake for weeks before ICU admission and hence may have a high risk for refeeding syndrome. Importantly, protein-wasting effect of hypocaloric (low carbohydrate) nutrition is minor if you provide adequate proteins (if at least 50% of energy is provided). With a normal body mass index, we also know that these patients can be given hypocaloric diet carefully. In fact, a study done by Zusman et al. calculated the percentage of administered calories by resting EE (%ADCal/REE): each patient was assigned one value representing the mean of the stay's delivered kcal. They report a U-shaped curve of mortality by %ADCal/REE, the lowest mortality being observed for 70% of the measured EE value. What has been practically seen is if we target at least 100%, possibly we may reach to 70% of the requirements, which may be beneficial.

Suggested Reading
1. Zusman O, Theilla M, Cohen J, Kagan I, Bendavid I, Singer P. Resting energy expenditure, calorie and protein consumption in critically ill patients: a retrospective cohort study. Crit Care. 2016;20(1):367.

Q.29. A 64-year-old male was admitted with exacerbation of COPD and needed noninvasive ventilator. It was decided to start nutrition for this patient immediately expecting catabolic state. However, all options mentioned below are false except one. Please choose the right option.
   a. It is advisable to start the patient on parenteral nutrition.
   b. Passing a nasogastric tube is contraindicated in patients on NIV.
   c. There is no need to start nutrition in a patient so early. We should wait.
   d. It is safer to feed using a nasojejunal tube in this patient.

Ans. c

Explanation: Critically ill patients when placed on NIV at the time of admission are expected to either improve within 1–2 days or deteriorate and require intubation as NIV is only a bridge to invasive ventilation or improvement. Passing a nasogastric tube though fraught with difficulties in such cases (desaturation and mask leak) can still be attempted, provided it is safe to disconnect the patient off the NIV for a while and primary problem has reduced and the patient is still not taking adequate nutrition (not able to achieve adequate energy provision even after 3–4 days). There is no indication to start this patient on nasojejunal feeds. One study has also demonstrated that enteral nutrition is an independent factor associated with airway complications, longer duration of NIV, and hospitalization. Importantly, enteral nutrition did not affect the mortality or rate of NIV failure.

Suggested Reading
1. Gay PC. Complications of noninvasive ventilation in acute care. Respir Care. 2009;54(2):246-57, discussion 257-8.
2. Kogo M, Nagata K, Morimoto T, Ito J, Sato Y, Teraoka S, et al. Enteral nutrition is a risk factor for airway complications in subjects undergoing noninvasive ventilation for acute respiratory failure. Respir Care. 2017;62(4):459-67.

Q.30. The patient mentioned in previous question further improved and the NIV was converted to high-flow nasal cannula (60% flow and 40% FiO_2), which was easily tolerated by the patients. At this point, what among the following is correct?
   a. Using the high-flow nasal cannula at higher flows increases the chances of aspiration.
   b. Such patients benefit with higher calorie intake in the long run.
   c. Usually patients on any form of NIV are poorly fed.
   d. These patients may benefit with a low-carbohydrate high-fat diet.

Ans. c

Explanation: There are no studies to suggest that high flows may lead to increased aspiration. In fact higher the flows, higher and more effective are the protective mechanisms in the larynx to prevent aspiration. However, this is a slightly increased difficulty in swallowing at high rates; however, this has not increased the chances of aspiration. However, there is data to suggest that these patients are generally poorly fed. In such COPD patients, a low-carbohydrate high-fat diet has been studied and some small studies have also shown some beneficial effects in pulmonary function in

COPD patients. However, this data is for stable COPD patient at home when compared with similar patients who were provided with high-carbohydrates and low-fat diets. Theoretically preferable is use of fats and production of ketone bodies will help in the reduction of lung inflammation. However, the data from preclinical and clinical studies in hospitalized patient with acute exacerbation of COPD about the most appropriate carbohydrate/fat substrate mixture for COPD patients is complicated and controversial and bigger randomized controlled trials are required.

Suggested Reading
1. Abd El Sabour Faramawy M, Abd Allah A, El Batrawy S, Amer H. Impact of high fat low carbohydrate enteral feeding on weaning from mechanical ventilation. Egyptian J Chest Dis Tuberc. 2014;63(4):931-8.
2. Allen K, Galek K. The influence of airflow via high-flow nasal cannula on duration of laryngeal vestibule closure. Dysphagia. 2021;36:729-35.
c. Cai B, Zhu Y, Ma Yi, Xu Z, Zao Yi, Wang J, et al. Effect of supplementing a high-fat, low-carbohydrate enteral formula in COPD patients. Nutrition. 2003;19(3):229-32.

CHAPTER

Endocrine and Metabolism

Madhava Reddy D, Nitika Yadav, Priya Gole

Q.1. A 32-year-old female presented with diarrhea for the past month with weight loss and recurrent events of bronchospasm. On further evaluation, she was found to have NET (neuroendocrine tumor). Considering the following statements, select the appropriate answer.
  a. The majority of the NETs are functional tumors.
  b. They are typically rapidly growing.
  c. Classic carcinoid syndrome is seen in >50% of the patients.
  d. Once the biochemical diagnosis is made, abdominal computed tomography (CT) scanning is the diagnostic procedure of choice for tumor identification.

Ans. d

Explanation: Neuroendocrine tumors are heterogeneous groups of rare tumors arising from various organs containing endocrine epithelium. Most of them are nonfunctional and rarely presented with classic carcinoid syndromes such as flushing, diarrhea, wheezing, bronchospasm, and right-sided heart disease.

An initial screening test is to measure 24-hour urinary excretion of 5-HIAA (5-hydroxyindoleacetic acid). Lungs and liver metabolize the majority of the substances released. Thus, in patients without carcinoid syndrome, this test is not useful. An abdominal CT scan is the diagnostic procedure of choice once the biochemical diagnosis is made to identify the tumor location and metastatic state. Somatostatin analogs (SSAs) are the mainstay of symptomatic treatment. For those without metastasis and local disease, surgical resection can be considered.

Suggested Reading
1. Bhattacharyya S, Davar J, Dreyfus G, Caplin ME. Carcinoid heart disease. Circulation. 2007;116(24):2860-5.
2. Jiao Y, Shi C, Edil BH, de Wilde RF, Klimstra DS, Maitra A, et al. DAXX/ATRX, MEN1, and mTOR pathway genes are frequently altered in pancreatic neuroendocrine tumors. Science. 2011;331:1199-203.
3. Modlin IM, Gustafsson BI, Moss SF, Pavel M, Tsolakis AV, Kidd M. Chromogranin A—biological function and clinical utility in neuroendocrine tumour disease. Ann Surg Oncol. 2010;17:2427-43.

4. Onaitis MW, Kirshbom PM, Hayward TZ, Quayle FJ, Feldman JM, Seigler HF, et al. Gastrointestinal carcinoids: characterization by the site of origin and hormone production. Ann Surg. 2000;232:549-56.
5. Vinik AI, Chaya C. Clinical presentation and diagnosis of neuroendocrine tumours. Hematol Oncol Clin North Am. 2016;30:21-48.

Q.2. A 22-year-old male presented to intensive care unit (ICU) with altered sensorium and fever with neck rigidity. Cerebrospinal fluid (CSF) analysis revealed bacterial meningitis. His last 24-hour urine output was 4 L with sodium going up from 148 to 156 mEq/L. Serum osmolality is 320 mOsm/kg. Urinary osmolality is 100 mOsm/kg. The next ideal step should be:
a. Start on DDAVP (arginine vasopressin).
b. Water deprivation test.
c. Start patient on indomethacin.
d. Start patient on thiazide diuretic.

Ans. a

Explanation: DDAVP (arginine vasopressin) is an ADH analog that has no vasopressor activity but has a higher duration of action compared to ADH. In the case of central DI, this replaces the ADH deficiency leading to the correction of polyuria or free water loss. Free water loss needs to be calculated in the setting of hypernatremia; accordingly, a correction needs to be started. In case of no response to DDAVP, nephrogenic DI could be probable cause. It can be treated with indomethacin in case of lithium-induced DI or thiazide diuretics to stimulate proximal tubular sodium and water reabsorption hence diminishing water delivery to ADH-sensitive collecting tubules.

Suggested Reading
1. Adrogué HJ, Madias NE. The challenge of hyponatremia. J Am Soc Nephrol. 2012;23(7): 1140-8.
2. Ball SG, Baylis PH. Vasopressin, diabetes insipidus, and syndrome of inappropriate antidiuresis. In: DeGroot LJ, Jameson JL (Eds). Endocrinology, 5th edition. Philadelphia, PA: Elsevier; 2006. 537-56.
3. Ellison DH, Berl T. Clinical practice. The syndrome of inappropriate antidiuresis. N Engl J Med. 2007;356(20):2064-72.
4. Robinson AG, Verbalis JG. Posterior pituitary. In: Melmed S, Polonsky KS, Larsen PR, Kronenberg HM (Eds). Williams Textbook of Endocrinology, 13th edition. Philadelphia, PA: Elsevier; 2016. pp. 313-24.
5. Sterns RH, Nigwekar SU, Hix JK. The treatment of hyponatremia. Semin Nephrol. 2009;29(3):282-99.

Q.3. A 78-year-old male with a history of traumatic fracture followed by hemiarthroplasty of the right hip 6 months back presented with altered sensorium for 5 days. On further evaluation, the noncontrast computed tomography (NCCT) head was found to be normal.
- *Serum calcium:* 17 mg/dL (toxicity), ionized calcium level 1.7 mmol/L
- *Intact parathyroid hormone (PTH) levels:* <20 pg/mL (suppressed)
- *Vitamin D levels:* 160 ng/mL (toxicity)

Considering the following statements regarding the management of this patient, choose the incorrect statement.
a. Aggressive hydration with normal saline as tolerated over the first 24–48 hours to increase excretion of urinary calcium.
b. Bisphosphonate therapy needs to be initiated immediately.
c. Calcitonin injection is a highly potent temporizing measure to control serum calcium.
d. Denosumab can be considered in case of acute kidney injury or resistance to bisphosphonate therapy.

Ans. c

Explanation: The two most common causes of hypercalcemia are primary hyperparathyroidism and malignancy-associated hypercalcemia. Other significant causes are vitamin D toxicity, lithium therapy, and granulomatous diseases. Certain medications can cause hypercalcemia such as thiazide diuretics, excessive intake of vitamin A, estrogens, growth hormones, and ganciclovir.

In general, calcium levels up to 12 mg/dL are asymptomatic. Levels >15 mg/dL can cause severe symptoms such as drowsiness and cardiac arrest.

Once hypercalcemia is identified, evaluation should be started to identify intact PTH levels. If they are suppressed, further evaluation should be done to identify whether vitamin D levels are elevated or not. If not elevated, look for PTH-related peptide/bone resorption/decreased calcium excretion. In case of vitamin D toxicity, it should be discontinued and appropriate therapy should be initiated.

In case of elevated intact PTH, further evaluation should be directed at primary hyperparathyroidism/familial hypocalciuric hypercalcemia, etc.

The primary focus of treating acute hypercalcemia is to increase urinary calcium excretion by adequate hydration. Loop diuretics can be employed only after adequate hydration with limited effect. In case of severe symptoms, the patient should be considered for urgent hemodialysis. Once the cause is identified, reversible calcium-lowering therapy can be initiated immediately. Bisphosphonate treatment provides long-term effects in reducing serum calcium levels, but they have maximum effect at 2–4 days and last for 3–4 weeks. Two agents are FDA-approved—pamidronate and zoledronic acid. Vitamin D being fat soluble will take a long time to get eliminated from the body. Ketoconazole can inhibit its hydroxylation of 25-hydroxy vitamin D to 1,25-hydroxyvitamin D. Calcitonin is a relatively weak, rapidly acting agent. Acquired resistance often develops within the first 48 hours, but it can be considered a temporary measure before the effect of bisphosphonates comes into effect.

Suggested Reading
1. Dietzek A, Connelly K, Cotugno M, Bartel S, McDonnell AM. Denosumab in hypercalcemia of malignancy: a case series. J Oncol Pharm Pract. 2015;21(2):143-7.
2. LeGrand SB, Leskuski D, Zama I. Narrative review: Furosemide for hypercalcemia: an unproven yet common practice. Ann Intern Med. 2008;149(4):259-63.
3. Lumachi F, Brunello A, Roma A, Basso U. Cancer-induced hypercalcemia. Anticancer Res. 2009;29(5):1551-5.

4. Major P, Lortholary A, Hon J, Abdi E, Mills G, Menssen HD, et al. Zoledronic acid is superior to pamidronate in the treatment of hypercalcemia of malignancy: a pooled analysis of two randomized, controlled clinical trials. J Clin Oncol. 2001;19(2):558-67.

Q.4. A 29-year-old young lady came to the hospital with a complaint of weight loss of 5 kg in the last 15 days, agitational behavior, and irregular menstruation. On further evaluation, she was having tremors and a large thyroid mass. On auscultation, it showed bruit. Thyroid-stimulating hormone (TSH) receptor antibodies report is awaited. Considering the following statements, choose the incorrect statement.
   a. Beta-blocker therapy was initiated immediately notwithstanding the TSH receptor antibody status.
   b. Glucocorticoids inhibit the conversion of T4 to T3 and also reduce thyroid gland secretion.
   c. Methimazole is the primary drug for Graves' disease and can be continued into the pregnancy.
   d. Radioiodine therapy can be considered 6 months before the pregnancy.

Ans. c

Explanation: The clinical presentation correlates with Graves' disease, suggested by thyroid mass with bruit—large hyperactive thyroid hormone-producing tumor. Typically, patients with Graves' disease show anti-TSH receptor antibodies, which stimulate thyroid gland growth, and increased hormone secretion. The mainstay of treatment in case of hyperthyroidism is a beta-blocker to alleviate the symptoms including tachycardia, palpitations, tremors, and agitational behavior if there are no contraindications even if the primary diagnosis of Graves' disease is not confirmed. Thionamides, which interfere with thyroid hormone production along with beta-blockers, are an effective primary modality of treatment. Methimazole is the preferred agent in view of single daily dosing and minimal side effects. In case of pregnancy, methimazole should be discontinued during the first trimester in view of teratogenicity. Propylthiouracil (PTU) is considered safe during the first trimester. Radioiodine therapy can be considered for definitive therapy in nonpregnant females/those who refused to have surgery as it has minimal side effects. In case of a planned pregnancy, it should be given at least 6 months before. Glucocorticoids can be used as adjunctive agents to inhibit the conversion of T4 to T3 and also to reduce thyroid hormone secretion.

Suggested Reading
1. Geffner DL, Hershman JM. Beta-adrenergic blockade for the treatment of hyperthyroidism. Am J Med. 1992;93:61.
2. Ma C, Xie J, Wang H, Li J, Chen S. Radioiodine therapy versus antithyroid medications for Graves' disease. Cochrane Database Syst Rev. 2016;(2):CD010094.
3. Pearce SHS, Dayan C, Wraith DC, Barrell K, Olive N, Jansson L, et al. Antigen-specific immunotherapy with thyrotropin receptor peptides in Graves' hyperthyroidism: A Phase I Study. Thyroid. 2019;29:1003.
4. Ross DS, Burch HB, Cooper DS, Greenlee MC, Laurberg P, Maia AL, et al. 2016 American Thyroid Association Guidelines for Diagnosis and Management of Hyperthyroidism and Other Causes of Thyrotoxicosis. Thyroid. 2016;26:1343-1421.

5. Ross DS. Radioiodine therapy for hyperthyroidism. N Engl J Med. 2011;364:542.
6. Tagami T, Yambe Y, Tanaka T, Tanaka T, Ogo A, Yoshizumi H, et al. Short-term effects of β-adrenergic antagonists and methimazole in new-onset thyrotoxicosis caused by Graves' disease. Intern Med 2012; 51:2285-90.

Q.5. An 85-year-old bedridden male presented with a history of poor oral intake and confusion in the ICU. On evaluation, the patient is found to have electrolyte deficiencies—hypophosphatemia and hypomagnesemia. The patient was treated with electrolyte supplementation. After adequate careful fluid resuscitation, he was started on enteral nutrition at lower calories. Within 12 hours, patient became tachypneic with tachycardia. Considering the following statements, choose the incorrect statement.
a. Signs of heart failure after initiating feeding suggestive of refeeding syndrome, feeding should be discontinued immediately.
b. Repeated measures of electrolytes are needed once feeding is initiated.
c. Thiamine supplementation before initiating feeding decreases the risk of refeeding syndrome.
d. Respiratory failure is a rare phenomenon in refeeding syndrome.

Ans. d

Explanation: The refeeding syndrome is a life-threatening complication of initiating feeding in critically ill malnourished patients via oral, enteral, or parenteral route. It is characterized primarily by neurological, muscular, and hematological changes. The initiation of feeding leads to a profound fall in plasma concentrations of phosphorous, potassium, and magnesium leading to serious electrolyte imbalances causing heart failure, confusion, encephalopathy, arrhythmias, respiratory failure, rhabdomyolysis, etc.

Any malnourished patient is at risk of refeeding syndrome. Patients need to be thoroughly investigated for hypophosphatemia, hypokalemia, hypomagnesemia, hyperglycemia, thiamine deficiency, and trace element deficiency (Zn, Fe, and Se). The patient should be provided with adequate supplementation of deficient elements. Fluid resuscitation should be judicious to avoid any fluid overload. Cautious and gradual restoration of energy should be considered with frequent measurements of electrolytes. Any suspected complications need to be addressed with promptness. In the case of refeeding syndrome, feeding should be stopped immediately. After correcting deficient electrolytes and thiamine supplementation, feeding can be restarted after 12–24 hours at lower calories.

Suggested Reading
1. Brooks MJ, Melnik G. The refeeding syndrome: an approach to understanding its complications and preventing its occurrence. Pharmacotherapy. 1995;15:713-26.
2. Hayek ME, Eisenberg PG. Severe hypophosphataemia following the institution of enteral feedings. Arch Surg. 1989;124:1325-8.
3. Matz R. Parallels between treated uncontrolled diabetes and the refeeding syndrome with emphasis on fluid and electrolyte abnormalities. Diabetes Care. 1994;17:1209-13.

4. Solomon SM, Kirby DF. The refeeding syndrome: a review. J Parenter Enteral Nutr. 1990;14:90-7.
5. Vaszar LT, Culpepper-Morgan JA, Winter SM. Refeeding syndrome induced by cautious enteral alimentation of a moderately malnourished patient. Gastroenterologist. 1998;6:79-81.

Q.6. Which of the following statements is wrong regarding the endocrine management of a brain-dead patient who is a potential donor?
   a. Central diabetes insipidus (DI) should be treated with desmopressin or vasopressin.
   b. Persistent blood glucose levels above 180 mg/dL must be controlled.
   c. Steroids can be considered in case of persisting hemodynamic instability post adequate volume resuscitation.
   d. Regular thyroid hormone replacement should be initiated in all.

Ans. d

Explanation: Brain-dead donors have hypothalamus–pituitary axis dysfunction, leading to reduced vasopressin levels, leading to diabetes insipidus of central origin. It usually presents with polyuria, hypernatremia, low urinary-specific gravity, and hyperosmolarity. Initial management includes low sodium-containing fluids for replacement followed by desmopressin or vasopressin. Brain death leads to hormonal imbalance and insulin resistance leading to hyperglycemia. Hyperglycemia should be controlled by targeting blood sugars under 180 mg/dL. The presumed reason for corticosteroid deficiency is hypothalamus–pituitary axis dysfunction and the hemodynamic instability that follows it. This could also lead to the release of proinflammatory and immunological mediators. This is associated with reduced graft function. High doses of steroids may reduce brainstem death-induced inflammation and help to modulate immune function. Steroids are generally considered in case of hemodynamic instability post adequate volume resuscitation. Thyroid hormone replacement as a routine practice in all brain-dead donors has no strong recommendation. It should be considered in brain-dead donors with hemodynamic instability requiring vasopressor support.

Suggested Reading
1. Kotloff RM, Blosser S, Fulda GJ, Malinoski D, Ahya VN, Angel L, et al. Management of the potential organ donor in the ICU: Society of Critical Care Medicine/American College of Chest Physicians/Association of Organ Procurement Organizations Consensus Statement. Crit Care Med. 2015;43(6):1291-325.
2. Kotsch K, Ulrich F, Reutzel-Selke A, Pascher A, Faber W, Warnick P, et al. Methylprednisolone therapy in deceased donors reduces inflammation in the donor's liver and improves outcome after liver transplantation: a prospective randomized controlled trial. Ann Surg. 2008;248(6):1042-50.
3. Powner DJ, Kellum JA. Maintaining acid-base balance in organ donors. Prog Transplant. 2000;10(2):95-8.
4. Salim A, Martin M, Brown C, Belzberg H, Rhee P, Demetriades D. Complications of brain death: frequency and impact on organ retrieval. Am Surg. 2006;72(5):377-81.
5. Wood KE, Becker BN, McCartney JG, D'Alessandro AM, Coursin DB. Care of the potential organ donor. N Engl J Med. 2004;351(26):2730-9.

A 19-year-old male with a history of intermittent headaches presented to the emergency with complaints of palpitations and sweating. On examination, the patient was found to have a blood pressure of 190/120 mm Hg. The patient was shifted to ICU for further management. Answer the following questions (7–9) regarding the above clinical scenario.

Q.7. Which of the following statements is incorrect?
  a. Plasma-free metanephrines and 24-hour urinary metanephrines are highly sensitive to the diagnosis.
  b. Beta-blockers, phenoxybenzamine, and tricyclic antidepressants are associated with false-positive urinary metanephrines.
  c. Contrast-enhanced computed tomography (CECT) is a radiological investigation of choice.
  d. CT is favored over MRI in patients with suspected metastasis.

Ans. d

Explanation: Pheochromocytomas are neuroendocrine tumors arising from catecholamine-producing chromaffin cells of the adrenal medulla. Tumors arising from the extra-adrenal medulla are paragangliomas. The most common presenting clinical features are headache, palpitations, sweating, pallor, fatigue, and weight loss. Patients with pheochromocytoma could be completely asymptomatic also. Definitive diagnosis of pheochromocytoma is made by a biochemical evaluation followed by anatomical and functional imaging to localize. Biochemical evaluation includes highly sensitive tests to detect plasma and urinary metanephrines. A negative test usually excludes the diagnosis, but a positive test could be a false positive due to beta-blockers, phenoxybenzamine, tricyclic antidepressants, theophylline, and monoamine oxidase (MAO) inhibitors.

Anatomical evaluation of the tumor should start with CECT chest and abdomen. In case of metastatic disease, skull base and neck paragangliomas and patients with surgical clip artifacts MRI are favored over CT.

Suggested Reading
1. Borhani AA, Hosseinzadeh K. Quantitative versus qualitative methods in evaluation of T2 signal intensity to improve accuracy in the diagnosis of pheochromocytoma. Am J Roentgenol. 2015;205(2):302-10.
2. Castinetti F, Taieb D, Henry JF, Walz M, Guerin C, Brue T, et al. Management of endocrine disease: Outcome of adrenal sparing surgery in heritable pheochromocytoma. Eur J Endocrinol. 2016;174(1):R9-R18.
3. Eisenhofer G, Keiser H, Friberg P, Mezey E, Huynh TT, Hiremagalur B, et al. Plasma metanephrines are markers of pheochromocytoma produced by catechol-O-methyltransferase within tumours. J Clin Endocrinol Metab. 1998;83(6):2175-85.
4. Lenders JW, Duh QY, Eisenhofer G, Gimenez-Roqueplo AP, Grebe SK, Murad MH, et al. Pheochromocytoma and paraganglioma: an endocrine society clinical practice guideline. J Clin Endocrinol Metab. 2014;99(6):1915-42.
5. Lenders JW, Pacak K, Walther MM, Linehan WM, Mannelli M, Friberg P, et al. Biochemical diagnosis of pheochromocytoma: which test is best? JAMA. 2002;287(11):1427-34.
6. Lenders JWM, Eisenhofer G. Update on modern management of pheochromocytoma and paraganglioma. Endocrinol Metab (Seoul). 2017;32(2):152-61.

Q.8. Identify the correct statement regarding pheochromocytoma.
   a. Preoperative volume replacement, heart rate, and blood pressure normalization are associated with low perioperative mortality.
   b. Patients with familial pheochromocytoma are associated with a lower incidence of bilateral disease.
   c. Beta-blockers and alpha-blockers should be started simultaneously.
   d. Labetalol is the initial beta-blocker of choice to control hypertensive crisis.

Ans. a

Explanation: The main goal of preoperative management is to normalize blood pressure, heart rate, and restore volume and prevent surgery-induced catecholamine storm. With appropriate preoperative preparation, the mortality during the perioperative period could come to <1% from 30 to 45%. Patients with familial pheochromocytoma are associated with bilateral disease and need bilateral adrenalectomy. Alpha-blocker initiation leads to tachycardia, which needs beta-blockers to control. Using beta-blockers like labetalol with a predominant beta-blocker than alfa-blocking action can lead to uncontrolled hypertension and should not be started until after adequate alpha-adrenergic blockage is achieved to prevent a paradoxical rise in the blood pressure due to unopposed alpha-adrenergic receptor stimulation.

Suggested Reading
1. Niemeijer ND, Alblas G, van Hulsteijn LT, Dekkers OM, Corssmit EP. Chemotherapy with cyclophosphamide, vincristine and dacarbazine for malignant paraganglioma and pheochromocytoma: systematic review and meta-analysis. Clin Endocrinol (Oxf). 2014;81(5):642-51.
2. Sawka AM, Jaeschke R, Singh RJ, Young WF Jr. A comparison of biochemical tests for pheochromocytoma: Measurement of fractionated plasma metanephrines compared with the combination of 24-hour urinary metanephrines and catecholamines. J Clin Endocrinol Metab. 2003;88(2):553-8.
3. Schieda N, Alrashed A, Flood TA, Samji K, Shabana W, McInnes MD. Comparison of quantitative MRI and CT washout analysis for differentiation of adrenal pheochromocytoma from adrenal adenoma. Am J Roentgenol. 2016;206(6):1141-8.
4. van Hulsteijn LT, Niemeijer ND, Dekkers OM, Corssmit EP. (131)I-MIBG therapy for malignant paraganglioma and phaeochromocytoma: systematic review and meta-analysis. Clin Endocrinol (Oxf). 2014;80(4):487-501.
5. Wiseman GA, Pacak K, O'Dorisio MS, Neumann DR, Waxman AD, Mankoff DA, et al. The usefulness of 123I-MIBG scintigraphy in the evaluation of patients with known or suspected primary or metastatic pheochromocytoma or paraganglioma: results from a prospective multicenter trial. J Nucl Med. 2009;50(9):1448-54.

Q.9. Regarding pheochromocytoma in pregnancy, choose the incorrect statement.
   a. Urinary metanephrines and localization of tumor with MRI are considered for diagnosis.
   b. Phenoxybenzamine followed by beta-blockers is necessary to control blood pressure and tachycardia.

c. Surgical resection is not considered at any stage.
d. Combined cesarean delivery and tumor resection are performed.

Ans. c

Explanation: Pheochromocytoma is a rare but potentially lethal cause of hypertension in pregnancy. Diagnosis is usually made with biochemical testing and MRI for tumor localization. Women should be prepared for surgery after adequate preparation by phenoxybenzamine followed by beta-blockage as necessary if the presentation is within 24 weeks, preferably during the second trimester. If the diagnosis is made after 24 weeks of gestation, medical management is continued until fetal maturation, and then combined cesarean delivery and tumor resection are performed.

Suggested Reading
1. Lenders JW. Pheochromocytoma and pregnancy: a deceptive connection. Eur J Endocrinol 2012;166(2):143-150.
2. Pearl J, Price R, Richardson W, Fanelli R; Society of American Gastrointestinal Endoscopic Surgeons. Guidelines for diagnosis, treatment, and use of laparoscopy for surgical problems during pregnancy. Surg Endosc. 2011;25(11):3479-92.

Q.10. A 30-year-old psychiatric patient presents with nausea, lethargy, and fits. She is on no medication and is previously well. She has post-ictal with a Glasgow coma scale (GCS) of 11. Routine blood reveals a plasma sodium concentration of 113 mmol/L. Urinary sodium concentration is >20 mmol/L. Which one of the following statements is true?
a. Conn's syndrome is part of the differential diagnosis.
b. If due to psychogenic polydipsia then fluid restriction will be sufficient treatment.
c. A water deprivation test is indicated.
d. SIADH may cause this picture.

Ans. d

Explanation: The differential diagnosis of hyponatremia is broad and includes a syndrome of inappropriate antidiuretic hormone secretion (SIADH), drugs, GI tract losses, adrenocortical failure, diuretic therapy, renal, cardiac, and hepatic failure, and psychogenic polydipsia. A low-plasma sodium value may be accompanied by a low- or high-urinary sodium value. A water deprivation test can help to distinguish between diabetes insipidus and psychogenic polydipsia, but sodium of 113 mmol/L on presentation effectively excludes the former which is a failure to reabsorb free water in the collecting ducts causing a very dilute diuresis and consequent hypernatremia. Conn's syndrome (primary hyperaldosteronism) is characterized by renal sodium and water retention and causes hypertension but not hyponatremia. Nephrogenic diabetes insipidus may cause high-plasma osmolality and sodium, and inappropriately dilute urine. Regardless of the cause, this requires aggressive treatment to increase plasma sodium in a controlled fashion; this may include the judicious use of diuretics and hypertonic saline. A rise of 4–6 mmol/L plasma sodium should be enough to prevent fitting, after which fluid restriction and gradual sodium increase may be sufficient.

Suggested Reading
1. Adrogue HJ, Madias NE. Hyponatraemia. N Engl J Med. 2000;342(21):1581-9.

Q.11. A 44-year-old homeless alcoholic presents for detoxification in a generally debilitated state. After 4 days in the hospital, he is admitted to the high-dependency area with progressive respiratory failure, tachycardia, diarrhea, ataxia, and progressive renal impairment. Blood tests show sodium = 133 mmol/L, potassium = 5.1 mmol/L, urea = 14 mmol/L (39 mg/dL), creatinine = 244 µmol/L (2.76 mg/dL), albumin = 28 g/L, phosphate = 0.22 mmol/L (0.68 mg/dL), and creatine kinase = 2,500 U/L. Chest X-ray shows upper lobe diversion consistent with mild pulmonary edema. The most likely unifying diagnosis is:
   a. Silent myocardial infarction
   b. Wernicke's encephalopathy
   c. Refeeding syndrome
   d. Rhabdomyolysis

Ans. c

Explanation: The refeeding syndrome occurs when a chronically malnourished patient receives renutrition. It is characterized by a low-serum phosphate with a variety of clinical features including arrhythmias and cardiac failure, Wernicke's encephalopathy, leukocyte and platelet dysfunction, rhabdomyolysis, renal failure, and myopathy. All abnormalities are secondary to hypophosphatemia, which is a consequence of elevated levels of insulin which are part of the switch from a starvation state to carbohydrate metabolism. It may occur with either enteral or parenteral nutrition. At risk, patients should receive a calorie and carbohydrate-restricted diet, with daily electrolyte monitoring, prophylactic thiamine, and intravenous (IV) phosphate replacement if <0.5 mmol/L or symptomatic.

Suggested Reading
1. Fung AT, Rimmer J. Hypophosphataemia secondary to the oral refeeding syndrome in a patient with long-term alcohol misuse. MJA. 2005;183(6):324-6.

Q.12. Which of the following physiological changes does not contribute to stress hyperglycemia?
   a. Increased cortisol levels
   b. Increased corticotrophin-releasing hormone (CRH) levels
   c. Insulin resistance
   d. Increased glycogenesis

Ans. d

Explanation: Stress hyperglycemia is a term used to describe hyperglycemia and insulin resistance in critical illness, including surgical insults and trauma. The degree of hyperglycemia is related to the severity of insult to the body and is correlated with the severity of illness or injury scores and type of surgery. Perhaps unsurprisingly, the degree of stress hyperglycemia is also related to outcomes such as mortality, morbidity, and length of stay.

Physiological stress activates the hypothalamus–pituitary–adrenal (HPA) axis and sympathetic nervous system. Increased CRH, adrenocorticotrophic hormone

(ACTH), and cortisol are seen, along with greatly increased levels of circulating catecholamines. These act to increase glycogenolysis, gluconeogenesis, and insulin resistance, leading to increased glucose levels. This is an adaptive mechanism known as stress hyperglycemia.

Critical illness and stressors such as shock, sepsis, trauma, and surgery lead to activation of the HPA axis and the sympathetic adrenal system. Increased corticotrophin-releasing hormone (CRH) release from the hypothalamus leads to increased ACTH from the anterior pituitary and activation of the immune system. ACTH then stimulates cortisol release from the adrenal cortex. Activation of the locus coeruleus leads to increased epinephrine release from the adrenal medulla and norepinephrine release from sympathetic nerves.

Cortisol, epinephrine, and norepinephrine activate gluconeogenesis, glycogenolysis, and insulin resistance, which lead to hyperglycemia. Stress hyperglycemia is thought to be an adaptive response, freeing up fuel for the fight-or-flight response. In critical illness, mild stress hyperglycemia may be protective, but excessive or prolonged stress responses become maladaptive and harmful. This may be reflected in the fact that tight glycemic control (e.g., between 4 and 7 mmol/L) has been found to increase mortality (e.g., the NICE-SUGAR trial), while looser glycemic control is widely recommended (e.g. in sepsis, stroke, myocardial infarction, trauma, head injury, etc.).

Suggested Reading
1. Marik PE, Bellomo R. Stress hyperglycemia: an essential survival response! Crit Care Med. 2013;41:e93-4.

Q.13. In a case of hyperkalemia, which of the following ECG change is not seen?
   a. Presence of tented T waves is the first sign.
   b. Sine wave pattern
   c. The P wave is often absent.
   d. Short PR interval

Ans. d

Explanation: Although the ECG may be entirely normal in severe hyperkalemia, it is typically associated with several characteristic ECG changes. The QRS complex widens in hyperkalemia; it is narrowed in hypokalemia. Tented T waves are seen first on the ECG in hyperkalemia, followed by a prolonged PR interval and then flattened or absent P waves.

Suggested Reading
1. Webster A, Brady W, Morris F. Recognising signs of danger: ECG changes resulting from an abnormal serum potassium concentration. Emerg Med J. 2002;19:74-7.
2. Weisberg L. Management of severe hyperkalaemia. Crit Care Med 2008;36:3246-51.

Q.14. A 47-year-old gentleman with no comorbidities was admitted to ICU in a drowsy state. History was taken from attendants for anorexia, nausea, abdominal pain, and

significant weight loss. On examination, he appeared weak and dry, the following are his laboratory reports:
- *Sodium:* 137 mEq/L (mmol/L)
- *Blood urea nitrogen (BUN):* 11 mg/dL
- *Bicarbonate:* 28 mmol/L
- *Creatinine:* 1.0
- *Glucose:* 104 mg/dL (4.6 mmol/L)
- *Ca (ionized):* 1.5
- **Parathyroid hormone level 200 pg/mL**

About the assessment and management of severe hypercalcemia in this case, which of the following is incorrect?
a. Hypercalcemic crisis is most commonly caused by primary hyperparathyroidism.
b. Digoxin is the drug of choice for arrhythmias associated with hypercalcemia.
c. Acute kidney injury and anuria occur when calcium levels are >4 mmol/L.
d. Renal replacement therapy may be required if intravenous fluid resuscitation is unsuccessful.

Ans. b

Explanation: Hypercalcemia is usually a chronic condition managed in primary care. Patients present with vague symptoms such as lethargy, polydipsia, abdominal pains, and constipation. The most common cause for hypercalcemia is hyperparathyroidism caused by either parathyroid adenoma or gland hyperplasia. The usual treatment involves encouraging oral rehydration followed by referral to an endocrinologist and surgeon for definitive parathyroidectomy. Other causes include malignancies such as myeloma, breast cancer, prostate cancer, and lung cancer.

Once the calcium level rises above 3 mmol/L, the patient is often unable to take in adequate oral rehydration. Intravenous fluid should be administered, and furosemide can also be given to promote diuresis and reduce total body calcium levels. A hypercalcemic crisis develops when the calcium level reaches a critical level (usually >4 mmol/L). At this point, two organs are at risk: firstly the kidneys, because oliguria and anuria can develop, leading to renal failure; and secondly the brain, as drowsiness and coma will develop if the calcium remains untreated.

In addition to intravenous fluid resuscitation, bisphosphonates can be administered. The advice of the local endocrinologist should be sought, as care is required in patients with renal impairment. Pamidronate or zoledronate is the recommended drug. Renal replacement therapy may be required, and calcium-free or low-calcium dialysate should be used. Treatment may also require aggressive potassium and magnesium replacement, as these are often low and will fall further once rehydration is commenced. Corticosteroids can also be given to help lower calcium levels, and this is particularly effective in patients with myeloma.

Suggested Reading
1. Ramrakha P, Moore K. Endocrine emergencies. In: Oxford Handbook of Acute Medicine, 3rd edition. Oxford: Oxford University Press; 2010. pp. 515-72.
2. Ziegler R. Hypercalcemic crisis. J Am Soc Nephrol 2001;12 (Suppl 1):S3-9.

Q.15. A 43-year-old woman with a history of atrial fibrillation on digoxin was admitted to ICU after bariatric surgery, postoperatively she complains of recurrent vomiting, unable to pass motion, and flatus. On examination, the abdomen is soft on palpation, with no guarding or rigidity, on auscultation 1–2 bowel sounds per minute.

Laboratory parameters showed creatinine of 0.8, Na of 137, K of 1.9, Ca (ionized) of 1.1, and ECG showed U waves.

Which of the following statements regarding this case is incorrect?
a. Maximum potassium correction should not exceed 40 mmol/h.
b. U waves are small positive deflections seen after the T waves on the ECG.
c. The duration of the action potential and refractory period are increased.
d. Patients taking digoxin are relatively resistant to the effects of hypokalemia.

Ans. d

Explanation: Hypokalemia is a common electrolyte disturbance seen in hospital patients. There are many causes, including reduced intake of potassium (in food or fluids), vomiting and diarrhea, GI surgery, diuretics, or treatment for hyperkalemia. In mild cases, there are usually no ECG changes and the patient may be asymptomatic or feel weak and lethargic. As potassium levels fall, the resting membrane potential increases and repolarization is delayed. This results in an increase in the duration of the action potential and refractory period, which is potentially arrhythmogenic. The maximum rate of potassium infusion should not exceed 40 mmol/h, as this may cause arrhythmias and asystole.

The ECG changes that are seen are a reduction in the T-wave amplitude (T-wave flattening), depression of the ST segment, and the appearance of U waves. U waves are small positive deflections seen after the T wave. They are seen best in leads V2 and V3. Giant U waves are sometimes seen in severe cases and can be mistaken for peaked T waves. They are differentiated from T waves by being broad-based, and there is the apparent lengthening of the QT interval, which is a QU interval. Peaked T waves in hyperkalemia are usually narrow-based, with a prominent peak, and the QT interval is normal or decreased.

The risk of hypokalemia is that ventricular arrhythmia can occur. This is more likely to occur in patients who have had a recent myocardial infarction. There is also a risk of prolongation of the QT interval and torsades de pointes. Patients taking digoxin are more sensitive to the effects of hypokalemia, and ventricular arrhythmias are more likely to occur.

Suggested Reading
1. Alfonzo A, Isles C, Geddes C, Deighan C. Potassium disorders: clinical spectrum and emergency management. Resuscitation. 2006;70:10-25.
2. Bersten AD, Soni N. Oh's Intensive Care Manual, 5th edition. Edinburgh: Butterworth-Heinemann; 2003.
3. Webster A, Brady W, Morris F. Recognising signs of danger: ECG changes resulting from an abnormal serum potassium concentration. Emerg Med J. 2002;19:74-7.

Q.16. A 50-year-old gentleman presented to the emergency with a headache followed by vomiting, with a Glasgow Coma Scale of 5. CT scan revealed subarachnoid hemorrhage (SAH) in the basilar cisterns. He was managed with endovascular coiling. But, after 7 days, his urine output increased to 5 L/day and he became hypotensive. Considering the following laboratory data:
- *Sodium:* 130 mEq/L
- *Potassium:* 3.4 mEq/L
- *Plasma osmolality:* 270 mOsm/kg
- *Urine sodium concentration:* 71 mEq/L
- *Urine osmolality:* 93 mmol/L
- *Glucose:* 172 mg/dL
- *TSH:* 3.1 mIU/L
- *Triglyceride:* 118 mg/dL

Which of the following is the most likely cause of the above changes?
a. CSW syndrome
b. Central DI
c. Osmotic diuresis
d. SIADH

Ans. a

Explanation: Cerebral salt-wasting (CSW) syndrome and SIADH are usually present with similar laboratory data. Volume status differentiates them as separate entities. Patients with CSW syndrome tend to be hypotensive with low-extracellular fluid, whereas SIADH patients are usually euvolemic.

Cerebral salt wasting is caused by SAH, intracranial infections, and intracranial tumors. CSW is managed with adequate fluid resuscitation and mineralocorticoid therapy, whereas SIADH is managed with fluid restriction.

Cerebral salt wasting results from the release of natriuretic peptides from the brain and the disruption of sympathetic neural input leading to decreased activation of RAS (renin–angiotensin–aldosterone system) leading to decreased sodium absorption in the proximal tubules.

Suggested Reading
1. Maesaka JK, Imbriano L, Mattana J, Gallagher D, Bade N, Sharif S. Differentiating SIADH from cerebral/renal salt wasting: Failure of the Volume Approach and Need for a New Approach to Hyponatremia. J Clin Med. 2014;3(4):1373-85.
2. Momi J, Tang CM, Abcar A, Kujubu DA, Sim JJ. Hyponatremia–what is cerebral salt wasting? Perm J. 2010;12(2):62-5.

Q.17. A 32-year-old gentleman was admitted to ICU after a road traffic accident with a history of transient loss of consciousness, CT reveals subdural hemorrhage. His GCS is 4 on admission. He was started on 3% NS and underwent emergency craniotomy, postoperatively after 24 hours, his urine output was 350 mL/h.

Further laboratory evaluation found:
- *Serum sodium:* 155 mEq/L
- *Urine-specific gravity:* 1.013
- *Urine random sodium:* 55 mEq/L (mmol/L)
- *Urine random creatinine:* 51 mg/dL

- *Urine osmolality:* 199 mOsm/kg
- *Serum osmolality:* 300 mOsm/kg

Desmopressin administration caused an increase in urine osmolality. Which of the following is the most likely cause for increased urine output?
a. Syndrome of inappropriate antidiuretic hormone secretion (SIADH)
b. Central diabetes insipidus (DI)
c. Cerebral salt-wasting (CSW) syndrome
d. Psychogenic polydipsia

Ans. b

Explanation: Diabetes insipidus results in polyurea due to improper water balance and failure of kidney to retain water. This could result from inadequate secretion of antidiuretic hormone (ADH) from posterior pituitary gland or due to complete or partial resistance to ADH in kidney.

This leads to inability of kidney to concentrate urine above 300 mOsm/kg, and thus leading to loss of additional water from kidney.

Water deprivation test in case of primary polydipsia where kidney function and ADH production is adequate leads to concentration of urine in response to water deprivation and thus increasing the urine osmolality to >600 mOsm/kg.

Suggested Reading
1. Makaryus AN, McFarlane AI. Diabetes insipidus: diagnosis and treatment of a complex disease. Cleve Clin J Med. 2006;73(1):65-71.
2. Robertson GL. Diabetes insipidus. Endocrinol Metab Clin North Am. 1995;24(3):549-72.

Q.18. A 60-year-old male, chronic obstructive pulmonary disease (COPD) patient was admitted to the ICU for respiratory failure. He had a fever, cough, and loss of appetite for 1 week. He is intubated and sedated. Tube feeds are initiated. Electrolyte levels are as follows:
- *Serum calcium:* 7.0 mg/dL
- *Serum phosphorus:* 0.9 mg/dL
- *Serum magnesium:* 1.6 mg/dL
- *Serum potassium:* 3.6 mg/dL
- *Serum sodium:* 138 mg/dL

What replacement strategy should be initiated for this patient?
a. IV calcium followed by IV phosphorus
b. IV phosphorus followed by IV calcium
c. IV calcium followed by oral phosphorus replacement
d. Oral phosphorus replacement only

Ans. c

Explanation: This patient has hypophosphatemia from refeeding syndrome. This patient has concomitant low-serum calcium levels. Early replacement of phosphorus is warranted in refeeding syndrome; however, hypocalcemia can worsen with phosphorus replacement; therefore, calcium should be replaced before phosphorus correction.

It is recommended to replace phosphorus with IV supplementation instead of oral due to absorption issues often encountered in this patient group.

Suggested Reading
1. Mehanna HM, Moledina J, Travis J. Refeeding syndrome: what it is, and how to prevent and treat it. BMJ. 2008;336:1495-8.

Q.19. A 36-year-old G2P1 female at 34 weeks of gestation and with a history of chronic kidney disease develops hypertension and altered mental status followed by seizures. She is started on intravenous magnesium with seizure resolution. She becomes somnolent 3 hours later, and a physical examination reveals hyporeflexia. What is the immediate management for this symptom?
    a. Hypotonic IV fluids
    b. Calcium gluconate infusion
    c. Hemodialysis
    d. Furosemide

Ans. b

Explanation: Patients showed signs and symptoms consistent with hypermagnesemia. This patient is predisposed to higher levels of serum magnesium due to underlying renal impairment. Although hemodialysis will be the most definitive management for removing magnesium from the system in this patient with CKD (chronic kidney disease), immediate and first-line management of the central nervous system and cardiac side effects should be done by the administration of IV calcium which acts as a magnesium antagonist. Unless the patient is anuric, medical management with intravenous fluids and loop diuretics should also be initiated (choice D) after giving calcium, especially in severe or symptomatic cases.

Suggested Reading
1. Mordes JP, Wacker WE. Excess magnesium. Pharmacol Rev. 1977;29(4):273-300.

Q.20. A 19-year-old female with hyperthyroidism underwent total thyroidectomy for thyrotoxicosis with reimplantation of parathyroid glands. She was admitted to ICU on postoperative day 20 with complaints of tingling extremities and carpopedal spasms. Laboratory parameters showed hypocalcemia despite supplementation and normal parathyroid hormone (PTH) levels. Which of the following statements regarding her condition is *not* correct?
    a. The syndrome most often occurs in patients with chronic increases in bone resorption induced by high levels of PTH.
    b. Patients often present with hypocalcemia, hypophosphatemia, hypermagnesemia, and hypokalemia.
    c. Sudden withdrawal of PTH causes an imbalance between osteoblast-mediated bone formation and osteoclast-mediated bone resorption.
    d. It can occur despite normal or even elevated levels of PTH.

Ans. b

Explanation: Hypocalcemia is a common problem after parathyroidectomy or thyroidectomy. The acute withdrawal of PTH causes an increase in osteoblast-mediated bone formation and a decrease in osteoclast-mediated bone resorption. Hypocalcemia after surgery is usually transient, as the degree of bone disease is typically mild and normal parathyroid tissue recovers function within a few days. Severe or prolonged hypocalcemia is called the hungry bone syndrome, and most often occurs in patients with a chronic increase in bone resorption induced by high levels of PTH or in patients with high-bone turnover induced by excess thyroid hormone. Hungry bone syndrome can occur despite normal or even elevated levels of PTH.

Patients with hungry bone syndrome often present with concurrent hypophosphatemia, hypomagnesemia, and hyperkalemia. These imbalances reflect increased bone influx and efflux. Treatment consists of aggressive electrolyte supplementation and may necessitate a continuous infusion of calcium. Severe cases can be managed with dialysis with a high-calcium bath.

Suggested Reading
1. Brasier AR, Nussbaum SR. Hungry bone syndrome: clinical and biochemical predictors of its occurrence after parathyroid surgery. Am J Med. 1988;84:654.
2. Ho LY, Wong PN, Sin HK, Wong YY, Lo KC, Chan SF, et al. Risk factors and clinical course of the hungry bone syndrome after total parathyroidectomy in dialysis patients with secondary hyperparathyroidism. BMC Nephrol. 2017;18:12.
3. Tohme JF, Bilezikian JP. Diagnosis and treatment of hypocalcemic emergencies. Endocrinologist. 1996;6:10.

Q.21. A 54-year-old female patient has been on amiodarone tablet for the past 5 years with good compliance. The patient now comes to an emergency with complaints of palpitations, weight loss, and anxiety. The patient does not give any prior history of thyroidal illness but her thyroid function tests show suppressed TSH, elevated FT4, and normal FT3. Choose the incorrect answer.
a. The patient is suffering from amiodarone-induced thyrotoxicosis type 1.
b. Amiodarone can be continued.
c. Oral prednisolone is the preferred treatment.
d. Spontaneous remission can occur.

Ans. a

Explanation:

	AIT type 1	AIT type 2
Underlying thyroid abnormality	Yes	No
Onset after start amiodarone	Short (3 months)	Long (30 months)
Thyroid antibodies	Present in Graves	Usually absent
Color flow Doppler sonography	High vascularity	Low/absent vascularity
Thyroid radioiodine uptake	Low, normal, and high	Suppressed
Preferred treatment	Antithyroid drugs	Oral prednisone
Amiodarone continuation	No	Possible
Spontaneous remission	No	Frequent
Subsequent hypothyroidism	No	Possible (17%)
Subsequent definitive treatment	Generally yes	No

(AIT: amiodarone-induced thyrotoxicosis)

Suggested Reading
1. Ahmed S, Van Gelder IC, Wiesfeld AC, Van Veldhuisen DJ, Links TP. Determinants and outcome of amiodarone-associated thyroid dysfunction. Clin Endocrinol. 2011;75(3):388-94.
2. Bartalena L, Bogazzi F, Chiovato L, Hubalewska-Dydejczyk A, Links TP, Vanderpump M. 2018 European Thyroid Association (ETA) guidelines for the management of amiodarone-associated thyroid dysfunction. Eur Thyroid J. 2018;7(2):55-66.

Q.22. A 54-year-old woman has been treated for hypothyroidism for many years. While taking a levothyroxine dosage of 112 µg daily, she has maintained a stable serum TSH concentration of 1–4 mIU/L. She is hospitalized for abdominal pain and diagnosed with an aortic aneurysm. During recovery from her surgery, the patient develops paralytic ileus. Which of the following is an incorrect statement for thyroid hormone therapy for her?
a. Levothyroxine oral dose can be withheld for 1–2 days if the oral route is unavailable.
b. If oral therapy cannot be resumed within 3 days, intravenous levothyroxine should be administered.
c. IV dose equivalent to oral dose should be administered.
d. Neither oral nor intravenous T3 indicated.

Ans. c

Explanation: Hypothyroid patients should be continued on their outpatient L-T4 dose. Oral L-T4 is the preferred method for replacing thyroid hormone in a hypothyroid patient. Because of the long half-life of about 7 days of LT4, the L-T4 dose can be held for 1–2 days, if the oral route is unavailable. If oral therapy cannot be resumed within 3 days, intravenous L-T4 should be administered. Because <75% of an oral dose of LT4 is absorbed, the intravenous L-T4 dose should be ~75% less than the oral dose. Neither oral nor intravenous L-T3 is indicated in the hypothyroid patient in the absence of myxedema coma.

If hypothyroidism is diagnosed in the ICU setting and initiation of thyroid hormone replacement is required, special consideration should be given to patients with coronary artery disease. In patients with significant preexisting coronary artery disease, starting thyroid hormone may aggravate angina. It is recommended that the initial dose of L-T4 should not exceed 25 µg for those with known ischemic heart disease and 50 µg for patients aged 65 years or older without such a preexisting diagnosis.

The oral dose of L-T4 may differ in the ICU setting due to pharmacologic agents or gastrointestinal conditions that may decrease the absorption of L-T4. Patients with jejunoileal bypass surgery, bowel resection, malabsorptive disorders (such as celiac disease), and conditions that impair gastric acidity may need adjustment in the dose of L-T4. L-T4 should not be administered within 2–3 hours of calcium carbonate, bile acid sequestrants, ferrous sulfate, phosphate binders, sucralfate, and aluminum-containing antacids as they may interfere with the absorption of L-T4. Also by their effect of decreasing gastric acidity, proton pump inhibitors, if given for a long period, may decrease the absorption of L-T4.

Suggested Reading
1. Bello G, Paliani G, Annetta MG, Pontecorvi A, Antonelli M. Treating nonthyroidal illness syndrome in the critically ill patient: still a matter of controversy. Curr Drug Targets. 2009;10(8):778-87.
2. Jonklaas J, Bianco AC, Bauer AJ, Burman KD, Cappola AR, Celi FS, et al. Guidelines for treatment of hypothyroidism. Thyroid. 2014;24(12):1670-750.

Q.23. Which of the below statements is incorrect considering the management of myxedema coma?
a. T4 is the main thyroid hormone used for replacement.
b. It has a high-mortality rate of up to 50%.
c. Active rewarming should be started as soon as possible.
d. Glucocorticoid replacement is mandatory in these patients.

Ans. c

Explanation: Despite its gravity, the management of the hypothermia of myxedema coma differs from the treatment of exposure-induced hypothermia in euthyroid subjects. In a myxedema coma, the patient should be kept in a warm room and covered with blankets. Active rewarming should be avoided because it increases oxygen consumption and promotes peripheral vasodilation and circulatory collapse. Active rewarming is recommended only for situations of severe hypothermia in which ventricular fibrillation is an immediate threat.

Suggested Reading
1. Jonklaas J, Bianco AC, Bauer AJ, Burman KD, Cappola AR, Celi FS, et al. Guidelines for the treatment of hypothyroidism: prepared by the American Thyroid Association Task Force on thyroid hormone replacement. Thyroid. 2014;24(12):1670-751.
2. Wood-allum CA, Shaw PJ, Thyroid disease and the nervous system. In: José Biller, José M. Ferro (Eds). Handbook of Clinical Neurology. Elsevier, Volume 120, 2014; pp. 703-35, ISSN 0072-9752, ISBN 9780702040870

Q.24. A 50-year-old gentleman was brought to the emergency by ambulance with complaints of pain and numbness in both legs. At arrival, purple spots were evident on his neck and face. Examination of the vital sign indicated septic shock. Laboratory data and blood gas analysis revealed disseminated intravascular coagulation, multiple organ failure, and metabolic acidosis. Peripheral blood smears revealed Howell-Jolly's bodies. A rapid urinary pneumococcal antigen test was also found to be positive and CT abdomen was suggestive of small spleen size with bilateral adrenal hemorrhage.
Which of the following statements is true?
a. If treatment started early, most of the patients recover.
b. Almost always associated with meningococcal infection.
c. Treatment is parenteral administration of steroids.
d. Associated with hemorrhage in the pituitary gland.

Ans. c

Explanation: Waterhouse–Friderichsen syndrome (WFS) is an emergency condition, characterized by fever, cyanosis, bruises, and/or shock. It most commonly occurs with meningococcal infection but can occur with other infections also, e.g., *Streptococcus pneumoniae*, *Staphylococcus aureus*, and *Haemophilus influenzae*. Disseminated intravascular coagulation (DIC) is the phenomenon which leads to adrenal hemorrhage. It is treated with steroids along with treatment of underlying disease. Even if treatment is started early, mortality is very high.

Suggested Reading
1. Sonavane A, Baradkar V, Salunkhe P, Kumar S. Waterhouse-Friderichsen syndrome in an adult patient with meningococcal meningitis. Indian J Dermatol. 2011;56(3):326-8.
2. Vincentelli C, Molina EG, Robinson MJ. Fatal pneumococcal Waterhouse-Friderichsen syndrome in a vaccinated adult with congenital asplenia. Am J Emerg Med. 2009;27(6):751. e3-e5.

Q.25. A 49-year-old female patient with a history of Hashimoto thyroiditis presented to the hospital for the evaluation of dizziness, nausea, and vomiting. The patient was hypotensive. Darkening of the palmar creases and tongue was noted. Laboratory data showed serum sodium = 110 mEq/L, potassium = 5.1 mEq/L, serum osmolality = 239 mOsm/kg, urinary osmolarity = 381 mOsm/kg, and urinary sodium = 94 mEq/L.

What is the most likely diagnosis?
a. Dehydration
b. Syndrome of inappropriate antidiuretic hormone secretion
c. Primary adrenal insufficiency
d. Primary polydipsia

Ans. c

Explanation: Adrenal insufficiency (AI) is a relatively rare but serious condition characterized by reduced production of glucocorticoids and/or mineralocorticoids and adrenal androgens due to the destruction of the adrenal gland or lack of its stimulation. It can be divided into primary adrenal insufficiency (PAI), secondary adrenal insufficiency (SAI), and tertiary adrenal insufficiency (TAI), depending on whether the disease process affects the adrenal cortex, anterior pituitary gland, or the hypothalamus, respectively. Clinical features include fatigue and lethargy, weight loss, salt craving, postural dizziness, anorexia, abdominal discomfort, joint and muscle aches, increased pigmentation of the skin, and mucous membranes, especially on sun-exposed areas and those subject to friction, such as knuckles, skin creases, elbows, scars, breast areola (caused by stimulation of dermal melanocortin receptors due to high ACTH and other pro-opiomelanocortin peptides), low blood pressure, and orthostatic hypotension. Laboratory findings include hyponatremia, hyperkalemia, hypoglycemia, hypercalcemia, normochromic anemia, eosinophilia, and lymphocytosis.

- While dehydration (choice A) is a common cause of hyponatremia, associated urinary sodium is frequently <25 mEq/L.

- A syndrome of inappropriate antidiuretic hormone secretion is a diagnosis of exclusion (choice B).
- The patient did not have a history of excessive water intake (choice D).

Suggested Reading
1. Arlt W, Allolio B. Adrenal insufficiency. Lancet. 2003;361:1881-93.
2. Salvatori R. Adrenal insufficiency. JAMA. 2005;294:2481-8.

Q.26. A 24-year-old young male patient underwent laparoscopic adrenalectomy for recently diagnosed pheochromocytoma. The patient is shifted to ICU for postoperative management where he develops hypotension. Which of the following cannot be used for the correction of hypotension in this patient?
a. Norepinephrine
b. Intravenous fluids
c. Epinephrine
d. Phenylephrine

Ans. d

Explanation: Hypotension is a state of low perfusion where it leads to damage to end organs due to hypoperfusion. The most common reasons for hypotension following adrenalectomy in the postoperative settings are chronic or circulating volume state, sudden decrease in catecholamine levels, blood loss, downregulation of catecholamine receptors, and septic shock. Usual management includes adequate volume resuscitation and vasopressor support if needed. Norepinephrine is the drug of choice followed by epinephrine and vasopressin. Pure alpha agonists like phenylephrine are not recommended due to the remnant effect of preoperative alpha blockade.

Suggested Reading
1. Bravo EL. Pheochromocytoma. Cardiol Rev. 2002;10:44-50.
2. Namekawa T, Utsumi T, Kawamura K, Kamiya N, Imamoto T, Takiguchi T, et al. Clinical predictors of prolonged postresection hypotension after laparoscopic adrenalectomy for pheochromocytoma. Surgery. 2016:159;763-70.
3. Olson SW, Deal LE, Piesman M. Epinephrine-secreting pheochromocytoma presenting with cardiogenic shock and profound hypocalcemia. Ann Intern Med. 2004:140;849-51.

Q.27. A 54-year-old man with carcinoma of the bladder was scheduled for transurethral resection of a bladder tumor. He was obese and had a history of a prior stroke. He was very anxious about the procedure and refused a neuraxial block. The surgery, therefore, proceeded under general anesthesia. The operation duration was 75 minutes. Glycine 1.5% solution was used as irrigation fluid. Reversal of neuromuscular blockade was given when a train-of-four count of 3/4 was achieved. 4 hours after the surgery, the patient shows signs of confusion and begins to experience seizures. Which of the following is the most likely complication causing the patient's symptoms?
a. Hyponatremia
b. Hyperglycemia
c. Hypertension
d. Hypocalcemia

Ans. a

Explanation: Electrolyte-free hypotonic solutions such as glycine, mannitol, and sorbitol solutions are used as distending media to enable monopolar electrical systems to be used for coagulation and tissue resection. However, with the low viscosities, these irrigation fluids bear potential risks of rapid fluid absorption resulting in fluid overload, dilutional hyponatremia, and subsequent side effects. The rate of fluid absorption is driven primarily by the gradient between irrigation pressure and venous pressure (or the pressure of the operating cavity). In general, irrigation fluid is absorbed at a rate of 10–30 mL per minute during procedures. Fluid absorption increases with resection extent and longer operation time. The exposure of venous sinuses in the prostate provides ready access to irrigation fluid to the circulation, putting these patients at particular risk.

The presentation of transurethral resection of prostate (TURP) syndrome varies, with symptoms developing any time from 15 minutes to 24 hours after the operation. Symptoms include headache, burning sensation in the face and hands, restlessness, and tachypnea. Visual disturbances, such as blurred vision and transient blindness, can occur. If left untreated, patients can deteriorate with features of nausea and vomiting, respiratory distress, pulmonary edema, confusion, convulsions, and coma. Hypothermia is another important factor to consider in cases of suspected TURP syndrome, given the systemic absorption of large volumes of physiologically hypothermic solutions.

The treatment of TURP syndrome is largely supportive, with early recognition of the developing syndrome being critical to the best outcomes.

Suggested Reading
1. Jin Y, Tian J, Sun M, Yang K. A systematic review of randomised controlled trials of the effects of warmed irrigation fluid on core body temperature during endoscopic surgeries. J Clin Nurs. 2011;20:305-16.
2. O'Donnell AM, Foo ITH. Anaesthesia for transurethral resection of the prostate. Contin Educ Anaesth Crit Care Pain. 2009;9:92-6.

Q.28. A 45-year-old gentleman with a history of uncontrolled diabetes presented to the ICU with a history of shortness of breath and fever for the past 5 days and altered sensorium for 1 day. His blood glucose level is 380 mg/dL. pH is 7.02, with a bicarbonate of 4 and an anion gap of 22. The serum potassium value is 3.2 mmol/L, and sodium is 148 mmol/L. Urine ketone came positive for 3+. Which of the following statements is incorrect?
  a. The usual fluid deficit in DKA is around 4–6 L.
  b. Potassium correction needs to be started before insulin therapy.
  c. Bicarbonate therapy has an insignificant role in the above case.
  d. Once blood sugars are controlled, insulin therapy can be stopped.

Ans. d

Explanation: Diabetic ketoacidosis (DKA) is due to relative insulin deficiency, and excessive counterregulatory hormones such as glucagon and cortisol accompanied by dehydration.

Various exacerbating factors include infection, trauma, pregnancy, myocardial infarction, stroke, etc. Laboratory findings include hyperglycemia (glucose > 250 mg/dL), glycosuria, elevated anion gap, metabolic acidosis, and serum or urine ketones.

The typical total body water deficit is 4–6 L. Sodium deficit is 7–10 mEq/L and potassium deficit is 3–5 mEq/kg. When potassium is <5 mEq/L, potassium correction should be undertaken along with fluid resuscitation. Initial intravenous loading bolus insulin started at 0.1–0.15 U/kg of regular insulin followed by continuous infusion of 0.1 U/kg/h. Monitor blood glucose every hour, expected blood glucose decline to be 50–75 mg/dL/h. A slower response could indicate insulin resistance and inadequate fluid resuscitation. In case of <250 mg/dL serum glucose, add 5% dextrose to intravenous fluids and decrease insulin infusion rate by up to half. The criterion for resolution of DKA states that a glucose <200 mg/dL, serum bicarbonate of >18 mEq/L with a normal anion gap, and a venous pH of >7.3. Bicarbonate therapy in DKA is controversial and should not be routinely administered unless the serum pH is <7.0 or the patient has life-threatening hyperkalemia.

Suggested Reading
1. Fayfman M, Pasquel FJ, Umpierrez GE. Management of hyperglycemic crises. Med Clin North Am. 2016;101(3):587-606.
2. Joint British Diabetes Societies Inpatient Care Group. (2013). The management of diabetic ketoacidosis in adults, 2nd edition. [online] Available from: http://www.diabetologists-abcd.org.uk/jbds/jbds_ip_dka_adults_revised.pdf. [Last accessed June, 2023]
3. Naunheim R, Jang TJ, Banet G, Richmond A, McGill J. Point-of-care test identifies diabetic ketoacidosis at triage. Acad Emerg Med. 2006;13(6):683-5.

CHAPTER 12

Neurocritical Care

Indu Kapoor, Charu Mahajan, Hemanshu Prabhakar

Q.1. A 21-year-old male was brought to the emergency department (ED) with a history of a head injury following a road traffic accident. On examination, his Glasgow Coma Scale (GCS) was E1V2M3, blood pressure (BP)—140/90 mm Hg, pulse rate—55/min, respiratory rate—35/min, irregular and oxygen saturation—92% on oxygen by face mask. His trachea was secured with an endotracheal tube (8 mm ID). His computed tomographic (CT) scan revealed subdural hematoma (SDH), 15 mm in thickness with midline shift of 8 mm. He was taken up for decompressive craniectomy under general anesthesia. Intraoperative course was uneventful. On postoperative day 2, patients GCS deteriorated further with absence of cough reflex, corneal reflex, cough reflex, and gag reflex with dilated pupils which were nonreactive bilaterally. Apnea test was performed to confirm if the patient is brain dead. Which of the following sentence is true for apnea test?
a. Absence of respiration if partial pressure of carbon dioxide ($PaCO_2$) >60 mm Hg
b. Absence of respiration if PaO_2 of <60 mm Hg
c. Duration between two apnea tests should be 24 hours
d. Apnea test can be done if patient has mid-dilated pupils

Ans. a

Explanation: To determine the brain death, apnea test is a mandatory examination as it provides an essential sign of definitive loss of brainstem function. Patient is preoxygenated before performing an apnea test. There are several techniques to maintain sufficient oxygenation during apnea test. Some clinicians disconnect the patient from the ventilator and to insert a catheter or cannula into the endotracheal tube down to the level of the carina and provide pure oxygen at a rate of 4–10 L/min. Others do not disconnect from the ventilator but the minute volume is decreased to a very low level (0.5–2 L/min). Apnea test is positive when no breathing effort is observed at a $PaCO_2$ of 60 mm Hg or with a 20 mm Hg increment from baseline; thereby supporting the diagnosis of brain death.

Suggested Reading
1. Lang CJ, Heckmann JG. How should testing for apnea be performed in diagnosing brain death? Adv Exp Med Biol. 2004;550:169-74.
2. Machado C, Perez J, Scherle C, Areu A, Pando A. Brain death diagnosis and apnea test safety. Ann Indian Acad Neurol. 2009;12(3):197-200.

3. Tsai WH, Lee WT, Hung KL. Determination of brain death in children—a medicial center experience. Acta Paediatr Taiwan. 2005;46(3):132-7.

Q.2. The emergency department received a mass causality from a building collapse that happened in a factory. The victim sustained head injuries following this mishap. Most of the patients received were having very low GCS and were later on confirmed as brain-dead. Which of the following brain dead patient could not be taken up for organ donation?
a. Elderly
b. Pregnant
c. Female
d. Human immunodeficiency virus (HIV) positive

Ans. d

Explanation: Transmission of infectious disease through organ donor to recipient has been associated with severe complications and poor outcomes. In an attempt to prevent donor-derived infections, organ and tissue donors are evaluated to identify those that might be more likely to harbor transmissible pathogens. Donor testing includes the donor's microbial culture data (e.g., blood, urine, sputum), serologic assay results [e.g., antibodies against HIV, hepatitis B virus (HBV), and hepatitis C virus (HCV)], and increasingly, nucleic acid testing (NAT) results, including assays for HIV, HCV, or HBV.

Suggested Reading
1. Centers for Disease Control and Prevention (CDC). HIV transmitted from a living organ donor—New York City, 2009. MMWR Morb Mortal Wkly Rep. 2011;60(10):297-301.
2. Greenwald MA, Kuehnert MJ, Fishman JA. Infectious disease transmission during organ and tissue transplantation. Emerg Infect Dis. 2012;18(8):e1.

Q.3. A 45-year-old female was diagnosed with a left frontal contusion following a fall from height. During her stay in neurointensive care unit, she developed a fever on day 2 which was continuous in nature initially later it fluctuated from 37.5–38.5°. Fever was associated with tachypnea (RR 30–35/min), high heart rate (120–130/min), and hypertension (mean blood pressure 100–110 mm Hg). Her culture reports were nonconclusive and she did not respond to any empirical antibiotic therapy or antipyretic agents. She was diagnosed as a case of central fever. Which of the following could be the best option to treat central fever in a traumatic brain-injured patient?
a. Paracetamol
b. Cold sponging
c. Baclofen
d. Cold fluids

Ans. c

Explanation: The central fever is suspected if fever is occurring within 72 hours of admission following intracranial hemorrhage, tumor, or stroke along with negative cultures, and absent infiltrate on chest X-rays. Different drugs are used successfully to treat central fever which includes dantrolene, bromocriptine, amantadine, and baclofen. Baclofen acts directly on the raphe nuclei to suppress brown adipose tissue activation which leads to a decrease in body temperature.

Suggested Reading
1. Childers MK, Rupright J, Smith DW. Post-traumatic hyperthermia in acute brain injury rehabilitation. Brain Inj. 1994;8(4):335-43.
2. Lee H, Kim J, Lim J, Jo YS, Kim SK. Central Hyperthermia Treated With Baclofen for Patient With Pontine Hemorrhage. Ann Rehabil Med. 2014;38(2):269-72.
3. Sengupta D, Kapoor I, Mahajan C, Prabhakar H. Baclofen for neurogenic fever in a patient with cerebral contusion. J Clin Anesth. 2019;55:134-5.
4. Yung-Sung H, Ming-Chang H, Lee M, Huang Y-H, Lee J-D. Baclofen successfully abolished prolonged central hyperthermia in a patient with basilar artery occlusion. Acta Neurol Taiwan. 2009;18(2):118-22.

Q.4. A 65-year-old man met with an accident while driving a two-wheeler. He was brought to the emergency department a passerby. He was bleeding from ear, nose, and mouth. He also had blisters on front and back of the head. Neurosurgeon on call was informed by the emergency doctor as he was suspecting the head injury. Neurosurgeon on examination found his GCS E2V3M4. Neurosurgeon found the clinical signs of raised intracranial pressure which include high blood pressure, bradycardia, and unequal pupils sluggishly reactive to light. Which of the following diagnostic modality could not diagnose midline shift in a traumatic brain-injured patient?
a. Ultrasound (USG)
b. CT scan
c. Magnetic resonance imaging (MRI) scan
d. X-ray

Ans. d

Explanation: Midline shift (MLS) of the brain is a life-threatening condition that requires urgent diagnosis and treatment. There could be a two-fold increase in mortality when the MLS exceeded 1 cm. A MLS above 0.5 cm on the initial brain CT scan has been shown to predict poor neurological outcomes. The early detection of a MLS in neurocritically ill patients is therefore crucial because it allows the implementation of a timely and appropriate treatment plan. Apart from CT scan and MRI scan of the brain, transcranial ultrasonography (TCS) has been shown to visualize the intracranial structures. TCS could detect MLS with reasonable accuracy in neurosurgical intensive care unit (ICU) patients and that it could be used as a bedside tool to facilitate early diagnosis and treatment for patients with a significant intracranial mass effect.

Suggested Reading
1. Becker DP, Miller JD, Ward JD, Greenberg RP, Young HF, Sakalas R. The outcome from severe head injury with early diagnosis and intensive management. J Neurosurg. 1977;47(4):491-502.
2. Bogdahn U, Becker G, Winkler J, Greiner K, Perez J, Meurers B. Transcranial color-coded real-time sonography in adults. Stroke. 1990;21:1680-8.
3. Motuel J, Biette I, Srairi M, Mrozek S, Kurrek MM, Chaynes P, et al. Assessment of brain midline shift using sonography in neurosurgical ICU patients. Crit Care. 2014;18(6):676.
4. Quattrocchi KB, Prasad P, Willits NH, Wagner FC Jr. Quantification of midline shift as a predictor of poor outcome following head injury. Surg Neurol. 1991;35(3):183-8.

Q.5. A 19-year-old male was working in his farm when he was hit by a bull. He has a loss of consciousness associated with bleeding from nose. He was taken to a nearby hospital where first aid was given to him. He was referred to our hospital and received in ED after 5 hours of injury. His GCS was E3V3M5 with stable vitals (BP—138/70 mm Hg and PR—76/min). His CT scan head was suggestive of a small hemorrhagic contusion in the frontal and parietal region on right side. He was shifted to neurointensive care unit for further observation and monitoring. As per 4th edition Brain Trauma Foundation (BTF) guidelines, which neuromonitoring modality is not recommended in patients with traumatic brain injury (TBI)?
  a. Transcranial Doppler (TCD)
  b. Jugular bulb venous oxygen saturation ($SjVO_2$)
  c. Intracranial pressure (ICP)
  d. Cerebral perfusion pressure (CPP)

Ans. a

Explanation: As per 4th edition BTF guidelines, there is a level IIb recommendation for ICP monitoring in patients with TBI to reduce in-hospital and 2 weeks postinjury mortality. Intracranial pressure should be monitored in all salvageable patients with a TBI (GCS 3-8 after resuscitation) and an abnormal CT scan or in patients with severe TBI with a normal CT scan if ≥2 of the following features are noted at admission: age >40 years, unilateral or bilateral motor posturing, or SBP <90 mm Hg. There is a level IIb recommendation for CPP monitoring to decrease 2 weeks mortality. In advanced cerebral monitoring, level III recommendation is there to use $SjVO_2$ monitoring to reduce mortality and improve outcomes at 3 and 6 months postinjury.

Suggested Reading
  1. Carney N, Totten AM, O'Reilly C, Ullman JS, Hawryluk GW, Bell MJ, et al. Guidelines for the Management of Severe Traumatic Brain Injury, Fourth Edition. Neurosurgery. 2017;80(1):6-15.

Q.6. A 45-year-old lady presented to outpatient department (OPD) with complaints of headache for last few months. Her CT scan head was suggestive of a large supratentorial tumor measuring 4 × 3.8 × 5 cm. She is a known hypertensive since last 2 years on tablet amlodipine 5 mg OD. She was posted for elective craniotomy and excision of tumor under general anesthesia. Suddenly at night, she became drowsy with vitals suggestive of hypertension and bradycardia. A repeat CT scan head was planned and it showed gross peritumor edema with a midline shift of 7 mm. She was taken up for emergency decompressive craniectomy under general anesthesia. Which of the following is not a noninvasive method of ICP monitoring?
  a. Optic nerve sheath diameter
  b. Pupillometer
  c. Transcranial sonography
  d. Brain tissue oxygenation ($PbtO_2$)

Ans. d

Explanation: Intracranial pressure monitoring is important in many neurosurgical and neurological patients. The gold standard for ICP monitoring is the invasive procedure that includes insertion of catheter in the anterior horn of lateral ventricle. There are noninvasive methods of ICP monitoring that avoids the complications such as hemorrhage, infection, and pain that are associated with invasive method. Optic nerve sheath diameter (ONSD) is a commonly used surrogate for ICP. Rationale being, the communication of the subarachnoid space with the intracranial cavity, changes in cerebrospinal fluid (CSF) pressure could be transmitted along the optic nerve. Pupillometry is a useful tool for screening patients with possibly increased ICP; however, it cannot be suggested for continuous ICP monitoring. A relationship between ICP and TCD-derived flow velocities has been described in the literature. An increase in ICP correlates with a decrease in TCD-derived flow velocities and an increase in Pourcelot index or resistance index (RI), where RI = (systolic flow velocity – diastolic flow velocity)/(systolic flow velocity).

Suggested Reading
1. Chen JW, Gombart ZJ, Rogers S, Gardiner SK, Cecil S, Bullock RM. Pupillary reactivity as an early indicator of increased intracranial pressure: The introduction of the Neurological Pupil index. Surg Neurol Int. 2011;2:82.
2. Khan MN, Shallwani H, Khan MU, Shamim MS. Noninvasive monitoring intracranial pressure - A review of available modalities. Surg Neurol Int. 2017;8:51.
3. Kimberly HH, Shah S, Marill K, Noble V. Correlation of optic nerve sheath diameter with direct measurement of intracranial pressure. Acad Emerg Med. 2008;15(2):201-4.

Q.7. A 55-year-old male was brought to the emergency department with sudden weakness on left side of the body along with slurring of speech. He was last seen normal 2 hours back by his son. He was known hypertensive and diabetic for last 5 years. On examination, patient was fully conscious. His vitals showed blood pressure: 170/90 mm Hg, pulse rate: 76/min, oxygen saturation: 95%. His NCCT head showed an infarct in the left middle cerebral artery (MCA) territory. He was immediately shifted to neuroradiology laboratory for intravenous thrombolysis under monitored anesthesia care. After 3 hours patient complained of swollen face, difficulty in breathing with rashes all over the body. Clinicians made the diagnosis of angioedema in this patient and treated him accordingly. Angioedema is a side effect of which drug?
a. Tenecteplase
b. Alteplase
c. Noradrenaline
d. Tranexamic acid

Ans. b

Explanation: Angioedema is a sudden, transient swelling of well-demarcated areas of the dermis, subcutaneous tissue, mucosa, and submucosal tissues, which occurs with or without urticaria. It can progress rapidly, and may involve the mouth, tongue, larynx, lips, or face making it a medical emergency. It could be hereditary, acquired, idiopathic, and allergic because of the administration of drugs such as angiotensin-converting enzyme (ACE) inhibitors and thrombolytics. The incidence of angioedema after alteplase treatment was up to 5%, and concurrent use of ACE inhibitors and signs of ischemia on initial CT were the major risk factors for the development of angioedema.

Angioedema caused by alteplase treatment is usually mild. Most of the patients respond to antihistamines, steroids, and epinephrine. Sometimes endotracheal intubation is required if the airway is compromised.

Suggested Reading
1. Bernstein JA, Moellman J. Emerging concepts in the diagnosis and treatment of patients with undifferentiated angioedema. Int J Emerg Med. 2012;5(1):39.
2. Engelter ST, Fluri F, Buitrago-Tellez C, Marsch S, Steck AJ, Ruegg S, et al. Life-threatening orolingual angioedema during thrombolysis in acute ischemic stroke. J Neurol. 2005;252(10):1167-70.
3. Hill MD, Barber PA, Takahashi J, Demchuk AM, Feasby TE, Buchan AM. Anaphylactoid reactions and angioedema during alteplase treatment of acute ischemic stroke. CMAJ. 2000;162(9):1281-4.
4. Hill MD, Buchan AM. Thrombolysis for acute ischemic stroke: results of the Canadian alteplase for stroke effectiveness study. CMAJ. 2005;172(10):1307-12.

Q.8. Which of the following statement is true about brain heart crosstalk in a neurologically injured patient?
a. Only ascending pathways are involved in communication between brain and heart
b. Catecholamine theory is most widely accepted mechanism
c. Echocardiography will not show any specific finding
d. Brain heart crosstalk is less common in females

Ans. b

Explanation: There are number of mechanisms of stress cardiomyopathy have been discussed over many years which include microvascular dysfunction, multivessel coronary artery spasm, spontaneous coronary artery thrombus lysis, and increased level of catecholamine. The most widely accepted theory for stress cardiomyopathy is catecholamine theory. Catecholamine surge occurs following neurological injury and may dispose to repolarization abnormalities. This surge can occur within 48 hours of injury and might persist for even a week and more.

Suggested Reading
1. Boland TA, Lee VH, Bleck TP. Stress-induced cardiomyopathy. Crit Care Med. 2015;43(3):686-93.
2. Bybee KA, Prasad A. Stress-related cardiomyopathy syndromes. Circulation. 2008;118(4): 397-409.
3. Prabhakar H, Kapoor I. Brain and Heart Crosstalk, 1st edition. Singapore: Springer Nature Pte. Ltd.; 2020.

Q.9. A 35-year-old operated case of Basal ganglia bleed was admitted in neurointensive care unit for last 5 days. His present GCS was E2VtM4. Patient is on injection fentanyl and injection midazolam infusion as he is irritable and agitated. For sedation monitoring which of the following score can be used?
a. Visual analog scale (VAS) score
b. World Federation of Neurosurgeons (WFNS) score
c. Richmond Agitation and Sedation Scale (RASS) score
d. Likert score

Ans. c

Explanation: Richmond agitation and sedation score is a commonly used score for monitoring sedation in intensive care units. It is a 10-point score ranging from +4 to –5. The score of 0 indicates that patient is calm and alert. Other scores such as VAS score used for pain assessment, the WFNS score is used for grading of subarachnoid hemorrhage (SAH), and the Likert score is used for measuring patients satisfaction.

Suggested Reading
1. Imai K, Morita T, Yokomichi N, Mori M, Naito AS, Yamauchi T, et al. Association of the RASS Score with Intensity of Symptoms, Discomfort, and Communication Capacity in Terminally Ill Cancer Patients Receiving Palliative Sedation: Is RASS an Appropriate Outcome Measure? Palliat Med Rep. 2022;3(1):47-54.
2. Prabhakar H, Tripathy S, Gupta N, Singhal V, Mahajan C, Kapoor I, et al. Consensus Statement on Analgo-sedation in Neurocritical Care and Review of Literature. Indian J Crit Care Med. 2021;25(2):126-33.
3. Taran Z, Namadian M, Faghihzadeh S, Naghibi T. The Effect of Sedation Protocol Using Richmond Agitation-Sedation Scale (RASS) on Some Clinical Outcomes of Mechanically Ventilated Patients in Intensive Care Units: a Randomized Clinical Trial. J Caring Sci. 2019;8(4):199-206.

Q.10. A 55-year-old female presented with complaints of ascending weakness starting from lower limbs and progressing to upper limb gradually over last few days. She landed up in ED with difficulty in breathing. A clinical diagnosis of Guillain–Barré syndrome (GBS) was made and she was planned for emergency intubation. What would be the choice of neuromuscular blocking agent to use for rapid sequence intubation (RSI) in GBS patient?
a. Rocuronium
b. Succinylcholine
c. Pancuronium
d. Vecuronium

Ans. a

Explanation: In this case, rocuronium would be the choice of agent for RSI. Rocuronium dose @1 mg/kg will give optimal condition and time frame for intubation same as succinylcholine. Succinylcholine though provides rapid onset of action, it can exaggerate hyperkalemic response following degeneration in skeletal muscle. On the other hand, pancuronium and vecuronium will have slower onset of action.

Suggested Reading
1. Fokke C, van den Berg B, Drenthen J, Walgaard C, van Doorn PA, Jacobs BC. Diagnosis of Guillain—Barré syndrome and validation of Brighton criteria. Brain. 2014;137(Pt 1):33-43.
2. Willison HJ, Jacobs BC, van Doorn PA. Guillain—Barré syndrome. Lancet. 2016;388(10045): 717-27.

Q.11. A relative of a 67-year-old male brought him to the ED with low GCS (E2V2M4). The relative found him unconscious at the stairs. There is a past history of hypertension and diabetes given by the relative. In ED his blood sugar was 156 mg/dL. His airway was secured with ET cuffed tube 8.00 mm ID. His carotid angiography revealed >70% stenosis of right internal carotid artery. He was then scheduled for carotid

stenting under general anesthesia. Intraoperative period remained uneventful. His neuromuscular blockade was not reversed because of poor preoperative GCS. On postoperative day 2, patient had multiple episodes of seizures along with marker hypertension. What could be the possible cause:
a. Cerebral hyperperfusion syndrome
b. Uncontrolled blood pressure
c. Inadequate sedation
d. Severe pain

Ans. a

Explanation: Cerebral hyperperfusion syndrome (CHS) is a known complication that can occur in patients undergoing carotid stenting or carotid endarterectomy (CEA). It typically occurs 2-7 days postsurgery. This condition is characterized by neurological deficit, seizures, blurry vision, headache, and hypertension. Treatment of CHS includes blood pressure control and treatment of raised intracranial pressure.

Suggested Reading
1. Bharadwaj D, Kapoor I, Mahajan C, Prabhakar H. Cerebral hyperperfusion syndrome after external carotid artery-middle cerebral artery bypass for carotid artery giant aneurysm. J Clin Anesth. 2019;54:41-2.
2. Wu TY, Anderson NE, Barber PA. Neurological complications of carotid revascularisation. J Neurol Neurosurg Psychiatry. 2012;83(5):543-50.

Q.12. Which of the following statement regarding use of steroids in patients with traumatic brain injury is true?
a. Steroids are safe to be used in patients with traumatic brain injury
b. GUDHIS trial used hydrocortisone for patients with traumatic brain injury
c. There is a level II recommendation against use of steroids in patients with traumatic brain injury
d. Steroids can be used for adrenal insufficiency which is an adverse effect of traumatic brain injury

Ans. d

Explanation: As per the recent brain trauma foundation guidelines (4th edition), there is a level I recommendation against its use in patients with traumatic brain injury. However, this should not be used as a blanket statement regarding use of steroids in these patients. Adrenal insufficiency is a known adverse effect of traumatic brain injury. Its incidence is as high as 25% in these patients. Steroids can be used empirically in these patients using a stress dose.

Suggested Reading
1. Powner DJ, Boccalandro C. Adrenal insufficiency following traumatic brain injury in adults. Curr Opin Crit Care. 2008;14(2):163-6.
2. Prabhakar H, Rajan S, Kapoor I, Mahajan C. Problem Based Learning Discussions in Neuroanesthesia and Neurocritical Care, 1st edition. Singapore: Springer Nature Pte. Ltd.; 2020.

Q.13. A 10-month-old female child was brought to OPD with complaint of abnormal head shape. Her CT scan head confirmed the diagnosis of coronal synostosis. She was full term, delivered vaginally with no complications at birth or prior hospitalization history. She was planned for cranial vault remodeling surgery under general anesthesia. Her intraoperative course was uneventful with blood loss of around 100 mL, which was replaced in the operation theater. Her neuromuscular blockade was reversed successfully and was shifted to intensive care unit with spontaneous movements for further management and monitoring. What is the best option for postoperative pain management in this patient?
   a. Scalp block
   b. Fentanyl
   c. Paracetamol
   d. All of the above

Ans. d

Explanation: At present the literature is scarce in providing information describing various options for pain management after craniosynostosis repair surgery. Use of scalp block after induction of anesthesia or at the end of the surgery, provides an optimal postoperative pain relief in these patients. It also reduces the consumptions of opioids as well as other analgesics in intensive care unit. Opioids is another options which provides good pain relief, however vigilant monitoring would be required with opioids as it might cause respiratory depression. Paracetamol is one of the most commonly and safest analgesics being used in young children.

Suggested Reading
1. Kattail D, Macmillan A, Musavi L, Pedreira R, Faateh M, Cho R, et al. Pain Management for Nonsyndromic Craniosynostosis: Adequate Analgesia in a Pediatric Cohort? J Craniofac Surg. 2018;29(5):1148-53.
2. Pardey Bracho GF, Pereira de Souza Neto E, Grousson S, Mottolese C, Dailler F. Opioid consumption after levobupivacaine scalp nerve block for craniosynostosis surgery. Acta Anaesthesiol Taiwan. 2014;52(2):64-9.

Q.14. Which of the following is not true about postoperative concerns and complications in patients with craniopharyngioma?
   a. Incidence of diabetes insipidus (DI) is around 20–30%
   b. Hypovolemia should be maintained with the use of normal saline
   c. Postoperative pain is a minor concern
   d. Postoperative hypopituitarism incidence is around 50–100%

Ans. d

Explanation: In postoperative period signs and symptoms of hypopituitarism such as anterior and posterior pituitary dysfunction is seen 50–100% of patients. Steroid replacement is given to these patients. Some patients receive steroids even for long duration in order to balance hypothalamic-pituitary axis. The incidence of DI is around 70–90%. Intranasal desmopressin is effective to treat DI. Normovolemia should be maintained in the postoperative period. Pain is a major concern in these patients. Multimodal approach including scalp block, opioids, and acetaminophen are helpful.

Suggested Reading
1. Cohen M, Bartels U, Branson H, Kulkarni AV, Hamilton J. Trends in treatment and outcomes of pediatric craniopharyngioma, 1975–2011. Neuro Oncol. 2013;15(6):767-74.
2. Prabhakar H, Rajan S, Kapoor I, Mahajan C. Problem Based Learning Discussions in Neuroanesthesia and Neurocritical Care, 1st edition. Singapore: Springer Nature Pte. Ltd.; 2020.

Q.15. A 72-year-old man with a history of obstructive sleep apnea (OSA) was operated for a pituitary tumor. He had undergone transnasal transsphenoidal (TNTS) surgery under general anesthesia. In past, he often used continuous positive airway pressure (CPAP) at night for obstructive sleep apnea (OSA). In preoperative examination, his weight was around 85 kg, height was 156 cm, blood pressure was 140/88 mm Hg, pulse rate was 76/min, and oxygen saturation is 95% on room air. In postoperative period, he was shifted to intensive care unit with oxygen on a face mask @6 L/min with an oxygen saturation of 99%. After 2 hours patient complained of difficulty in breathing along with a fall in oxygen saturation to 92%. Looking at the present scenario, which method you would not recommend to build up his oxygen levels?
a. Face mask with reservoir bag
b. High-flow nasal cannula
c. Lateral position with oral airway
d. CPAP

Ans. d

Explanation: The use of CPAP in patients who have undergone TNTS surgery might increase the risk of pneumocephalus and meningitis. Moreover, it can also aggravate the edema of nasal as well as oral cavity with an already compromised airway. At present, there are no consensus statements or guidelines for management for patients with OSA following TNTS surgery.

Suggested Reading
1. Rahimi E, Mariappan R, Tharmaradinam S, Manninen P, Venkatraghavan L. Perioperative management and complications in patients with obstructive sleep apnea undergoing transsphenoidal surgery: Our institutional experience. J Anaesthesiol Clin Pharmacol. 2014;30(3):351-4.
2. Venkatraghavan L, Perks A. Postoperative management of obstructive sleep apnea after transsphenoidal pituitary surgery. J Neurosurg Anesthesiol. 2009;21(2):179-80.

Q.16. A 69-year-old female was admitted to neurointensive care unit with diagnosis of mild head injury with a fracture right tibia. The nurse attending the patient told the clinician that her patient is agitated and often has irrelevant talk. She was a known diabetic and hypertensive on regular medication. Which of the following could not be the possible cause of agitation in this patient admitted in neurointensive care unit?
a. Delirium
b. Hypotension
c. Hyperglycemia
d. Pain

Ans. c

Explanation: Pain is a common place in neurointensive care unit. Critically ill patients may experience more pain than healthy people due to hypernociception. Uncontrolled pain may increase agitation, and have a deleterious effect on the intracranial pressure (ICP) in patients with traumatic brain injury which can further result in delirium and post-traumatic stress disorder. Severe pain may also cause hemodynamic disturbances such as tachycardia, bradycardia, hypertension, and hypotension. As per an Indian Consensus statement on analgosedation in neurocritically ill patients, analgesics should be started before sedation in these patients (strong recommendation).

Suggested Reading
1. Fischer M, Jackson M, Abd-Elsayed A. Pain in the neurocritical care unit. In: Prabhakar H, Ali Z (Eds). Textbook of Neuroanesthesia and Neurocritical Care, 1st edition. Singapore: Springer; 2019. pp. 319-31.
2. Hannawi Y, Ziai WC. Analgesia, sedation, and paralysis in the neurocritical care Unit. In: Torbey MT (Ed). Neurocritical Care, 2nd edition. Cambridge: Cambridge University Press; 2019. pp. 33-49.
3. Prabhakar H, Tripathy S, Gupta N, Singhal V, Mahajan C, Kapoor I, et al. Consensus Statement on Analgo-sedation in Neurocritical Care and Review of Literature. Indian J Crit Care Med. 2021;25(2):126-33.

Q.17. The clinical manifestations of paroxysmal sympathetic hyperactivity (PSH) include all of the following, except for which of the following?
 a. Respiratory depression b. Tachypnea
 c. Hyperthermia d. Diaphoresis

Ans. a

Explanation: Paroxysmal sympathetic hyperactivity is a clinical condition characterized by paroxysmal episodes of sympathetic hyperactivity after traumatic brain injury. The core clinical features include tachycardia, hypertension, tachypnea, hyperthermia, sweating, and/or increased muscle tone with possible dystonic posturing. The pathophysiology of PSH is not clearly defined. The PSH is thought to be driven by the loss of the inhibition of excitation in the sympathetic nervous system without parasympathetic involvement.

Suggested Reading
1. Baguley IJ, Perkes IE, Fernandez-Ortega JF, Rabinstein AA, Dolce G, Hendricks HT, et al. Paroxysmal sympathetic hyperactivity after acquired brain injury: consensus on conceptual definition, nomenclature, and diagnostic criteria. J Neurotrauma. 2014;31(17):1515-20.
2. Perkes I, Baguley IJ, Nott MT, Menon DK. A review of paroxysmal sympathetic hyperactivity after acquired brain injury. Ann Neurol. 2010;68(2)126-35.
3. Zheng RZ, Lei ZQ, Yang RZ, Huang GH, Zhang GM. Identification and Management of Paroxysmal Sympathetic Hyperactivity After Traumatic Brain Injury. Front Neurol. 2020;11:81.

Q.18. A 19-year-old male was brought to the emergency department after he was hit by a four-wheeler while cycling back from the park. On examination, his GCS was

E1V2M5 (8/15). **Bilateral pupils were dilated and nonreactive to light. His CT scan head was suggestive of diffuse SAH following traumatic brain injury. His GCS-P score was 6. What in the abbreviation GCS-P, P refers to?**
a. Pupil
b. Pediatric
c. Ptosis
d. Pain

Ans. a

Explanation: The Glasgow Coma Scale-Pupil (GCS-P) is recently introduced for assessing traumatic brain injury. The range of GCS is from 3 to 15 whereas GCS-P score ranges from 1–15. The GCS-P score is calculated by subtracting the pupil score from the total GCS score. The pupil score includes—bilateral pupils not reactive to light: 2, unilateral pupil reactive to light: 1, and both pupils reactive to light: 0. The pupillary findings have been found to significantly affect the decision-making and outcome of patients with traumatic brain injury.

Suggested Reading
1. Kobata H, Ikawa F, Sato A, Kato Y, Sano H. Significance of Pupillary Findings in Decision Making and Outcomes of World Federation of Neurological Societies Grade V Subarachnoid Hemorrhage. Neurosurgery. 2023.
2. Mack WJ, Hickman ZL, Ducruet AF, Kalyvas JT, Garrett MC, Starke RM, et al. Pupillary reactivity upon hospital admission predicts long-term outcome in poor grade aneurysmal subarachnoid hemorrhage patients. Neurocrit Care. 2008;8(3):374-9.

Q.19. An intracranial pressure on more than X in a patient of traumatic brain injury requires treatment. Which of the following is *correct*?
a. X = 16 mm Hg
b. X = 18 mm Hg
c. X = 20 mm Hg
d. X = 22 mm Hg

Ans. d

Explanation: The 4th edition Brain Trauma Foundation (BTF) guidelines recommend (level IIb) treatment of intracranial pressure (ICP) >22 mm Hg as a value above this is associated with increased mortality. BTF guidelines also recommend (level III) that a combination of ICP values, clinical findings, and CT brain findings may be used to make management decisions.

Suggested Reading
1. Carney N, Totten AM, O'Reilly C, Ullman JS, Hawryluk GW, Bell MJ, et al. Guidelines for the Management of Severe Traumatic Brain Injury, Fourth Edition. Neurosurgery. 2017;80(1):6-15.

Q.20. The popular trials MR CLEAN, SWIFT PRIME, ESCAPE, and DAWN are related to which of the following neurologic conditions?
a. Traumatic brain injury
b. Status epilepticus
c. Stroke
d. Subarachnoid hemorrhage

Ans. c

Explanation: The endovascular treatment options for a patient with stroke include mechanical thrombectomy or intra-arterial thrombolysis. These options are considered in patients who are not eligible for intravenous tissue plasminogen activator (tPA). However, a patient planned for endovascular therapy should receive IV tPA. The above trials MR CLEAN, SWIFT PRIME, and ESCAPE are the randomized controlled trials (RCTs) on endovascular treatment of acute ischemic stroke using stent retrievers. These studies demonstrated the improved recanalization rate and outcome after acute ischemic stroke. The DAWN trial extended the time window for mechanical thrombectomy in large anterior circulation vessel occlusion to 6–24 hours in patients who had a mismatch between the severity of clinical deficit and the infarct volume.

Suggested Reading
1. Berkhemer OA, Fransen PS, Beumer D, van den Berg LA, Lingsma HF, Yoo AJ, et al. A randomized trial of intraarterial treatment for acute ischemic stroke. N Engl J Med. 2015;372(1):11-20.
2. Goyal M, Demchuk AM, Menon BK, Eesa M, Rempel JL, Thornton J, et al. Randomized assessment of rapid endovascular treatment of ischemic stroke. N Engl J Med. 2015;372(11):1019-30.
3. Nogueira RG, Jadhav AP, Haussen DC, Bonafe A, Budzik RF, Bhuva P, et al. Thrombectomy 6 to 24 hours after Stroke with a Mismatch between Deficit and Infarct. N Engl J Med. 2018;378(1):11-21.
4. Saver JL, Goyal M, Bonafe A, Diener HC, Levy EI, Pereira VM, et al. Stent-retriever thrombectomy after intravenous t-PA vs. t-PA alone in stroke. N Engl J Med. 2015;372(24): 2285-95.

Q.21. A 70-year-old patient presented with a complaint of weakness in left side of the body with loss of consciousness. The time when last seen normal is not known to the attendant. Patient's airway was secured with an endotracheal tube and was shifted for a CT scan head. His CT scan head revealed intracranial hemorrhage (ICH) in the right lobar region with volume of 45 mL. The functional outcome in patients with primary intracerebral hemorrhage (FUNC) score used for the likelihood of functional independence in patients with intracerebral hemorrhage includes all, except for which of the following?
 a. Age
 b. Glasgow Coma Score
 c. Pupillary reaction
 d. Location of bleed

Ans. c

Explanation: Intracranial hemorrhage (ICH) is the most fatal and disabling stroke subtype. Widely used tools for prediction of mortality are fundamentally limited in that they do not account for effects of withdrawal of care and are not designed to predict functional recovery. Functional outcome in patients with primary intracerebral hemorrhage score is a valid clinical assessment tool that identifies patients with ICH who will attain functional independence and thus, can provide guidance in clinical decision-making. It is a functional outcome risk stratification scale. The score ranged from 0 to 11 with a score of 11 indicating a strong likelihood of functional independence. The components of the FUNC score are—age, GCS, location of ICH, ICH volume, and pre-ICH cognitive impairment.

Suggested Reading
1. Broderick JP, Adams HP Jr, Barsan W, Feinberg W, Feldmann E, Grotta J, et al. Guidelines for the management of spontaneous intracerebral hemorrhage: a statement for healthcare professionals from a special writing group of the Stroke Council, American Heart Association. Stroke. 1999;30(4):905-15.
2. Gebel JM, Broderick JP. Intracerebral hemorrhage. Neurol Clin. 2000;18(2):419-38.
3. Rost NS, Smith EE, Chang Y, Snider RW, Chanderraj R, Schwab K, et al. Prediction of functional outcome in patients with primary intracerebral hemorrhage: the FUNC score. Stroke. 2008;39(8):2304-9.

Q.22. In the diagnostic workup of status epilepticus, which of the following should be done first?
a. MRI of brain
b. Electroencephalogram (EEG)
c. Blood gas analysis
d. Finger-stick glucose

Ans. b

Explanation: Continuous EEG monitoring is an indispensable tool for the management of status epilepticus in the intensive care unit. It helps in diagnosis of absence seizures and assessment of efficacy of treatment for status epilepticus or refractory status epilepticus. In a comatose patient, it is advised to do continuous EEG monitoring for at least 48 hours.

Suggested Reading
1. Claassen J, Taccone FS, Horn P, Holtkamp M, Stocchetti N, Oddo M. Recommendations on the use of EEG monitoring in critically ill patients: consensus statement from the neurointensive care section of the ESICM. Intensive Care Med. 2013;39(8):1337-51.
2. Herman ST, Abend NS, Bleck TP, Chapman KE, Drislane FW, Emerson RG, et al. Consensus statement on continuous EEG in critically ill adults and children, part II: personnel, technical specifications, and clinical practice. J Clin Neurophysiol. 2015;32(2):96-108.

Q.23. A 28-year-old female presented with complaints of involuntary movement of the body with a fever associated with vomiting. She is not able to stand since morning and had generalized tonic-clonic seizures 30 minutes ago. On examination her GCS was 12/15, RR: 25/min, SpO$_2$: 91% on room air. She was taken for a CT scan brain which was suggestive of meningitis with hydrocephalus. She was admitted to neurointensive care unit for further management. Her CSF to serum glucose ratio was found to be normal. What could be the possible diagnosis?
a. Tubercular meningitis
b. Bacterial meningitis
c. Fungal meningitis
d. Viral meningitis

Ans. d

Explanation: Many bacteria metabolize glucose, and because the blood-brain barrier minimizes transversal, the ratio can be useful in determining whether there is a bacterial infection in the CSF or not. The normal CSF to serum glucose ratio is 0.6. It is used to distinguish between bacterial and viral meningitis, as it is often lowered in bacterial meningitis and normal in viral meningitis. The CSF/blood glucose ratio may be a better single indicator for bacterial meningitis. Since the CSF glucose and blood glucose values are promptly and easily obtained from a lumbar puncture, the CSF/serum glucose ratio should be considered as a timely diagnostic indicator of bacterial meningitis. It may also help exclude the diagnosis of bacterial meningitis, especially in cases in which no microorganisms can be cultured. Again in the case of fungal meningitis, CSF/serum glucose ratio will be low.

Suggested Reading
1. Roos K. Principles of neurologic infectious diseases, 1st edition. New York: McGraw-Hill, Medical Pub. Division. 2005. p. 4.
2. Tamune H, Takeya H, Suzuki W, Tagashira Y, Kuki T, Honda H, et al. Cerebrospinal fluid/blood glucose ratio as an indicator for bacterial meningitis. Am J Emerg Med. 2014;32(3): 263-6.

Q.24. A 58-year-old female was operated (craniotomy and clipping) for right anterior cerebral artery (ACA) aneurysm under general anesthesia. On preoperative examination, her GCS was full (15/15), with no neurological deficit with stable vitals. Her intraoperative course remained uneventful with the total clipping time of 7 minutes. Her trachea was extubated and neuromuscular blockade was reversed at the end of the surgery. She was shifted to neurointensive care for further monitoring and management. On postoperative day 2, patient had a fall in GCS (10/15). On TCD examination, the velocities in the MCA was 170 cm/s. Patient was already on intravenous nimodipine. The ICU physician is now planning for intra-arterial nimodipine. Which of the following mode of treatment will not treat vasospasm in this patient?
a. Stellate ganglion block
b. Milrinone
c. Dexmedetomidine
d. Conivaptan

Ans. d

Explanation: The effect of stellate ganglion block (SGB) on cerebral hemodynamics has been assessed using transcranial Doppler (TCD), which showed a significant increase in cerebral perfusion pressure due to a decrease in cerebral vascular tone. The SGB is a simple and minimally invasive technique, effective in improving cerebral perfusion by relieving symptomatic cerebral vasospasm, however, large randomized trials are required to compare its efficacy with other treatment modalities. Intra-arterial milrinone is a safe and effective treatment modality for refractory cerebral vasospasm following aneurysmal subarachnoid hemorrhage. The α_2-adrenergic agonist dexmedetomidine (DEX) has huge potential for protecting against cerebral vasospasm, a leading cause of death and disability after subarachnoid hemorrhage. Biomarker assays for SAH have recently emerged as tools for predicting vasospasm and outcomes. Dexmedetomidine administration was found to reduce the severity of cerebral vasospasm and improved neurological function in SAH rats; this may be closely linked to reduced CSF IL-6 levels. Further human trials on this topic would be good to evaluate the effect of DEX on cerebral vasospasm.

Suggested Reading
1. Abulhasan YB, Ortiz Jimenez J, Teitelbaum J, Simoneau G, Angle MR. Milrinone for refractory cerebral vasospasm with delayed cerebral ischemia. J Neurosurg. 2020;134(3):971-82.
2. Gupta MM, Bithal PK, Dash HH, Chaturvedi A, Mahajan RP. Effects of stellate ganglion block on cerebral haemodynamics as assessed by transcranial Doppler ultrasonography. Br J Anaesth. 2005;95(5):669-73.
3. Jain V, Rath GP, Dash HH, Bithal PK, Chouhan RS, Suri A. Stellate ganglion block for treatment of cerebral vasospasm in patients with aneurysmal subarachnoid hemorrhage—A preliminary study. J Anaesthesiol Clin Pharmacol. 2011;27(4):516-21.
4. Song Y, Lim BJ, Kim DH, Ju JW, Han DW. Effect of Dexmedetomidine on Cerebral Vasospasm and Associated Biomarkers in a Rat Subarachnoid Hemorrhage Model. J Neurosurg Anesthesiol. 2019;31(3):342-49.

Q.25. A 41-year-old male underwent spinal instrumentation surgery for prolapsed intervertebral disc (PIVD) involving T11-L5 spine. On preoperative examination, power in bilateral lower limb was 4/5. He was doing his routine work with the help of an assistant for last 1 year. He had a history of diabetes mellitus for last 5 years on oral hypoglycemics. He was also a chronic smoker for last 20 years (2 packs/day). His intraoperative course was uneventful. On postoperative day 1, he complained of difficulty in breathing. Which of the following is not the risk factor for respiratory complications in this patient?

a. Multiple level instrumentation
b. Bilateral lower limb power 4/5
c. Diabetes mellitus
d. Chronic smoker

Ans. b

Explanation: It is widely accepted that respiratory complications are common after spinal surgeries. Patients who have a history of smoking, diabetes mellitus, or chronic obstructive pulmonary disease are at greater risk of respiratory depression following lumbar spine surgery. Also patients who undergo multiple-level spinal instrumentation surgeries have a higher respiratory complication rate compared to laminectomies or discectomies, especially among older patients. Deep vein thrombosis (DVT) is one of the major factors which could lead to disastrous respiratory or other hemodynamic complications if not diagnosed or treated timely. DVT is common in patients with prolonged immobility.

Suggested Reading
1. Al-Dujaili TM, Majer CN, Madhoun TE, Kassis SZ, Saleh AA. Deep venous thrombosis in spine surgery patients: incidence and hematoma formation. Int Surg. 2012;97(2):150-4.
2. Murgai R, D'Oro A, Heindel P, Schoell K, Barkoh K, Buser Z, et al. Incidence of Respiratory Complications Following Lumbar Spine Surgery. Int J Spine Surg. 2018;12(6):718-24.
3. Prabhakar H, Rajan S, Kapoor I, Mahajan C. Problem Based Learning Discussions in Neuroanesthesia and Neurocritical Care, 1st edition. Singapore: Springer Nature Pte. Ltd.; 2020.
4. Qaseem A, Snow V, Fitterman N, Hornbake ER, Lawrence VA, Smetana GW, et al. Risk assessment for and strategies to reduce perioperative pulmonary complications for patients undergoing noncardiothoracic surgery: a guideline from the American College of Physicians. Ann Intern Med. 2006;144(8):575-80.

Q.26. What postoperative complication can be expected in a 9-month-old child who underwent meningomyelocele repair surgery under general anesthesia?
   a. Laryngospasm
   b. Latex allergy
   c. Apnea
   d. All of the above

Ans. d

Explanation: Laryngospasm is the sustained closure of vocal cords. Children are more predisposed to this complication as slightest noxious stimulus could aggravate it. Under a light plane of anesthesia, it can cause desaturation or even respiratory arrest. Treatment includes—jaw thrust, deepen the plane of anesthesia and succinylcholine as a drug of choice @dose of 0.1–0.2 mg/kg body weight. Latex allergy is quite common in young children with meningomyelocele. Latex is used in many in hospital equipment which increases the exposure risk to young children. Treatment options for latex allergy are, simply removing the irritant, steroids, antihistamines, and sometimes airway support too. Postoperative apnea is a major concern with surgery in neonates and infants. It is imperative that these children should be strictly monitored for 12–24 hours.

Suggested Reading
1. Chand MB, Agarwal J. Anesthetic challenges and management of meningocele repair. Postgrad Med J NAMS. 2011;11:41-5.
2. Cochrane DD, Adderley R, White CP, Norman M, Steinbok P. Apnea in patients with myelomeningocele. Pediatr Neurosurg. 1990;16(4-5):232-9.
3. Rendeli C, Nucera E, Ausili E, Tabacco F, Roncallo C, Pollastrini E, et al. Latex sensitisation and allergy in children with myelomeningocele. Childs Nerv Syst. 2006;22(1):28-32.

Q.27. Which of the following is not a component of the Burdenko Respiratory Insufficiency Scale (BRIS)?
   a. Mental score using RASS
   b. Swallowing, cough
   c. End-tidal carbon dioxide ($EtCO_2$)/$PaCO_2$ ratio
   d. Index PaO_2/FiO_2

Ans. c

Explanation: In stroke patients, there is no acceptable scale that would help in making decision regarding intubation. Burdenko Respiratory Insufficiency Scale is a useful scale in such cases. The scale evaluates mental status with RASS, swallowing, coughing, airway patency, and PaO_2/FiO_2 ratio. Each component has been given a score from 0 to 4. BRIS minimal score is 0 (healthy person) and maximal score is 12 with normal weight. Scoring is increased by 1 point in patients with obesity (body mass index: 30 kg/m^2). BRIS score of ≤3 means patient can breathe spontaneously, whereas a score ≥4 is a gray zone.

Suggested Reading
1. O'Neil KH, Purdy M, Falk J, Gallo L. The Dysphagia Outcome and Severity Scale. Dysphagia. 1999;14(3):139-45.

2. Prabhakar H, Rajan S, Kapoor I, Mahajan C. Textbook of Neuroanesthesia and Neurocritical Care, 1st edition. In: Prabhakar H, Ali Z (Eds). Singapore: Springer Nature Pte. Ltd.; 2019.
3. Wijdicks EF, Scott JP. Causes and outcome of mechanical ventilation in patients with hemispheric ischemic stroke. Mayo Clin Proc. 1997;72(3):210-3.

Q.28. Which of the following statement is not true for nutritional assessment and management in a neurologically ill patient admitted in intensive care unit?
a. Enteral nutrition should be started within 24–48 hours
b. NRS-2202 score is used to assess nutritional risk
c. Nimodipine use in SAH patients may exacerbate poor nutritional status
d. Enteral feeding is not safe during moderate hypothermia after intracranial hemorrhage

Ans. d

Explanation: Enteral nutrition should be started early in neurologically ill patients to combat hypermetabolic state and prevent secondary complications. The Society of Critical Care Medicine recommends enteral nutrition within 24–48 hours. It has also been observed that early enteral nutrition is associated with reduced mortality, less infection rate, and decreased length of hospital stay. The nutritional risk predictors such as Nutritional Risk Screening 2002 (NRS 2002) and Nutrition Risk in Critically ill (NUTRIC) are most widely used scores in intensive care unit. NRS 2002 considers both disease severity and malnutrition with scores ranging from 0 to 3 in each component. Patient with score a >3 is considered at risk and score >5 at high risk. Use of nimodipine in SAH patients for prevention of delayed cerebral ischemia may exacerbate the poor nutritional status of the patient as the drug commonly causes diarrhea. The use of loperamide can help prevent this side effect. The use of enteral feeding in patients with intracranial hemorrhage during active hypothermia has not shown any gastrointestinal adverse effects.

Suggested Reading
1. Dobak S, Rincon F. "Cool" Topic: Feeding During Moderate Hypothermia After Intracranial Hemorrhage. JPEN J Parenter Enteral Nutr. 2017;41(7):1125-30.
2. Marik PE, Zaloga GP. Early enteral nutrition in acutely ill patients: a systematic review. Crit Care Med. 2001;29(12):2264-70.
3. McClave SA, Taylor BE, Martindale RG, Warren MM, Johnson DR, Braunschweig C, et al. Guidelines for the Provision and Assessment of Nutrition Support Therapy in the Adult Critically Ill Patient: Society of Critical Care Medicine (SCCM) and American Society for Parenteral and Enteral Nutrition (A.S.P.E.N.). JPEN J Parenter Enteral Nutr. 2016;40(2):159-211.
4. Prabhakar H, Rajan S, Kapoor I, Mahajan C. Textbook of Neuroanesthesia and Neurocritical Care, 1st edition. In: Prabhakar H, Ali Z (Eds). Singapore: Springer Nature Pte Ltd.; 2019.

Q.29. A 25-year-old female was operated for frontal high-grade glioma under general anesthesia. On preoperative examination, she was fully conscious with stable vitals. Her intraoperative course was uneventful. At the end of the surgery, when patient was planned for neuromuscular blockade reversal, there was sudden jittery

movement in whole body. Injection phenytoin loading dose was given to the patient and shifted to neuro intensive care unit with an endotracheal tube in situ. She continued to have seizures in the postoperative period for 24 hours and beyond. She also received midazolam, sodium valproate, thiopentone, and ketamine infusion for 24 hours but without any attenuation of seizure episodes. Finally, a volatile inhalational anesthetic agent (isoflurane) was added to the treatment. Within 20 minutes of administration of isoflurane, seizure activity ceased. What is the diagnosis?
  a. Status epilepticus
  b. Drug refractory status epilepticus
  c. Super-refractory status epilepticus
  d. Residual effect of anesthetic agents

Ans. c

Explanation: Super-refractory status epilepticus (SRSE) is a life-threatening state of persisting seizure activity defined as SE that continues up to or beyond 24 hours after the start of anesthetic medications, and this includes those cases where SE recurs on the reduction or withdrawal of anesthetic medications. Treatment of such a condition is still not clear. General anesthesia with volatile anesthetic agent is considered to be the last reserved resort in the management of SRSE.

Suggested Reading
  1. Tomar GS, Kapoor I, Mahajan C, Prabhakar H. Volatile Anesthetic for Management of Super-refractory Status Epilepticus. Indian J Crit Care Med. 2017;21(3):183.
  2. Shorvon S, Trinka E, Schmutzhard E. Complications of the management of status epilepticus. In: Shorvon S, Trinka E (Eds). The 3rd London-Innsbruck Colloquium on Status Epilepticus. Epilepsia: Cambridge University Press; 2011.

Q.30. **Which of the following sentence is true about kidney dysfunction after traumatic brain injury (TBI)?**
  a. Interleukin-6 (IL-6) levels are strongly associated with renal dysfunction
  b. Acute kidney injury may aggravate TBI
  c. About 12% of the patients with TBI develop AKI during first week of ICU admission
  d. All of the above

Ans. d

Explanation: The pathophysiology of renal dysfunction in TBI is not fully understood. Traumatic brain injury leads to an inflammatory response, with the release of cytokines in the cerebrospinal fluid and serum. Interleukin-6 has been studied extensively in several diseases, and increased IL-6 levels have been associated with acute kidney injury in patients who underwent cardiac surgery and septic patients. In patients with TBI and in animal models of TBI, IL-6 increases within 1 hour after injury, and a high IL-6 level is associated with poor outcomes. A preplanned subanalysis of Collaborative European NeuroTrauma Effectiveness Research in Traumatic Brain Injury (CENTER-TBI) in patients with an ICU stay of >72 hours showed that 12% developed acute kidney injury (AKI) based on the serum creatinine criteria of Kidney Disease Improving Global Outcomes (KDIGO) during the first week of ICU stay.

Suggested Reading

1. Chawla LS, Seneff MG, Nelson DR, Williams M, Levy H, Kimmel PL, et al. Elevated plasma concentrations of IL-6 and elevated APACHE II score predict acute kidney injury in patients with severe sepsis. Clin J Am Soc Nephrol. 2007;2(1):22-30.
2. Robba C, Banzato E, Rebora P, Iaquaniello C, Huang CY, Wiegers EJA, et al. Acute kidney injury in traumatic brain injury patients: results from the Collaborative European NeuroTrauma Effectiveness Research in traumatic brain injury study. Crit Care Med. 2021;49(1):112-26.
3. Woodcock T, Morganti-Kossmann MC. The role of markers of inflammation in traumatic brain injury. Front Neurol. 2013;4-18.
4. Zhang WR, Garg AX, Coca SG, Devereaux PJ, Eikelboom J, Kavsak P, et al. Plasma IL-6 and IL-10 concentrations predict AKI and long-term mortality in adults after cardiac surgery. J Am Soc Nephrol. 2015;26(12):3123-32.

CHAPTER 13

Trauma

Khusrav Bajan, Budhaditya Chattopadhyay

SPINE TRAUMA

Q.1. You have been asked to give a teaching session to a group of medical students attached to the emergency department. The topic of the session is "spinal cord injuries in the emergency department". You are discussing the spinal tracts and their patterns of injury. Regarding the lateral corticospinal tract, which of the following is true?
  a. Located in the anterolateral aspect of the cord
  b. Controls contralateral motor power
  c. Transmits contralateral pain and temperature sensation
  d. Transmit ipsilateral proprioception and light touch sensation
  e. Located in the posterolateral aspect of the cord

Ans. e

Explanation: The origin point of spinal cord starts from the medulla oblongata at the level of foramen magnum and it ends at the L1 level in the adult group which is called the conus medullaris. Beyond this point lies the cauda equina which can withstand certain level of injuries initially.

Spinal cord tracts that are examined clinically:
- The lateral corticospinal tract
- Spinothalamic tract
- Dorsal columns

The spinal cord tracts are paired ones and can be unilaterally or bilaterally injured. When both sensory and the motor functions are not elicited on examination below a certain level of injury then it is termed as complete spinal injury. However, when a certain degree of these functions are still intact then it is termed as incomplete spinal cord injury and the recovery prognosis remains better compared to complete cord injuries.

Tract	Location	Function
Dorsal columns	Posteromedial aspect of cord	Transmits ipsilateral proprioception, vibration, and light-touch sensation
Spinothalamic tract	Anterior and lateral aspect of cord	Conveys pain, crude touch, and temperature sensation to the opposite side
Lateral corticospinal tract	Posterolateral aspect of cord	Controls ipsilateral motor power

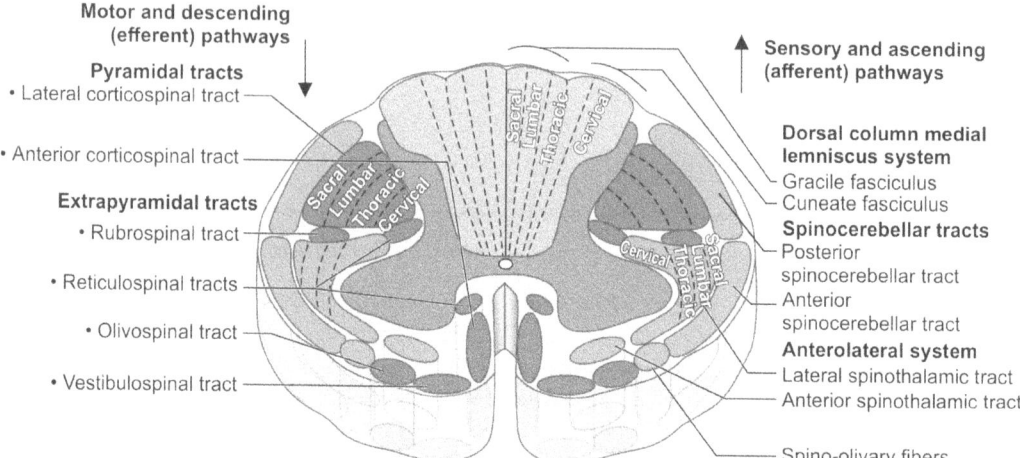

Q.2. A 16-year-old boy is brought to the emergency department with spine motion restriction and placed on a spine board for transport. During a sporting event, the patient collided with another player resulting in patient experiencing significant neck pain, but on further examination, he revealed to not have any paresthesia and can move all his extremities. A computed tomography (CT) cervical was done which showed signs of fractures of the first cervical vertebra.

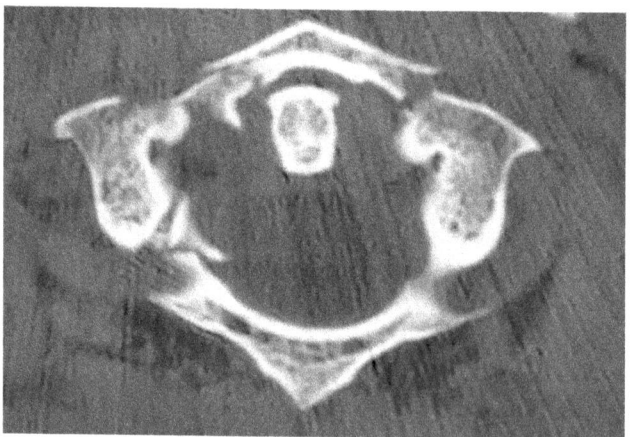

Which of the following best describes this fracture?
a. Odontoid fracture
b. Hangman fracture
c. Teardrop fracture
d. Jefferson fracture
e. Clay-shoveler's fracture

Ans. d

Explanation:
- Fracture of the superior articular surfaces of the lateral masses of the first cervical vertebra (C1) is known as the Jefferson fracture. It is also termed as a C1 burst fracture. Most of the time can be associated with a C2 fracture which should be evaluated at the same time. These fractures are considered to be unstable and

thorough spine motion restriction should be maintained during management in the emergency department.
- Fracture of the odontoid part of C2 vertebra is termed as odontoid fracture which is also another unstable cervical fracture.
- Traumatic defects of the C2 pars interarticularis occur when the cervicocranial is thrown into extreme hyperextension secondary to abrupt deceleration observed in high-speed motor vehicle clashes. This kind of injuries is termed as Hangman's fracture, which is also a variant of unstable cervical injury.
- Injuries due to assault to the back of the neck leading to avulsion fracture of the spinous process occurring due to cervical hyperextension or direct impact are termed as clay-shoveler's fracture.
- Diving accidents in certain cases lead to teardrop fracture, which is disruption of all the cervical ligaments leading to a triangular-shaped fracture of the vertebral body. Such fractures are deemed unstable and observed in condition like anterior cord syndrome.

Q.3. A 33-year-old man is brought to the emergency department by the paramedics after being stabbed in the back on roadside in a rally riot. His blood pressure (BP) is 124/82 mm Hg, heart rate (HR) is 115 beats/min, respiratory rate (RR) is 16 breaths/min, and oxygen saturation is 96% on room air. On the secondary survey, you note motor weakness of his right lower extremity and the loss of pain sensation in the left lower extremity. Which of the following is the most likely diagnosis?
   a. Spinal shock
   b. Brown–Sequard syndrome
   c. Central cord syndrome
   d. Anterior cord syndrome
   e. Cauda equina syndrome

Ans. b

Explanation:
- Brown–Sequard syndrome is commonly associated with penetrating trauma in which a patient presents on clinical examination with same side motor paralysis and opposite side loss of pain and temperature sensation recorded below the level of the injury sustained. Among the several cord lesions, this has a better overall recovery prognosis.
- Spinal shock is associated with loss of autonomic tone including neurologic functions below the level of injury associated with flaccid paralysis, loss of reflex activity, and bladder involvement.
- Characteristic finding in central cord syndrome is sign of sensorimotor weakness more in the upper extremities than the lower extremities.
- Anterior cord syndrome is exhibited with sparing of components supplied by dorsal column such as proprioception and vibratory sensation and loss of pain sensation with motor paralysis below the level of lesion.
- Cauda equina syndrome features saddle anesthesia with bowel and bladder irregularities along with motor and sensory loss in the lower extremities.

Brown-Sequard syndrome:

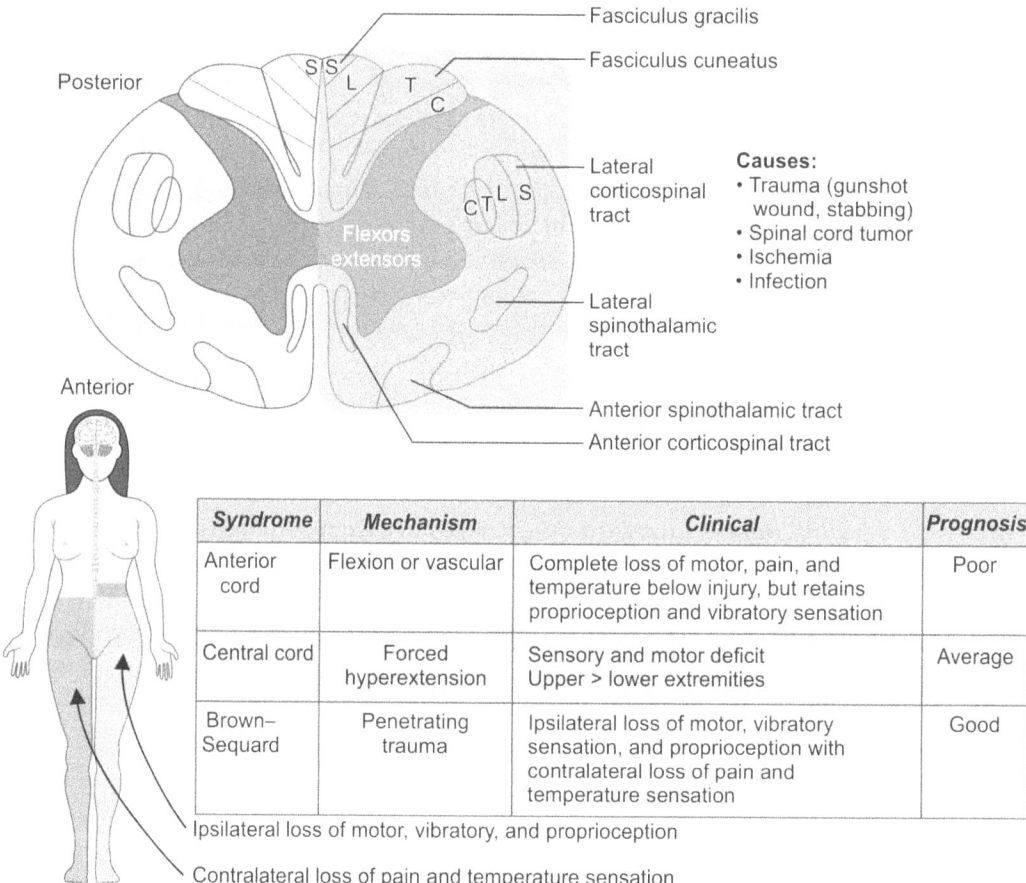

Q.4. A 68-year-old man is brought to the emergency department (ED) after falling on the pavement landing on his face while walking to his house. Patient was brought by the paramedics with adequate spine motion restriction. On evaluation in the ED, patient had absent sensory and motor functions in the upper extremities and reduced in the lower extremities compared to the upper. Rectal examination showed reduced rectal tone. Which of the following is the most likely diagnosis?
  a. Transverse myelitis
  b. Brown–Sequard syndrome
  c. Central cord syndrome
  d. Parkinson disease
  e. Anterior cord syndrome

Ans. c

Explanation:
- Central cord syndrome is observed in injuries involving forced hyperextension of the neck resulting in contusions to the central part of the cord. As a result, it leads to motor and sensory deficits more in the upper extremities compared to the

lower extremities. In addition, it is also associated with reduced rectal tone and disproportionate sensory deficits.
- Anterior cord syndrome is exhibited with sparing of components supplied by dorsal column like proprioception and vibratory sensation and loss of pain sensation with motor paralysis below the level of lesion.
- Brown-Sequard syndrome is commonly associated with penetrating trauma in which a patient presents on clinical examination with same side motor paralysis and opposite side loss of pain and temperature sensation recorded below the level of the injury sustained. Among the several cord lesions, this has a better overall recovery prognosis.
- Transverse myelitis exhibits loss of entire motor and sensory functions below the level of lesion but associated with an inflammatory involvement.
- Parkinson disease does not exhibit with the above symptoms in such acute phase including no symptoms of paralysis, and the disease slowly progresses over an extended period of time.

Central cord syndrome:

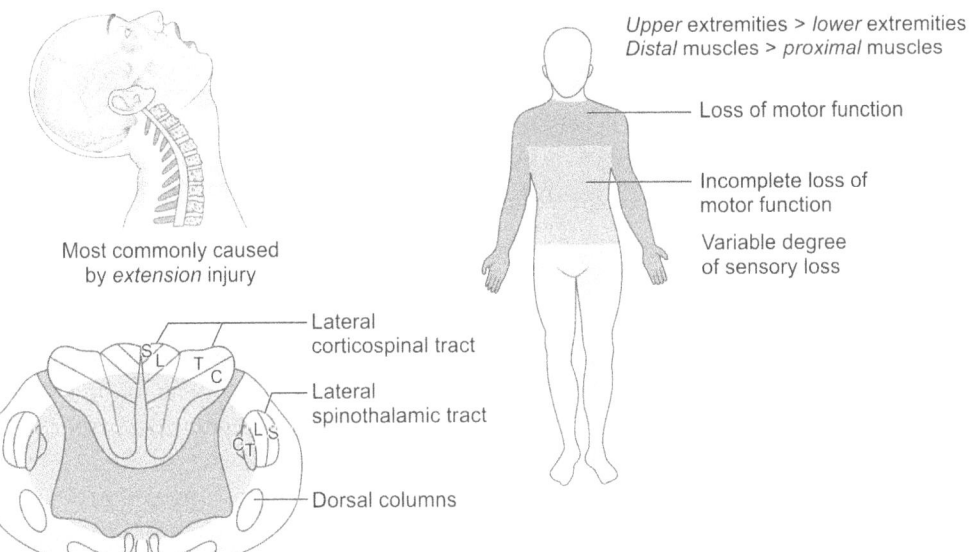

Syndrome	Mechanism	Clinical	Prognosis
Anterior cord	Flexion or vascular	Complete loss of motor, pain, and temperature below injury, but retains proprioception and vibratory sensation	Poor
Central cord	Forced hyperextension	Sensory and motor deficit Upper > lower extremities	Average
Brown–Sequard	Penetrating trauma	Ipsilateral loss of motor, vibratory sensation, and proprioception with contralateral loss of pain and temperature sensation	Good

Q.5. A 60-year-old male patient comes to the emergency department with complaints of lower back pain after falling from stairs in his home a day before. On examination, he points out that the pain extends down to his lower limbs. Also, he is having difficulties to pass urine since yesterday night. Rectal examination shows reduced tone. On sensory examination, he is revealed to have absent plantar flexion. Which of the following is the most likely diagnosis?
   a. Disk herniation
   b. Spinal stenosis
   c. Osteomyelitis
   d. Abdominal aortic aneurysm
   e. Cauda equina syndrome

Ans. e

Explanation:
- Cauda equina syndrome is an acute condition which should be identified at the earliest and correction needed promptly. Key features being saddle anesthesia, lower limb tenderness, impaired bladder and bowel function, and loss of motor and sensory components in the lower extremities. Condition requires prompt magnetic resonance imaging (MRI) and neurosurgical reference.
- Disk herniation does not exhibit bowel or bladder dysfunction. It is associated with peripheral nerve root compression.
- Spinal stenosis resulting due to narrowing of the canal exhibits increased cord compression with extension of back but relieved on flexion.
- Osteomyelitis is associated with fever leading to infection in the bone.
- Abdominal aortic aneurysm is usually identified with beside POCUS assessment and further CT studies. It does not usually associate with neurological compromise.

Q.6. A 28-year-old male patient was brought to the emergency department with history of fall from a two-wheeler after hitting an obstacle on the road near the pavement. Patient was transported on a spine board with spine motion restriction. On arrival to ED, patient was conscious. On examination, patient complained of weakness in all his four extremities. He did not have any other external injuries or deformities. On taking the vitals, it was documented as bradycardic and hypotensive with normal body temperature and oxygen saturation on room air. Bedside extended focused assessment with sonography for trauma (e-FAST) and chest X-ray and pelvis X-ray showed normal findings. On physical examination, he showed significant reduced motor strength but intact peripheral sensations in his all four extremities. Which of the following is the most likely diagnosis?
   a. Hypovolemic shock
   b. Neurogenic shock
   c. Cardiogenic shock
   d. Anaphylactic shock
   e. Septic shock

Ans. b

Explanation:
- Neurogenic shock represents with opposed sympathetic outflow tracts and unopposed vagal tone resulting in bradycardia and hypotension. This condition

must be treated with strict spine motion restriction and resuscitation should include fluid initially and then vasopressors, if needed, if patient is nonresponder to fluid administration.
- Hypovolemic shock is associated with circulatory volume deficit due to internal or external hemorrhagic causes leading to decreased oxygen delivery at the tissue level.
- Cardiogenic shock is associated with reduced cardiac output and results in restricted tissue perfusion.
- Hypersensitivity reaction at the systemic level with hemodynamic instability is observed in anaphylactic shock. Patient may also exhibit impending respiratory failure due to compromised airway which should be managed promptly.
- Septic shock represents as a hemodynamic instability like hypotension with hypoperfusion ultimately leading to multiorgan failure resulting from local or systemic infection.

HEAD TRAUMA (TBI)

Q.1. You are assessing a medical student as she examines a 32-year-old man who has been assaulted. The medical student believes the patient has features suggestive of a basal skull fracture. Which of the following features is suggestive of a basal skull fracture?
a. Epistaxis
b. Subconjunctival hemorrhage with no posterior border seen
c. Preauricular bruising
d. Oculomotor nerve palsy
e. Septal hematoma

Ans. b

Explanation:
- Skull base fractures are based on morphology, which can be linear or stellate and depressed or nondepressed.
- *Basilar skull fracture is associated with the following key features:*
  - Cerebrospinal fluid (CSF) leak detected through nose or ear (rhinorrhea or otorrhea)
  - Cranial nerve defects such as the 6th nerve leading to facial paralysis or 7th nerve leading to hearing defects
  - Unilateral or bilateral ear bleed (hemotympanum)
  - Ocular trauma like subconjunctival hemorrhage (with no posterior border seen)
  - Bruising around the mastoid process (Battle's sign)
  - Pooling of blood around the eyes causing periorbital ecchymosis (raccoon eyes)

Q.2. A 40-year-old male patient is transported to the emergency department with history of fall on the street due to a slippery surface. Patient was initially unconscious post fall for approximately 1 minute after which he regained consciousness. On arrival to the ED, vitals were recorded as heart rate of 70 beats/min and blood pressure of 160/90 mm Hg and oxygen saturation of 97% on room air. On examination, he had a 5-cm lacerated wound on the temporal aspect of his scalp with active bleeding. Patient exhibited retrograde amnesia (having no memories of the event). Patient repeatedly enquired about the event and his current whereabouts. En route to the CT scan, patient has one episode of vomiting but remained stable. Scan report came back as normal. Which is the probable diagnosis?
a. Cerebral contusion
b. Post-traumatic epilepsy
c. Trauma-induced Alzheimer
d. Cerebral concussion
e. Diffuse axonal injury

Ans. d

Explanation:
- Cerebral concussion is usually associated with patients having episodes of amnesia of the event with insistent questioning about the details of the incident. Also, patients may exhibit symptoms of headache with or without episodes of vomiting with no focal neurological deficits. Symptoms like loss of consciousness are observed due to impairment of the reticular activating system. These patients improve over time and have normal CT brain findings.
- Diffuse axonal injury happens due to shearing of nerve fibers in the brain and patients present in unconscious state and remain in extended period of coma.
- Cerebral contusion has similar findings to cerebral concussion but is also associated with significant neurological impairment including occasional focal sensory and motor deficits.
- In certain scenarios with depressed skull fractures or intracranial bleed, patient may exhibit episodes of post-traumatic epilepsy within the first week of the traumatic brain injury.

Q.3. A 60-year-old man was brought to the emergency department from his home where he was found lying on the ground. His vitals in the ED were recorded as heart rate of 130 beats/min with blood pressure of 94/66 mm Hg and oxygen saturation of 96% at room air. Primary survey suggests that his eyes were opening to sound and limb movement to pain. On further examination, clear fluid was detected leaking from his right ear and there was minimal bruising around the mastoid bone. Which of the following is the most likely diagnosis?
a. Le Fort fracture
b. Basilar skull fracture
c. Otitis interna
d. Otitis externa
e. Tripod fracture

Ans. b

Explanation:
- Basilar skull fractures features key elements like battle sign which is ecchymosis around the mastoid bone, raccoon eyes which is periorbital ecchymosis, CSF leakage from nose (rhinorrhea) and ear (otorrhea) and lastly blood detected behind the tympanic membrane suggestive of hemotympanum. The common locations of basilar skull fractures are the tympanic membrane, petrous part of the temporal bone, and the external auditory canal.
- Le fort fractures are associated with high-velocity trauma involving the face. It is categorically classified into three types which are as follows:
  1. Le Fort type I is a transverse fracture at the level of the nasal fossa.
  2. Le Fort type II is a pyramidal shaped fracture involving the infraorbital rims, its apex being just above the bridge of the nose.
  3. Le Fort type III is categorized as a complete craniofacial disruption.

Q.4. A 30-year-old male is brought to the emergency department by the paramedics. History suggests that he was involved in a four-wheeler accident which had head-on collision with a tree. Prior to the arrival of the paramedics to the accident site, according to the bystanders, patient exited himself from the vehicle and collapsed shortly after a while. On arrival to the ED, vitals were documented as heart rate of 56 beats/min with blood pressure of 170/84 mm Hg. Oxygen saturation was noted to be 94% on room air. Patient remained unconscious with sonorous breathing pattern. On primary survey, left pupil was noted to be fixed and dilated. Due to poor airway patency, drug-assisted intubation with spine motion restriction was done and patient was shifted for a head CT which is shown as:

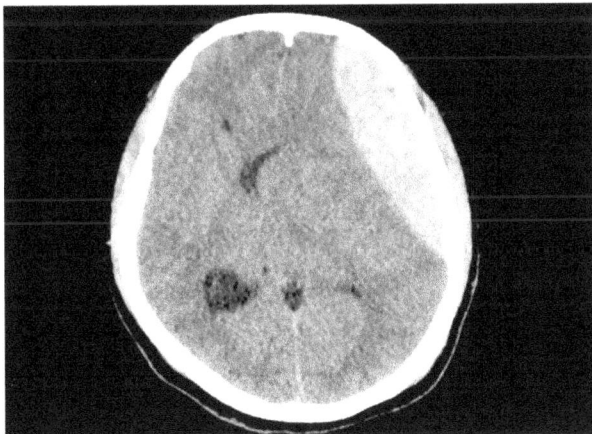

Which of the following is the most likely diagnosis?
a. Epidural hematoma
b. Subdural hematoma
c. Subarachnoid hemorrhage
d. Intracerebral hematoma
e. Cerebral contusion

Ans. a

Explanation:
- Epidural hematoma commonly presents with the disruption of the middle meningeal artery involving the temporal or the temporoparietal area mostly associated with or without depressed skull fractures. A common element observed in epidural hematomas is the lucid interval following loss of consciousness in patients. It usually appears as a biconvex hyperdense area on CT. Early detection and evacuation is a key structure in the management of such conditions.
- Subdural hematomas occur due to bridging of emissary veins in the subdural space and appear as crescent-shaped hyperdense areas on the CT scans. These tend to cross the suture lines, which is a distinguishing factor when compared to extradural hematomas.
- The intracerebral hematomas or the cerebral contusions are usually observed in the frontotemporal and occipital areas and can be seen on the same side of impact or on the opposite side of the brain termed as contrecoup injuries.

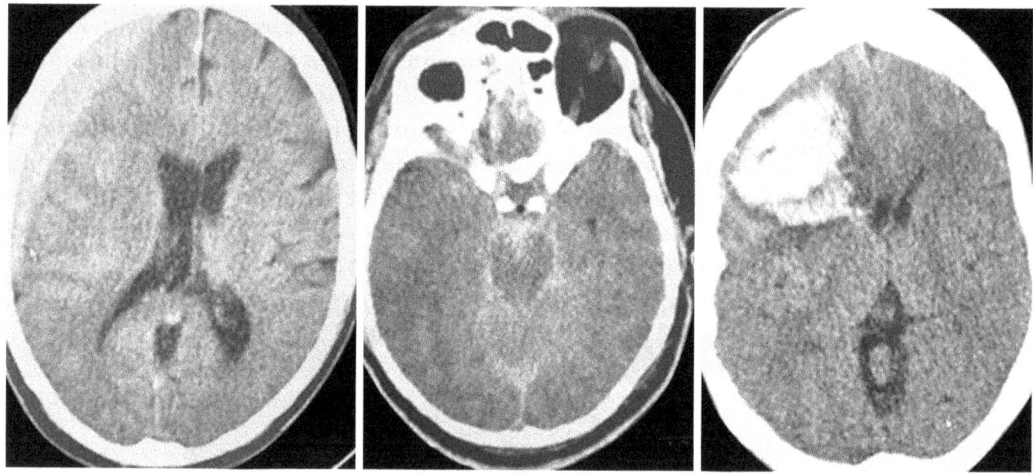

Q.5. A 65-year-old male patient is transported to the emergency department by the paramedics with a history of collision with a two-wheeler while walking. On arrival to ED, vitals were recorded as heart rate of 68 beats/min and blood pressure of 170/84 mm Hg. Primary survey was done and GCS was documented as no eye opening to any response, no verbal sounds, and withdrawing only to pain. Bilateral pupils were unequal and not responding to light stimulus. Which is the most common sign of increasing intracranial pressure leading to impending brain herniation?
  a. Ipsilateral pupillary dilation
  b. Sudden change in the GCS level
  c. Sudden significant elevation of blood pressure
  d. Contralateral pupillary dilation
  e. Motor weakness of both upper and lower extremities on one side

Ans. a

Explanation: Cerebral herniation is associated with progressive increase in the intracranial pressure leading to disruption of the cerebral autoregulation resulting in detrimental injuries to the brain. Most commonly observed is the uncal herniation which is associated with extracranial bleeding in traumatic brain injuries. The classical signs of the uncal herniation are the same side pupillary dilation and opposite side hemiparesis. Usually, the medial part of the temporal lobe, which is known as uncus, is involved in herniation. It causes compression of the pyramidal tract giving rise to signs of motor weakness of the opposite side of the body. The third cranial nerve which is the oculomotor nerve also gets compressed during temporal lobe herniation leading to unopposed sympathetic activity resulting in pupillary dilation.

ADVANCED TRAUMA LIFE SUPPORT

Q.1. A 27-year-old male patient is transported to the emergency department after being involved in a road traffic accident between a two-wheeler and a four-wheeler. Patient was driving the two-wheeler, which was found to be badly damaged and victim was found approximately 10 feet away from his vehicle. On arrival to the ED, his vitals were recorded as tachycardic with blood pressure of 90/60 mm Hg, tachypneic, and oxygen saturation of 98% with 15 L of oxygen support. What is the minimum percentage of blood loss required to cause a drop in the systolic blood pressure?

a. Loss of <10% of blood volume
b. Loss of >5% of blood volume
c. Loss of 10-30% of blood volume
d. Loss of 30-40% of blood volume
e. Loss of >40% of blood volume

Ans. d

Explanation:

Parameter	Class I	Class II (mild)	Class III (moderate)	Class IV (severe)
Approximate blood loss	<15%	15–30%	31–40%	>4–0%
Heart rate	↔	↔/↑	↑	↑/↑↑
Blood pressure	↔	↔	↔/↓	↓
Pulse pressure	↔	↓	↓	↓
Respiratory rate	↔	↔	↔/↑	↑
Urine output	↔	↔	↓	↓↓
Glasgow Coma Scale score	↔	↔	↓	↓
Base deficit*	0 to −2 mEq/L	−2 to −6 mEq/L	−6 to −10 mEq/L	−10 mEq/L or less
Need for blood products	Monitor	Possible	Yes	Massive transfusion protocol

*Base excess is the quantity of base (HCO_3^-, in mEq/L) that is above or below the normal range in the body. A negative number is called a base deficit and indicates metabolic acidosis.
Source: Mutschler M, Nienaber U, Brockamp T, Wafaisade A, Wyen H, Peiniger S, et al. A critical reappraisal of the ATLS classification of hypovolaemic shock: does it really reflect clinical reality? Resuscitation. 2013;84(3):309-13.

Q.2. A 32-year-old male patient was brought late night to the emergency department by the paramedics. He was earlier involved in a fight at a club where he was repeatedly being punched in his abdomen and face and also being hit on the head. On arrival to ED, his vitals were recorded as heart rate of 84 beats/min with blood pressure of 164/82 mm Hg and oxygen saturation of 94% with 15 L of oxygen support through a nonrebreather mask. He was having shallow breaths with grunting sounds with suspected tongue fall. He was not opening his eyes to pain stimulus, with no response to vocal commands and withdrawing only to pain stimulus. On further examination, he has a deep laceration to the temporal region with active bleeding. Which of the following is the most appropriate next step in management?

a. Control of bleeding from the lacerated wound in the scalp.
b. Perform rapid sequence induction and orotracheal intubation.
c. Start IV fluid resuscitation.
d. Administer hypertonic saline.
e. Perform an emergency bedside burr hole procedure of the cranium.

Ans. b

Explanation: The Glasgow coma scale is used as an objective scale to assess the severity of traumatic head injuries and graded as mild (GCS score of 13–15), moderate (GCS score of 9–12), and severe (GCS score of 3–8) traumatic brain injury. In the above case scenario, patient had a GCS of <9 and falls under the classification of severe traumatic brain injury. With the impending risk of raised intracranial pressure and incidence of herniation leading to respiratory compromise, it is recommended for an early drug-assisted intubation for airway protection; then after hemodynamic stabilization, transfer the patient for an emergent CT brain scan and further management.

Q.3. A 40-year-old male patient was brought to the emergency department following a road traffic accident involving a head-on collision between two four-wheeler vehicles. Extrication of the patient from the vehicle was difficult and took an extended period of time. En route to the hospital, the paramedics placed a wide bore intravenous cannula and started fluid resuscitation in view of hypotension. On arrival to ED, the vitals were recorded as tachycardic and hypotensive with oxygen saturation of 98% with 15 L of oxygen support through nonrebreather mask (NRBM). Patient was conscious but diaphoretic. Patient continued to remain hypotensive even with initial fluid resuscitation and massive transfusion protocol was initiated. On abdominal examination, the patient grimaced, and a lacerated wound was found on the arm with active bleeding which was managed accordingly. As part of the primary survey, bedside FAST was performed which is shown below:

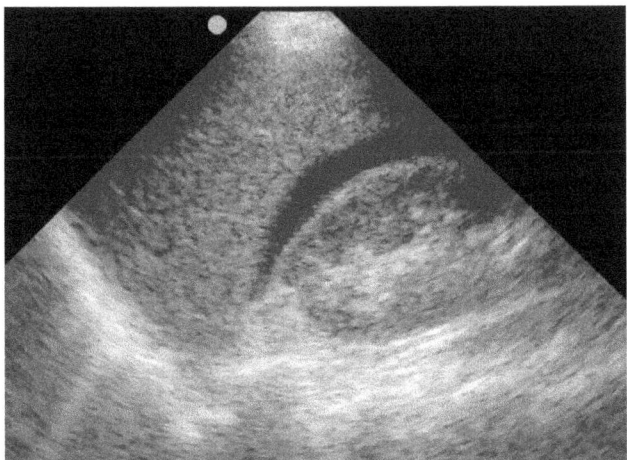

What is the next recommended step in the management of the patient?
a. Initiate massive transfusion protocol and continue with fluid resuscitation.
b. Transfer the patient for an urgent CT scan of abdomen and pelvis.
c. Transfuse 4 units of whole blood immediately.
d. Transfer the patient promptly to OT for emergency laparotomy after discussing with the on-call surgical team.
e. Perform a diagnostic peritoneal lavage bedside.

Ans. d

Explanation: Focused assessment by sonography for trauma (FAST) examination is a key component of the primary survey in trauma patients. It is effectively used primarily in the suspected blunt abdomen trauma with persistent hypotension post fluid resuscitation to rule out need for emergent exploratory laparotomy after discussion with the surgical team. The four zones, which are seen, are the right and left upper quadrant followed by suprapubic area and the subcostal view. The right upper quadrant shows the hepatorenal space (Morrison pouch) and the left upper quadrant is the space between the left spleen and left kidney. In female patients, positive FAST findings can be found in the pouch of Douglas which is the space between the anterior wall of the rectum and the posterior wall of the uterus. It makes the corresponding space relates to the rectovesical pouch.

Q.4. A 27-year-old male patient is brought to the emergency department following a road traffic accident which happened approximately an hour ago involving head-on collision between a two-wheeler and a four-wheeler vehicle. Patient was initially mobile and complaining of neck pain on movement and difficulty in respiration due to tenderness on the right side of chest particularly on inspiration. On arrival to ED, his vitals were checked and recorded as heart rate of 110 beats/min with blood pressure of 100/70 mm Hg with oxygen saturation of 95% on room air. In the primary survey, unequal chest rise was observed, reduced on the right side with significant reduced air entry. On palpation, patient complained of tenderness on the right side of chest. Patient continued to be tachypneic and a bedside e-FAST was done promptly with the linear probe on the chest wall along with M-mode. The image of the scan is shown below:

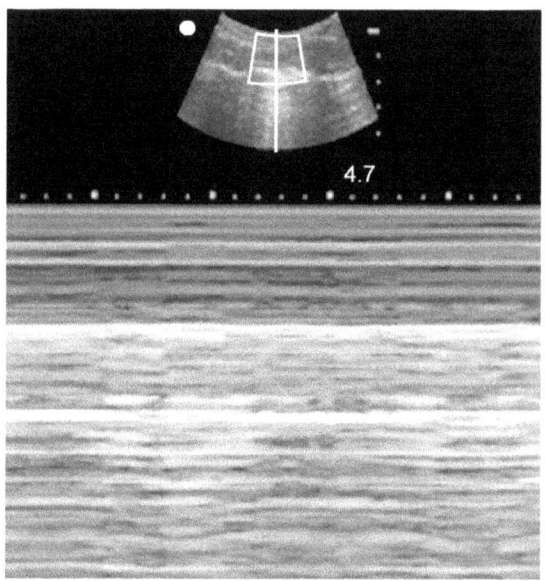

Which of the following diagnoses does the ultrasound finding support?
a. Massive hemothorax
b. Multiple rib fractures
c. Pneumothorax
d. Pleural effusion
e. Aortic dissection

Ans. c

Explanation: Extended FAST is a key component of the primary survey and is used to rule out pneumothorax. A linear probe is used to perform the scan. In M-mode or motion mode, two specific signs are observed. One is the seashore sign and the other is stratosphere sign or the barcode sign. A stratosphere sign with presence of lung point is a diagnostic criterion for pneumothorax. The lung point is defined as the point where the pneumothorax ends, and the normal lung starts. On M-mode, a lung point will show stratosphere sign with small periods of seashore sign as the visceral pleura slides into view. A positive sliding sign suggests movement of the visceral pleura as it slides over the fixed parietal pleura. However, only the absence of sliding sign does not confirm for pneumothorax as other conditions such as pulmonary contusions or bullous emphysema can show similar findings. Hence, observing the lung point gives a 100% specific confirmation for pneumothorax.

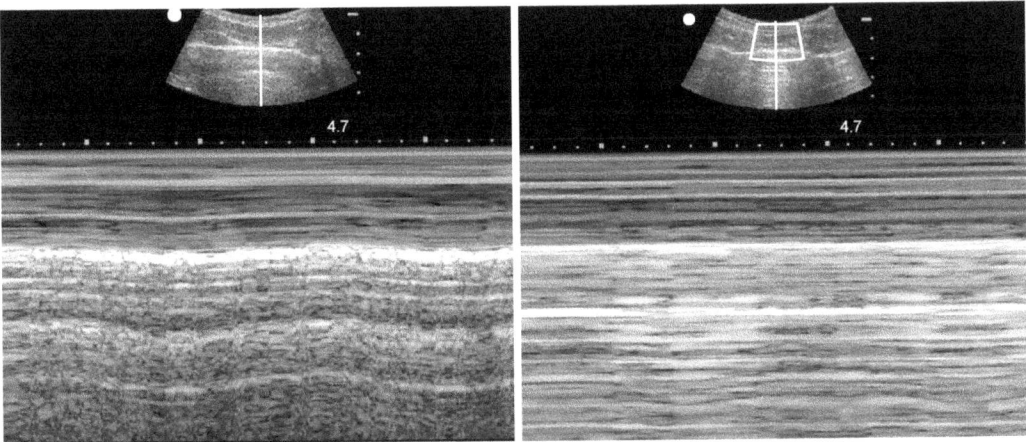

Human lung —no pneumothorax Human lung —pneumothorax

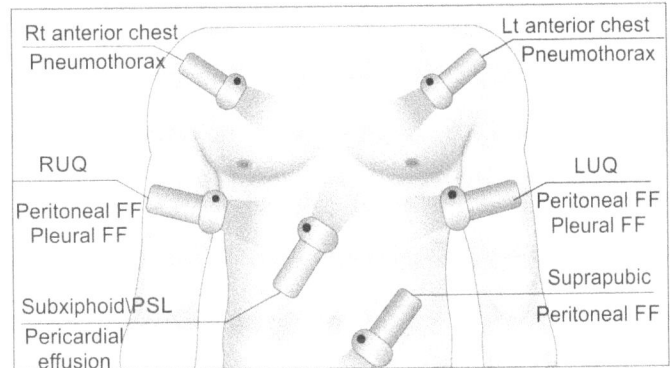

(FF: free fluid; Lt: left; LUQ: left upper quadrant; PSL: parasternal long;
Rt: right; RUQ: right upper quadrant)

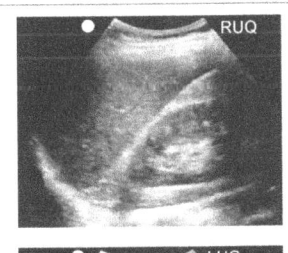

RUQ
- Longitudinal plane view
- Demonstrate hepatorenal interface
- Labeled RUQ

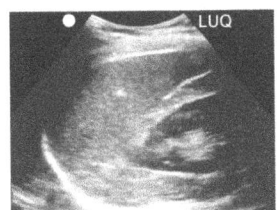

LUQ
- Longitudinal plane view
- Demonstrate splenorenal interface
- Labeled LUQ

Contd...

Contd...

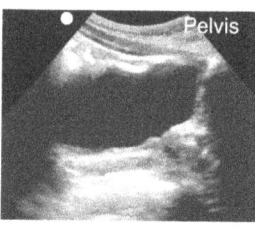

Pelvis
- Longitudinal view
- *Female*: Demonstrate bladder, uterus, pouch of Douglas, rectum
- *Male*: Demonstrate bladder, prostate, rectovesical pouch, rectum
- Labeled pelvis

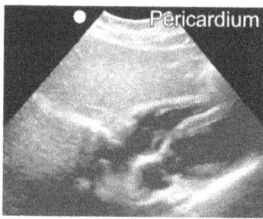

Pericardium
- Subxiphoid, parasternal long axis of apical plane alternative view
- Demonstrate pericardium, ventricles, atria
- Labeled pericardium

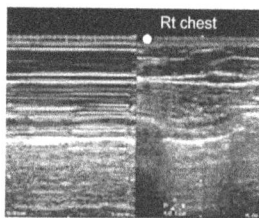

RT chest
- Longitudinal plane anterior view
- Demonstrate lung sliding with M-mode trace
- Labeled RT chest

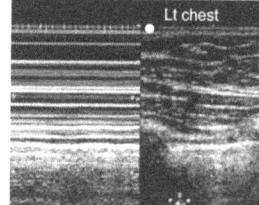

LT chest
- Longitudinal plane anterior view
- Demonstrate lung sliding with M-mode trace
- Labeled LT chest

(Lt: left; LUQ: left upper quadrant; Rt: right; RUQ: right upper quadrant)

POLYTRAUMA

Q.1. A 32-year-old man is brought to the emergency department after being stabbed during a fight in a nearby club. He has one wound to the right side of the chest that the paramedics described as bubbling with blood on scene. They have placed an occlusive dressing over the wound. The paramedics tell you that en route the patient's heart rate has normalized and he "looked better". On arrival to the emergency department, he suddenly becomes hypotensive and unresponsive. What diagnosis is the likely responsible for the patient's current condition?
a. Cardiac tamponade
b. Tension pneumothorax
c. Massive hemothorax
d. Flail chest
e. Pulmonary contusion

Ans. b

Explanation: Open pneumothorax can be managed in a prehospital setup by applying a three-way occlusive dressing at the site of the wound. The dressing is to be taped on three sides around the wound to give a flutter-like valve effect. By doing this when patient is inspiring the dressing occludes the wound, preventing air from entering and during the expiration phase, the open end of the dressing aids in the escape of the air. This is a temporary measure till the patient can be transferred to an emergency department for further management. However, if a dressing is applied with all four ends sealed then an open pneumothorax is converted to a tension pneumothorax with hemodynamic instability. In such scenario, emergent chest tube placement is required as soon as possible. Following placement of tube, surgical closure of the wound could be done.

Q.2. A 26-year-old male patient is brought to the emergency department from a nearby political rally where he was involved in an altercation. According to the paramedics, he was stabbed multiple times on his chest. He also has a small laceration on his forehead and a deformity in the thigh region. On arrival to ED, his vitals were checked and recorded as extremely tachycardic with a heart rate of 134 beats/min along with hypotension, blood pressure of 80/60 mm Hg, and oxygen saturation of 94% with 15 L of oxygen support through NRBM. Two wide-bore cannulas were immediately placed and started on fluid resuscitation. On further examination in the primary survey, patient remained drowsy and moaning to pain stimulus only. On chest examination, patient has equal chest rise and bilateral equal breath sounds and had jugular venous distention. Suddenly the nurse shouts for help as monitor showed asystole and patient became unresponsive with no pulse. Which of the following is the most appropriate next step in management?
   a. Shift patient to OT immediately.
   b. Initiate cardiopulmonary resuscitation (CPR) and consider for ED thoracotomy
   c. Consider emergency pericardiocentesis
   d. Administer injection adrenaline
   e. Consider placement of ICD tubes on both sides

Ans. b

Explanation: The above scenario is suggestive of a penetrating injury to the chest region leading to a traumatic arrest. Usually in such an incidence, in presence of significant hemodynamic instability on presentation leading to cardiac arrest in prehospital or hospital setup, ED thoracotomy should be considered as the most effective tool of treatment. Patient showed a triad of signs such as hypotension, jugular venous distention, and muffled heart sounds suggestive of Beck's triad leading to cardiac tamponade. Tachycardia and marked hypotension also play a significant role and in certain cases; jugular venous distention is not observed in view of marked hypovolemia. The recommended method of treatment in the presence of ongoing cardiac arrest is promptly relieving of the tamponade through thoracotomy to attain possibility of a better clinical outcome.

Q.3. A 32-year-old man is brought to the emergency department by the paramedics after being stabbed in his neck. The patient is able to speak full sentences. His breath sounds are equal bilaterally. His blood pressure is 140/76 mm Hg, HR is 104 beats/min, RR is 18 breaths/min, and oxygen saturation is 97% on room air. The stab wound is located between the angle of the mandible and the cricoid cartilage and violates the platysma. There is blood oozing from the site although there is no expanding hematoma.

A 40-year-old male patient is wheeled into the emergency department by the paramedics with a history of stab injury to the neck region approximately 30 minutes before. On arrival to ED, vitals were recorded as heart rate of 112 beats/min with blood pressure of 134/78 mm Hg and oxygen saturation of 97% on room air. Patient is not tachypneic and is able to converse with the ED doctor without any difficulty. On examination, it was found out that the stab injury is located below the angle of mandible but above the cricoid cartilage and the depth of the wound is beyond the platysma. There was active oozing of blood but no hematoma detected in the neck region.

What is the preferred next step in management?
a. Apply a tight compression bandage to stop the bleed.
b. Examine the active bleeder and clamp the site if possible.
c. Plan to shift the patient promptly to OT for a zone I injury after applying direct pressure on the wound.
d. Plan to shift the patient promptly to OT for a zone II injury after applying direct pressure on the wound.
e. Plan to shift the patient promptly to OT for a zone III injury after applying direct pressure on the wound.

Ans. d

Explanation:
- The neck region is one of the vulnerable spots for trauma leading to life-threatening complications. Most common mechanisms being penetrating or blunt trauma to the neck region or strangulation. Each of these mechanisms can affect the patient's airway or the esophagus or any vascular anatomy. For effective management of trauma to the neck, it has been divided into three zones which are shown in the image below.
  - Zone I represents the area between the cricoid cartilage and the clavicle and sternal notch.
  - Zone II represents the area between the angle of mandible and the cricoid cartilage.
  - Zone III represents the area between the base of the skull and the angle of mandible.
- Usually Zone II injuries need to be managed by surgical exploration and hence patients should be transferred to the OT immediately.

- Zone I and Zone III can be managed with the combination of angiography, CT scanning, or bronchoscopy or esophagoscopy.
- Critical component one needs to keep in mind in managing a neck trauma is the need of airway management if needed at the earliest.

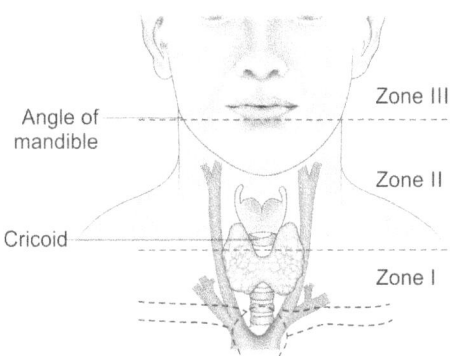

Q.4. A 37-year-old construction worker is brought to the emergency department by the paramedics from the construction site after falling approximately from 30 feet from a scaffold. His vital signs include BP = 82/52 mm Hg, HR = 136 beats/minute, and oxygen saturation = 91% on 100% oxygen via face mask. On examination, he has obvious head trauma with a 6-cm scalp laceration overlying a skull fracture on his occiput. He has no response to vocal stimulus, his respirations are shallow, and you can hear gurgling with each attempted breath. Auscultation of the chest reveals diminished breath sounds on the right. There is no jugular venous distention (JVD) or anterior chest wall crepitus. His pelvis is unstable with movement laterally to medially, and you note blood at the urethral meatus. His left leg is grossly deformed at the thigh region, and there is an obvious fracture of his right arm.

A 35-year-old male patient is brought to the emergency department by the paramedics. The patient is a construction worker, working in a high-rise building which is under construction. History suggests that the patient lost his balance and fell down from approximately 20 feet onto a hard concrete surface. On arrival to ED, patient's vitals were recorded as heart rate of 124 beats/min with hypotension, blood pressure of 80/50 mm Hg, and oxygen saturation of 90% with 15 L of oxygen support through an NRBM. On examination, it was noted that patient had a 5-cm deep laceration in the occipital region with obvious signs of head and cervical injuries. Primary survey shows patient to be obtunded and respiration being sonorous. There is reduced breath sound on the left side of the chest with crepitus on palpation. Pelvic compression is positive and visible deformity of the left thigh is noted.

Which of the following is the immediate intervention needed to be done in these patients?
a. Transfer the patient for an urgent CT scan of head.
b. Apply pelvic binder and Thomas splint in the left lower limb.

c. Place two wide-bore cannulas and start rapid transfusion protocol.
d. Proceed with urgent drug-assisted intubation with spine motion restriction.
e. Insert an ICD on the left side of the chest wall.

Ans. d

Explanation:
- According to Advanced Trauma Life Support (ATLS) principle, primary survey is the initial step to approach a trauma patient. The components of the primary survey are airway with spine motion restriction, breathing with ventilation, circulation with hemorrhagic control, disability, and exposure. The primary goal of the primary survey is to identify potential life-threatening injuries and subsequent steps to stabilize the patient, and to proceed with the primary adjuncts and then onto secondary survey. The above scenario shows the patient's airway is not patent and having signs of impending respiratory distress, and hence airway stabilization with strict spine motion restriction is the first priority to proceed with the management of this trauma victim.
- Need for chest tube insertion for suspected hemothorax and/or pneumothorax (PTX) demonstrated by decreased breath sounds and oxygen saturation of 90%.
- Extremity injuries are typically not life threatening and are assessed after the ABC are evaluated.

Q.5. In the previous question, the patient is immediately intubated and receives 1 L of warm crystalloid. Patient's vitals were checked again and patient continued to be tachycardic and hypotensive in spite of initial fluid resuscitation and no improvement in the oxygen saturation even after orotracheal intubation and providing a fraction of inspired oxygen (FiO_2) of 100%. On repeat auscultation of the chest, you continue to hear diminished breath sounds on the left. Which of the following is the next preferred treatment protocol in this patient?
a. Perform bedside focused abdominal sonography for trauma (FAST) examination.
b. Place a pelvic binder to stabilize the pelvis.
c. Transfer the patient for CT scans of the patient's head and cervical spine.
d. Perform needle thoracostomy of the left chest.
e. Administer 100 cc of 3% hypertonic saline.

Ans. d

Explanation:
- In the ABCDEs of trauma, after the airway is secured, attention should be turned to the patient's breathing. The patient remains hemodynamically unstable and hypoxic after endotracheal intubation and has decreased breath sounds on the right. These are signs of tension PTX. Tension PTX is a life-threatening condition that develops when air is trapped in the pleural cavity and expands to compress the mediastinum and compromises cardiopulmonary function. The diagnosis is based on clinical assessment and should not be delayed for further diagnostic testing. In

the unstable patient, treatment for a tension PTX is accomplished by performing a needle thoracostomy.
- The FAST examination is performed to screen the abdomen for hemoperitoneum. This is an appropriate part of the trauma evaluation, but airway patency takes more priority in this patient.
- Pelvic binders are a tamponade device used in trauma patients with suspected pelvic injury potentially associated with major hemorrhage. This intervention would take place after addressing the airway and breathing in this patient.
- CT scans of the patient's head and cervical spine may play a role in evaluation of this patient; however in view of hemodynamic instability, patient cannot be transported for CT scan.
- 3% hypertonic saline is an osmotic agent given to patients with concern for increased intracranial pressure. This may be considered in this patient given the signs of head trauma and decreased mental status, but this is not the most immediate next action to be performed.

Q.6. A 43-year-old man is brought by the paramedics to the emergency department following a fall from stairs. In the ED, on examination, patient is awake but tachypneic. Patient has a deformity of the left shoulder with pain and restricted movement. Patient is complaining of pain in the right side of chest more on inspiration and the right lower limb appears to be rotated externally with apparent shortening. Vital signs were stable and primary survey was done and patient stabilized. During secondary survey, a shoulder X-ray is taken and the image is shown below:

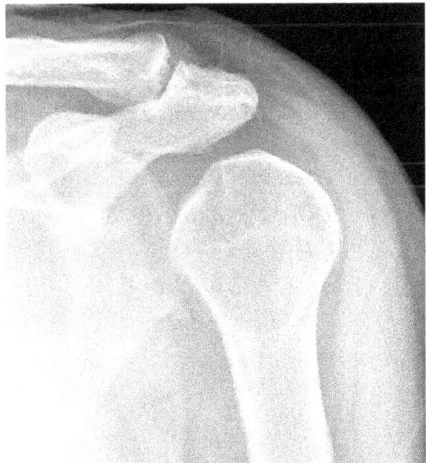

What is the diagnosis?
a. Anterior shoulder dislocation
b. Posterior shoulder dislocation
c. Fracture of humeral neck
d. Distal clavicular fracture
e. Acromioclavicular joint disruption

Ans. b

Explanation: This is uncommon injury and is easy to miss. It results from a blow onto the anterior shoulder or a fall onto the internally rotated arm. It may also occur during seizures or after an electric shock (when other injuries and medical problems may be partly responsible for it being initially overlooked).

The patient presents with the shoulder internally rotated. Anteroposterior (AP) shoulder X-ray may appear normal, but careful inspection reveals an abnormally symmetrical appearance of the humeral head ("light bulb sign") and loss of congruity between the humeral head and the glenoid. A modified axial shoulder X-ray (from above) or a translateral view confirms posterior dislocation.

Manipulate under sedation: Apply traction and external rotation to the upper limb at 90° to the body. If difficult, refer for reduction under general anesthesia (GA). Treat and follow-up postmanagement.

TRANSFUSION IN TRAUMA

Q.1. A 27-year-old woman is being brought to the emergency department after being ejected from her vehicle following a high-speed road traffic accident. Upon arrival, her BP is 80/52 mm Hg and HR is 146 beats/min. Two large-bore IVs are placed, and 1 L of IV fluids has been administered.

A 30-year-old female patient is brought to the emergency department after being involved in a high-speed road traffic accident. Vitals were recorded as heart rate of 146 beats/min and blood pressure of 80/52 mm Hg and oxygen saturation of 95% with 10 L of oxygen delivered by NRBM. Immediately two wide-bore intravenous cannulas were placed and fluid resuscitation started with 1 L of warm crystalloids.

Which of the following statements is the most appropriate regarding management of these hypotensive trauma patients who fail to respond to initial volume resuscitation?

a. It is important to wait for fully cross-matched blood prior to transfusion.
b. Begin an epinephrine infusion.
c. Blood group Type O with RH-negative should be considered for blood transfusion.
d. Until adequate fluid resuscitation is not done, blood transfusion should not be initiated.
e. Blood group Type O with RH-positive should be considered for blood transfusion.

Ans. c

Explanation:

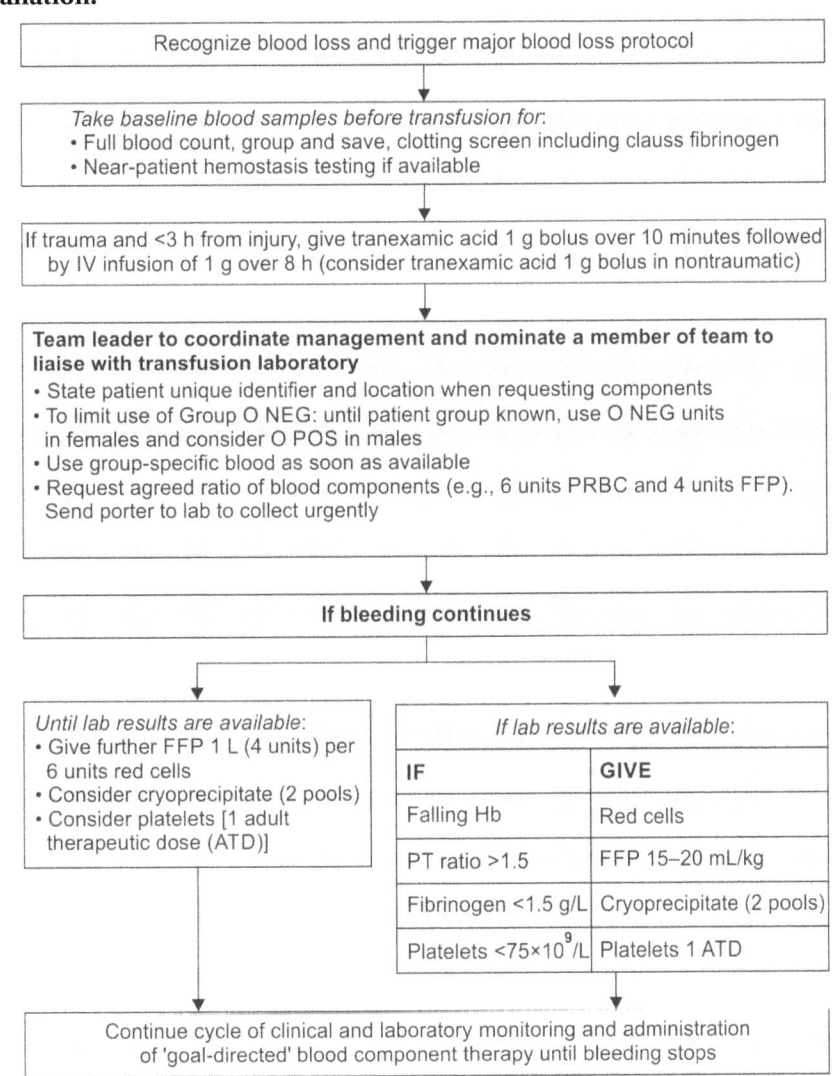

(FFP: fresh frozen plasma; IV: intravenous; PT: prothrombin time; PRBC: packed red blood cell)

TRANSPORT IN TRAUMA

Q.1. Paramedics are being called to a local cricket coaching club following an event during a cricket match. One young player is unresponsive to verbal stimuli after a head-on collision with the nonstriker player (both wearing helmets) while attempting to take a run. Vitals were recorded as heart rate of 58 beats/min with blood pressure of 98/64 mm Hg. There is a small crack at the top of the helmet, but it is otherwise intact and strapped tightly to the patient's head.

Paramedics called up the nearest trauma center to enquire regarding whether to remove his helmet in order to assess for head trauma. What is the recommended prehospital treatment for this patient?

a. Do not attempt to remove the helmet, maintain cervical spine precautions, and transfer the patient on a backboard to the hospital.
b. While maintaining cervical spine precautions, carefully remove the helmet and assess for head injury.
c. Check the patient's pupils and if there is asymmetry, remove the helmet with cervical spine precautions.
d. Wait at the scene for a physician to arrive with an electric saw for removal of the helmet and further on-scene assessment.
e. Do not remove the helmet but assess the cervical spine for step-off or any signs of obvious injury before transfer.

Ans. a

Explanation:
- A properly fitted helmet holds the head in a position of neutral spinal alignment; field removal of these devices is not recommended. Instead, the helmet and shoulder pads should remain on as the athlete is immobilized and transported on a rigid backboard. Simultaneous removal of the helmet should be done after clinical assessment and radiographs at the hospital. Radiographs can be repeated after removal of the helmet as clinically indicated. The proper removal of a helmet requires four people and should not be attempted out of hospital.
- Even with pupil asymmetry, the emergency medical team's (EMT's) best course of action is to expeditiously transport the patient to the ED for definitive care because paramedics are not trained to perform any techniques to relieve impending uncal herniation.
- The use of an electric saw is not indicated, and unnecessary prehospital delays should be avoided.
- Adequate cervical spine assessment is unreliable and potentially dangerous in the prehospital setting and would also unnecessarily delay transport.

CHAPTER

14

Cardiovascular System

Harish Mallapura Maheshwarappa, Robert James Premkumar, Ganesh KM

Q.1. A 66-year-old male patient in the intensive care unit (ICU) was resuscitated successfully after a witnessed cardiac arrest. An electrocardiogram (ECG) showed ST elevations in the anteroseptal lead, and an echocardiography revealed a left ventricular ejection fraction of 25%. An emergency coronary angiogram was performed, and the left anterior descending artery was revascularized. Due to persistent cardiogenic shock during the procedure, the patient was initiated on venoarterial extracorporeal membrane oxygenation (VA-ECMO) via the femoral vein and femoral artery. The patient's oxygenation and hemodynamic status showed an improving trend, but on day 3 of ECMO, a saturation of 80% was noted in the right upper limb, while it remained at 100% in the lower limbs. The settings on ECMO were as follows—flow 4 lumped-parameter model (LPM), rpm 3,000, sweep gas 4 LPM, and FiO_2 100%. The postoxygenator pO_2 was 400 mm Hg, and a repeat echocardiography showed an EF of 40%. Which of the following is the most appropriate next line of management?
a. Increase ECMO flow
b. Change the oxygenator
c. Add an extra oxygenator
d. Convert to venoarteriovenous (VAV) ECMO
e. Push the return cannula proximally

Ans. d

Explanation: The patient is presenting with differential hypoxemia due to Harlequin or North-South syndrome. In the setting of peripheral VA-ECMO, venous blood is drained from the right atrium and returned in a retrograde manner through the femoral or iliac artery back toward the thoracic aorta. As a result, patients on peripheral VA-ECMO have an area of watershed in the aorta where the two bloodstreams meet, which can be located anywhere between the aortic root and diaphragm. The location of this watershed region depends on the LV output relative to ECMO flow, with a more distal location when LV output is high and a more proximal location when LV output is low. While blood from the ECMO circuit is typically well-oxygenated, blood from the LV is dependent on adequate pulmonary gas exchange, which may be compromised in acute cardiogenic shock and pulmonary edema. As the LV output improves, the watershed region is pushed distally. However, if this region is situated distal to the left subclavian artery, there is a significant risk of profound hypoxemia to the brain, heart, and upper extremities, leading to Harlequin or North-South syndrome. The initial management for this condition involves treating pulmonary pathology and increasing ventilator support to enhance oxygenation of blood exiting the LV. Increasing ECMO flow can further strain the LV and worsen pulmonary edema and blood oxygenation, making it an unsuitable option. Additionally, replacing or adding an oxygenator is not required, as the existing one is functioning efficiently, as indicated by the postoxygenator pO_2. The recommended solution is to convert to VAV ECMO, where the arterial return cannula is split using a Y connector to deliver oxygenated blood into the venous system and pulmonary circulation. Alternatively, a central VA ECMO can be used, which eliminates the watershed region. If hemodynamics allow, weaning to veno-venous (VV) ECMO may also be considered.

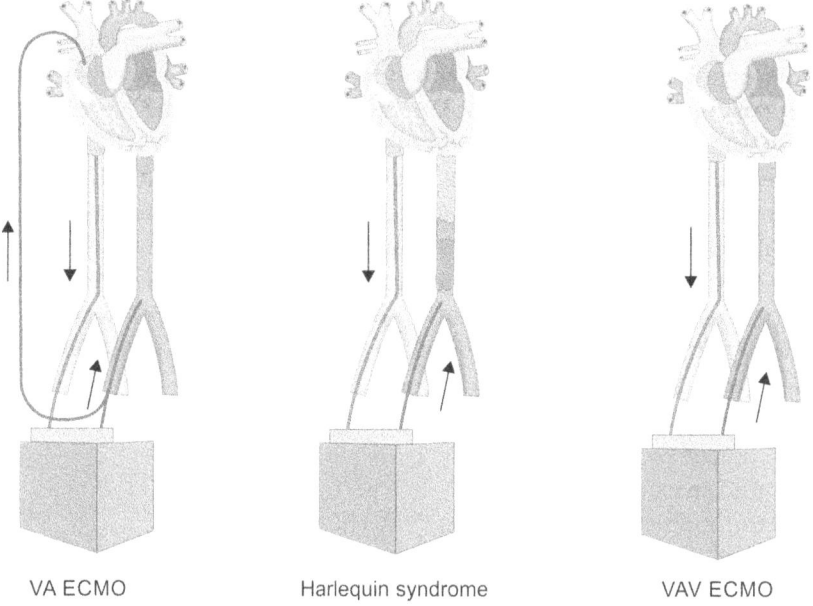

VA ECMO   Harlequin syndrome   VAV ECMO

(ECMO: extracorporeal membrane oxygenation; VA: venoarterial; VAV: venoarteriovenous)

Suggested Reading
1. Rao P, Khalpey Z, Smith R, Burkhoff D, Kociol RD. Venoarterial extracorporeal membrane oxygenation for cardiogenic shock and cardiac arrest. Circ Heart Fail. 2018;11(9):e004905.

Q.2. **A 77-year-old male patient who recently underwent coronary artery bypass grafting has been transferred to your ICU and is currently in the control mode of mechanical ventilation. During the handover process, you observe that the patient is experiencing bradycardia with a heart rate of 40/min and hypotension with a blood pressure (BP) of 80/50 mm Hg, accompanied by a SaO_2 of 94% with a FiO_2 of 0.4 and positive end-expiratory pressure (PEEP) of 5 cmH_2O. The patient has a temporary pacemaker via epicardial wires, and the ECG shows wide QRS complexes at a rate of 40 beats per minute (BPM), while pacing spikes are seen at a rate of**

80 BPM. Upon review of the pacemaker's settings, you note that it is in VVI mode with a sensitivity of 2 mV, voltage output of 5 mA, and a set rate of 80 BPM. Which of the following is the most appropriate step?
a. Increase the set pacemaker rate
b. Replace the pacemaker battery
c. Increase the pacemaker output voltage
d. Increase the pacemaker sensitivity
e. Change to VOO mode

Ans. c

Explanation: The common problems encountered with pacemakers are failure to capture, failure to pace, failure to sense, and oversensing. In the case of failure to capture, the pacemaker fires as expected but fails to depolarize the myocardium. Although a pacer spike is observed on the ECG, no QRS complex immediately follows it. Fibrosis around the pacemaker lead, improper programming of voltage, electrolyte abnormalities, and antiarrhythmic drugs can increase resistance at the wire/myocardium interface and cause this condition. Increasing the output voltage may result in capture. Failure to pace, on the other hand, is suspected when the heart rate is below the programmed lower rate of the pacemaker and no pacer electrical output is observed on the electrocardiogram. Lead malfunction, battery failure, cross-talk inhibition, or oversensing can cause this issue. In the case of failure to sense, also known as undersensing, the pacemaker fails to detect spontaneous myocardial depolarization, leading to asynchronous pacing. Atrial or ventricular pacing spikes arise regardless of P waves or QRS complex, resulting in too many pacing spikes. This condition can occur due to improper programming of sensing threshold, lead malfunction, myocardial fibrosis, and electrolyte abnormalities. Lastly, oversensing occurs when the pacemaker senses external electrical signals such as those from electrocautery, resulting in inappropriate inhibition of the pacing stimulus.

Suggested Reading
1. Safavi-Naeini P, Saeed M. Pacemaker troubleshooting: common clinical scenarios. Tex Heart Inst J. 2016;43(5):415-8.

Q.3. A 55-year-old female with poor left ventricular systolic function status postcoronary artery bypass grafting is currently admitted to the ICU. She required mechanical ventilation and inotropic support guided by pulmonary artery catheter (PAC) and was on DDD mode of pacemaker via epicardial wires. After successful weaning off mechanical ventilator support, the patient was extubated, taken off pacemaker support, and inotropes were tapered and discontinued. On the third postoperative day, the patient develops a new onset hypotension. The patient's vitals include HR: 110/min, BP: 70/50 mm Hg, saturation: 94% on face mask 5 LPM, and respiratory rate (RR): 30/min. Cardiac output monitor reveals a cardiac index (CI) of 1.8, central venous pressure (CVP) of 17 mm Hg, right ventricular pressure (RVP) of 27/18 mm Hg, pulmonary artery pressure (PAP) of 28/18 mm Hg, and pulmonary artery wedge pressure (PCWP) of 17 mm Hg. Given the patient's medical history and current presentation, what is the most probable cause for the hypotension?

a. Cardiogenic shock
b. Pulmonary embolism
c. Septic shock
d. Cardiac tamponade
e. Hypovolemic shock

Ans. d

Explanation: One of the key diagnostic criteria for cardiac tamponade is the elevation and equalization of diastolic pressures in all cardiac chambers, which is observed in this case. The PAC provides direct measurements of several important hemodynamic parameters, including [right atrial pressure (RAP) normal range 1-10 mm Hg], RVP normal range 15-30/0-8 mm Hg, PAP normal range 15-30/5-15 mm Hg, [pulmonary capillary wedge pressure (PCWP) normal range 5-15 mm Hg], and [mixed venous oxygen saturation (SvO$_2$) normal range 70-75%], as well as derived parameters such as CI normal range 2.6–4.2 L/min/m^2, [systemic vascular resistance (SVR) normal range 900–1,400 dynes/s/cm^5], and [pulmonary vascular resistance (PVR) normal range 150–250 dynes/s/cm^5]. The patterns of these parameters can be used to identify different types of shock, including cardiogenic, hypovolemic, obstructive, and septic shock.

Pulmonary artery catheter (PAC) parameters in various types of shock:

Type of shock	CI	SVR	PVR	SvO$_2$	RAP	RVP	PAP	PAOP
Cardiogenic	↓	↑↑	N	↓	↑	↑	↑	↑
Hypovolemic	↓	↑	N	↓	↓	↓	↓	↓
Distributive shock	N-↑	↓	N	N-↑	N-↓	N-↓	N-↓	N-↓
Obstructive	↓	N-↑	↑	N-↓	↑	↑	↑	N-↓

(CI: cardiac index; PAP: pulmonary artery pressure; PAOP: pulmonary artery occlusion pressure; PVR: pulmonary vascular resistance; RAP: right atrial pressure; RVP: right ventricular pressure; SvO$_2$: mixed venous oxygen saturation; SVR: systemic vascular resistance)

Suggested Reading
1. Kaplan JA. In: Augoustides JGT, Manecke GR, Maus T Jr, Reich DL (Eds). Kaplan's Cardiac Anesthesia: for Cardiac and Noncardiac Surgery, 7th edition. Amsterdam: Elsevier; 2017.
2. Marine HK, Warren I, Cole BC, Vladimir ND. Washington Manual of Critical Care, 2nd edition. Philadelphia: Wolters Kluwer Health; 2015.

Q.4. A 44-year-old male patient underwent percutaneous coronary intervention and revascularization for an occlusion in the proximal left anterior descending artery yesterday. Due to cardiogenic shock, the patient was initiated on intra-aortic balloon pump (IABP) support. The patient's condition had been improving, with saturation of 94% with 2 LPM O$_2$ via nasal prongs and HR 90/min and BP 130/80 mm Hg on minimal inotropic support, earlier today. However, the patient's oxygen requirement has now increased along with a drop in blood pressure. The following IABP balloon pressure trace has been noted. Based on the information provided, what is the most likely cause of these changes in the patient's condition?

Normal intra-aortic balloon pump (IABP) balloon pressure waveform:

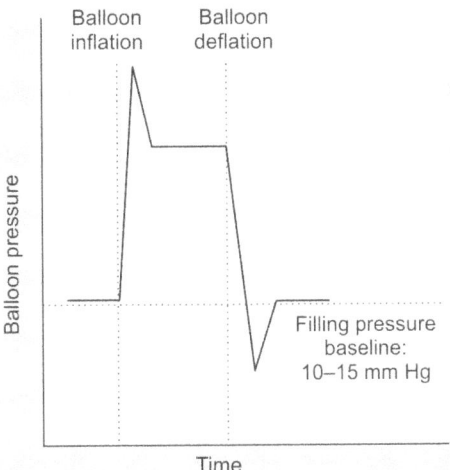

a. The balloon is too small for the patient
b. The balloon is disconnected
c. The balloon catheter is kinked
d. There is a leak in the balloon
e. There is an early balloon inflation

Ans. c

Explanation: The IABP console displays the balloon pressure waveform below the arterial pressure waveform. A normal balloon pressure waveform begins at the baseline, increases during inflation has a positive overshoot at peak inflation, and plateaus throughout the balloon's duration of inflation (diastole). The waveform then decreases during deflation, has a negative overshoot at peak deflation, and returns to baseline. A rounded balloon pressure waveform without a plateau may be caused by a kink in the catheter tubing, improper catheter placement, an oversized catheter for the aorta, or insufficient sheath retraction to allow for proper inflation of the IABP. Additional alterations in the balloon pressure waveform may result from gas loss, which can cause the balloon pressure to fall below baseline; prolongation, shortening, or variability in the duration of the plateau, which can occur in the presence of bradycardia, tachycardia, or arrhythmias such as atrial fibrillation, respectively. In hypertension, the amplitude increases, whereas in hypotension, it decreases.

Suggested Reading
1. www.scribd.com. IABP Learning Package. [online] Available from: https://www.scribd.com/document/415255974/IABP-Learning-Package [Last accessed June, 2023].

Q.5. A male athlete, aged 40 years old, who recently recovered from coronavirus disease 2019 (COVID-19) pneumonia, presents with sudden onset of central chest pain that has persisted for the past 8 hours. The pain was exacerbated by sitting in a recliner chair and alleviated by leaning forward. The patient denied any history of fever. He was alert and oriented with a heart rate of 90 beats per minute, blood pressure of 130/90 mm Hg in both upper limbs, respiratory rate of 20 breaths/min, oxygen saturation of 97% in room air, and afebrile. His chest X-ray showed normal findings, and his troponin T level was negative. Echocardiography findings were within normal limits. The patient's ECG is provided below. Given the patient's clinical presentation, what is the most appropriate line of management?

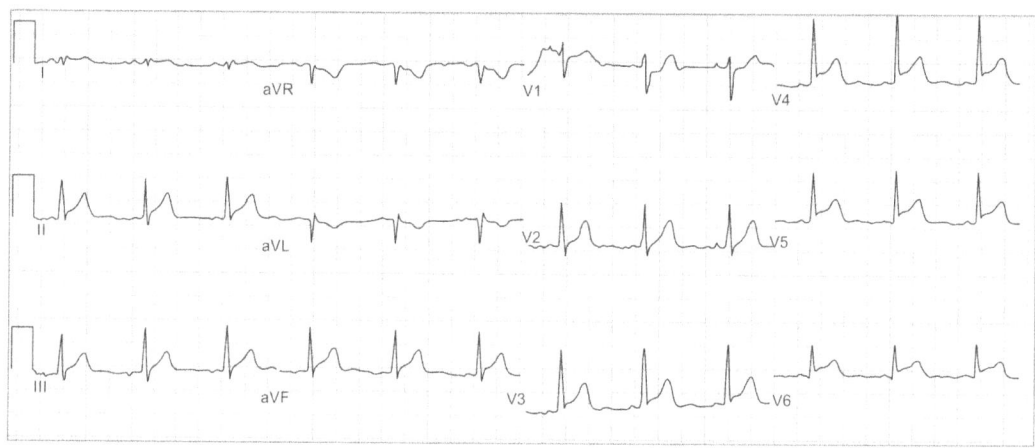

a. Corticosteroids
b. Coronary angiogram
c. CT angiogram
d. Reassurance
e. Nonsteroidal anti-inflammatory drugs (NSAIDs) with colchicine

Ans. e

Explanation: The patient's clinical presentation is suggestive of viral pericarditis, which may be related to a recent COVID-19 infection. As per the 2015 European Society of Cardiology (ESC) guidelines, a clinical diagnosis of acute pericarditis is based on the presence of at least two of the following criteria: (i) pericarditic chest pain (sharp/pleuritic which improves on sitting up or leaning forward); (ii) pericardial pleural rub; (iii) new-onset widespread ST-elevation or PR-depression; and (iv) new or worsening pericardial effusion. Inflammatory markers such as C-reactive protein (CRP) may be elevated, providing supportive evidence and monitoring therapy. Additionally, markers of myocardial injury, such as troponin, may be elevated in the case of myocarditis. Therefore, there is a class 1 recommendation for performing an ECG, transthoracic echocardiogram, chest X-ray, and CRP/troponin. Targeted testing is necessary to rule out other potentially life-threatening conditions such as acute coronary syndrome, pulmonary embolism, and aortic dissection. Treatment of acute pericarditis caused by a viral infection typically involves aspirin or NSAIDs as first-line agents, along with colchicine as an adjuvant. Specific targeted therapy is required for other etiologies. When pericarditis recurs after a symptom-free period of

>4–6 weeks it is termed recurrent pericarditis and when pericarditis lasts >3 months, it is termed chronic pericarditis.

Suggested Reading
1. Adler Y, Charron P, Imazio M, Badano L, Barón-Esquivias G, Bogaert J, et al. ESC Guidelines for the diagnosis and management of pericardial diseases: The Task Force for the Diagnosis and Management of Pericardial Diseases of the European Society of Cardiology (ESC) Endorsed by: The European Association for Cardio-Thoracic Surgery (EACTS). Eur Heart J. 2015;36(42):2921-64.

Q.6. A 68-year-old male who is a known case of interstitial lung disease with severe pulmonary hypertension, on ambrisentan and tadalafil, and is admitted in your ICU with complaints of fever, cough, and breathing difficulty for the past 3 days. Computed tomography (CT) scan of chest revealed consolidation. A diagnosis of community-acquired pneumonia was made and he was initiated on antibiotics, bronchodilators, and other supportive care. In view of worsening respiratory distress, he was intubated and mechanically ventilated. He is on control mode of ventilation with FiO$_2$ 0.5, PEEP 8 mm Hg, RR 18, and tidal volume 420 mL. His vitals are heart rate (HR) of 90/min, BP of 90/50, and saturation of 96%. Arterial blood gas analysis shows a rising trend of lactates. You also note that he has cold peripheries with bilateral pitting pedal edema. You are faced with the dilemma of whether to give fluids or not. Which of the following gadgets is least preferable?
a. Passive leg raise
b. Central venous pressure
c. Pulse pressure variation
d. Pulmonary arterial catheter
e. Stroke volume variation

Ans. b

Explanation: The assessment of fluid responsiveness involves both static and dynamic indices. Static indices comprise measurements such as CVP, pulmonary capillary wedge pressure, heart rate, and blood pressure. Dynamic indices, on the other hand, encompass measures such as pulse pressure variation, stroke volume variation, inferior vena cava (IVC) collapsibility, and response to passive leg raise. Dynamic indices are deemed superior to static indices. Left ventricular end diastolic volume (LVEDV) is related to left ventricular end-diastolic pressure (LVEDP) by the left ventricular compliance. The LVEDP, in turn, is related to the left atrial pressure (LAP) by the diastolic pressure gradient across the mitral valve. The PCWP is associated with LAP by the pulmonary capillary resistance. The pulmonary artery diastolic (PAD) pressure is an estimate of PCWP, whereas CVP reflects the PAD pressure if right ventricular function is normal. Hence, in patients with pulmonary hypertension and tricuspid regurgitation, CVP may not be an accurate measure of systemic preload. Among the static indices, pulmonary artery wedge pressure represents a better measure of systemic preload in such cases.

Relationship between CVP and LVEDV:

CVP ∝	PAD ∝	PCWP ∝	LAP ∝	LVEDP ∝	LVEDV
↑	↑	↑	↑	↑	
Right ventricle	Pulm vasc resistance	Airway pressure	Mitral valve	Left ventricular compliance	

(CVP: central venous pressure; LVEDV: left ventricular end-diastolic volume)

Suggested Reading
1. Cherpanath TGV, Geerts BF, Lagrand WK, Schultz MJ, Groeneveld ABJ. Basic concepts of fluid responsiveness. Neth Heart J. 2013;21(12):530-6.
2. Kaplan JA. In: Augoustides JGT, Manecke GR, Maus T Jr, Reich DL (Eds). Kaplan's Cardiac Anesthesia: for Cardiac and Noncardiac Surgery, 7th edition. Amsterdam: Elsevier; 2017.

Q.7. An 88-year-old male patient has been admitted to the intensive care unit following coronary artery bypass grafting. The patient was initially on IABP support for cardiogenic shock, which has now been discontinued. The patient had been receiving unfractionated heparin infusion for the same and has now been transitioned to subcutaneous injections of unfractionated heparin at 5,000 U every 6 hours. On the fifth day of hospitalization, the patient's platelet count has dropped to 90,000/μL from an initial count of 280,000/μL, and a preliminary diagnosis of heparin-induced thrombocytopenia (HIT) is being considered. What would be the appropriate next line of management for this patient?
a. Stop unfractionated heparin and give enoxaparin
b. Stop unfractionated heparin and transfuse four random donor platelets
c. Stop unfractionated heparin and give fondaparinux
d. Withhold all anticoagulation
e. Confirm with HIT antibody reports before stopping heparin

Ans. c

Explanation: Heparin-induced thrombocytopenia is a prothrombotic condition due to immunoglobulin G antibodies that target complexes of platelet factor 4 (PF4) and heparin. It is more common with unfractionated heparin (UFH) than with low-molecular-weight heparin (LMWH) with the incidence ranging from <0.1% to 7%. About half the cases of HIT are complicated by thrombosis, which may be venous or arterial and may be limb or life-threatening. The 4Ts score is used to estimate the probability of HIT. In those with intermediate to high risk of HIT, heparin should be discontinued immediately; a nonheparin anticoagulant is initiated and it is recommended to obtain an immunoassay. Those with a positive immunoassay are suggested to obtain a functional assay. Nonheparin anticoagulants suggested are argatroban, bivalirudin, danaparoid, and fondaparinux, and direct oral anticoagulant (DOAC). The choice of anticoagulant is influenced by drug factors such as availability, cost, and ability to monitor the anticoagulant effect, route of administration, and half-life and patient factors such as renal function, liver function, bleeding risk, and clinical stability and experience of the clinician. Platelet transfusion may be an option only for patients with active bleeding or at high risk of bleeding.

Suggested Reading
1. Cuker A, Arepally GM, Chong BH, Cines DB, Greinacher A, Gruel Y, et al. American Society of Hematology 2018 guidelines for management of venous thromboembolism: heparin-induced thrombocytopenia. Blood Adv. 2018;2(22):3360-92.
2. Pishko AM, Cuker A. Heparin-induced thrombocytopenia in cardiac surgery patients. Semin Thromb Hemost. 2017;43(7):691-8.

Q.8. A 25-year-old female patient who suffered a right femur fracture in a road traffic accident (RTA) is under postoperative care in your ICU. On the second postoperative day, the patient was alert and pain-free with a heart rate of 70 beats per minute, blood pressure of 100/70 mm Hg, saturation of 97% on room air, and respiratory rate of 18 breaths/min. However, after mobilization, the patient experiences desaturation and hypotension that requires oxygen support via a facemask and inotropic therapy. To further assess the patient's condition, you perform a bedside echocardiogram. In cases of acute pulmonary embolism, echocardiographic findings may include:
a. Left ventricular apical ballooning with hypercontractile basal segments
b. Right ventricular free wall hypokinesia with hyperdynamic apex
c. Diastolic collapse of right ventricle
d. Systolic right atrial collapse
e. Septal deviation toward right ventricle

Ans. b

Explanation: Echocardiography can play a significant role in the evaluation of known or suspected pulmonary embolism. Its potential applications include diagnosis, assessment of hemodynamic consequences, determination of management, evaluation of cardiopulmonary responses to therapeutic interventions, and exclusion of other entities that may present similarly to pulmonary embolism. Acute pulmonary embolism may present with direct or indirect echocardiographic findings. Direct findings include visualization of the thrombus in the pulmonary artery. Indirect features include McConnell's sign, which is characterized by right ventricular free wall hypokinesia with hyperdynamic apex, D sign with ventricular septal flattening toward the left ventricle, right atrial and ventricular dilatation, an unusual degree of pulmonary or tricuspid regurgitation, and pulmonary artery hypertension. Other choices that are given are not seen in pulmonary embolism. Left ventricular apical ballooning with hypercontractile basal segments is seen in Takotsubo's cardiomyopathy. Diastolic collapse of the right ventricle and systolic collapse of the right atrium are seen in cardiac tamponade.

Suggested Reading
1. Goldstein SA, Kronzon I, Khandheria B, Mor-Avi V. ASE's Comprehensive Echocardiography, 2nd edition. Amsterdam: Elsevier Health Sciences; 2015.

Q.9. A 20-year-old gentleman who is a known case of depression is admitted in your ICU with acute gastroenteritis. His ECG is shown below. Which of the following conditions is least likely?

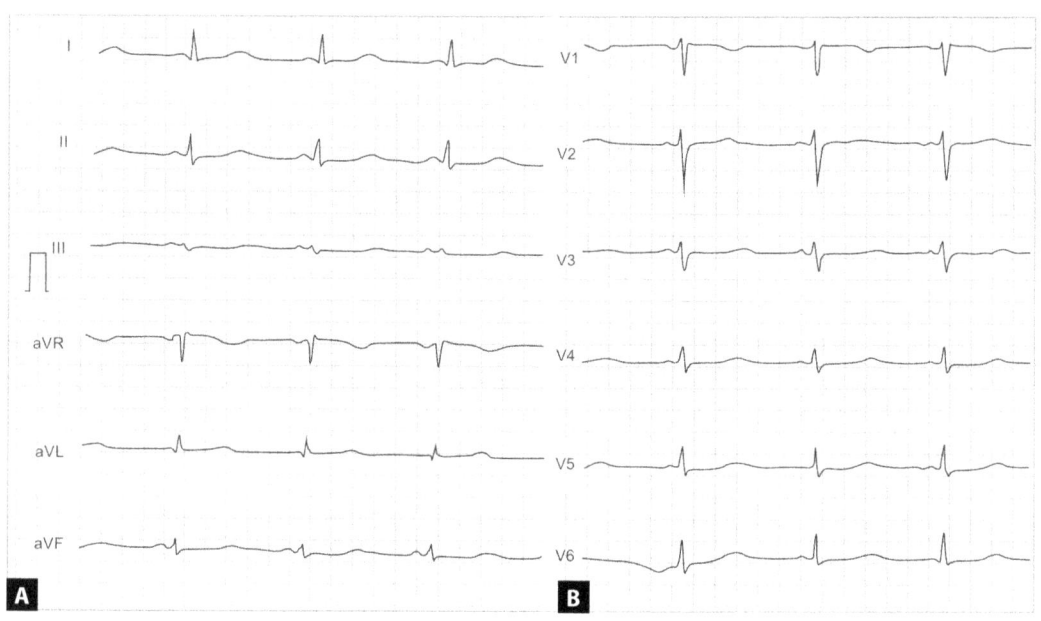

a. Hypothermia
b. Tricyclic antidepressant usage
c. Hypocalcemia
d. Hypokalemia
e. Hypermagnesemia

Ans. e

Explanation: This patient exhibits a prolonged QT interval, a condition attributed to various factors. These factors include hypothermia, which may be accompanied by Osborn waves (positive deflection of the J point); sodium channel blocking drugs such as tricyclic antidepressants, hypocalcemia, and hypokalemia which may be accompanied by prominent U waves; hypomagnesemia but not hypermagnesemia; acute myocardial infarction; raised intracranial pressure, which may be accompanied by cerebral T waves (widespread deep T wave inversions) and congenital QT syndromes. It is noteworthy that the QT prolongation associated with hypothermia and hypocalcemia is unique in that it is completely due to the prolongation of the ST-segment, with the T-waves remaining unchanged.

Suggested Reading
1. Mattu A. In: Brady WJ (Ed). ECGs for the Emergency Physician 1, 1st edition. London: BMJ Books; 2003.

Q.10. A 55-year-old female who had lost her son in an RTA recently presents with complaints of sudden onset chest discomfort. Electrocardiogram showed ST elevations in inferolateral leads and cardiac enzymes were elevated. Echocardiography showed a left ventricular ejection fraction of 25%; left ventricular apical ballooning with hypercontractile basal segments. She underwent coronary angiography but no significant coronary artery disease was found. Which of the following is contraindicated in this patient?
a. Beta-blockers
b. Diuretics
c. Inotropes
d. Calcium channel blockers

Ans. c

Explanation: The patient exhibits features consistent with Takotsubo cardiomyopathy, a form of acute heart failure that mimics acute myocardial infarction. Also known as stress-induced cardiomyopathy or broken heart syndrome, its underlying pathophysiology is not fully understood but is believed to be related to the excessive release of catecholamines in response to a stressor, such as an emotional or medical condition like subarachnoid hemorrhage. The ECG may show widespread ST/T wave abnormalities, while cardiac enzymes such as troponin and B-type natriuretic peptides may be elevated. Echocardiography may reveal left ventricular apical ballooning with hypercontractile basal segments, while coronary angiogram may show normal coronaries or nonobstructive coronary artery disease. Despite its transient nature, Takotsubo cardiomyopathy carries a high risk of morbidity and mortality. Treatment is currently based on expert consensus and extrapolation from the management of myocardial infarction (MI), as there are no established guidelines. Inotropes such as adrenaline, noradrenaline, and dobutamine should be avoided, as excess catecholamines can exacerbate the condition. In cases of pulmonary edema, diuretics, and nitroglycerin may be used, provided there is no left ventricular outflow tract obstruction. Left ventricular assist devices (LVAD), IABP, and VA ECMO may be employed in cases of shock, while intravenous fluids, β-blockers, and LVADs may be used in cases of LVOT obstruction.

Suggested Reading
1. Singh T, Khan H, Gamble DT, Scally C, Newby DE, Dawson D. Takotsubo syndrome: pathophysiology, emerging concepts, and clinical implications. Circulation. 2022;145(13):1002-19.

Q.11. A 25-year-old young lady presents to you with complaints of palpitation and breathing difficulty. She is a known case of trigeminal neuralgia on carbamazepine. Now, she is conscious and oriented. Her heart rate is 150/min and blood pressure is 110/70 mm Hg, respiratory rate is 24 breaths/min and her oxygen saturation is 98% on 2 L/min via nasal prongs. ECG is taken immediately which is shown below. There is an 18 G peripheral venous cannula. What is the most appropriate next line of management?

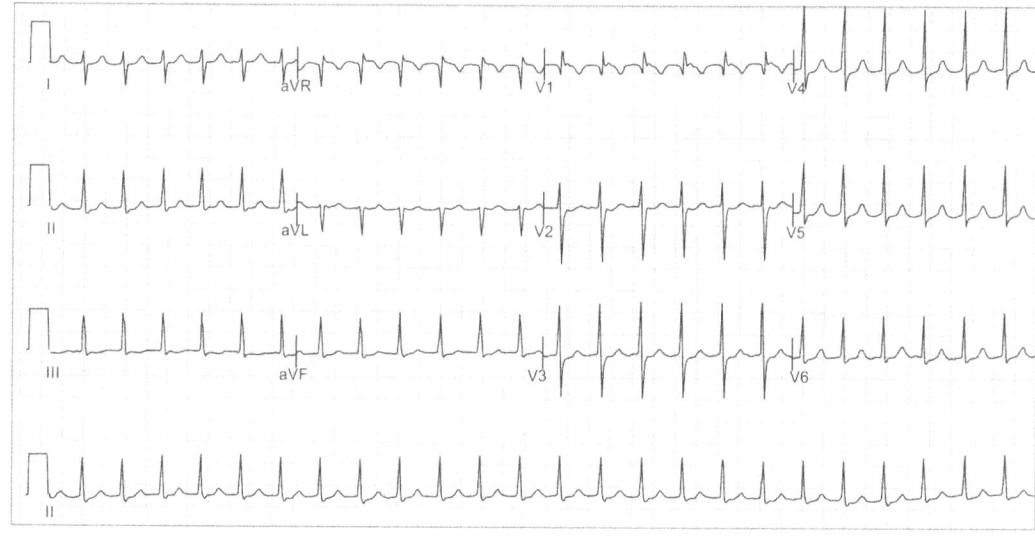

a. Adenosine 3 mg IV rapid bolus
b. Adenosine 6 mg IV rapid bolus
c. Synchronized cardioversion
d. Amiodarone 150 mg IV bolus
e. Amiodarone 300 mg IV bolus

Ans. a

Explanation: This patient has supraventricular tachycardia without hemodynamic instability. In accordance with the 2019 European Society of Cardiology guidelines, a vagal maneuver is recommended as a first-line treatment (class I recommendation). If this is unsuccessful, an intravenous bolus of adenosine (6–18 mg) is recommended as a Class I treatment option. Adenosine acts on the atrioventricular (AV) node, decreasing conduction, with its effects further enhanced by carbamazepine. Hence, the standard dose of adenosine should be reduced in patients on carbamazepine or dipyridamole; those who have undergone cardiac transplant, or in those where adenosine is administered through a central line. Denervation of the sinoatrial (SA) and AV nodes makes cardiac transplant patients more sensitive to adenosine. Amiodarone is not suitable for treating supraventricular tachycardia. Synchronized cardioversion is not recommended in the absence of hemodynamic instability, but it is a class I recommendation for cases where drug therapy fails to convert or control the tachycardia or when hemodynamic instability is present.

Suggested Reading
1. Brugada J, Katritsis DG, Arbelo E, Arribas F, Bax JJ, Blomström-Lundqvist C, et al. 2019 ESC Guidelines for the management of patients with supraventricular tachycardiaThe Task Force for the management of patients with supraventricular tachycardia of the European Society of Cardiology (ESC). Eur Heart J. 2020;41(5):655-720.

Q.12. A male patient, 70 years of age, is receiving IABP support after experiencing cardiogenic shock postpercutaneous coronary intervention for the acute coronary syndrome. The IABP pressure tracing is shown below. Please recommend the next course of action in light of these observations.

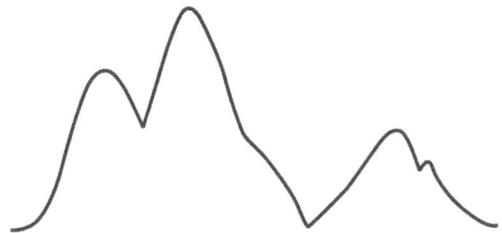

a. Get a repeat chest X-ray to reconfirm IABP balloon position
b. Set the balloon pump to inflate early
c. Set the balloon pump to deflate late
d. Set the balloon pump to deflate early
e. Maximize augmentation

Ans. d

Explanation: The IABP is a mechanical device used for hemodynamic support in patients with cardiogenic shock and acute decompensated heart failure. The inflation of the balloon during diastole leads to increased aortic root pressure and coronary perfusion pressure, resulting in increased myocardial oxygen supply. Conversely, deflation just before the next systolic ejection reduces aortic pressure, improving forward ejection from the heart and decreasing myocardial work and oxygen demand. When electrocardiography is used as a trigger, in patients with sinus rhythm, the IABP is programmed to inflate during the mid-T wave and deflate at the peak of the R wave, which corresponds to the start of diastole and systole, respectively. When arterial pressure waveform is used as a trigger, the balloon should inflate with the dicrotic notch, which corresponds to aortic valve closure, and should deflate before the systolic arterial upstroke which corresponds to aortic valve opening. A properly timed and functioning balloon pump can increase cardiac output by 20–30% and decrease afterload by up to 15%. These benefits are lost when the balloon is inflated or deflated early or late. In our patient, the peak for diastolic augmentation is wider; the assisted aortic end-diastolic blood pressure is not lower than the unassisted aortic end-diastolic blood pressure and the rise of assisted systolic blood pressure is slow and prolonged. All these indicate that the balloon deflation is delayed which increases afterload and therefore oxygen demand. The balloon pump needs to be set to deflate early.

Suggested Reading
1. Kaplan JA. In: Augoustides JGT, Manecke GR, Maus T Jr, Reich DL (Eds). Kaplan's Cardiac Anesthesia: for Cardiac and Noncardiac Surgery, 7th edition. Amsterdam: Elsevier; 2017.

Q.13. Which of the following is an inappropriate diagnostic method for evaluating left ventricular diastolic function in a 69-year-old man admitted to the ICU with acute pulmonary edema? His ECG shows atrial fibrillation with a rapid ventricular rate with no significant ST/T changes.
a. Mitral wave E/A ratio
b. Tissue Doppler E/e'
c. Mitral E wave deceleration time (DT)
d. Isovolumetric relaxation time (IVRT)

Ans. a

Explanation: Although the mitral E/A ratio is commonly employed to evaluate diastolic dysfunction, its application is limited in certain clinical conditions such as sinus tachycardia, atrial fibrillation, and first-degree atrioventricular block. To comprehend this limitation, it is crucial to understand the methodology for assessing diastolic dysfunction, which employs the E/A ratio. The E/A ratio is calculated using pulse wave Doppler across the mitral valve in the apical four-chamber view. In individuals without diastolic dysfunction, there is a brisk flow of blood from the left atrium to the left ventricle during early diastole, which results in a peak mitral flow velocity known as the E wave. During the latter phase of diastole, the atrial kick facilitates the transfer of the remaining blood from the left atrium to the left ventricle, resulting in a peak mitral flow velocity known as the A wave, which is substantially smaller than the E wave, thus producing an E/A ratio >1 **(see below Figure A)**. However, as left ventricular relaxation becomes impaired and left ventricular stiffness increases, the left atrium to left ventricle gradient decreases, resulting in a more prominent A wave and an E/A ratio <1 (grade 1) **(see below Figure B)**. Subsequently, as an adaptive mechanism to restore a "pseudonormal" left atrium to left ventricle gradient, left atrial pressures to increase, leading to an E/A ratio of 1-1.5 (grade 2) **(see below Figure C)**. As left ventricular stiffness further increases, adaptive mechanisms fail, resulting in a very high E wave and low A wave, with an E/A ratio >2 (grade 3) **(see below Figure D)**. In patients with atrial fibrillation, the E and A waves are fused, rendering them less useful for diagnostic purposes **(see below Figure E)**. All the other methods mentioned may be used.

Grades of diastolic dysfunction:

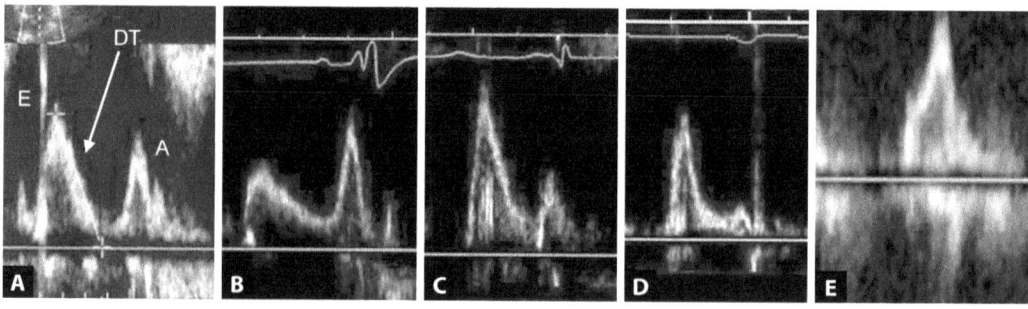

Suggested Reading
1. Goldstein SA, Kronzon I, Khandheria B, Mor-Avi V. ASE's Comprehensive Echocardiography, 2nd edition. Amsterdam: Elsevier Health Sciences; 2015.

2. Mottram PM, Marwick TH. Assessment of diastolic function: what the general cardiologist needs to know. Heart. 2005;91(5):681-95.

Q.14. **In the absence of a cardiac output monitor, passive leg raising combined with the measurement of the change in aortic velocity time integral (VTI) using echocardiography has been selected to assess fluid responsiveness in a patient. Which of the following views is best suited for obtaining the necessary images? What is the formula to calculate stroke volume from aortic VTI?**
  a. Transthoracic parasternal long axis, SV = $D^2 \times 0.785 \times$ LVOT VTI
  b. Transthoracic subcostal 4-chamber, SV = $\pi (D/2)^2 \times$ LVOT VTI
  c. Transthoracic parasternal short axis (aortic valve level), SV = $\pi (D/2)^2 \times$ LVOT VTI
  d. Transthoracic apical five-chamber, SV = $D^2 \times 0.785 \times$ LVOT VTI

Ans. d

Explanation: Transthoracic apical five-chamber view is the widely used view for measuring aortic VTI. To obtain accurate measurements, the pulse wave Doppler gate is carefully placed in the left ventricular outflow tract (LVOT) at a distance of approximately 1 cm from the aortic valve. The resulting waveform corresponds to the flow through the LVOT during systole, and the downward wave is traced to obtain the VTI. In healthy individuals, aortic VTI values >18 cm are considered normal. Following a passive leg raising (PLR) maneuver, an increase in VTI of 10–15% suggests volume responsiveness. Cardiac output can be calculated using the formula, CO = Stroke volume (SV) × heart rate (HR). SV = LVOT area × LVOT VTI. LVOT area = $\pi \times$ (LVOT diameter/2)^2 = $D^2 \times 0.785$. Therefore, CO = $D^2 \times 0.785 \times$ LVOT VTI × HR. LVOT diameter is obtained from a transthoracic parasternal long-axis view.

Transthoracic apical five-chamber view:

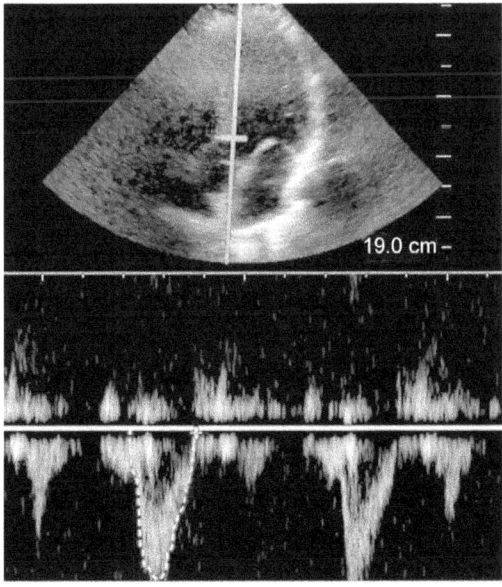

Suggested Reading
1. Goldstein SA, Kronzon I, Khandheria B, Mor-Avi V. ASE's Comprehensive Echocardiography, 2nd edition. Amsterdam: Elsevier Health Sciences; 2015.
2. www.tampaemergencymedicine.org. (2020). Cardiac VTI—The New IVC for Fluid Responsiveness? [online]. Available from: https://www.tampaemergencymedicine.org/blog/cardiac-vti-the-new-ivc-for-fluid-responsiveness [Last accessed June, 2023].

Q.15. A 24-year-old football player sustained a sudden cardiac arrest on the field. He was successfully resuscitated after 20 minutes of cardiopulmonary resuscitation (CPR). He was diagnosed with hypertrophic cardiomyopathy with left ventricular outflow tract obstruction. He is on mechanical ventilation and hemodynamic support guided by a pulmonary artery catheter. His vitals are HR: 100/min, BP: 84/42 (56) mm Hg, saturation: 94% on FiO_2 0.4, and PEEP 5 cmH_2O. Cardiac output monitor reveals a cardiac output of 6 L/min, CVP of 8 mm Hg, PAP of 28/12 mm Hg, and PCWP of 12 mm Hg. Which agent will you use?
a. Phenylephrine
b. Adrenaline
c. Noradrenaline
d. Dopamine
e. Dobutamine

Ans. a

Explanation: Hypertrophic cardiomyopathy (HCM) is an inherited cardiac disorder characterized by increased thickness of the left ventricular (LV) wall, which cannot be explained by abnormal loading conditions. Resting systolic anterior motion (SAM) of the anterior mitral leaflet, causing left ventricular outflow tract (LVOT) obstruction, is seen in one-third of HCM patients. Similarly, another one-third of patients experience LVOT obstruction during exercise or maneuvers such as Valsalva. Approximately 25% of HCM patients are symptomatic and are at increased risk of sudden cardiac death. LVOT obstruction is triggered by factors that decrease afterload (such as septic shock and vasodilators); decrease preload (hypovolemia and hemorrhage), increase heart rate (pain, arrhythmias, inotropic agents, and fever), or increase contractility (inotropes). Therefore, treatment involves addressing the precipitating cause. Inotropes, β-agonists, nitrates, and diuretics should be discontinued or reduced, hypovolemia addressed with intravenous fluids, and nonvasodilating β-blockers may be titrated to the maximum tolerated dose. In this patient, SVR calculated using the given parameters of mean arterial pressure (MAP), central venous pressure, and cardiac output (CO) using the formula SVR = 80 × (MAP − CVP)/CO, yields a value of 640 $dynes/s/cm^5$ (normal range 900–1,400 $dynes/s/cm^5$), indicating decreased afterload. Therefore, the preferred agent would be phenylephrine, a pure α-agonist, to increase SVR.

Suggested Reading
1. Slama M, Tribouilloy C, Maizel J. Left ventricular outflow tract obstruction in ICU patients. Curr Opin Crit Care. 2016;22(3):260-6.

Q.16. A 30-year-old male presented to the emergency room with sudden onset chest pain and shortness of breath. He has a history of smoking two cigarette packs daily for the last 6 years. His blood pressure is 180/100 mm Hg, his heart rate is 90 beats per minute, and his respiratory rate is 26 breaths/min. Computed tomography scan done shows the following image. Regarding the management of this patient, all are true except which of the following?

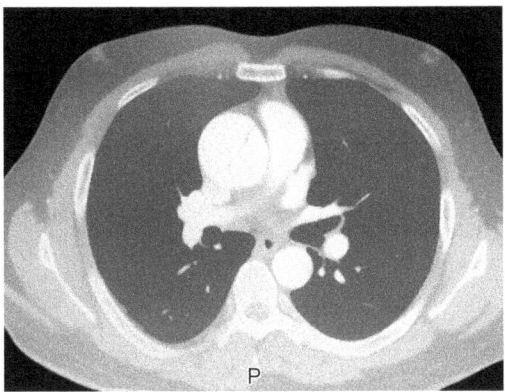

a. Finding a normal chest X-ray does not rule out dissection
b. Acutely lowering the blood pressure with vasodilators will reduce the chances of the dissection propagating further
c. Surgical management is always required in type A dissection
d. The incidence of spinal cord ischemia is similar between the open surgical approach and TEVAR

Ans. b

Explanation: Tight blood pressure control and reduction of the rate of pressure rise during systole is vital to reduce the chances of dissection propagation. The shear force within the aorta is defined as the change in pressure over time, dP/dt. If you look at the picture below, the first one is the baseline arterial waveform, where the dP/dt represents the shear forces, and the second one is where the addition of vasodilators in isolation has caused reflex tachycardia and in fact, increased the dP/dt now the last one is where the addition of β-blocker has reduced the dP/dt. Stanford type A always requires surgical management, whereas type B it is medical management unless it is complicated. For complicated type B endovascular approach with TEVAR is preferred. Type B is complicated when there is refractory pain, malperfusion, rupture or leak, and rapid expansion after 48 hours. The incidence of spinal cord ischemia is similar when either approach is used, which is between 2 and 10%. In up to 20% of patients, the chest X-ray is normal with type A dissection.

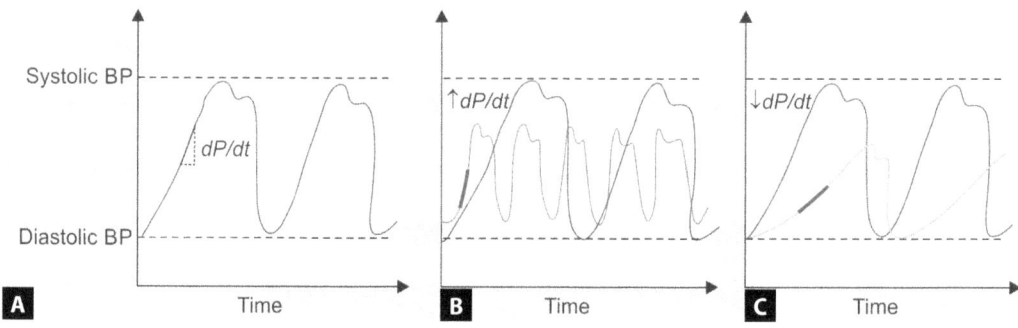

Suggested Reading
1. Chen SW, Lee KB, Napolitano MA, Murillo-Berlioz AE, Sattah AP, Sarin S, et al. Complications and management of the thoracic endovascular aortic repair. Aorta (Stamford). 2020;8(3):49-58.
2. Flower L, Arrowsmith JE, Bewley J, Cook S, Greco R, Sadeque S, et al. Management of acute aortic dissection in critical care. J Intensive Care Soc. 2023;1-10.

Q.17. A 25-year-old male presents to the emergency room with a history of profuse watery diarrhea since 2 days. His vitals are as follows heart rate of 130 beats per minute, blood pressure of 100/60 mm Hg, respiration of 24 breaths/min, and temperature of 98.9°F. The patient is given an IV bolus of 2 L balanced crystalloid. Which cardiac parameter is expected to increase from this intervention?
a. Chronotropy
b. Inotropy
c. Lusiotropy
d. Dromotropy

Ans. b

Explanation: Frank–Starling law is based on the link between the initial length of the myocardial fibers and the force generated by contraction. The left ventricular performance curves relate preload, measured as left ventricular end-diastolic volume (EDV) or end-diastolic pressure (EDP) to cardiac performance, measured as ventricular stroke volume or cardiac output. In this patient, as he is fluid depleted, with fluid resuscitation, his preload (volume status) will improve. In other words, the EDV will increase so will the cardiac output. Cardiac contractility is also known as inotropy. Chronotropy increases the heart rate, lusiotropy increased effectiveness of active diastolic relaxation, dromotropy means an increased speed of electrical conduction and bathmotropy means a modification of the degree of excitability.

Suggested Reading
1. Delicce AV, Makaryus AN. Physiology, Frank Starling Law. In: StatPearls [Internet]. Treasure Island (FL): StatPearls Publishing; 2023.

Q.18. Regarding finerenone, all are true except for which of the following?
a. It is a nonsteroidal mineralocorticoid receptor antagonist (MRA)
b. It exhibits anti-inflammatory and antifibrotic activity

c. When used with angiotensin-converting enzyme (ACEI) or angiotensin II receptor blockers (ARBs), life-threatening hyperkalemia may occur
d. It significantly slows down the chronic kidney disease (CKD) progression and reduces cardiovascular events

Ans. c

Explanation: Based on FIDELIO-DKD (Finerenone in Reducing Kidney Failure and Disease Progression in Diabetic Kidney Disease), FIGARO-DKD (Finerenone in Reducing Cardiovascular Mortality and Morbidity in Diabetic Kidney Disease), and FIDELITY pooled analysis, finerenone is a novel, nonsteroidal MR antagonist, MR overactivity is seen in diabetes and CKD. Mineralocorticoid receptor overactivity in diabetes triggers inflammation and fibrosis in kidneys, and in CKD it is one of the reasons for the progression of CKD and increased cardiovascular events. The evidence from the above studies points toward a significant slowing of CKD progression and reduced cardiovascular events. Finerenone also exhibits protection from new-onset atrial fibrillation in CKD patients. All the patients in the two randomized controlled trials (RCTs) were on ARBs and ACEI, hyperkalemia did occur in a small group of patients which was managed by alerting the regimes of therapy but no deaths due to hyperkalemia were reported.

Q.19. A 56-year-old lady presents to the emergency room with complaints of profuse sweating and giddiness since the last hour. She was diagnosed with tachycardia bradycardia syndrome and underwent permanent pacemaker insertion 10 years back. She is a hypothyroid patient and is on thyroxine supplements and hypertensive on β-blocker and angiotensin receptor antagonist therapy. On examination, her vitals are—heart rate 48 beats per minute, blood pressure 90/50 mm Hg, respiratory rate 22 breaths/min. An ECG is done, which reveals ST-segment depression which is concordant with QRS complexes. What is the next step in managing the patient?
a. Pacemaker interrogation
b. Injection of atropine 0.6 mg IV stat
c. Chest X-ray to look for lead fracture
d. Coronary angiogram
e. Injection glucagon/high dose insulin therapy along with dextrose

Ans. d

Explanation: Right ventricular pacing (RVPR) results in an intraventricular conduction delay similar to that seen with left bundle branch block (LBBB). The Sgarbossa criteria have been used to diagnose ST-elevation myocardial infarction (STEMI) in patients with RVPR and are the following: (i) concordant ST-segment elevation ≥1 mm for leads with a predominantly positive QRS complex (score 5); (ii) concordant ST depression ≥1 mm in leads V1, V2, or V3 (score 3); and (iii) excessively discordant ST-segment elevation ≥5 mm in leads with negative QRS complexes (score 2). A total score of ≥3 suggests the patient is having anterior wall myocardial infarction (AWMI). Based on this criteria this patient is likely suffering from MI and needs a coronary angiogram.

Pacemaker interrogation if the battery life is expired or to look for problems associated with capture is required if the patient had symptomatic bradycardia. Atropine would actually worsen ischemia. Lead fracture would result in symptomatic bradycardia. Glucagon or insulin therapy would be required in β-blocker toxicity.

Suggested Reading
1. Vrettos A, Panoulas V. Diagnosing STEMI in the presence of paced rhythm: dispelling the myth of the 'uninterpretable paced ECG'. BMJ Case Rep. 2021;14(7):e242546.

Q.20. A 32-year-old lady with a history of second vaginal delivery 4 weeks back presents with shortness of breath which is gradually worsening since 2 weeks to the extent of limiting her daily activity. Her only medication is a multivitamin. Her vitals are heart rate of 110 beats per minute, blood pressure of 104/60 mm Hg, and respiratory rate of 32 breaths/min. Echocardiogram reveals LV function of 35%. Given the likely diagnosis regarding the disease, all are true except for which of the following?
   a. Preeclampsia and hypertension are common risk factors and will cause diastolic heart failure
   b. Risk of thromboembolic disorders is high
   c. Addition of bromocriptine to standard heart failure treatment regimens will improve myocardial recovery
   d. Patients may benefit from implantable cardioverter-defibrillator (ICD) and cardiac resynchronization therapy (CRT)

Ans. a

Explanation: Peripartum cardiomyopathy (PPCM) is a form of systolic LV dysfunction [left ventricular ejection fraction (LVEF) <45%] that develops during the end of pregnancy or up to 5 months postpartum. In 2010 ESC defined PPCM as heart failure that develops toward the end of pregnancy or in the months of delivery where no other cause of heart failure is found. When the LVEF <30% or associated with LV dilatation, there is an increased risk of LV clot formation and is associated with thromboembolic events. Treatment with bromocriptine along with diuretics, ACEI/ARBS, and β-blockers has shown an improvement in LV function. Prolactin mediates PPCM a 2007 study concluded. Ventricular arrhythmias and sudden death contribute greatly to morbidity and mortality, with incidence being 2%. Since most women recover early implantation of ICD is discouraged.

Suggested Reading
1. Davis M, Arany Z, McNamara DM, Goland S, Elkayam U. Peripartum Cardiomyopathy: JACC State-of-the-Art Review. J Am Coll Cardiol. 2020, 75(2):207-21.
2. Honigberg MC, Givertz MM. Peripartum cardiomyopathy. BMJ. 2019;364:k5287.

Q.21. A 32-year-old male survives a motor vehicle crash and sustains multiple injuries, which include blunt force trauma to the thoracic cavity. Regarding blunt cardiac injury (BCI), all are true except for which of the following?
   a. About >70% of patients have associated sternal fractures
   b. Endovascular approach is preferred over open surgical approach of aortic injuries

c. Commotio cordis is associated with VF
d. LBBB is more common with BCI

Ans. d

Explanation: Cardiac trauma is a less common consequence of blunt injury but is often associated with high morbidity and mortality. Blunt cardiac injury often occurs due to forceful impact, rapid deceleration, or crush injuries without penetration of the chest and heart. The most common causes of BCT include motor vehicle accidents (MVA) (~50% of BCT), pedestrians being struck by a motor vehicle (~35%), motorcycle crashes (~9%), and falls from a significant height. In one series, 76% of BCI sternal fractures were noted. Apart from heart rate control and blood pressure control for aortic injuries endovascular approach for aortic injuries when ascending aorta is spared. Commotio cordis is when there is sudden cardiac death induced by VF usually seen in male athletes. Right bundle branch block (RBBB) is the most common arrhythmia associated with BCI due to its anterior location of the right side of the heart.

Suggested Reading
1. El-Andari R, O'Brien D, Bozso SJ, Nagendran J. Blunt cardiac trauma: a narrative review. Mediastinum. 2021;5:28.
2. Nair L, Winkle B, Senanayake E. Managing blunt cardiac injury. J Cardiothorac Surg. 2023;18(1):71.

Q.22. A 70-year-old male presents with heaviness in his chest and nausea. He is a diabetic and hypertensive on regular medications. An ECG is done and is given below. The patient is hemodynamically stable. Which is the best line of management?

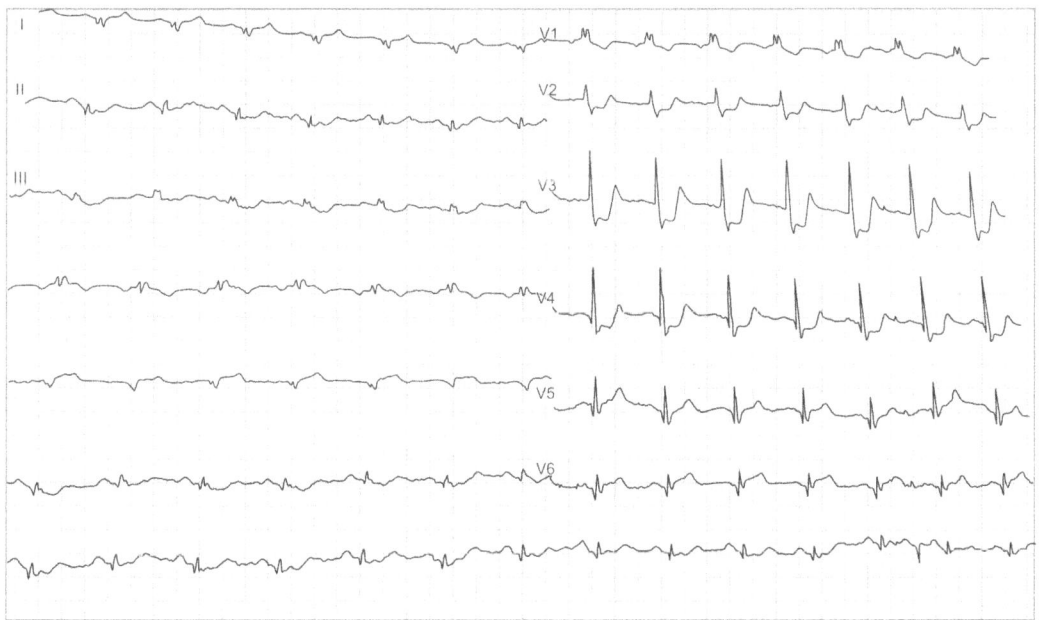

a. Patient has got RBBB, evaluate for myocardial ischemia
b. Patient has unstable angina, treat with nitrates, antiplatelets, and anticoagulation
c. Patient will benefit from a coronary angiogram
d. Patient will benefit from ICD

Ans. c

Explanation: This patient is suffering from posterior wall MI. He will benefit from an emergency coronary angiogram and stenting of the culprit vessel, usually left circumflex artery and in a few cases right coronary artery. When RBBB is associated with ST depression in V2–V4, 15 lead ECG will reveal ST elevation in V7, V8, and V9 which are more specific for posterior MI. ST-segment elevation in posterior leads of >0.5 mm is significant for diagnosing posterior wall MI. Brugada syndrome will be associated with coved ST elevation in V1–V3 and T wave inversion; these patients will have a high risk of VT and VF and will benefit from ICD.

Suggested Reading
1. Lizzo JM, Chowdhury YS. Posterior myocardial infarction. In: StatPearls [Internet]. Treasure Island (FL): StatPearls Publishing; 2023.
2. Ramjaun A, Garg A, Klaiman M, Sibbald M, Dong J. ECG changes in a case of posterior myocardial infarction in the presence of right bundle branch block. Cureus. 2021;13(2):e13281.

Q.23. Regarding HCM all are true except for which of the following?
a. One-third of patients have a nonobstructive form which predisposes to refractory heart failure
b. The common cause of sudden cardiac death in athletes
c. When patients present with acute decompensated heart failure (ADHF), diuretics, vasodilator, and rate control regime often reduces morbidity and mortality
d. LVOT gradient >50 mm Hg is an indication for septal myomectomy

Ans. c

Explanation: Hypertrophic cardiomyopathy has important features of LV outflow obstruction and concomitant MR. In critical care units, it forms a differential when patients present with systolic murmur and hypotension, syncope, and exercise-induced hypotension. Approximately one-third of patients with HCM have heart failure refractory to treatment. Ventricular tachyarrhythmias are common and a resting gradient >30 mm Hg predisposes patients for arrhythmias. It is a common cause of sudden death in athletes. During episodes of heart failure, optimizing LV volumes is the core principle in therapy, increasing preload and maintaining afterload and sinus rhythm rather than decreasing preload and afterload, which can precipitate LVOT obstruction. Drugs with negative inotropic effects such as β-blocker and verapamil have favorable hemodynamic outcomes. A LVOT gradient >50 mm Hg at rest or physiologic provocation is an indication of surgical myomectomy or septal alcohol ablation for relieving the symptoms of LVOT obstruction.

Suggested Reading
1. Basit H, Brito D, Sharma S. Hypertrophic cardiomyopathy. In: StatPearls [Internet]. Treasure Island (FL): StatPearls Publishing; 2023.

Q.24. A 50-year-old female presents to emergency room with shortness of breath since 2 hours, an ECG is obtained.

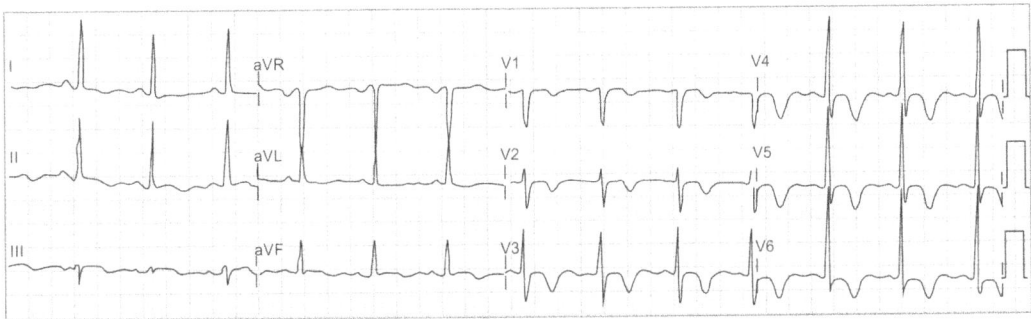

Which is the next best step in the management of this patient?
a. Repeat ECG in 30 minutes
b. Get an immediate ECHO cardiogram
c. Plan a stress ECHO
d. Get CT coronary angiogram

Ans. a

Explanation: This ECG is not diagnostic of STEMI but shows T-wave inversions that suggest myocardial ischemia and it is common for such patients to develop STEMI on subsequent ECGs. American Heart Association (AHA) recommends serial ECG monitoring if the initial ECG is not diagnostic.

Suggested Reading
1. Gulati M, Levy PD, Mukherjee D, Amsterdam E, Bhatt DL, Birtcher KK, et al. 2021 AHA/ACC/ASE/CHEST/SAEM/SCCT/SCMR Guideline for the Evaluation and Diagnosis of Chest Pain: A Report of the American College of Cardiology/American Heart Association Joint Committee on Clinical Practice Guidelines. Circulation. 2021;144(22):e368-454.

Q.25. A 30-year-old male presents to the emergency room with gradual worsening of shortness of breath for 1 week. He gives a history of flu-like symptoms 2 weeks prior to the onset of breathing difficulty. On evaluation, he is dyspneic at rest, Heart rate of 110 beats per min with a blood pressure of 100/60 mm Hg. He has pedal edema. An urgent echocardiogram is done, which revealed an LVEF of 20%. Regarding the management of this patient, which one of the following is best avoided?
a. Digoxin
b. Lisinopril
c. Furosemide
d. ICD

Ans. a

Explanation: This patient has features suggestive of viral myocarditis, as the history of viral illness is preceded by acute heart failure. Treatment of which is usually supportive. Diuretics for symptomatic relief, ACEI/ARBs in case of left ventricular failure. Digoxin and NSAIDs are best avoided. Digoxin is known to worsen myocardial injury by increasing the production of proinflammatory cytokines. Though NSAIDs are the drugs of choice for pericardial diseases in contrast, they increase inflammation and myocardial necrosis in myocarditis. As these patients are at high risk for developing arrhythmias, ICD implantation might be prudent. Patients with refractory heart failure may require LVAD or cardiac transplantation.

Suggested Reading
1. Kindermann I, Barth C, Mahfoud F, Ukena C, Lenski M, Yilmaz A, et al. Update on myocarditis. J Am Coll Cardiol. 2012;59(9):779-92.

Q.26. A 50-year-old male underwent percutaneous transluminal coronary angioplasty (PTCA) for AWMI and is in ICU for monitoring. The staff nurse transduces the radial sheath line, and the following waveform is noted. Which one of the following best describes the condition?

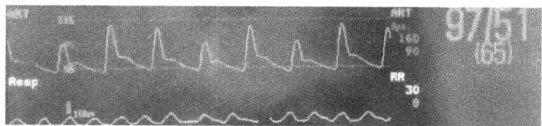

a. It is pulsus paradoxus and consistent with cardiac tamponade—the patient should undergo pericardiocentesis
b. It is pulsus alternans and consistent with pericardial effusion or poor LV function
c. It is consistent with sinus arrhythmia—just observe the patient
d. It is seen with hypovolemia following MI; the patient will benefit from volume expansion

Ans. b

Explanation: The pulse waveform suggests of pulsus alternans associated with low LV function of pericardial effusion. If the beat-to-beat variation is seen on ECG, it is referred to as electrical alternans. Pulsus paradoxus is an exaggerated fall in the BP during inspiration, >12 mm Hg or 10% of the baseline, it is 80% sensitive in cardiac tamponade. Sinus arrhythmia is usually seen in young adults due to respiratory variations in vagal nerve firing which result in irregular heart rate with R-R interval longer than 0.12 seconds but with a monomorphic P wave. In hypovolemia, pulse pressure variation (PPV) >13% suggests fluid responsiveness, and especially in this patient volume expansion should be done cautiously.

Suggested Reading
1. Henery D, Tummala R. Pulsus alternans. In: StatPearls [Internet]. Treasure Island (FL): StatPearls Publishing; 2023.

2. Yartsev A. (2021). Cardiac-tamponade. [online] Available from: https://derangedphysiology.com/main/required-reading/cardiac-arrest-and-resuscitation/Chapter%20221/cardiac-tamponade [Last accessed June, 2023].

Q.27. **A 40-year-old lady with severe acute respiratory distress syndrome (ARDS) is initiated on VV ECMO; on day 5, one of your juniors notices "CHATTER" of the circuit and you are called to assess the situation and troubleshoot. All are true except which one of the following statements?**
  a. This could indicate a problem with preload, increase the speed of the pump initially and transfuse blood if Hb <7 g/dL and crystalloids to increase the preload
  b. Look for a source of bleeding, especially the retroperitoneum
  c. Measure the intra-abdominal pressure (IAP) and take steps to reduce the IAP
  d. It could be an early sign of sepsis, reculture, and escalate the antibiotics

Ans. a

Explanation: Chattering is in patients on VV ECMO when there is an issue with the preload. The first step is to reduce the pump speed so that the blood flow is optimized. Transfusion of blood and blood products and crystalloids to restore preload. Bleeding is always a concern in patients on ECMO, you need to examine all the cannulation sites, rule out upper GI bleed, and especially look for retroperitoneal bleed. Pneumothorax and abdominal compartment syndrome can as well cause chattering due to a reduction in preload. Vasodilation and sepsis will cause chattering on ECMO and is an early sign of sepsis as fever may not be obvious as the temperature will be controlled by ECMO.

Suggested Reading
  1. Krishnamurthy V, Karanth S. Rational approach to chatter in venovenous extracorporeal membrane oxygenation to limit fluid administration: An algorithmic description. Indian J Crit Care Med. 2022;26(2):244-5.
  2. Zakhary B, Vercaemst L, Mason P, Lorusso R, Brodie D. How I manage drainage insufficiency on extracorporeal membrane oxygenation. Crit Care. 2020;24(1):151.

Q.28. **A 70-year-old male who is a diabetic, hypertensive, and diagnosed as ischemic heart disease. He develops sudden cardiac arrest and dies. Regarding out-of-hospital cardiac arrest (OHCA) which one is true?**
  a. He would have developed ventricular fibrillation
  b. He would have developed ventricular tachycardia
  c. He would have pulseless electrical activity
  d. He would have had atrial fibrillation

Ans. c

Explanation: About 30 years ago, in most sudden cardiac arrest (SCD) the initial cardiac rhythm was identified as VT/VF, and more recent data suggests that the initial rhythm is OHCA; in SCD the initial rhythm was found to be nonshockable rhythms, pulseless electrical activity (PEA), and asystole. The patient would unlikely have SCD due to AF.

Suggested Reading
1. Katritsis DG, Gersh BJ, Camm AJ. A clinical perspective on sudden cardiac death. Arrhythm Electrophysiol Rev. 2016;5(3):177-82.
2. Myerburg RJ, Halperin H, Egan DA, Boineau R, Chugh SS, Gillis AM, et al. Pulseless electric activity: definition, causes, mechanisms, management, and research priorities for the next decade: report from a National Heart, Lung, and Blood Institute workshop. Circulation. 2013;128(23):2532-41.

Q.29. A 70-year-old man, with a past medical history of congestive heart failure, atrial fibrillation, and hypertension presents with exertional dyspnea and lower limb swelling for the last 3 days. The patient's LVEF is 20%. On admission to the cardiac failure unit, he is started on dobutamine infusion with a blood pressure of 70/50 mm Hg. 4 hours later; you are called as the patient has developed atrial fibrillation with a fast ventricular response. Which of the following measures could have prevented the episode?
a. Metoprolol after dobutamine administration
b. Amiodarone at any time during the episode
c. Atropine along with dobutamine
d. Digoxin before dobutamine administration

Ans. d

Explanation: Dobutamine administration is useful for patients who present with systolic heart failure, infusion via large veins can be reasonably given during hospitalization. Dobutamine increases the risk of atrial fibrillation, especially in patients with preexisting AF. A regimen of digoxin given prior to reducing the risk of rapid ventricular rate in patients with preexisting AF. Beta-blockers cannot be administered along with dobutamine as it is sympathomimetic.

Suggested Reading
1. David S, Zaks JM. Arrhythmias associated with intermittent outpatient dobutamine infusion. Angiology. 1986;37(2):86-91.

Q.30. Regarding infective endocarditis (IE), all are true except which of the following?
a. Majority are caused by the staphylococcal group of organisms
b. As per Duke criteria, diagnosis is confirmed with positive blood culture of a typical IE organism, fever >38°C
c. Aortic lesions are more common
d. Risk of stroke is high when the vegetation is >10 mm

Ans. b

Explanation: Dukes criteria for diagnosis of IE is mentioned underneath.

Modified Duke criteria for the clinical diagnosis of infective endocarditis.*

- *Major clinical criteria*
  - *Positive blood culture:*
    - Typical microorganisms [*Staphylococcus aureus,* viridans streptococci, *Streptococcus gallolyticus, Haemophilus* species, *Aggregatibacter* (formerly *Actinobacillus*) species, *Cardiobacterium* species, *Eikenella corrodens,* and *Kingella* species (HACEK), and community-acquired enterococci in the absence of a primary focus] consistent with infective endocarditis from two separate blood cultures
    - Microorganisms consistent with infective endocarditis from persistently positive blood cultures, defined as ≥2 positive cultures from blood samples drawn >12 hours apart or all of three or a majority of ≥4 separate cultures of blood (with first and last sample drawn at least 1 hour apart)
    - Single positive blood culture for *Coxiella burnetii* or phase 1 immunoglobulin G (IgG) antibody titer >1:800
  - *Positive echocardiography:*
    - Vegetation (defined as an oscillating intracardiac mass on a valve or supporting structure), abscess, or new partial dehiscence of a prosthetic valve
    - New valvular regurgitation (an increase or change in preexisting murmur is not sufficient)
- *Minor clinical criteria:*
  - Presence of predisposing cardiac condition or intravenous drug use
  - Temperature ≥38.0°C (100.4°F)
  - Vascular phenomena such as systemic arterial emboli, septic pulmonary emboli, mycotic aneurysm, intracranial hemorrhage, conjunctival hemorrhages, or Janeway lesions
  - Immunologic phenomena such as glomerulonephritis. Osler nodes. Roth spots, or rheumatoid factor
  - Positive blood cultures that do not meet major criteria or serologic evidence of active infection with organism consistent with infective endocarditis

*The three main indications of surgery in patients with infective endocarditis are heart failure due to valvular dysfunction or perforation, uncontrolled endocardial infection and prevention of systemic embolization especially to the brain. In a recent RCT early surgery significantly reduced inhospital death and embolization at 6 weeks. Thus option B is correct answer as it is necessary for 2 positive cultues with microorganisms consistent with infective endocarditis.

Suggested Reading

1. Chambers HF, Bayer AS. Native-valve infective endocarditis. N Engl J Med. 2020;383(6):567-76.

CHAPTER 15

Renal/Fluids/Electrolyte

Saumitra Misra

Q.1. Which one of the following is *incorrect* regarding acid-base approaches?
a. Boston approach is the descriptive approach which is based on base excess.
b. Stewart approach is the quantitative approach which is based on strong ion difference.
c. Copenhagen's semiquantitative approach is based on buffer-base concept.
d. pH stat hypothesis deals with temperature-corrected blood gases

Ans. a

Explanation: The Boston Method of arterial blood gas (ABG) analysis is based on six bicarbonate-based bedside rules to assess compensation. The Copenhagen method is based on the use of Standard Base Excess for acid-base analysis.

Suggested Reading
1. Kishen R, Honoré PM, Jacobs R, Joannes-Boyau O, De Waele E, De Regt J, et al. Facing acid-base disorders in the third millennium—the Stewart approach revisited. Int J Nephrol Renovasc Dis. 2014;7:209-17.

Q.2. Regarding fluid therapy on the intensive care unit (ICU) which of the following is *correct*?
a. Human albumin solution is the preferred resuscitation fluid in traumatic brain injury.
b. The use of hydroxyethyl starch has been shown to increase mortality in critically ill patients.
c. The Saline versus Albumin Fluid Evaluation (SAFE) study suggests that the use of albumin as a primary resuscitation fluid is generally associated with worse outcomes in critically ill patients.
d. The Fluid Expansion As Supportive Therapy (FEAST) trial supports the use of a 20 mL/kg initial crystalloid bolus strategy in acutely ill children.

Ans. b

Explanation: In critically ill patients requiring acute volume resuscitation, use of hydroxyethyl starch compared with other resuscitation solutions was associated with an increase in mortality and acute kidney injury (AKI). Resuscitation with albumin was associated with increased intracranial pressure (ICP) and mortality in traumatic brain injury (TBI) patients. SAFE trial showed that use of 4% albumin or 0.9% sodium chloride for fluid resuscitation had similar outcomes at 28 days. FEAST trial showed that children with severe febrile illnesses and impaired perfusion, who were treated with fluid boluses, had a significantly increased mortality compared with controls in resource-limited settings in Africa.

Suggested Reading
1. Cooper DJ, Myburgh J, Heritier S, Finfer S, Bellomo R, Billot L, et al. Albumin resuscitation for traumatic brain injury: is intracranial hypertension the cause of increased mortality? J Neurotrauma. 2013;30(7):512-8.
2. Finfer S, Bellomo R, Boyce N, French J, Myburgh J, Norton R, et al. A comparison of albumin and saline for fluid resuscitation in the intensive care unit. N Engl J Med. 2004;350(22):2247-56.
3. Hartog CS, Natanson C, Sun J, Klein HG, Reinhart K. Concerns over use of hydroxyethyl starch solutions. BMJ. 2014;349:g5981.
4. Maitland K, Kiguli S, Opoka RO, Engoru C, Olupot-Olupot P, Akech SO, et al. Mortality after fluid bolus in African children with severe infection. N Engl J Med. 2011;364(26):2483-95.

Q.3. An 89-year-old man is found on the floor of his house. He is confused and complaining of lethargy and tingling of his hands and feet. While being transferred to hospital he suffers a brief and self-terminating seizure. On arrival, examination shows muscle weakness with positive Chvostek's and Trousseau's signs. ECG a QTc of 500 ms. Which primary electrolyte disturbance best explains all these findings?
   a. Hypokalemia.
   b. Hypocalcemia.
   c. Hyponatremia.
   d. Hypercalcemia

Ans. b

Explanation: Hypocalcemia usually presents as an asymptomatic laboratory finding but sometimes as a severe, life-threatening condition. Distinguishing acute from chronic hypocalcemia and asymptomatic from severely symptomatic hypocalcemia is critical for determining appropriate therapy. In the setting of acute hypocalcemia, rapid treatment may be necessary.

Suggested Reading
1. Steele T, Kolamunnage-Dona R, Downey C, Toh CH, Welters I. Assessment and clinical course of hypocalcemia in critical illness. Crit Care. 2013;17:R106.

Q.4. In which of the following, Cairo–Bishop classification is used?
   a. Rhabdomyolysis
   b. Tumor lysis syndrome (TLS)
   c. Abdominal compartment syndrome
   d. Hepatorenal syndrome

Ans. b

Explanation: Tumor lysis syndrome is described as the metabolic derangements that occur with tumor breakdown after the initiation of chemotherapy. TLS results from the rapid destruction of malignant cells and causing the release of intracellular ions, nucleic acids, proteins, and their metabolites. These metabolites can overwhelm the body's normal homeostatic mechanisms and cause hyperuricemia, hyperkalemia, hyperphosphatemia, hypocalcemia, and uremia. TLS can lead to acute kidney and can be life-threatening. Early recognition of patients at risk and initiation of therapy for TLS is essential.

Suggested Reading
1. Cairo MS, Bishop M. Tumour lysis syndrome: new therapeutic strategies and classification. Br J Haematol. 2004;127(1):3-11.

Q.5. A patient with intra-abdominal sepsis develops progressive uremia and oliguria after 5 days on the ICU. He requires renal replacement therapy (RRT), and continuous venovenous hemodiafiltration is instituted. The following are appropriate initial settings *except*:
   a. Blood flow rate of 25 mL/min
   b. A bicarbonate-buffered replacement fluid
   c. Ultrafiltration rate of 35 mL/kg/hour
   d. Replacement solution added to blood before passage through the filter

Ans. c

Explanation: Continuous renal replacement therapy (CRRT) dose is essentially quantified by the effluent flow rate and there is no survival benefit at a dose >20–25 mL/kg/hour. The target blood flow rate in a stepwise manner starting at 25 mL/min and increasing slowly (over 10–15 min) to 100–150 mL/min. Net ultrafiltration rates are usually <2 mL/kg/hour. Bicarbonate-buffered solutions are preferred over lactate-buffered solutions to prevent iatrogenic hyperlactatemia. The replacement fluid is delivered prefilter to ensure the prescribed dose.

Suggested Reading
1. See EJ, Bellomo R. How I prescribe continuous renal replacement therapy. Crit Care. 2021;25(1):1.

Q.6. A 55-year-old long-stay patient develops hypophosphatemia, hypomagnesemia, and hypokalemia following the introduction of enteral nutrition. What is the most appropriate next management step?
   a. Electrolyte replacement and continue enteral feeding
   b. Electrolyte replacement and stop enteral feeding
   c. Electrolyte replacement and reduce enteral feeding
   d. Electrolyte replacement and convert enteral feed to parenteral nutrition

Ans. c

Explanation: Refeeding syndrome is defined as the potentially fatal shifts in fluids and electrolytes that may occur in malnourished patients receiving artificial refeeding (whether enterally or parenterally). The hallmark biochemical feature of refeeding syndrome is hypophosphatemia. However, the syndrome is complex and may also feature abnormal sodium and fluid balance; changes in glucose, protein, and fat metabolism; thiamine deficiency; hypokalemia; and hypomagnesemia. If the syndrome is detected, the rate of feeding should be slowed down and essential electrolytes should be replenished.

Suggested Reading
1. Mehanna HM, Moledina J, Travis J. Refeeding syndrome: what it is, and how to prevent and treat it. BMJ. 2008;336(7659):1495-8.

Q.7. Which of the following is not *true* about Warburg effect?
a. It causes type B lactic acidosis (LA)
b. It is observed in patients with malignancy with a high tumor burden
c. It does not have a good prognosis
d. It causes type A LA

Ans. d

Explanation: Lactic acidosis is classified on the basis of presence or absence of tissue hypoxia. In type A LA, there is impaired tissue oxygenation. In type B LA, there is no evidence of tissue hypoxia. Warburg effect is a type B LA that could be suspected in patients with malignancy having a significant tumor burden. It occurs when malignant cells take up glucose and convert it to lactate despite the presence of sufficient oxygen. There is no well-defined treatment for patients with malignancy presenting with Warburg effect and type B LA. Thiamine supplementation is suggested to improve the mitochondrial function, since it acts as cofactor for many enzymes in Krebs cycle.

Suggested Reading
1. Liberti MV, Locasale JW. The Warburg Effect: How Does it Benefit Cancer Cells? Trends Biochem Sci. 2016;41(3):211-8.

Q.8. Which of the following is not *true* about syndrome of inappropriate antidiuretic hormone (SIADH)?
a. It is a type of euvolemic hypotonic hyponatremia
b. Urine osmolality >100 mOsm/kg
c. Urine sodium <20 mEq/L in untreated SIADH
d. Urine sodium >40 mEq/L in untreated SIADH

Ans. c

Explanation: Hyponatremia is the most frequent electrolyte disorder and the SIADH accounts for approximately one-third of all cases. In the diagnosis of SIADH it is important to ascertain the euvolemic state of extracellular fluid volume, both clinically and by laboratory measurements.

Suggested Reading
1. Ellison DH, Berl T. Clinical practice. The syndrome of inappropriate antidiuresis. N Engl J Med. 2007;356(20):2064-72.

Q.9. Which of the following condition is usually not associated with hypophosphatemia?
a. Tumor production of fibroblast growth factor 23 (FGF23)
b. Secondary hyperparathyroidism

c. Vitamin D deficiency
d. Respiratory alkalosis

Ans. b

Explanation: Acute hypophosphatemia is common in critically ill patients. It should be promptly evaluated and the underlying causes evaluated. It is associated with significant morbidity and mortality. Secondary hyperparathyroidism causes hyperphosphatemia.

Suggested Reading
1. Felsenfeld AJ, Levine BS. Approach to treatment of hypophosphatemia. Am J Kidney Dis. 2012;60(4):655-61.

Q.10. Prerenal AKI and renal AKI can be differentiated on the basis of:
a. Creatinine clearance
b. Plasma bicarbonate
c. Urine output
d. Fractional excretion of sodium (FENa)

Ans. d

Explanation: The FENa measures the percent of filtered sodium that is excreted in the urine. This calculation is widely used to differentiate prerenal disease (decreased kidney perfusion) from acute tubular necrosis (ATN) as the cause of AKI.

Suggested Reading
1. Lima C, Macedo E. Urinary Biochemistry in the Diagnosis of Acute Kidney Injury. Dis Markers. 2018;2018:4907024.

Q.11. Which of the following is not a buffer in commercially available commonly used balanced crystalloids?
a. Succinate
b. Malate
c. Acetate
d. Gluconate

Ans. a

Explanation:

Fluid	Osmolality (mOsm/L)	Na	K	Ca	Mg	Cl	Lactate	Malate	Gluconate	Acetate
RL	273	131	4.5	2.7	-	109	28	-	-	-
Plasmalyte A	294	140	5	-	3.0	98	-	-	23	27
Sterofundin ISO	309	145	4	2.5	1.0	127	-	5	-	24

All values in mEq/L except osmolality.

Suggested Reading
1. Semler MW, Kellum JA. Balanced Crystalloid Solutions. Am J Respir Crit Care Med. 2019;199(8):952-60.

Q.12. In which of the following cardiorenal syndrome (CRS) subtype, the acute worsening of renal function causes cardiac dysfunction?
  a. CRS type 1
  b. CRS type 2
  c. CRS type 3
  d. CRS type 4

Ans. c

Explanation:

Type 1 (acute cardiorenal)	Acute worsening of heart function leading to acute kidney injury and/or dysfunction	Cardiogenic shock and AKI, acute decompensated heart failure (ADHF) resulting in AKI
Type 2 (chronic cardiorenal)	Chronic abnormalities in heart function leading to cardiorenal) progressive kidney injury and/or dysfunction	Chronic heart failure with left ventricular remodeling and dysfunction leading to chronic kidney disease (CKD)
Type 3 (acute renocardiac)	Acute worsening of kidney function leading to acute heart injury and/or dysfunction	Heart failure in the setting of AKI from volume overload, inflammatory surge (e.g., pericarditis), and accompanying metabolic disturbances
Type 4 (chronic renocardiac)	Chronic kidney disease leading to heart injury, disease, and/or dysfunction	Myocardial remodeling and heart failure from CKD-associated cardiomyopathy
Type 5 (secondary cardiorenal)	Systemic conditions leading to simultaneous injury and/or dysfunction of heart and kidney	Diabetes, amyloidosis, sepsis, cirrhosis, and vasculitis

Suggested Reading
1. Prastaro M, Nardi E, Paolillo S, Santoro C, Parlati ALM, Gargiulo P, et al. Cardiorenal syndrome: Pathophysiology as a key to the therapeutic approach in an under-diagnosed disease. J Clin Ultrasound. 2022;50(8):1110-24.

Q.13. Which of the following statement is not *true* about AKI biomarkers?
  a. A combination of stress, damage, and functional biomarkers, along with clinical information, are being researched to identify high-risk patient groups and improve the diagnostic accuracy of AKI.
  b. None of the biomarkers currently being investigated/researched, can identify the severity of AKI
  c. These biomarkers are being identified/researched in urine and plasma.
  d. Acute kidney disease (AKD) is described as acute or subacute damage and/or loss of kidney function for a duration as long as 90 days.

Ans. b

Explanation: Acute kidney injury is common in ICU patients and causes significant morbidity as well as mortality. Currently two functional biomarkers, (1) serum creatinine (sCr) and (2) urine output, are used to define AKI, but these markers are limited by delayed changes following kidney injury and have low sensitivity and specificity. Several novel biomarkers have been shown to detect AKI earlier and are more sensitive than sCr. For any prevention strategies to be effective, patients with high risk need to be identified before kidney insults result in kidney damage, and AKI needs to be diagnosed as early as possible.

Suggested Reading
1. Ostermann M, Zarbock A, Goldstein S, Kashani K, Macedo E, Murugan R, et al. Recommendations on Acute Kidney Injury Biomarkers From the Acute Disease Quality Initiative Consensus Conference: A Consensus Statement. JAMA Netw Open. 2020;3(10):e2019209.

Q.14. Magnesium (Mg^{2+}) binds to which channels/receptors present in distal convoluted tubule (DCT) to prevent Potassium (K^+) secretion?
a. NKCC
b. Na-K-ATPase
c. BK
d. ROMK

Ans. d

Explanation: K^+ is the most abundant intracellular cation, creating a large chemical gradient that favors the outward flow of K^+ through ROMK. Normally, Mg^{2+} binds to a cytosol exposed site in ROMK to limit this outward flow. During hypomagnesemia, fewer Mg^{2+} ions can bind to this site, and K^+ is secreted more freely. Thus, Mg^{2+} deficiency causes K^+ wasting. This likely explains why magnesium repletion is required to efficiently restore potassium concentrations to normal during concomitant hypomagnesemia and hypokalemia.

Suggested Reading
1. Subramanya AR, Ellison DH. Distal convoluted tubule. Clin J Am Soc Nephrol. 2014;9(12):2147-63.

Q.15. Which of the following drugs is not commonly associated with high anion gap metabolic acidosis (HAGMA)?
a. Tenofovir
b. Isoniazid
c. Aspirin
d. Ethylene glycol

Ans. a

Explanation: Drugs causing HAGMA: GOLD MARK (Mnemonic)
- Glycols (propylene glycol and ethylene glycol)
- Oxoproline—5-oxoproline (or pyroglutamic acid) is associated with chronic acetaminophen use, often by malnourished women.
- L-lactate
- D-lactate—D-lactic acid can occur in some patients with short bowel syndromes
- Methanol
- Aspirin
- Renal failure (versus uremia)
- Ketoacidosis

Drugs causing Normal Anion Gap Metabolic acidosis (NAGMA): USED PART (Mnemonic)
- *U:* Ureteroenterostomy
- *S:* Small bowel fistula

- *E:* Extra chloride
- *D:* Diarrhea
- *P:* Pancreatic fistula
- *A:* Addison's disease, Acetazolamide
- *R:* RTA
- *T:* Tenofovir and Topiramate

Suggested Reading

1. Pham AQ, Xu LH, Moe OW. Drug-Induced Metabolic Acidosis. 2015;4:F1000 Faculty Rev-1460.

Q.16. A 47-year-old male, known case of (k/c/o) chronic liver disease secondary to alcohol, presented to the emergency department because of a 1-week history of progressively severe ascites. He has not had any fevers, chills, or abdominal pain. He has noted a mild decrease in his urine output. At his outpatient department (OPD) visit last week, his sCr was 1.2 mg/dL. On examination, his pulse is 90 bpm and his blood pressure (BP) is 98/54 mm Hg. He has jaundice and a nontender, distended abdomen with tense ascites. On presentation, his hemoglobin—9.5 g/dL, total leukocyte count—5.6×10^3 cells/mm^3, creatinine is 3.2 mg/dL, and he has no proteinuria or hematuria. Which of the following is not *correct* as part of his management?

a. 20% albumin infusion started at a dose of 1 g/kg/day
b. Diuretics may be withdrawn initially
c. Octreotide/terlipressin started
d. Hemodialysis will have a good long-term prognosis.

Ans. d

Explanation: The occurrence of AKI in patients with end-stage liver disease constitutes one of the most challenging clinical scenarios in critical care medicine. Prerenal azotemia, ATN, and hepatorenal syndrome type 1 (HRS-1) could be responsible for sudden worsening in renal function. HRS-1 which is a specific type of AKI that occurs in the context of advanced cirrhosis and portal hypertension, is associated with particularly high mortality.

Suggested Reading

1. Velez JCQ, Therapondos G, Juncos LA. Reappraising the spectrum of AKI and hepatorenal syndrome in patients with cirrhosis. Nat Rev Nephrol. 2020;16(3):137-55.

Q.17. A 20-year-old boy presented in the emergency with status epilepticus. His BP readings were in the range from 180–200/110–120 mm Hg. His seizures were controlled with IV midazolam. He was transferred to the ICU where his BP still remain high. His investigations show microscopic hematuria, proteinuria, and a sCr of 2.8 mg/dL. Which of the following would be the antihypertensive of choice in this scenario?

a. IV nitroglycerin
b. IV furosemide
c. IV nicardipine
d. IV sodium nitroprusside

Ans. c

Explanation: Hypertensive emergency has to be treated promptly. IV nitroglycerin may not be a good choice to control BP because of risk of raised intracranial pressure (ICP). IV sodium nitroprusside should be avoided because of deranged renal function. IV furosemide may be tried later to correct volume overload. IV nicardipine has good efficacy to control the BP.

Suggested Reading
1. Peacock WF, Varon J, Baumann BM, Borczuk P, Cannon CM, Chandra A, et al. CLUE: a randomized comparative effectiveness trial of IV nicardipine versus labetalol use in the emergency department. Crit Care. 2011;15:R157.

Q.18. A 70-year-old man k/c/o chronic kidney disease (CKD) [glomerular filtration rate (GFR)—45 mL/min/1.73 m^2] on routine follow-up has an Hb—8.0 g/dL. What type of anemia would most likely be found on evaluation?
  a. Microcytic hypochromic
  b. Normocytic normochromic
  c. Macrocytic hyperchromic
  d. Pancytopenia

Ans. b

Explanation: The anemia of CKD is hypoproliferative, usually normochromic and normocytic. In this regard, it is morphologically indistinguishable from the anemia of chronic disease. Folate or vitamin B$_{12}$ deficiencies may lead to macrocytosis, whereas iron deficiency or inherited disorders of Hb formation (e.g., α- or β-thalassemia) may produce microcytosis. Iron deficiency, especially if long-standing, is associated with hypochromia.

Suggested Reading
1. KDIGO Clinical Practice Guideline for Anemia in Chronic Kidney Disease. Kidney Int Suppl. 2012;2(4):288-335.

Q.19. Which of the following is a nonthrombotic microangiopathy (non-TMA) cause of obstetric emergency?
  a. HELLP syndrome
  b. Atypical hemolytic uremic syndrome (aHUS)
  c. Thrombotic thrombocytopenic purpura (TTP)
  d. Acute fatty liver of pregnancy (AFLP)

Ans. d

Explanation: HELLP syndrome is an extreme presentation of gestational hypertension in which a peripartum patient presents with thrombocytopenia and microangiopathic hemolytic anemia (MAHA) with end-organ injury. Other less common TMA disorders in pregnancy that present with thrombocytopenia, MAHA, and end-organ damage include aHUS and TTP. AFLP is a rare non-TMA obstetric emergency that can present with acute liver failure and is very challenging to manage in the critically ill obstetric patient.

Suggested Reading
1. Szczepanski J, Griffin A, Novotny S, Wallace K. Acute Kidney Injury in Pregnancies Complicated With Preeclampsia or HELLP Syndrome. Front Med (Lausanne). 2020;7:22.

Q.20. A 35-year-old man presented to the emergency with progressive worsening dyspnea and productive cough. He has had recurrent sinusitis in the past 1 year. On physical examination, mild tenderness over the bilateral frontal region and pedal edema are noted. Laboratory studies show sCr level of 3.5 mg/dL and blood urea nitrogen (BUN) of 56 mg/dL. Result of antiglomerular basement membrane antibody test is negative and result of antineutrophil cytoplasmic antibody test is positive. Urine microscopy shows 2+ protein and 2+ blood. Red blood cells are visible in the urine sediment. Chest X-ray (CXR)—bilateral pleural effusion. Which of the following is the most likely diagnosis?
  a. Allergic interstitial nephritis
  b. Goodpasture syndrome
  c. Immunoglobulin A (IgA) nephropathy
  d. Wegener granulomatosis

Ans. d

Explanation: The patient has sinusitis, hematuria with deranged renal function, pleural effusions, and positive result of antineutrophil cytoplasmic antibody test, all of which are seen in Wegener granulomatosis. In allergic interstitial nephritis, eosinophils are noted on urinalysis and there is no history of recent drug therapy that could have precipitated allergic interstitial nephritis. In Goodpasture syndrome, antiglomerular basement membrane antibody is present. IgA nephropathy is not associated with a positive result of antineutrophil cytoplasmic antibody test.

Suggested Reading
  1. Semple D, Keogh J, Forni L, Venn R. Clinical review: Vasculitis on the intensive care unit—part 1: diagnosis. Crit Care. 2005;9(1):92-7.
  2. Semple D, Keogh J, Forni L, Venn R. Clinical review: Vasculitis on the intensive care unit—part 2: treatment and prognosis. Crit Care. 2005;9(2):193-7.

Q.21. A 60-year-old woman (postrenal transplant 5 years back) was admitted to the ICU for severe hypoxemic respiratory failure. She had a 6-month history of fatigue and dyspnea without fever. High-resolution computed tomography (HRCT) chest scan shows bilateral asymmetrical consolidations, ground-glass opacities, and bilateral pleural effusion. Microbiological evaluation of bronchoalveolar lavage (BAL) fluid was negative. Analysis of BAL cells showed intrapulmonary hemorrhage. Which of the following statement is not *correct*?
  a. Sirolimus-associated pneumonitis could present with above clinical features and findings.
  b. Sirolimus should be discontinued and high-dose corticosteroids started.
  c. Invasive mechanical ventilation must be avoided at all costs.
  d. Sirolimus trough concentrations may be checked.

Ans. c

Explanation: Sirolimus-associated pneumonitis has been observed after solid organ transplants. Diagnosis is made after exclusion of infective and other toxic causes of lung injury. The pneumonitis responds to drug withdrawal, however, regression of pneumonitis has also been described after dose reduction of sirolimus. Factors that may be related to the risk for sirolimus-related pneumonitis may include late switch to sirolimus, age, underlying disease, concomitant immunosuppressive treatment, and serum levels of sirolimus. A patient of sirolimus-induced pulmonary toxicity should be managed as any other patient of hypoxemic respiratory failure. Indications of invasive mechanical ventilation remain the same and it should not be delayed, if the clinical condition so demands.

Suggested Reading
1. Weiner SM, Sellin L, Vonend O, Schenker P, Buchner NJ, Flecken M, et al. Pneumonitis associated with sirolimus: clinical characteristics, risk factors and outcome—a single-centre experience and review of the literature. Nephrol Dial Transplant. 2007;22(12):3631-7.

Q.22. Which of the following is not *true* about denosumab?
a. It is indicated for treatment of hypercalcemia of malignancy refractory to denosumab
b. It is a monoclonal antibody to the receptor activator of nuclear factor-kappa B ligand (RANKL)
c. It may be used in postmenopausal women with osteoporosis at high risk of fracture.
d. It does not cause symptomatic hypocalcemia.

Ans. d

Explanation: Hypercalcemia of malignancy is an oncological emergency. It should be promptly identified and treated (hydration, bisphosphonate, and calcitonin). Treatment of the underlying cancer gets delayed in patients having recurrent or refractory hypercalcemia because of the avoidance of chemotherapeutic agents during hypercalcemia. Denosumab, a fully human monoclonal antibody against RANKL, inhibits the maturation, function, and survival of osteoclasts. Denosumab has been recently approved as a treatment option of hypercalcemia of malignancy. It can cause symptomatic hypocalcemia especially in patients with renal insufficiency.

Suggested Reading
1. Thosani S, Hu MI. Denosumab: a new agent in the management of hypercalcemia of malignancy. Future Oncol. 2015;11(21):2865-71.

Q.23. A 55-year-old woman with a history of hypertension and type 2 diabetes mellitus (DM) presents to the emergency department with high-grade fever, recurrent vomiting, and altered sensorium. On admission, she is febrile (temperature of 39.4°C), has tachycardia [heart rate (HR)—120 bpm] and BP 120/62 mm Hg. She has right-sided costovertebral angle tenderness. She is transferred to the ICU. Her investigations show TLC 22,000 cells/mm^3, sCr 2.5 mg/dL (baseline 0.8 mg/dL), and >50 pus cells/hpf on urine microscopy. Noncontrast computed tomography (NCCT) of the abdomen and pelvis shows right perinephric stranding but no calculi or hydronephrosis bilaterally. Blood and urine cultures are awaited. Which of the following statements about this patient's management is not *correct*?
a. She should receive pre-emptive RRT in view of her AKI-III
b. Appropriate antimicrobial therapy should be immediately started.

c. The patient's AKI puts her at increased risk for secondary infections during her hospitalization.
d. Acute pyelonephritis (APN) could be a likely cause of her condition.

Ans. a

Explanation: Acute pyelonephritis is characterized by dysuria, flank pain with costovertebral tenderness and high-grade fever (≥38.5°C) with chills. Routine urine examination in APN shows pus cells (WBC ≥ 5/hpf) or positive nitrite test or presence of bacteria on microscopy. Urine culture is positive (≥100,000 CFU/mL) which usually confirms the diagnosis in patients having typical clinical presentation. Abdominal imaging—ultrasonography/computed tomography (CT) is helpful to look for obstructive features in kidney. Complicated APN is defined when the patient has the presence of at least one risk factor such as pregnancy, DM, an immunocompromised state, urologic anatomical abnormalities, and urinary calculi. AKI associated with APN has been reported. Furthermore, increasing data suggest that AKI is a risk factor for subsequent sepsis or secondary infections. There is no role of pre-emptive RRT

Suggested Reading
1. Griffin BR, Liu KD, Teixeira JP. Critical Care Nephrology: Core Curriculum 2020. Am J Kidney Dis. 2020;75(3):435-52.
2. Jeon DH, Jang HN, Cho HS, Lee TW, Bae E, Chang SH, et al. Incidence, risk factors, and clinical outcomes of acute kidney injury associated with acute pyelonephritis in patients attending a tertiary care referral center. Ren Fail. 2019;41(1):204-10.

Q.24. A 64-year-old man is brought to emergency department with history of productive cough, fever, and worsening dyspnea on exertion since 7 days. He is tachypneic [respiratory rate (RR)—30/min] with use of accessory muscles of respiration. He has hypoxemic respiratory failure on admission. His respiratory distress worsens and invasive mechanical ventilation is instituted. Chest X-ray shows diffuse bilateral pulmonary opacities. Blood gas reveals a PaO_2 of 130 mm Hg on 100% FiO_2. Bedside echocardiography shows normal left ventricular (LV) systolic function. A nasopharyngeal swab comes back positive for coronavirus disease 2019 (COVID-19). He has deranged renal function (BUN—60 mg/dL and sCr—2.0 mg/dL). Which of the following statements is not *correct* about management of this patient's fluid balance?
   a. Fluid overload has consistently been shown to be associated with adverse outcomes in the critically ill.
   b. The combination of AKI and acute respiratory distress syndrome (ARDS) portends worse outcomes including higher mortality and increased hospital length of stay.
   c. Conservative fluid management in patients with ARDS is associated with increased risk of dialysis requiring AKI.
   d. Maintain euvolemia in patients with ARDS with AKI results in more ventilator and ICU-free days.

Ans. c

Explanation: Acute kidney injury is a common complication in critically ill patients, and is particularly problematic when coexisting with ARDS. Several studies have highlighted that AKI is an independent predictor for death in patients who are critically ill with acute lung injury. Clinical and experimental data indicate that there is significant crosstalk between injured kidneys and the lung. AKI exerts a multitude of deleterious effects on the lung via fluid overload leading to cardiogenic pulmonary edema as well as cytokine excess leading to noncardiogenic pulmonary edema.

Suggested Reading
1. Park BD, Faubel S. Acute Kidney Injury and Acute Respiratory Distress Syndrome. Crit Care Clin. 2021;37(4):835-49.

Q.25. Which of the following is not *correct* about rhabdomyolysis?
a. McMahon score is used to predict the risk of progression to AKI.
b. Hypocalcemia should be aggressively corrected in asymptomatic patient.
c. Creatine kinase (CK) is the standard biomarker of rhabdomyolysis.
d. Aspartate aminotransferase (AST) may be elevated.

Ans. b

Explanation: Rhabdomyolysis ranges in severity from asymptomatic elevations in CK levels to a life-threatening disorder characterized by severe AKI requiring RRT. McMahon score is a prognostic score generated from epidemiological data and laboratories available on admission. A score of six or greater indicates risk of AKI and need of dialysis. There is no consensus on the value of CK.

Suggested Reading
1. McMahon GM, Zeng X, Waikar SS. A risk prediction score for kidney failure or mortality in rhabdomyolysis. JAMA Intern Med. 2013;173(19):1821-8.

Q.26. Which of the following IV fluids has the least osmolality?
a. 0.9% NS
b. 0.45% NS
c. 5% D
d. RL

Ans. b

Explanation:

IV fluids	Osmolality (mOsm/L)
0.9% NS	308
0.45% NS	154
5% D	253
RL	273

Suggested Reading
1. Hoorn EJ. Intravenous fluids: balancing solutions. J Nephrol. 2017;30(4):485-92.

Q.27. Filtration fraction (FF) should not exceed ____ to avoid degradation of filter performance?
a. 5–10%
b. 20–25%
c. 45–50%
d. 60–65%

Ans. b

Explanation: The FF is defined as the ratio between the ultrafiltration flow rate (QUF) and the plasma flow rate (QP).

$$FF = QUF/QP.$$

Clinically, the FF should be kept ideally below 30%.

Suggested Reading
1. Karkar A, Ronco C. Prescription of CRRT: a pathway to optimize therapy. Ann Intensive Care. 2020;10(1):32.

Q.28. Which of the following electrolyte and acid-base disorders are not commonly seen as a complication with regional citrate anticoagulation (RCA)?
 a. Hypocalcemia
 b. High anion gap metabolic acidosis
 c. Metabolic alkalosis
 d. Hyponatremia

Ans. d

Explanation: Regional citrate anticoagulation (RCA) when incorporated with CRRT has to be monitored very carefully because it can significantly alter the metabolic milieu. It can cause metabolic alkalosis due to high citrate load getting converted to bicarbonate. It may cause metabolic acidosis if there is liver dysfunction (accumulation of citrate). RCA requires strict monitoring of calcium because it can lead to either hypocalcemia (inadequate replacement of calcium) or hypercalcemia (excess infusion of calcium). RCA may cause hypernatremia (if hypertonic trisodium citrate is used) and usually does not cause hyponatremia. The KDIGO guidelines suggest RCA rather than heparin in patients without any contraindication for citrate.

Suggested Reading
1. Karkar A, Ronco C. Prescription of CRRT: a pathway to optimize therapy. Ann Intensive Care. 2020;10(1):32.

Q.29. Which of the following is *incorrect* about diabetes insipidus (DI)?
 a. Recognizing diabetes insipidus is not easy in the critically ill.
 b. Diagnostic test of water deprivation is not feasible in the ICU settings.
 c. Polyuria, hypotonic urine, hypernatremia, and plasma hyperosmolality are seen.
 d. Serum arginine-vasopressin (AVP) measurements can be easily done for diagnosis because of its large half-life.

Ans. d

Explanation: The diagnosis of DI is not easy in the ICU because polyuria and hypernatremia may be seen during the course of stay of a critically patient. Central DI in a critically ill patient, with a background of an acute cerebral insult, should be suspected when there is polyuria and hypernatremia beyond the expected range.

The clues for diagnosis of DI in patients in the ICU:
- *Polyuria:* A critically ill adult patient having urine output of >300 mL/hour for at least 2 hours. An intensivist should be careful whenever urine output of the patient is >3 mL/kg/hour is observed. In neurocritical units, urine output ranging from 2 to 5 mL/kg/hour has also been observed in DI patients.

- *Hypotonic urine:* A critically ill patient with a background of acute cerebral injury and now having polyuria with a urine osmolality of <300 mOsm/kg. Urine osmolality helps to differentiate DI from polyuria due to a solute (osmotic) diuresis (urine osmolality >300 mOsm/kg).
- *Plasma hyperosmolality:* A serum sodium concentration of >145 mmol/L and a serum osmolality of >300 mOsm/kg may be used in the diagnosis of DI. However, an increase in serum sodium, rather than the absolute level, might be more relevant in patients in the ICU.

The measurement of serum AVP levels has been proposed to aid in the diagnosis of DI. However, due to the short half-life of the molecule, it remains very challenging. Copeptin, a prohormone of AVP, can be used as a substitute for AVP and has shown good results.

Suggested Reading
1. Harrois A, Anstey JR. Diabetes Insipidus and Syndrome of Inappropriate Antidiuretic Hormone in Critically Ill Patients. Crit Care Clin. 2019;35(2):187-200.

Q.30. Hyperkalemia is seen in which RTA?
a. Type I RTA
b. Type II RTA
c. Type III RTA
d. Type IV RTA

Ans. d

Explanation:

Type	Site	Urinary pH	Cause	Presentation	Potassium level
RTA type I	Distal tubular	>5.5	Failure of H^+ secretion	• Osteomalacia • Renal calculi	Hypokalemia
RTA type II	Proximal tubular	<5.5	Bicarbonate wasting	Muscle weakness	Hypokalemia
RTA Type IV	Distal tubular	<5.5	Hypoaldosteronism	Reduced aldosterone production or aldosterone resistance	Hyperkalemia

Suggested Reading
1. Brunner R, Drolz A, Scherzer TM, Staufer K, Fuhrmann V, Zauner C, et al. Renal tubular acidosis is highly prevalent in critically ill patients. Crit Care. 2015;19(1):148.

CHAPTER 16

Toxicology

Deven Juneja, Prashant Nasa

Q.1. A 24-year-old female presented to emergency room with an alleged history of consumption of multiple unknown tablets from her grandmother's medicine cabinet. She developed nausea, vomiting, abdominal pain, yellowish vision, and scotomas. She was brought to the hospital by her parents after 3–4 hours of ingestion. On examination, she was dull and confused. Heart rate was 98/min, respiratory rate 22/min, and blood pressure of 80/44 mm Hg. Electrocardiograph was suggestive of accelerated junctional rhythm. Arterial blood gases (ABGs) showed pH—7.28, pCO_2—35.6 mm Hg, pO_2—72 mm Hg, HCO_3—20.2 mEq/L, Na—138 mEq/L, K^+—5.6 mEq/L. What is the most likely drug consumed?
a. Amitriptyline
b. Beta-blockers
c. Calcium channel blockers
d. Digoxin

Ans. d

Explanation: Gastrointestinal (GI) symptoms are common and may be present in up to 70% of patients. Commonly reported symptoms include anorexia, abdominal pain, and nausea, but vomiting is uncommon. Digoxin toxicity has been reported to cause blurred or hazy vision but rarely patients may report seeing halos, flashing lights, or even color disturbances with yellow/green patterns. Presence of hyperkalemia suggests severe digoxin toxicity. Certain arrhythmias which are typically associated with digoxin toxicity include nonparoxysmal atrial tachycardia with atrioventricular (AV) block, new-onset Mobitz type I AV block, accelerated junctional rhythm with or without high-degree AV block, and bidirectional ventricular tachycardia. Patients with life-threatening toxicity may present with ventricular tachycardia, ventricular fibrillation, symptomatic high-degree AV block, or sinus arrest. Antidigoxin Fab fragments are indicated in the management of serious and life-threatening toxicity.

Suggested Reading
1. Bauman JL, Didomenico RJ, Galanter WL. Mechanisms, manifestations, and management of digoxin toxicity in the modern era. Am J Cardiovasc Drugs. 2006;6(2):77-86.
2. Kanji S, MacLean RD. Cardiac glycoside toxicity: more than 200 years and counting. Crit Care Clin. 2012;28(4):527-35.
3. Palatnick W, Jelic T. Calcium channel blocker and beta blocker overdose, and digoxin toxicity management. Emerg Med Pract. 2020;22(Suppl 9):1-42.
4. Pincus M. Management of digoxin toxicity. Aust Prescr. 2016;39(1):18-20.

Q.2. A 35-year-old male worker presents to emergency room in an unconscious state after a fire in a plastics factory. On examination, there are superficial burns involving the chest and upper limbs. His heart rate is 38/min and his systolic blood pressure is 55 mm Hg. He is immediately intubated for airway protection and fluid resuscitation is started with large-bore intravenous (IV) cannulas. Which of the following statements is FALSE regarding the further management of this patient?
   a. Cyanide toxicity should be suspected as the patient was a fire victim in plastics factory
   b. Cyanosis is hallmark of cyanide toxicity
   c. Cyanide levels are not useful in the acute management of patients
   d. There is high oxygen content in the venous blood in patients with cyanide poisoning

Ans. b

Explanation: Cyanide exposure can occur through various sources. However, smoke inhalation remains the most common source, especially when burning of products such as plastics, synthetic fibers, and polymers are involved. It should also be suspected when some industrial or factory worker suddenly collapses or presents with unexplained coma or severe metabolic acidosis and hyperlactatemia. In the initial stages, patients will have tachypnea and hyperpnea, which may be followed by respiratory depression or apnea. Even though patient is hypoxic, cyanosis is absent. Neurological involvement may present with altered mental status, syncope, unconsciousness, coma, seizures, or encephalopathy. Cherry-red complexion and bright red retinal veins, described with cyanide toxicity is uncommon and late findings. Concomitant carbon monoxide (CO) poisoning should be suspected in fire victims, especially in severe cyanide toxicity with cyanide levels >10 mmol/L. Because of inhibition of aerobic metabolism, the oxygen content of venous blood becomes abnormally high causing "arterialization" of venous blood. Hence, the difference between arterial and venous blood oxygen levels becomes <10 mm Hg. Acute management does not depend on the cyanide concentrations. Hydroxocobalamin is the treatment of choice. It acts by binding cyanide to form cyanocobalamin, which is further excreted by the kidneys. It is given in the dose of 70 mg/kg intravenously, with a maximum dose of 5 g. It may be administered along with sodium thiosulfate, which may aid in biotransformation of cyanide to thiocyanate. Sodium thiosulfate may be given intravenously in a dose of 12.5 g over 30 minutes. It has delayed onset of action. Further, thiocyanate may get accumulated in patients with renal dysfunction and lead to neurotoxicity. Other antidotes for cyanide poisoning include amyl nitrite or sodium nitrite, which act by inducing methemoglobinemia, which binds with cyanide to form cyanmethemoglobin. Amyl nitrite ampules may be given through inhalation if intravenous access is not available.

Suggested Reading
1. Barillo DJ. Diagnosis and treatment of cyanide toxicity. J Burn Care Res. 2009;30(1):148-52.
2. Baud FJ, Barriot P, Toffis V, Riou B, Vicaut E, Lecarpentier Y, et al. Elevated blood cyanide concentrations in victims of smoke inhalation. N Engl J Med. 1991;325(25):1761-6.
3. Borron SW. Recognition and treatment of acute cyanide poisoning. J Emerg Nurs. 2006;32(4 Suppl):S12-8.

4. Fortin JL, Ruttiman M, Domanski L, Kowalski JJ. Hydroxocobalamin: treatment for smoke inhalation-associated cyanide poisoning. Meeting the needs of fire victims. JEMS. 2004;29(8):suppl 18-21.
5. Hall AH, Saiers J, Baud F. Which cyanide antidote? Crit Rev Toxicol. 2009;39(7):541-52.
6. Mégarbane B, Delahaye A, Goldgran-Tolédano D, Baud FJ. Antidotal treatment of cyanide poisoning. J Chin Med Assoc. 2003;66(4):193-203.
7. Persson SA, Cassel G, Sellström A. Acute cyanide intoxication and central transmitter systems. Fundam Appl Toxicol. 1985;5(6 Pt 2):S150-9.
8. Shepherd G, Velez LI. Role of hydroxocobalamin in acute cyanide poisoning. Ann Pharmacother. 2008;42(5):661-9.

Q.3. Which of the following statements regarding lethal dose fifty (LD_{50}) for a substance is false?
   a. It is defined as the calculated dose which is expected to result in the death of 50% of the defined experimental animal population.
   b. It is not valid when the route of exposure is inhalational.
   c. It can be applied to both acute and chronic poisonings.
   d. As it is a single value, it is not indicative of toxic effects at different levels.

Ans. c

Explanation: Several dose-response terms have been defined to assess and predict the effect of exposure to various substances. Lethal dose fifty has been simply defined as the calculated dose which is expected to result in the death of 50% of the defined experimental animal population. It can be determined for all kinds of exposure except inhalational. It is also not valid for chronic exposure and may be determined only after an acute exposure to the particular substance. Even though these dose-response terms are frequently used in toxicology practice, they have several limitations. As they are determined in experimental animal populations, they may not entirely be applicable to human populations as many poisons act differently in humans. Additionally, as LD_{50} and lethal concentration fifty, depict single values; they may not be indicative of toxic effects at different doses or concentrations.

Suggested Reading
1. National Institute for Occupational Safety and Health. Registry of Toxic Effects of Chemical Substances. Washington, DC: DHHS (NIOSH) Publication; 1983.

Q.4. Which of the following is not true regarding snake bites?
   a. Krait bites present with neurotoxic symptoms but no local symptoms
   b. Cobra bites present with local swelling and necrosis along with neurotoxic symptoms
   c. Russell's viper bites may present with local, neurological, and coagulopathic symptoms
   d. Cobra bites do not respond to neostigmine

Ans. d

Explanation: Venomous snakes can be broadly classified into two families: *Elapidae* (cobras, kraits, and coral snakes) and *Viperidae* (Russell's viper, saw-scaled viper, pit vipers, hump-nosed vipers, and green pit vipers). The snakes of the Elapidae family primarily produce neurotoxic venom which leads to paralysis of muscles by blocking the neuromuscular junction. On the other hand, snakes from Viperidae family produce venom which has procoagulant enzymes and may lead to coagulopathy. The bite from Russell's viper cause local swelling, neurotoxicity (ptosis, external ophthalmoplegia, dysphagia, respiratory paralysis, and limb and muscle weakness), coagulopathy (hematuria, hematemesis, and gum bleeding), and even myotoxicity (myalgia and rhabdomyolysis). Rhabdomyolysis may also cause acute kidney injury. Cobra bites may also cause local symptoms such as swelling, blistering, and tissue necrosis, along with neurotoxicity but no coagulopathy. However, krait bite primarily causes only neurotoxic symptoms with no local effects or coagulopathy. Antisnake venom serum may be useful in all these bites but anticholinesterase effects of neostigmine may be helpful in reversing the paralytic effects of cobra bites. Data from case reports suggest that the postsynaptic blockage of neuromuscular junction may be competitive and reversible which may be reversed with neostigmine. However, atropine must be given prior to neostigmine to prevent muscarinic effects.

Suggested Reading
1. Ariaratnam CA, Sheriff MH, Arambepola C, Theakston RD, Warrell DA. Syndromic approach to treatment of snake bite in Sri Lanka based on results of a prospective national hospital-based survey of patients envenomed by identified snakes. Am J Trop Med Hyg. 2009;81(4):725-31.
2. Ariaratnam CA, Sheriff MH, Theakston RD, Warrell DA. Distinctive epidemiologic and clinical features of common krait (Bungarus caeruleus) bites in Sri Lanka. Am J Trop Med Hyg. 2008;79(3);458-62.
3. Warrell DA. WHO/SEARO guidelines for the clinical management of snake bites in the Southeast Asian Region. SE Asian Trop Med Pub Heath. 1999;30:1-85.

Q.5. A 35-year-old man was brought to the emergency department with an alleged history of consuming a bottle of homemade alcoholic beverage with his friends last night. He was in an inebriated state, confused, and had difficulty maintaining his balance while walking. He complained of severe abdominal pain, nausea, and vomiting. His blood pressure was 88/60 mm Hg, heart rate 118 beats/min, and respiratory rate 25 breaths/min. His blood glucose was 110 mg/dL. On examination, the patient had a fruity odor to his breath. The fundoscopic examination revealed bilateral optic disk edema. The initial laboratory investigations showed metabolic acidosis with a pH of 7.2 and, an anion gap of 24 mEq/L, and lactate of 2.4 mmol/L. Which of the following is not appropriate in the management of this patient?
a. Administration of fomepizole
b. Activated charcoal through a nasogastric tube
c. Hemodialysis
d. Intravenous fluids
e. Send ethanol, ethylene glycol, and methanol levels

Ans. b

Explanation: The clinical presentation and laboratory findings are consistent with methanol poisoning. Charcoal has no role in alcohol intoxication as it does not absorb alcohol. Methanol is metabolized by alcohol dehydrogenase to formaldehyde and then to formic acid, which are toxic metabolites and can cause metabolic acidosis and optic nerve damage. Treatment involves administering fomepizole or ethanol (if fomepizole is not available) initially to inhibit (or saturate) the alcohol dehydrogenase and to prevent the formation of toxic metabolites. Hemodialysis is indicated in patients in later stages to eliminate metabolites. It is indicated in patients with severe acidosis or end-organ damage. Three or more cases of methanol poisoning within 3 days from the same geographic area should be considered as a possible "outbreak." Intravenous fluids and observation alone are not sufficient treatments for methanol poisoning.

Suggested Reading
1. Beauchamp GA, Valento M, Kim J. Toxic alcohol ingestion: prompt recognition and management in the emergency department [digest]. Emerg Med Pract. 2016;18(9 Suppl Points & Pearls):S1-2.
2. Ng PCY, Long BJ, Davis WT, Sessions DJ, Koyfman A. Toxic alcohol diagnosis and management: an emergency medicine review. Intern Emerg Med. 2018;13(3):375-83.

Q.6. Extracorporeal toxin removal (ECTR) may be attempted in cases of severe toxicity with all of the following drugs except for?
 a. Digoxin
 b. Metformin
 c. Lithium
 d. Methanol

Ans. a

Explanation: There is emerging clinical evidence related to utility of ECTR in the management of acute poisonings. For any toxin to be amenable for ECTR, ideally it should have a low molecular weight, protein binding, and volume of distribution. As data from large-scale randomized control trials is lacking, the current evidence is largely based on case series and reports. For this reason, the Extracorporeal Treatments in Poisoning (EXTRIP) workgroup was formed with an aim to assess the evidence and make recommendations for use of ECTR in the management of acute toxicity. As per the EXTRIP recommendations, ECTR should be considered in cases of severe poisoning with methanol, lithium, metformin, salicylates, acetaminophen, and certain other toxins. However, ECTR is not recommended for certain agents such as calcium channel blockers, tricyclic antidepressants, and digoxin. However, it is imperative to understand the basic characteristics of the suspected poison and the intricacies of the available modalities of extracorporeal therapies to choose the right patient, the right time, and the right modality of ECTR.

Suggested Reading
1. Calello DP, Liu KD, Wiegand TJ, Roberts DM, Lavergne V, Gosselin S, et al. Extracorporeal treatment for metformin poisoning: systematic review and recommendations from the Extracorporeal Treatments in Poisoning Workgroup. Crit Care Med. 2015;43(8):1716-30.
2. Decker BS, Goldfarb DS, Dargan PI, Friesen M, Gosselin S, Hoffman RS, et al. Extracorporeal treatment for lithium poisoning: systematic review and recommendations from the EXTRIP Workgroup. Clin J Am Soc Nephrol. 2015;10(5):875-87.

3. Ghannoum M, Nolin TD, Lavergne V, Hoffman RS; EXTRIP workgroup. Blood purification in toxicology: nephrology's ugly duckling. Adv Chronic Kidney Dis. 2011;18(3):160-6.
4. Juneja D, Singh O, Bhasin A, Gupta M, Saxena S, Chaturvedi A. Severe suicidal digoxin toxicity managed with resin hemoperfusion: a case report. Indian J Crit Care Med. 2012;16(4):231-3.
5. Juneja D, Singh O. Extracorporeal therapies: Specific poisons. In: Singh O, Juneja D (Eds). Principles and Practice of Critical Care Toxicology, 1st edition. New Delhi: Jaypee Brothers Medical Publishers (P) Ltd; 2019. pp. 274-87.
6. Mowry JB, Burdmann EA, Anseeuw K, Ayoub P, Ghannoum M, Hoffman RS, et al. Extracorporeal treatment for digoxin poisoning: systematic review and recommendations from the EXTRIP Workgroup. Clin Toxicol (Phila). 2016;54(2):103-14.
7. Roberts DM, Yates C, Megarbane B, Winchester JF, Maclaren R, Gosselin S, et al. Recommendations for the role of extracorporeal treatments in the management of acute methanol poisoning: a systematic review and consensus statement. Crit Care Med. 2015;43(2):461-72.

Q.7. All the following drug overdoses may present with alveolar hemorrhage, except?
  a. Anticoagulants
  b. Amiodarone
  c. Opioids
  d. Cocaine

  Ans. c

  Explanation: Lungs may be directly involved in several poisonings. However, rarely some drug overdoses may lead to alveolar hemorrhage and patients may present with hemoptysis and progressive shortness of breath. Apart from anticoagulants, and thrombolytics other drugs which may lead to alveolar hemorrhage include cocaine, amiodarone, nitrofurantoin, penicillamine, and toluene.

  Suggested Reading
  1. Schwarz MI, Fontenot AP. Drug-induced diffuse alveolar hemorrhage syndromes and vasculitis. Clin Chest Med. 2004;25(1):133-40.
  2. Singh O, Nasa P, Juneja D. Approach to a poisoned patient. In: Singh O, Juneja D (Eds). Principles and Practice of Critical Care Toxicology, 1st edition. New Delhi: Jaypee Brothers Medical Publishers (P) Ltd; 2019. pp. 3-18.

Q.8. A 34-year-old male presents to the emergency department with an altered mental status and a decreased level of consciousness. He had multiple episodes of vomiting and seizures. His family found him lying on his bed in an inebriated state with two empty bottles of locally procured alcohol. On examination, his vital signs are stable. His initial laboratory investigations show a metabolic acidosis with an anion gap of 24, an osmolal gap of 11 mmol, and serum calcium of 6 mg/dL. Which of the following is against the diagnosis of ethylene glycol intoxication?
  a. Elevated anion gap
  b. Serum lactate <5 mmol/L
  c. Serum level of ethylene glycol 12 mg/dL
  d. Normal osmolal gap
  e. Hypocalcemia

  Ans. c

Explanation: All other features are observed in ethylene glycol intoxication. The standard osmolal gap is 10–20 mOsm/L but has a wide range span of ~20 mOsm/L (e.g., from −10 mOsm to +10 mOsm). An ethylene glycol level >20 mg/dL is regarded as potentially toxic. However, it is elevated only in early intoxication. Ethylene glycol 20 mg/dL corresponds to an osmolal shift of only 3 mOsm/L. If the baseline osmolality of the patient was at the lower end of normal, a clinically significant ethylene glycol intoxication can occur with a normal osmolal gap. Additionally, in the later phase of intoxication, after the metabolism of ethylene glycol to glycolic acid or oxalic acid, the osmolal gap will invariably be absent. Hence, a high anion gap (progressively increasing on trend) is more suggestive of toxic alcohol intoxication. Finally, an elevated osmolal gap has low specificity and may be elevated in various other conditions:
- Toxic alcohols (ethylene glycol, methanol, and isopropyl alcohol)
- Other alcohols (mannitol, glycerol, and ethanol)
- Ketoacidosis (due to acetone generation)
- Renal failure
- Shock
- Contrast dye and intravenous immunoglobulin
- Hypermagnesemia, hypercalcemia, and lithium intoxication
- Pseudohyponatremia (e.g., due to hyperproteinemia or hyperlipidemia)

Suggested Reading
1. Farkas J. (2020). Ethylene glycol & methanol poisoning. [online] Available from: https://emcrit.org/ibcc/alcohols/#osmolal_gap [Last assessed June, 2023].
2. Gallagher N, Edwards FJ. The Diagnosis and Management of Toxic Alcohol Poisoning in the Emergency Department: A Review Article. Adv J Emerg Med. 2019;3(3):e28.
3. Ross JA, Borek HA, Holstege CP, King JD. Toxic alcohol poisoning. Emerg Med Clin North Am. 2022;40(2):327-41.

Q.9. Multidose-activated charcoal (MDAC) may be used for gastric decontamination in selected patients with all the following poisonings, except?
 a. Digoxin
 b. Amitriptyline
 c. Organophosphates
 d. Opioids

Ans. c

Explanation: Activated charcoal may be used for gastric decontamination if the patient presents within 1 hour of ingestion. Further, it should be ensured that the airway is protected before attempting gastric decontamination. Multidose activated charcoal is not routinely indicated but may be considered in patients who have ingested agents with a significant enterohepatic circulation (e.g., opioids and digoxin), drugs that decrease GI transit (anticholinergics, tricyclic antidepressants, and opioids), and sustained release formulations. An initial dose of 50–100 g is given which is followed by a repeated dose of 12.5 g every 2–4 hourly. However, certain agents such as alcohols, acids, and pesticides such as organophosphates and carbamates, iron, and lithium are not absorbed by activated charcoal and hence it may not be useful in such poisonings.

Suggested Reading
1. Bonilla-Velez J, Marin-Cuero DJ. The use of activated charcoal for acute poisonings. Int J Med Students. 2017;5(1):45-52.
2. Chyka PA, Seger D, Krenzelok EP, Vale JA; American Academy of Clinical Toxicology; European Association of Poisons Centres and Clinical Toxicologists. Position paper: Single-dose activated charcoal. Clin Toxicol (Phila). 2005;43(2):61-87.
3. Singh O, Nasa P, Juneja D. Approach to a poisoned patient. In: Singh O, Juneja D (Eds). Principles and Practice of Critical Care Toxicology, 1st edition. New Delhi: Jaypee Brothers Medical Publishers (P) Ltd; 2019. pp. 3-18.
4. Tenenbein M. Multiple doses of activated charcoal: time for reappraisal II. Ann Emerg Med. 2003;42(4):597-8.

Q.10. A 55-year-old male, with a history of deep vein thrombosis on enoxaparin, presents to emergency room with sudden onset right side weakness which developed 2 hours ago. Urgent computed tomography scan of the brain shows left intracranial bleed with a midline shift. Last dose of enoxaparin was administered 6 hours before the presentation. Which of the following statements regarding use of protamine sulfate is incorrect?
   a. At high doses protamine may have some weak anticoagulant activity
   b. Protamine does not completely neutralize factor Xa activity
   c. Dose of protamine is dependent on time since administration of enoxaparin
   d. Recombinant factor VIIa has no role in managing bleeding secondary to enoxaparin administration

Ans. d

Explanation: Protamine sulfate is the drug of choice for treating bleeding associated with ultrafractionated heparin (UFH) and low molecular weight heparins (LMWHs). Protamine is recommended for reversing the effects of LMWH in patients with intracranial hemorrhage receiving therapeutic doses of LMWH. For neutralization of 100 units of UFH, 1 mg protamine is required. For LMWHs, the dose of protamine is dependent on the dose and time since administration of LMWH. For every 1 mg of enoxaparin, 1 mg of protamine is required for neutralization, if enoxaparin was taken within the last 8 hours. If >8 hours have elapsed, only 0.5 mg of protamine is required for every 1 mg of enoxaparin administered. Protamine should be given slowly, over 10 minutes of intravenous infusion, as rapid bolus may lead to hypotension. No hepatic or renal dose modification is necessary. However, protamine can only partially neutralize the antifactor Xa activity. Protamine, at high doses, may have a weak anticoagulation effect. Recombinant factor VIIa (90 µg/kg IV) may have some efficacy in neutralizing the effects of LMWH and hence, may be considered if protamine is not available or contraindicated.

Suggested Reading
1. Caravati EM. Protamine sulfate. In: Dart RC (Ed). Medical Toxicology, 3rd edition. Philadelphia, PA: Lippincott Williams and Wilkins; 2004. pp. 243-4.
2. Frontera JA, Lewin JJ, Rabinstein AA, Aisiku IP, Alexandrov AW, Cook AM, et al. Guideline for Reversal of Antithrombotics in Intracranial Hemorrhage: A Statement for Healthcare

Professionals from the Neurocritical Care Society and Society of Critical Care Medicine. Neurocrit Care. 2016;24(1):6-46.
3. Pai M, Crowther MA. Neutralization of heparin activity. Handb Exp Pharmacol. 2012;(207):265-77.

Q.11. A 28-year-old woman was brought to the emergency department by her friends after a college party. According to her friends, she had been drinking alcohol and taking drugs called "liquid ecstasy" [gamma hydroxybutyrate (GHB)]. She was "high" for some duration. Upon arrival, she was found to be unresponsive, with shallow breathing and constricted pupils. Her vital signs were stable, and her oxygen saturation was 95% on room air. The ABG showed mild respiratory acidosis. In view of the altered mental status and respiratory acidosis, the decision for tracheal intubation was taken. She became violent and agitated during the laryngoscopy. The following statements are correct for GHB, except?
   a. GHB is a central nervous system (CNS) depressant and causes respiratory depression
   b. Management is primarily supportive with airway management and cardio-respiratory support
   c. Flumazenil can be helpful in respiratory depression
   d. GHB toxicity is a clinical diagnosis, as drug assays are not readily available
   e. Sudden loss of consciousness and abrupt awakening in 2-4 hours is typical with isolated GHB overdose

Ans. c

Explanation: Gamma hydroxybutyrate is a precursor of the inhibitory neurotransmitter gamma-aminobutyric acid (GABA). Lower doses stimulate dopamine release with an initial period of euphoria, while higher doses inhibit dopamine release through agonist action on GABA-B receptors. This is responsible for the central nervous system (CNS) and respiratory depression. It is abused for sleep aid, rave parties, and weight-loss supplement, but is banned in the United States. It is used for illicit purposes because of its colorless and odorless nature, and hence, can be used to spike any drink, resulting in its "date-rape" drug label. The diagnosis is mainly clinical based on the history and its symptoms. Urine and blood drug assays should be sent to identify coingestion of alcohol or other drugs of abuse. Gas chromatography and mass spectrometry are confirmatory tests but are not readily available. There is no antidote for GHB toxicity. Treatment is mainly supportive with airway, breathing, and circulatory support. As it is a short-acting drug and there may be rapid improvement in consciousness, a higher threshold for intubation may be warranted. In suspected opioid overdose, IV naloxone can be tried. However, IV flumazenil does not have any role in GHB toxicity.

Suggested Reading
1. Carlier L, Van Belleghem V, Croes K, Hooft F, Desmet M, Heylen O, et al. Gamma-hydroxybutyrate (GHB), an unusual cause of high anion gap metabolic acidosis. CJEM. 2018;20(S2):S2-5.

2. Le JK, Richards JR. Gamma-Hydroxybutyrate Toxicity. In: StatPearls [Internet]. Treasure Island (FL): StatPearls Publishing; 2022.
3. O'Connell T, Kaye L, Plosay JJ 3rd. Gamma-hydroxybutyrate (GHB): a newer drug of abuse. Am Fam Physician. 2000;62(11):2478-83.

Q.12. Which of the following statements regarding the use of Rumack–Matthew nomogram in patients with paracetamol overdose is not true?
a. It may be used for both acute and chronic ingestions
b. It may be misleading if the exact time of ingestion is unknown in cases of acute overdose
c. Its role is unclear if the patient has consumed sustained release preparations
d. In patients presenting 24 hours after acute ingestion, the risk of hepatotoxicity cannot be ruled out even if the paracetamol levels are below the nomogram line

Ans. a

Explanation: Uses of Rumack–Matthew nomogram has been advocated in evaluating the risk of complications and deciding on therapy in patients with acute paracetamol overdose. It has no role in patients with chronic ingestions. Even in patients with acute ingestion, there are several limitations to using Rumack–Matthew nomogram. It may be misleading in patients who have ingested sustained-release tablets and in those in whom the exact time of ingestion is unknown. Moreover, if the patients present after 24 hours of ingestion, the risk of hepatotoxicity cannot be ruled out even if the paracetamol levels are below the nomogram line.

Suggested Reading
1. Bateman DN. Paracetamol poisoning: beyond the nomogram. Br J Clin Pharmacol. 2015;80(1):45-50.
2. Ferner RE, Dear JW, Bateman DN. Management of paracetamol poisoning. BMJ. 2011;342:d2218.
3. Wong A, Graudins A. Risk prediction of hepatotoxicity in paracetamol poisoning. Clin Toxicol (Phila). 2017;55(8):879-92.

Q.13. A 24-year-old college student was brought to the emergency department by friends. She took a pill at a party and started behaving erratically. On examination, she is found to be agitated, obtunded, has dilated pupils, febrile (temperature 38°C), with a heart rate of 128/min, blood pressure of 220/118, and has profuse sweating. She is unable to provide any coherent information about the pill she took. All of the following can be used for the management of this patient except?
a. Labetalol
b. Lorazepam
c. Intubation and ventilation
d. Metoprolol
e. Phentolamine

Ans. d

Explanation: Ecstasy [3,4-methylenedioxymethamphetamine (MDMA)] is a sympathomimetic drug that is a common drug of abuse in parties and raves because of its neurostimulatory (euphoric) effects. The tablet available in the market is a mixture of various neurostimulants such as MDMA, 3,4-methylenedioxyamphetamine (MDA), ephedrine, ketamine, and paracetamol. Hence, considerable adverse effects and toxicity may be observed in patients with a single dose or after first-time ingestion due to random dose and composition. Ecstasy has amphetamine and has hallucinogenic effects due to an increase in the overall concentration of norepinephrine, dopamine, and serotonin at the synaptic cleft. The symptoms of ecstasy intoxication include dilated pupils, increased heart rate and blood pressure, profuse sweating, disorientation, seizures, and agitation. It can cause fulminant hepatic failure, cardiac dysrhythmias, intracranial hemorrhages, rhabdomyolysis, and renal failure. Agitation should be controlled with benzodiazepines such as lorazepam and diazepam. Airway control, along with stabilization of breathing and circulation should be the initial approach. Intravenous hydration with active cooling to control hyperthermia should be done. However, caution with overzealous fluids should be exercised in patients with hyponatremia and myocardial infarction. Beta-blocker alone without alpha blockade may worsen the crisis. Hence, labetalol is the drug of choice for blood pressure control due to adrenergic crisis.

Suggested Reading
1. Figurasin R, Maguire NJ. 3,4-Methylenedioxy-Methamphetamine Toxicity. In: StatPearls [Internet]. Treasure Island (FL): StatPearls Publishing; 2023.
2. Steinkellner T, Freissmuth M, Sitte HH, Montgomery T. The ugly side of amphetamines: short- and long-term toxicity of 3,4-methylenedioxymethamphetamine (MDMA, 'Ecstasy'), methamphetamine and d-amphetamine. Biol Chem. 2011;392(1-2):103-15.

Q.14. **A 69-year-old female who had undergone a left hip replacement surgery was discharged on oral dabigatran 110 mg once a day. Her other comorbidities included diabetes and hypertension, which were controlled with metformin and amlodipine. Now she presented with sudden onset right side weakness and altered mental status. In the emergency room, she had to be intubated for airway protection. All her baseline laboratory parameters including coagulopathy markers are within normal range. Urgent computed tomography scan showed left intracranial hemorrhage with midline shift. All the following form important components of clinical management except for?**
a. Intravenous tranexamic acid 500 mg
b. Intravenous andexanet infusion
c. Urgent hemodialysis
d. Prothrombin complex concentrate (PCC), if an antidote is not available

Ans. b

Explanation: In patients with dabigatran-induced bleeding, idarucizumab, a monoclonal antibody fragment that binds with dabigatran and its metabolites, is the drug of choice. The dose is 5 g intravenously, which may be repeated once if the bleeding continues. Its onset of action is 10–30 minutes and it may achieve a complete reversal of dabigatran activity within minutes of administration. Dabigatran is dialyzable and may be removed by hemodialysis or hemadsorption. Andexanet is the antidote for bleeding associated with apixaban and rivaroxaban use. Even though antifibrinolytic agents such as tranexamic acid and epsilon-aminocaproic acid may not be very effective in reversing the effects of dabigatran, they may be used in patients with life-threatening bleeding. Similarly, PCC has not been shown to be effective in managing bleeding associated with any direct-acting oral anticoagulants and are not FDA approved for this indication, but may be used in patients with life-threatening bleeding where specific antidotes are not available. No coagulation test can accurately predict the risk of bleeding in patients taking dabigatran. However, diluted thrombin time (dTT) may be more sensitive than prothrombin time or thromboplastin time in monitoring the efficacy of direct thrombin inhibitors such as dabigatran, argatroban, and bivalirudin.

Suggested Reading
1. Allison TA, Lin PJ, Gass JA, Chong K, Prater SJ, Escobar MA, et al. Evaluation of the use of low-dose 4-factor prothrombin complex concentrate in the reversal of direct oral anticoagulants in bleeding patients. J Intensive Care Med. 2020;35(9):903-8.
2. Douxfils J, Ageno W, Samama C-M, Lessire S, Cate HT, Verhamme P, et al. Laboratory testing in patients treated with direct oral anticoagulants: a practical guide for clinicians. J Thromb Haemost. 2018;16(2):209-19.
3. Frontera JA, Lewin JJ III, Rabinstein AA, Aisiku IP, Alexandrov AW, Cook AM, et al. Guideline for reversal of antithrombotics in intracranial hemorrhage: a statement for healthcare professionals from the Neurocritical Care Society and Society of Critical Care Medicine. Neurocrit Care 2016;24(01):6-46.
4. Gosselin RC, Adcock DM, Bates SM, Douxfils J, Favaloro EJ, Gouin-Thibault I, et al. International Council for Standardization in Haematology (ICSH) recommendations for laboratory measurement of direct oral anticoagulants. Thromb Haemost. 2018;118(3):437-50.
5. Koscielny J, Rutkauskaite E, Sucker C, von Heymann C. How do I reverse oral and parenteral anticoagulants? Hamostaseologie. 2020;40(2):201-13.
6. Levy JH, Ageno W, Chan NC, Crowther M, Verhamme P, Weitz JI, et al. When and how to use antidotes for the reversal of direct oral anticoagulants: guidance from the SSC of the ISTH. J Thromb Haemost. 2016;14(3):623-7.

Q.15. A 32-year-old woman with a history of depression presented to the emergency department after ingesting an unknown amount of iron tablets. On arrival, she was alert and oriented but complained of abdominal pain, nausea, and vomiting. Serum iron performed 4 hours after the ingestion confirmed the presence of iron, with iron levels of 569 µg/dL. Which of the following is the most appropriate next step in the management of this patient?
a. Administer activated charcoal
b. Begin intravenous fluid resuscitation
c. Order a gastric lavage
d. Administer chelating agent and deferoxamine
e. Wait and monitor closely

Ans. d

Explanation: Iron overdose is a common toxic ingestion and constitutes a medical emergency. After initial gastrointestinal symptoms (nausea, vomiting, diarrhea, hematemesis, and hematochezia), multiorgan failure, coagulopathy, hepatic dysfunction, myocardial dysfunction, renal failure shock, and death can happen. Activated charcoal does not bind iron and is ineffective. Whole bowel irrigation with polyethylene glycol can help in elimination of pills and reduce absorption. Gastric lavage is risky because of risk of aspiration and perforation. The management of iron toxicity includes stabilizing the patient's vital signs, and administering a chelating agent such as deferoxamine, to remove excess iron from the body. Indications of deferoxamine (which can cause hypotension) are metabolic acidosis, systemic toxicity, worsening symptoms, and serum iron level >350 µg/dL. Intravenous fluid resuscitation may be necessary to maintain the patient's blood pressure and prevent shock, but it does not directly address the toxicity of iron. Waiting and monitoring closely is not appropriate in cases of iron overdose, as the toxicity can progress rapidly and lead to life-threatening complications.

Suggested Reading
1. Yuen HW, Becker W. Iron Toxicity. In: StatPearls [Internet]. Treasure Island (FL): StatPearls Publishing; 2023.
2. Yu D, Giffen MA Jr. Suicidal iron overdose: A case report and review of literature. J Forensic Sci. 2021;66(4):1564-9.

Q.16. Which of the following statements regarding carbon monoxide poisoning is not true?
a. Most common symptoms are related to the central nervous and cardiovascular systems
b. Hyperbaric oxygen is indicated in all patients with carbon monoxide poisoning
c. Coexisting cyanide poisoning should be suspected in patients caught in fires
d. Long-term follow-up is indicated in all patients

Ans. b

Explanation: Exposure to carbon monoxide leads to formation of carboxyhemoglobin (COHb) which has 250 times more affinity to oxygen than normal hemoglobin. Patients may present with mild symptoms such as headache and dizziness but severe poisoning may lead to coma and death. The earliest symptoms are neurological but patients generally die because of cardiac toxicity. However, overall mortality remains low, ranging from 1 to 3%. Patients with moderate and severe poisoning may present with cardiac symptoms including left ventricle systolic dysfunction, arrhythmias, and even myocardial infarction. The typical "cherry red" discoloration of skin is rarely present but signifies severe toxicity. The mainstay of therapy remains delivery of 100% oxygen with an aim to reduce COHb concentration to below 3%. Use of 100% oxygen reduces the half-life of CO from 320 minutes to 74 minutes. Use of hyperbaric oxygen may further reduce the half-life to 20–30 minutes, but is not easily available. As CO poisoning may lead to long-term neurological sequelae, patients at risk of developing these long-term effects are candidates for hyperbaric oxygen therapy. These include patients with advanced age (>55 years), significant loss of consciousness, coma, persistent neurological deficit, severe metabolic acidosis with hyperlactatemia, pregnant patients, and those with myocardial ischemia or cardiogenic shock. However, long-term follow-up is indicated in all patients with CO poisoning as even a low level of exposure may have long-term neurological effects.

Suggested Reading
1. Hampson NB, Piantadosi CA, Thom SR, Weaver LK. Practice recommendations in the diagnosis, management, and prevention of carbon monoxide poisoning. Am J Respir Crit Care Med. 2012;186(11):1095-101.
2. Rose JJ, Wang L, Xu Q, McTiernan CF, Shiva S, Tejero J, et al. Carbon monoxide poisoning: Pathogenesis, management, and future directions of therapy. Am J Respir Crit Care Med. 2017;195(5):596-606.
3. Weaver LK, Hopkins RO, Chan KJ, Churchill S, Elliott CG, Clemmer TP, et al. Hyperbaric oxygen for acute carbon monoxide poisoning. N Engl J Med. 2002;347(14):1057-67.

Q.17. A 38-year-old male was airlifted from his mountain trekking trip in the Himalayas for severe stomach cramps, vomiting, and diarrhea. He reports that symptoms started after consuming a dinner of wild mushrooms from the forest. On physical examination, he appears dehydrated and has mild epigastric tenderness, a heart rate of 124/min, and a blood pressure of 94/56 mm Hg. Mushroom poisoning was suspected. Which of the following findings about mushroom poisoning is incorrect?
a. Hepatotoxicity is one of the dreadful complications
b. *Amanita phalloides* is the most common species responsible for the poisoning
c. Management is mainly supportive, and no specific antidotes are available
d. Toxicity is unaffected by cooking
e. Liver transplantation is contraindicated

Ans. e

Explanation: *Amanita phalloides* poisoning is the most likely type of mushroom poisoning in this case. It is a common cause of mushroom poisoning worldwide, and its symptoms typically develop 6–24 hours after ingestion. The two main toxins include phallotoxins and amatoxins. Phallotoxins bind to the cell membrane of erythrocytes and cause gastrointestinal symptoms like diarrhea. Amatoxin is primarily responsible for organ failure such as liver, kidney, pancreas, adrenal glands, and testes. It causes severe gastrointestinal symptoms, including nausea, abdominal cramp, vomiting, diarrhea, and liver and kidney failure. The diagnosis is mainly clinical and the management is mainly supportive. The management includes intravenous fluid hydration, correction of electrolytes, and metabolic acidosis. Fulminant acute liver failure is an indication of liver transplantation. Gastric lavage and multidose charcoal reduce gastrointestinal absorption. Early administration of drugs such as silibinin (silymarin derivative) and penicillin G can prevent the binding of amatoxins to plasma protein and its hepatic uptake. N-acetylcysteine has also been tried but its efficacy is unproven.

Suggested Reading
1. Verma N, Bhalla A, Kumar S, Dhiman RK, Chawla YK. Wild mushroom poisoning in north India: case series with review of literature. J Clin Exp Hepatol. 2014;4(4):361-5.

2. Wennig R, Eyer F, Schaper A, Zilker T, Andresen-Streichert H. Mushroom poisoning. Dtsch Arztebl Int. 2020;117(42):701-8.
3. Xue J, Lou X, Ning D, Shao R, Chen G. Mechanism and treatment of α-amanitin poisoning. Arch Toxicol. 2023;97(1):121-31.

Q.18. A previously healthy 26-year-old male presented with a 1-week history of productive cough, progressive dyspnea, malaise, nausea, and vomiting but no history of fever. He was a chronic smoker but had switched over to e-cigarettes a year ago. However, he had stopped using e-cigarettes two months ago. On examination, he is afebrile, conscious, and oriented but in respiratory distress. His heart rate is 111/min, respiratory rate 29/min, and blood pressure 145/76 mm Hg. His chest X-ray shows bilateral pulmonary infiltrates. Which of the following statements regarding electronic cigarette or vaping use-associated lung injury (EVALI) is true?
   a. There is no specific test and it is a diagnosis of exclusion
   b. It should not be considered in the present patient as he had stopped using e-cigarettes months ago
   c. There is no role of bronchoscopy
   d. Corticosteroids are contraindicated

Ans. a

Explanation: Electronic cigarettes or e-cigarette are commercially available battery-operated devices that contains varying amounts of nicotine along with other chemicals including humectants (propylene glycol and glycerin) and flavoring agents. Even though they are promoted as "safe," inhalation of e-cigarette fumes has been associated with significant toxicities. Several harmful chemicals such as diacetyl and vitamin E acetate (VEA), found in e-cigarettes and vape cartridges, have been found to be associated with EVALI. Patients with EVALI may present with primarily respiratory and gastrointestinal symptoms along with some constitutional symptoms. Patients with advanced age and preexisting respiratory and cardiac disease are at higher risk of severe disease and higher mortality. The case definition for EVALI includes use of an e-cigarette or dabbing up to 90 days prior to onset of symptoms, presence of pulmonary infiltrates on chest X-ray or ground glass haziness on computed tomography scan, and absence of any underlying pulmonary infection. Hence, EVALI is a diagnosis of exclusion and extensive work-up to rule out any other cause for lung pathology must be undertaken. Bronchoscopy and respiratory panels may also be done to rule out any viral, fungal, or other opportunistic or atypical infections. Treatment is generally supportive. Corticosteroids may be beneficial but should be initiated only after ruling out infective pathology.

Suggested Reading
1. Billa R, Tigges C, Vijayakumar N, Radke J, Pedati C, Weiner R, et al. E-cigarette, or Vaping, Product Use Associated Lung Injury (EVALI) with Acute Respiratory Failure in Three Adolescent Patients: A Clinical Timeline, Treatment, and Product Analysis. J Med Toxicol. 2020;16(3):248-54.
2. Blount BC, Karwowski MP, Morel-Espinosa M, Rees J, Sosnoff C, Cowan E, et al. Evaluation of Bronchoalveolar Lavage Fluid from Patients in an Outbreak of E-cigarette, or Vaping,

Product Use–Associated Lung Injury-10 states, August-October 2019. MMWR Morb Mortal Wkly Rep. 2019;68(45):1040-1.
3. Bozier J, Chivers EK, Chapman DG, Larcombe AN, Bastian NA, Masso-Silva JA, et al. The Evolving Landscape of E-Cigarettes: A Systematic Review of Recent Evidence. Chest. 2020;157(5):1362-90.
4. Cao DJ, Aldy K, Hsu S, McGetrick M, Verbeck G, De Silva I, et al. Review of health consequences of electronic cigarettes and the outbreak of electronic cigarette, or vaping, product use-associated lung injury. J Med Toxicol. 2020;16(3):295-310.
5. Werner AK, Koumans EH, Chatham Stephens K, Salvatore PP, Armatas C, Byers P, et al. Hospitalizations and deaths associated with EVALI. N Engl J Med. 2020;382(17):1589-98.

Q.19. A 35-year-old farmer was brought to the emergency department after an alleged history of ingestion of two tablets of pesticide [aluminum phosphide (ALP)]. On arrival, he was found to be conscious, in severe respiratory distress, and had vomited multiple times. On examination, his blood pressure was 78/46 mm Hg, heart rate 138 beats/min, and oxygen saturation was 82% on room air. His pupils were dilated and sluggishly reactive to light. The electrocardiogram (ECG) showed sinus tachycardia with no ST segment changes. After initial fluid bolus, the patient was immediately intubated and started on mechanical ventilation and vasopressors. The bedside 2-D echocardiography showed global hypokinesia with a left ventricle ejection fraction of 25%. What is the mechanism of toxicity of aluminum phosphide?
a. Inhibition of acetylcholinesterase enzyme
b. Inhibition of cytochrome C oxidase
c. Inhibition of sodium-potassium adenosine triphosphatase (ATPase) pump
d. Inhibition of calcium channels
e. Inhibition of ligand ion channels

Ans. b

Explanation: Aluminum phosphide is a highly toxic pesticide that kills insects and rodents. The lethal dose is 1–1.5 g, however, deaths have been reported even with smaller doses of 150–500 mg. On ingestion, ALP liberates phosphine gas, which causes noncompetitive inhibition of cytochrome C oxidase in mitochondria, blocking oxidative phosphorylation and leading to cellular hypoxia and metabolic acidosis. The inhibition of oxidative phosphorylation produces an energy crisis in the cells, affecting multiple organs, including the heart, lungs, and the liver. The clinical manifestations of ALP poisoning include profound hypotension (cardinal feature), refractory metabolic acidosis, cardiac arrhythmias, and cardiovascular collapse. No specific antidote is available, and management is mainly supportive.

Suggested Reading
1. Farahani MV, Soroosh D, Marashi SM. Thoughts on the current management of acute aluminum phosphide toxicity and proposals for therapy: An Evidence-based review. Indian J Crit Care Med. 2016;20(12):724-30.
2. Nasa P, Gupta A, Mangal K, Nagrani SK, Raina S, Yadav R. Use of continuous renal replacement therapy in acute aluminum phosphide poisoning: a novel therapy. Ren Fail. 2013;35(8):1170-2.

Q.20. All the following statements regarding use of pralidoxime (2-PAM) are true except for?
   a. When indicated in the management of organophosphorus poisoning, it should always be administered in conjunction with atropine.
   b. PAM is *not* indicated for the treatment of poisoning with substances with no anticholinesterase activity such as phosphorus, inorganic phosphates, and organophosphates.
   c. Use with caution as it may precipitate a myasthenic crisis
   d. PAM is contraindicated for carbamate poisoning as acetylcholinesterase is weakly affected by carbamates

Ans. d

Explanation: Role of 2-PAM in the management of organophosphorus poisoning has always been a matter of debate. The rationale behind using 2-PAM is that atropine only works on muscarinic receptors and 2-PAM may be useful in reversing the nicotinic effects of organophosphorus compounds. When indicated in management of organophosphorus poisoning, it should always be administered in conjunction with atropine to prevent precipitation of muscarinic symptoms. Preferably, it should be given within the first 48 hours of exposure. A bolus dose of 30 mg/kg over 30 minutes should be followed by an infusion of 8 mg/kg/h, which may be continued for several days, at least till the time patient is on invasive mechanical ventilation or until atropine is no longer required. Earlier, 2-PAM was contraindicated in patients with carbamate poisoning as studies conducted on patients with carbaryl toxicity showed poor clinical outcomes. However, subsequent reports with other carbamates showed positive results and hence, 2-PAM may be considered in poisoning with carbamates other than carbaryl.

Suggested Reading
  1. Gupta R, Parmar M. Pralidoxime. In: StatPearls [Internet]. Treasure Island (FL): StatPearls Publishing; 2023.
  2. Myhrer T, Aas P. Choice of approaches in developing novel medical countermeasures for nerve agent poisoning. Neurotoxicology. 2014;44:27-38.
  3. Walton EL. Pralidoxime and pesticide poisoning: A question of severity? Biomed J. 2016;39(6):373-5.

Q.21. A 65-year-old male presents to emergency room with an alleged history of ingestion of 10 tablets of extended-release metoprolol (50 mg) three hours ago. On examination, he is dull, and afebrile and has a heart rate of 35/min, systolic blood pressure of 60 mm Hg, and respiratory rate of 15/min. Immediate fluid resuscitation is started and an electrocardiogram is taken which shows sinus bradycardia with prolonged QRS. Which of the following statements regarding further management is false?
   a. Whole bowel irrigation (WBI) may be attempted for gastric decontamination
   b. Intravenous calcium chloride 10 mL of 10% solution, may be given through peripheral line

c. High-dose insulin euglycemic therapy should be instituted in severe toxicity
d. Pacing should be considered in patients with persistent shock secondary to unstable bradycardia or high-grade conduction disturbances

Ans. b

Explanation: Whole bowel irrigation may be attempted for gastric decontamination even though >3 hours have elapsed, as the patient had consumed extended-release preparation. However, it should be ensured that the patient's airway is protected before attempting WBI. Calcium gluconate may be given through a peripheral line in a dose of 30 mL of 10% solution (3 g) followed by an infusion of 0.6–1.2 mL/kg/h. However, calcium chloride should preferably be given through a central line, in a dose of 10 mL of 10% solution (1 g) followed by an infusion of 0.2–0.4 mL/kg/h. High-dose insulin euglycemic therapy is an important component of management of β-blocker toxicity. It is especially indicated in patients with severe toxicity with myocardial dysfunction. The onset of effect occurs within 15–60 minutes; hence it should be initiated early, especially when there is a history of high-dose ingestion, even in the absence of profound hemodynamic instability. Glucagon is also recommended in a dose of 5–10 mg bolus followed by 1–10 mg/h, because of its positive inotropic and chronotropic actions. However, it does not have much role in improving blood pressure. Lipid emulsion therapy may also be considered as salvage therapy in patients with refractory shock, not responding to routine therapy. Cardiac pacing should be considered in patients with persistent shock secondary to unstable bradycardia or high-grade conduction disturbances, which does not respond to vasopressors, glucagon, and high-dose insulin euglycemic therapy.

Suggested Reading
1. Cave G, Harvey M. Intravenous lipid emulsion as antidote beyond local anesthetic toxicity: a systematic review. Acad Emerg Med. 2009;16:815-24.
2. Kerns W 2nd. Management of beta-adrenergic blocker and calcium channel antagonist toxicity. Emerg Med Clin North Am. 2007;25(2):309-31.
3. Palatnick W, Jelic T. Emergency department management of calcium-channel blocker, beta blocker, and digoxin toxicity. Emerg Med Pract. 2014;16(2):1-19;quiz 19-20.
4. Thanacoody R, Caravati EM, Troutman B, Höjer J, Benson B, Hoppu K, et al. Position paper update: whole bowel irrigation for gastrointestinal decontamination of overdose patients. Clin Toxicol (Phila). 2015;53(1):5-12.

Q.22. A 45-year-old farmer was brought to the emergency department by his family members with complaints of altered sensorium, nausea, vomiting, and diarrhea. According to the family, he accidentally sprayed an insecticide on his body while working in the field. On examination, his pulse rate was 114 beats/min and blood pressure was 130/74 mm Hg, pupils were pinpoint and he was drooling saliva from the corner of his mouth. Organophosphorus poisoning was suspected and treatment was initiated. The patient was started on supportive treatment with atropine and pralidoxime. The following statements are correct for organophosphorus poisoning except?

a. Red blood cell cholinesterase activity correlates with the severity of exposure and can guide treatment
b. In adults, muscarinic symptoms predominate, and in children, symptoms are predominated by stimulation of nicotinic receptors
c. Organophosphorus can be absorbed via the skin, inhalation, and gastrointestinal tract
d. Intermediate neurological symptoms are not observed before 72 hours of ingestion
e. Atropine should be administered before administration of pralidoxime to avoid worsening of muscarinic-mediated symptoms

Ans. d

Explanation: Organophosphorus poisoning can occur due to ingestion, inhalation, or dermal contact with pesticides. The first step in the management involves donning personal protective equipment to avoid cross-contamination to healthcare workers. Second step is decontaminating the patient by removing and destroying skin clothing and flushing the skin with water. Acute clinical features are a mix of muscarinic and nicotinic symptoms. Muscarinic symptoms such as salivation, lacrimation, urination, defecation/diaphoresis, gastrointestinal cramps, and emesis (SLUDGE) are most frequently followed by symptoms related to central nervous and nicotinic receptors. Intermediate (or delayed) symptoms such as neck flexor weakness, proximal muscle weakness, cranial nerve involvement, depressed deep tendon reflexes, and respiratory failure are typically observed 24–96 hours after exposure. The diagnosis is mainly clinical, with symptoms and a history of contact with organophosphorus insecticides. Red blood cells cholinesterase and not plasma cholinesterase levels correlate with neuronal cholinesterase levels, used to confirm the diagnosis, and levels correlate with severity.

Suggested Reading
1. Peter JV, Sudarsan TI, Moran JL. Clinical features of organophosphate poisoning: A review of different classification systems and approaches. Indian J Crit Care Med. 2014;18(11):735-45.
2. Robb EL, Baker MB. Organophosphate Toxicity. In: StatPearls [Internet]. Treasure Island (FL): StatPearls Publishing; 2023.

Q.23. Lipid emulsion therapy (LET) may be tried in all the following cases of severe toxicity as salvage therapy, except?
a. Lithium
b. Amlodipine
c. Carbamazepine
d. Metoprolol
e. Amitriptyline

Ans. a

Explanation: Lipid emulsion therapy has been accepted as standard therapy in the management of severe local anesthetic systemic toxicity (LAST). Additionally, it is now increasingly being used in patients with less severe forms of LAST and in patients with other systemic toxicities as salvage therapy. It has now been tried in >65 different drugs overdoses and has shown to have probable benefits in severe toxicities related to calcium channel blockers, β-blockers, certain antiepileptics and antipsychotics, barbiturates, and tricyclic antidepressants. However, in these patients, its utility is largely restricted to patients with cardiac arrest or life-threatening arrhythmias who are not responding to the standard medical therapies. It is suggested that when high doses of lipids are administered intravenously, they form a "lipid sink," where lipophilic drugs may get accumulated and are therefore removed from the circulation. This may reduce their harmful effects and prevent the development of complications related to their high systemic levels. About 20% of lipids are given in a bolus dose of 1.5 mL/kg followed by a maintenance dose at a rate of 0.25 mL/kg/min.

Suggested Reading
1. Cave G, Harvey M. Intravenous lipid emulsion as antidote beyond local anesthetic toxicity: a systematic review. Acad Emerg Med. 2009;16(9):815-24.
2. Jamaty C, Bailey B, Larocque A, Notebaert E, Sanogo K, Chauny JM. Lipid emulsions in the treatment of acute poisoning: a systematic review of human and animal studies. Clin Toxicol (Phila). 2010;48(1):1-27.
3. Picard J, Ward SC, Zumpe R, Meek T, Barlow J, Harrop-Griffiths W. Guidelines and the adoption of 'lipid rescue' therapy for local anaesthetic toxicity. Anaesthesia. 2009;64(2):122-5.
4. Weinberg GL. Lipid emulsion infusion: resuscitation for local anesthetic and other drug overdose. Anesthesiology. 2012;117(1):180-7.

Q.24. A 32-year-old farmer was brought to the emergency department by his family members after he was found unconscious in his field. According to the family members, the patient had been spraying herbicide in his fields for the past two days. On examination, the patient was unresponsive, had difficulty breathing, and had blue discoloration of his lips and nails. The patient's blood pressure was 78/46 mm Hg, and his pulse rate was 125 beats/min. The patient was suspected of paraquat poisoning and was immediately intubated and transferred to the intensive care unit. Which of the following statements about paraquat poisoning is true?
   a. Principal organ of involvement is the gastrointestinal tract
   b. The main mechanism of action is through blockage of voltage-gated sodium channels
   c. Most typical route of poisoning is dermal contact with an intact skin
   d. Supplemental oxygen to keep peripheral oxygen saturation above 95%
   e. Kidneys are the primary route of excretion for paraquat

Ans. e

Explanation: Paraquat is a highly toxic herbicide with structural similarity to polyamines and is preferentially concentrated in type I and type II alveolar cells responsible for its high lung concentration. Dermal contact does not cause poisoning, except if the skin is broken or there is prolonged exposure to contaminated clothes. Paraquat is actively secreted by kidneys, accumulates in proximal tubes, and is excreted unchanged. These are also the two primary organs of toxicity for paraquat. The mechanism of toxicity is an intracellular generation of free oxygen radicals leading to cellular damage. Paraquat poisoning can cause severe lung damage, kidney failure, and liver damage. Treatment of paraquat poisoning is mainly supportive, and there is no specific antidote. Charcoal hemoperfusion has been tried to remove paraquat, but rapid absorption and extensive tissue distribution are the barriers to its efficacy. Supplemental oxygen is avoided because of the increased production of free oxygen radicals, responsible for its cytotoxicity. The management of acute respiratory distress syndrome (ARDS) is similar to ARDS of any other etiology.

Suggested Reading
1. Gil HW, Hong JR, Jang SH, Hong SY. Diagnostic and therapeutic approach for acute paraquat intoxication. J Korean Med Sci. 2014;29(11):1441-9.
2. Sukumar CA, Shanbhag V, Shastry AB. Paraquat: The poison potion. Indian J Crit Care Med. 2019;23(Suppl 4):S263-6.

Q.25. Which of the following statements regarding cocaine-induced cardiac dysfunction is false?
   a. Chest pain is the most common manifestation
   b. Cocaine has a positive chronotropic and inotropic effect
   c. Beta-blockers should be avoided in patients with cocaine-induced myocardial ischemia
   d. Aspirin has no clinical role in the management of cocaine-induced acute coronary syndrome (ACS)

Ans. d

Explanation: Cocaine commonly leads to cardiotoxicity which is secondary to coronary vasoconstriction and accelerated atherosclerosis. It also stimulates platelet aggregation, which may increase the risk of thrombosis. The most common presentation of cardiotoxicity is chest pain. Further investigations must be carried out to rule out ACS and myocardial ischemia. Rarely, cocaine abuse may also lead to aortic dissection and rupture. Acute intoxication may also present with tachyarrhythmias or conduction blocks. The mainstay of therapy for cocaine-induced ACS is aspirin, nitrates, and benzodiazepines. Beta-blockers should be avoided in these patients as their use may cause unopposed alpha-adrenergic stimulation which may lead to further coronary vasoconstriction and worsening of myocardial ischemia.

Suggested Reading
1. Hollander JE. Cocaine intoxication and hypertension. Ann Emerg Med. 2008;51(3 Suppl):S18-20.
2. McCord J, Jneid H, Hollander JE, de Lemos JA, Cercek B, Hsue P, et al. Management of cocaine-associated chest pain and myocardial infarction: a scientific statement from the American Heart Association Acute Cardiac Care Committee of the Council on Clinical Cardiology. Circulation. 2008;117(14):1897-907.

Q.26. A 30-year-old male patient was brought to the emergency department with complaints of dry mouth, blurred vision, confusion, and disorientation. His friends reported that he had ingested some unidentified substance (seeds) and initially was in euphoria before developing an altered sensorium. On physical examination, the patient was febrile (38°C), had flushed dry skin, his pupils were dilated and unresponsive to light, and had a dry mouth with slurred speech. Patient's heart rate was 118/min, and blood pressure was 187/99 mm Hg. The medical history was unremarkable, and he was not taking any medications. What is the most likely diagnosis for the patient's symptoms?

a. Meningitis
b. Carbon monoxide poisoning
c. Acute alcohol intoxication
d. *Datura* poisoning
e. Mushroom poisoning

Ans. d

Explanation: The patient has symptoms of anticholinergic syndrome, including dry mouth, dry skin, hyperpyrexia, dilated pupils, delirium, confusion, and disorientation, which the ingestion of plants such as *Datura* can cause. The tachycardia and dilated, unresponsive pupils are also characteristic of *Datura* poisoning. Meningitis would present with symptoms such as fever, headache, and neck stiffness. Carbon monoxide poisoning would present with symptoms such as headache, nausea, and confusion. Acute alcohol intoxication would present with symptoms such as slurred speech, unsteady gait, and impaired judgment. Mushroom poisoning has mainly gastrointestinal symptoms. Diagnosis is mainly clinical. Failure to produce miosis with 2–3 drops of 1% pilocarpine can also be used for the bedside diagnosis. Physostigmine is the antidote. However, due to toxic side effects such as seizures, bradyarrhythmias, asystole, and hypotension, physostigmine is reserved for only severe toxicity, hypertensive emergency, convulsions, coma, arrhythmias, or severe hallucinations.

Suggested Reading
1. Krenzelok EP. Aspects of Datura poisoning and treatment. Clin Toxicol (Phila). 2010;48(2):104-10.
2. Pillay VV, Sasidharan A. Oleander and Datura poisoning: An Update. Indian J Crit Care Med. 2019;23(Suppl 4):S250-5.

Q.27. A 67-year-old female, presented with accidental ingestion of 12 tablets of 75 mg amitriptyline two hours before presentation. All the following statements regarding further management are true except?

a. Phenytoin is the drug of choice for tricyclic antidepressant (TCA) induced seizures
b. Sodium bicarbonate can reverse TCA-induced arrhythmias
c. Hypomagnesemia may precipitate TCA toxicity
d. There is no role for extracorporeal therapies

Ans. a

Explanation: Tricyclic antidepressant overdose is associated with significant cardiovascular and neurological symptoms. TCAs lead to sodium channel blockade which may prolong PR interval, QRS duration, and QTc and hence, behave like class Ia antiarrhythmic agents. Even though they are considered to be relatively safe in first-degree heart block and patients with right bundle branch block, they are contraindicated in second and third-degree, bifascicular, and alternating bundle branch blocks.

Neurological symptoms may range from delirium, agitation, altered mental status, seizures, and coma. Seizures are secondary to anticholinergic and GABA-A antagonism. However, deaths are generally secondary to cardiovascular complications. Electrolyte abnormalities including hypokalemia and hypomagnesemia may exacerbate TCA toxicity. Sodium bicarbonate is the treatment of choice, which increases plasma protein binding of TCAs and reduces their plasma levels and toxicity. Intravenous magnesium sulfate may be tried in patients with arrhythmias not responding to sodium bicarbonate therapy. Phenytoin's mechanism of action is similar to class Ia antiarrhythmic agents and hence, may worsen TCA toxicity and is therefore contraindicated. Benzodiazepines are the preferred agents for managing seizures in these patients. Even though some case reports suggested clinical utility of extracorporeal therapies in TCA removal, but current evidence suggests that TCAs are not dialyzable and hence extracorporeal therapies are not presently indicated.

Suggested Reading
1. Body R, Bartram T, Azam F, Mackway-Jones K. Guidelines in Emergency Medicine Network (GEMNet): guideline for the management of tricyclic antidepressant overdose. Emerg Med J. 2011;28(4):347-68.
2. Yates C, Galvao T, Sowinski KM, Mardini K, Botnaru T, Gosselin S, et al. Extracorporeal treatment for tricyclic antidepressant poisoning: recommendations from the EXTRIP Workgroup. Semin Dial. 2014;27(4):381-9.
3. Zima AV, Qin J, Fill M, Blatter LA. Tricyclic antidepressant amitriptyline alters sarcoplasmic reticulum calcium handling in ventricular myocytes. Am J Physiol Heart Circ Physiol. 2008;295(5):H2008-16.

Q.28. Four members of same family (husband, wife, and two sons) presented to the emergency department with complaints of nausea, vomiting, and abdominal pain for the past 12 hours. They reported accidentally consuming the Kaner plant (yellow oleander) seeds with "herbal tea." On examination, the husband (45 years/male) was conscious but anxious, had a heart rate of 72/min with Mobitz type II AV block, blood pressure of 90/60 mm Hg, and serum potassium of 6.8 mEq/L. Which of the following is the most appropriate management for the patient?
a. Administer digoxin-specific antibody
b. Administer atropine
c. Administer adrenaline
d. Administer sodium bicarbonate
e. Urgent hemodialysis

Ans. a

Explanation: Kaner, or yellow oleander (*Thevetia peruviana*), is a toxic plant found in many parts of the world, including India. All parts of the plant, especially seeds and roots, are cardiotoxic and contain cardiac glycosides, which can cause severe toxicity when ingested. It is used in traditional medicine for various minor ailments and as a cytotoxic agent for the treatment of cancer. The gastrointestinal symptoms are most common in yellow oleander poisoning, followed by cardiac arrhythmias (AV block and other bradyarrhythmias), hypotension, lethargy, and drowsiness. Digoxin assays are positive for suspected poisoning. Serum hyperkalemia is common and severe hyperkalemia (>6.5 mEq/L) is an indication for digoxin-specific antibody therapy. Other antihyperkalemic measures such as insulin-dextrose and calcium chloride should be administered, till antibodies are procured. Atropine can be used to treat bradycardia and AV conduction abnormalities, but it is not the initial treatment of choice. Cutaneous or temporary venous pacemaker is indicated for symptomatic AV blocks or higher degree AV blocks, who fail to respond to atropine.

Digoxin-specific antibodies (digoxin-specific Fab fragments) are the treatment of choice for severe symptomatic bradyarrhythmia with hypotension unresponsive to atropine, severe hyperkalemia, and life-threatening ventricular arrhythmias. Hypotension can be corrected with careful crystalloid administration. Adrenaline and sodium bicarbonate are not indicated in the management of yellow oleander poisoning. Hemodialysis or hemoperfusion is ineffective for cardiac glycoside poisoning because of its large volume of distribution and high protein binding.

Suggested Reading
1. Krenzelok EP. Aspects of Datura poisoning and treatment. Clin Toxicol (Phila). 2010;48(2):104-10.
2. Pillay VV, Sasidharan A. Oleander and Datura poisoning: An update. Indian J Crit Care Med. 2019;23(Suppl 4):S250-5.

Q.29. A 35-year-old woman with a history of depression is brought to the emergency department after being found in a confused state at her home, with a swollen face, and difficulty in speaking. The patient was recently going through a tough divorce. Her family members found an empty bottle of Super Vasmol hair dye next to her. On examination, the patient is confused, with swollen face and neck, difficulty in opening mouth and swollen tongue, dilated pupils, and shallow breathing. The initial blood workup reveals high anion gap metabolic acidosis. Her peripheral oxygen saturation (SpO_2) is 95% on room air, her blood pressure is 146/78 mm Hg, and her pulse rate is 110/min. Which of the following is the most immediate management of the patient in the emergency department?
a. Immediate tracheostomy/cricothyrotomy
b. Rapid-sequence induction and intubation
c. Intravenous (IV) sodium bicarbonate
d. IV hydrocortisone
e. High-flow oxygen therapy

Ans. a

Explanation: The active ingredients of Super Vasmol hair dye contains paraphenylenediamine (PPD), resorcinol, propylene glycol, and cetostearyl alcohol. PPD is the key ingredient for toxicity. It causes free-radical-induced cytotoxicity and local irritation by its metabolites (quinone diamine) causing bullous edema limited to the face and neck. Quinone diamine also induces rhabdomyolysis and acute kidney injury (AKI) due to myoglobin casts.

The patient's presentation needs emergency surgical management of life-threatening airway obstruction. Tracheostomy is preferred over cricothyroidotomy for an emergency surgical airway because of extensive neck swelling and difficulty in identifying landmarks. Early endotracheal intubation before edema is overwhelming, or prophylactic intubation can avoid tracheostomy. Antihistaminics and steroids do not help in life-threatening airway emergencies and take time. IV hydration is required to reduce myoglobin cast-induced AKI. There is no role of hemodialysis in the elimination of PPD. High anion-gap metabolic acidosis is caused by propylene glycol and may need fomepizole or hemodialysis in case of central pathology.

Suggested Reading
1. Senthilkumaran S, Jena NN, Thirumalaikolundusubramanian P. Super Vasmol Poisoning: Dangers of darker shade. Indian J Crit Care Med. 2019;23(Suppl 4):S287-9.
2. Yadla M, Sailaja S, Ahmed N, Uppin M, Arlappa N. An unusual case of insecticide poisoning presenting as acute kidney injury. Saudi J Kidney Dis Transpl. 2017;28(6):1432-4.

Q.30. A 32-year-old woman with a history of bipolar disorder was brought to the emergency department by her family after they found her unconscious at home. She was prescribed sodium valproate by a psychiatrist for 3 months. According to the family, she had been very depressed and anxious for the past few days and took sodium valproate irregularly. On examination, the patient was comatose, with shallow breathing; pupils were bilaterally constricted but reacting to light. Her blood pressure was 84/60 mm Hg, and her SpO$_2$ was 95% on a high-flow oxygen mask at 10 L/min. Arterial blood gas showed respiratory and metabolic acidosis. She was immediately intubated and resuscitated with intravenous fluids. Blood tests revealed a serum valproic acid level of 1,060 µg/mL (therapeutic range: 50–125 µg/mL), and serum ammonia levels of 98 µg/dL (normal, 9–33). What is the most appropriate management for this patient?
a. Administer activated charcoal
b. Perform gastric lavage
c. Administer naloxone
d. Administer intravenous fluids and supportive care
e. Urgent hemodialysis

Ans. e

Explanation: Sodium valproate (2-propylpentanoic acid) is a branched-chain carboxylic acid used to treat epilepsy (partial and generalized seizures), acute mania, and bipolar disorders and is also prescribed as prophylaxis for migraine headaches. The overdose can lead to severe central nervous system depression, respiratory depression, hepatotoxicity, and hypotension. The laboratory abnormalities include hypernatremia, hypocalcemia, hyperammonemia, and high anion-gap metabolic acidosis. The first step in managing this patient is stabilizing her vital signs and providing supportive care, including airway management, oxygenation, and intravenous fluids to maintain blood pressure. Activated charcoal and gastric lavage may be considered within the first hour of ingestion, but their effectiveness decreases with time, and the risk of complications may outweigh the benefits. Naloxone is not indicated in sodium valproate overdose as it does not reverse its effects. Carnitine binds to valproic acid, forming valproylcarnitine that is renally excreted, and should be considered in patients with coma, hepatoxicity, and severe hyperammonemia. Valproate has a low molecular weight and low volume of distribution. Hemodialysis is very effective for the elimination of sodium valproate. The indications include coma, shock, cerebral edema, or valproate concentration >1,300 µg/mL.

Suggested Reading
1. Murty S. Antiepileptic overdose. Indian J Crit Care Med. 2019;23 (Suppl 4):S290-5.
2. Nasa P, Sehrawat D, Kansal S, Chawla R. Effectiveness of hemodialysis in a case of severe valproate overdose. Indian J Crit Care Med. 2011;15(2):120-2.

CHAPTER

Obstetric Critical Care

Manu MK Varma, Karun Mahesh KP, Impashree CM

Questions 1–6
A postpartum mother is shifted to intensive care unit (ICU). The obstetrician is anticipating that the patient is at high risk for postpartum hemorrhage as it requires instrumentation for delivery. The patient is coconscious and oriented but has complains of pain in pelvic region. She has a functioning epidural catheter that was inserted just over an hour ago upon admission with spontaneous rupture of amniotic membranes. All prior deliveries were spontaneous and uncomplicated. She has intravenous cannula in each arm, an oxygen face mask, continuous pulse oximetry readings show >95% saturation and blood pressure is 90/50 mm Hg with a pulse rate at 115 bpm; an indwelling urine catheter with clear-colored urine.

Q.1. Which of the following timeline, from delivery of the fetus, is close to the clinical definition of primary postpartum hemorrhage (PPH) and secondary PPH?
  a. Primary PPH occurs in <12 hours of delivery and secondary PPH occurs after 12 hours.
  b. Primary PPH occurs in <24 hours of delivery and secondary PPH occurs between 24 hours.
  c. Primary PPH occurs in <48 hours of delivery and secondary PPH occurs between 48 hours.
  d. Primary PPH occurs within the first 72 hours of delivery and secondary PPH occurs between 72 hours.

  Ans. b

Q.2. The gravid mother is more efficient to adapt to acute blood loss due to the following hemodynamic changes except:
  a. Increase in the total red cell mass
  b. Increase in the plasma volume
  c. Increase in the cardiac output
  d. Increase in the systemic vascular resistance

  Ans. d

Q.3. What is the least appropriate step in the management of the above patient?
  a. Ringer lactate fluid bolus
  b. Epidural analgesia with 0.25% bupivacaine

c. Oxytocin infusion
d. Tranexamic acid intravenous injection

Ans. b

Q.4. Epidemiologically what would be the most probable cause of PPH in the above described patient?
   a. Retained placenta
   b. Defects in coagulation
   c. Vaginal laceration
   d. Uterine atony

Ans. d

Q.5. In the medical management of the above patient, which of the following should be avoided if she was to be asthmatic?
   a. Oxytocin
   b. Methergine
   c. Mesoprost
   d. Carboprost

Ans. d

Q.6. Which of the following parameters is least likely to be affected in pregnancy?
   a. Systolic blood pressure
   b. Cardiac output
   c. Systemic vascular resistance
   d. Serum colloid oncotic pressure

Ans. a

Explanation (Q.1–6): Primary PPH occurs in <24 hours of delivery of the fetus. The secondary PPH can occur up to 6 weeks after delivery. Though many risk factors have been identified, uterine atony is the most common cause. The hemodynamic changes in pregnancy include increase in the blood volume (both red blood cells and plasma), heart rate, and cardiac output. Characteristically the systemic vascular resistance will reduce to facilitate the increase in the cardiac output. Administration of uterotonics along with fluid resuscitation remains the first line in the management of PPH. If the hemorrhage is not controlled in next 30 minutes, then the next line of management includes balloon tamponade, arterial embolization and/or laparotomy. The results from World Maternal Antifibrinolytic (WOMAN) trial, has shown the beneficial effects of tranexamic acid.

Suggested Reading
1. Dobos NM, Crozier TM, McLintock C. Peripartum hemorrhage. In: Einav S, Weiniger CF, Landau R (Eds). Principles and Practice of Maternal Critical Care. Cham: Springer; 2020. pp. 59-74.
2. Liu S, Jassal DS, Zelop CM. Cardiovascular changes in pregnancy. In: Einav S, Weiniger CF, Landau R (Eds). Principles and Practice of Maternal Critical Care. Cham: Springer; 2020. pp. 101-8.

Q.7. Nonstress test (NST) is primarily a test of fetal distress. It describes fetal heart rate acceleration in response to fetal movement perceived by the mother. The following are the abnormal NST, except:
   a. Baseline oscillation of <5 bpm
   b. Absent accelerations as well as beat-to-beat variability

c. Late decelerations with spontaneous uterine contractions
d. >15 bpm above baseline for >15 seconds, but <2 minutes, and all occurring within 20 minutes of beginning the test

Ans. d

Explanation: The range of normal baseline fetal heart rate (bFHR) is between 110 and 160. This is the mean level of fetal heart rate over 10-minute period. Normally there is a swing of heart rate above and below this baseline known as baseline variability. Characteristically it varies from 5 to 25 beats over a minute. The decrease in FHR to less than bFHR by at least 15/minute lasting at least 15 seconds is referred to as deceleration and is usually signals fetal distress. Prolonged nonvariable deceleration lasting more than contraction period is an indicator of pathological fetal hypoxemia.

Suggested Reading
1. Enabudoso E. Electronic fetal monitoring. In: Okonofua F, Balogun JA, Odunsi K, Victor N. Chilaka VN (Eds). Contemporary Obstetrics and Gynecology for Developing Countries, 2nd edition. Switzerland AG: Springer Nature; 2021. pp. 159-73.

Questions 8–11
A 30-year-old primigravida with 32 weeks of gestation is brought to hospital following a road traffic accident. She was the restrained driver of a vehicle driving on a skiddy road at around 50 mph (80 km/hour), when she lost control and had a frontal impact collision with another vehicle. She is a booked pregnancy and had an unremarkable pregnancy till date. On arrival, she is alert but appears anxious and uncomfortable. Her cervical spine is immobilized with a cervical collar and she is on a spinal board. She complains of pain in her chest and lower abdomen. There is a bruise across her right forehead. Her vital signs show a sinus tachycardia of 115 bpm, blood pressure 87/62 mm Hg, pulse oximetry 94% on room air, and respiratory rate 28/minute. She is being monitored with invasive central line and arterial catheters.

Q.8. Which of the following about initial management is false?
  a. As with all trauma patients, the initial assessment of the airway, breathing, circulation disability, and extremities takes precedence.
  b. Fetal heart rate should be assessed in primary survey.
  c. Tranexamic acid should be considered in the setting of trauma hemorrhage.
  d. Anti-D immunoglobulin G (IgG) should be administered within 72 hours to all Rh-negative mothers who present to the hospital after trauma.

Ans. b

Suggested Reading
1. Lopez CE, Salloum J, Varon AJ, Toledo P, Dudaryk R. The management of pregnant trauma patients: a narrative review. Anesth Analg. 2023;136(5):830-40.

Q.9. After a primary survey, you decide to administer analgesic for the mild headache that she complains. Which of the following is the analgesic of choice?
  a. Paracetamol
  b. Diclofenac
  c. Fentanyl
  d. Morphine

Ans. a

Q.10. The monitor is showing decrease in oxygen saturation. She is drowsy and does not obey simple commands. What is the best approach to improve oxygenation?
   a. Initiate noninvasive ventilation
   b. Initiate invasive positive pressure ventilation
   c. Initiate high flow nasal cannula
   d. Continue spontaneous ventilation on the room air

   Ans. b

Q.11. The patient develops hypotension, a bolus of crystalloid is administered. Which of the following is false about the resuscitation of this patient?
   a. Supine the patient and rise the leg
   b. Norepinephrine is the first choice of vasopressor.
   c. Vasopressin is uterotonic, hence not used as first line vasopressor in pregnancy.
   d. Ephedrine has favorable effect on uterine blood flow but increases risk of fetal acidosis.

   Ans. a

   Explanation (Q.8–11): As in any critically ill patients, if the respiratory distress is expected to be reversed in short time, noninvasive ventilation can be attempted in gravid mother only if she is able to protect airway with good spontaneous ventilation. But the risk of gastric distension and aspiration is relatively higher. Due to progressive increase in size of the uterus, supine positioning will lead to compression of inferior vena cava and hence hypotension. To avoid this supine hypotension, a 15° tilt or displacement of uterus to left should be done.

   Opioids cause neonatal respiratory depression, benzodiazepines have the risk of withdrawal syndrome in neonates. Nonsteroidal anti-inflammatory drugs (NSAIDs) are at the high risk for delayed closure of ductus arteriosus. Relatively paracetamol is safer analgesic in pregnancy.

   Vasopressor agents can alter uterine blood flow and can have effects on uterine contractions and fetal pH. Vasopressin in uterotonic, ephedrine decrease fetal pH, adrenaline can cause fetal dysrhythmias. Noradrenaline is relatively safer vasoconstrictor in pregnancy.

Suggested Reading
1. Banerjee A, Cantellow S. Maternal critical care: part I. BJA Educ. 2021;21(4):140-7.
2. Lopez CE, Salloum J, Varon AJ, Toledo P, Dudaryk R. The management of pregnant trauma patients: a narrative review. Anesth Analg. 2023;36(5):830-40.
3. Sela HY, Rottenstreich M. Trauma during pregnancy. In: Einav S, Weiniger CF, Landau R (Eds). Principles and Practice of Maternal Critical Care. Cham: Springer; 2020. pp. 465-83.
4. Teoh WH. Airway management during pregnancy and the peripartum period. In: Principles and Practice of Maternal Critical Care. New York: Springer; 2020:285-304.

Questions 12–14
A 30-year-old primigravida at 32 weeks gestation is admitted to the ICU with sepsis secondary to suspected pneumonia.

Obstetric Critical Care   **337**

Q.12. The family expresses its concerns on the effects of medications, investigations on the fetus. What should be the most appropriate advice to the family?
  a. Necessary investigations and drugs to save the mother should not be withheld.
  b. Investigations with adverse fetal effects will be avoided.
  c. Drugs with adverse fetal effects will be avoided.
  d. None of the above.

Ans. a

Q.13. Which of the following statement about the maternal sepsis is false?
  a. The physiology of normal pregnancy and response to labor can mask the presence of sepsis.
  b. Obstetric infections are usually monomicrobial.
  c. Chorioamnionitis should be suspected if there is foul-smelling liquor, pyrexia, maternal and fetal tachycardia.
  d. Termination of pregnancy is not indicated in pregnancy because of sepsis.

Ans. b

Q.14. Which of the following scores has shown to be better mortality prediction in septic obstetric patients?
  a. Acute Physiology and Chronic Health Evaluation II (APACHE II)
  b. Modified Obstetric Early Warning Scoring Systems (MOEWS)
  c. Sequential Organ Failure Assessment (SOFA)
  d. Sepsis in Obstetrics Score (SOS)

Ans. c

Explanation (Q.12–14): The physiological changes in pregnancy are bound to cover up the inflammatory response seen in sepsis. Tachypnea, tachycardia, leukocytosis, hyperlactatemia and increase in temperature are common in pregnancy. Obstetric infections are usually polymicrobial with group A *Streptococcus* and *Escherichia (E.) coli* being the most common organisms associate with maternal mortality. The sepsis detection scores are based on organ failures and not on inflammatory response and seem to be predicting mortality. But there are limited validated studies available.

Suggested Reading
1. Banerjee A, Cantellow S. Maternal critical care: part I. BJA Educ. 2021;21(4):140-7.
2. Banerjee A, Cantellow S. Maternal critical care: part II. BJA Educ. 2021;21(5):164-71.
3. Friedman AM, Ananth CV. Maternal deaths in developed countries: epidemiology and preventable causes. In: Principles and Practice of Maternal Critical Care. New York: Springer; 2020. pp. 3-12.

Q.15. Which of the following positions has highest functional residual capacity (FRC) in the pregnant woman?
  a. Upright position
  b. Supine position
  c. Supine with 30° head up position
  d. All of the above have same FRC

Ans. a

Q.16. Which of the following positions has the least cardiac output in the pregnant woman?
   a. Knee chest position
   b. Supine position
   c. Sitting position
   d. Standing position

   Ans. d

   Explanation (Q.15–16): The physiological respiratory changes in pregnancy include decrease in functional residual capacity (FRC), with increase in the tidal volume. The FRC reduces in supine position than in upright position. A pregnant woman in distress will benefit from supine with head-end elevation.

   Suggested Reading
   1. Izakson A, Cohen Y, Landau R. Physiologic changes in the airway and the respiratory system affecting management in pregnancy. In: Einav S, Weiniger CF, Landau R (Eds). Principles and Practice of Maternal Critical Care. Cham: Springer; 2020. pp. 271-83.

Q.17. All of the following patients meet clinical criteria for antiphospholipid syndrome (APS) testing except:
   a. A 29-year-old with a deep vein thrombosis (DVT) who is 36 weeks pregnant.
   b. A 60-year-old with retinal arterial thrombosis.
   c. An 18-year-old with three missed abortions at 6 weeks.
   d. A 30-year-old with a history of severe preeclampsia requiring delivery at 35 weeks gestation.

   Ans. d

Q.18. Which of the following is true regarding lupus anticoagulant?
   a. It is an anticoagulant.
   b. Testing involves screening and then a second confirmatory test.
   c. Results are reported as low, medium, or high levels.
   d. It can be tested while the patient is treated with anticoagulation.

   Ans. b

   Explanation (Q.17–18): APS is characterized by clinical features of recurrent venous and arterial thrombosis and/or pregnancy loss along with presence of anticardiolipin antibody and lupus anticoagulant. The lupus anticoagulant is a misnomer. It has a laboratory artefact that causes increase in activated partial thromboplastin time (aPTT) with minimal to no effect on prothrombin time.

   Suggested Reading
   1. Patel SN, Shander A. Physiology and pathology of coagulation in pregnancy. In: Einav S, Weiniger CF, Landau R (Eds). Principles and Practice of Maternal Critical Care. Switzerland: Springer; 2020. pp. 47-57.

Questions 19–23
A healthy 25-year-old primigravida at 27 weeks of gestation presents to the obstetric outpatient with 2–3 days history of intermittent right lower limb swelling and pain. While

waiting in the OPD, the woman has develops giddiness and becomes unresponsive. The rapid response team is activated and cardiopulmonary resuscitation (CPR) is initiated as central pulse was absent.

Q.19. Which of the following is not the standard practices of CPR in this patient?
   a. Chest compressions should be aimed at midsternal area.
   b. The chest compression to breathing ratio without a definitive airway is 30:2.
   c. Left lateral displacement of uterus.
   d. Defibrillation (if required) to be administered in standard energy levels.

   Ans. a

Q.20. On evaluation, a deep vein thrombus in the right lower limb was seen and a possibility of pulmonary thromboembolism was suspected. Even after return of spontaneous circulation (ROSC), the blood pressure does not improve with fluids and vasopressors. There are no obvious features of hemorrhage. The team decides to administer thrombolytic agent. Which of the following is the best approach?
   a. The diagnosis should be confirmed with D-dimer levels.
   b. Patient should be shifted to CT pulmonary angiogram (CTPA) for confirmation of diagnosis.
   c. Thrombolysis should be administered as soon as possible.
   d. Warfarin is the immediate choice of anticoagulation.

   Ans. c

Q.21. The patient is shifted to medical ICU (MICU) for further management. What is the therapy of choice for anticoagulation?
   a. Warfarin
   b. LMWH
   c. Oral Ecosprin
   d. Rivaroxaban

   Ans. b

Q.22. A possibility of autoimmune disease was suspected in this patient. Which of the following autoimmune diseases may flare up during pregnancy?
   a. Rheumatoid arthritis
   b. Psoriasis
   c. Graves' disease
   d. Systemic lupus erythematosus (SLE)

   Ans. d

Q.23. Which of the following disease-modifying drugs can be used for autoimmune diseases in pregnancy?
   a. Mycophenolate mofetil
   b. Leflunomide
   c. Sulfasalazine
   d. Cyclophosphamide

   Ans. c

Explanation (Q.19–23): The position of the heart is not affected in pregnancy. As in adult cardiopulmonary resuscitation (CPR) the hand position for chest compressions should be the center of the chest. But possibility of vena caval compression should be considered and uterus should be displaced while CPR. In a patient with pulmonary embolism, hemodynamic instability is marker of right heart dysfunction and the obstruction should be relieved by thrombolysis as soon as possible.

Anticoagulation is the mainstay of treatment in venous thromboembolism. In a gravid woman, long acting should be avoided. Warfarin is associated with increased risk for hemorrhage. Also, it can cause fetal abnormalities if used in early pregnancy. Heparin and low molecular weight heparin are relatively safer in pregnancy as they have better pharmacokinetics and pharmacodynamics.

The changes in immunological system are well described in pregnancy. The first trimester is characterized by proinflammation, which facilitates implantation, placentation, and protection against infection. Next comes the stage of immunological tolerance with anti-inflammatory Th2-predominant stage allowing rapid growth and development of the fetus. In third trimester, the proinflammatory stage returns to facilitate uterine contractions. The diseases with Th1 response such as rheumatoid arthritis, multiple sclerosis, psoriasis, and Graves' disease have a tendency to improve with pregnancy. However in the postpartum period, with sudden fall of estrogen levels, can flare up these diseases, whereas the diseases with Th2 response such as atopic eczema, SLE, and systemic sclerosis have a tendency to flare up.

Immunosuppressants such as methotrexate, mycophenolate mofetil, leflunomides, and cyclophosphamide are known to have teratogenic effects and should be avoided. Disease-modifying drugs such as hydroxychloroquine, sulfasalazine, mesalazine and azathioprine, and the calcineurin inhibitors ciclosporin and tacrolimus have favorable profile in pregnancy.

Suggested Reading
1. Jeejeebhoy FM, Zelop CM, Lipman S, Carvalho B, Joglar J, Mhyre JM, et al. Cardiac arrest in pregnancy: a scientific statement from the American Heart Association. Circulation. 2015;132(18):1747-73.
2. Narayan B, Nelson-Piercy C. Physiological changes of the immune system during pregnancy. In: Einav S, Weiniger CF, Landau R. (Eds). Principles and Practice of Maternal Critical Care. Cham: Springer; 2020. pp. 201-13.
3. Peltola L, Plaat F. Maternal resuscitation. In: Einav S, Weiniger CF, Landau R (Eds). Principles and Practice of Maternal Critical Care, 1st edition. Switzerland: Springer; 2020. pp. 373-82.
4. Simcox LE, Ormesher L, Tower C, Greer IA. Pulmonary thrombo-embolism in pregnancy: diagnosis and management. Breathe. 2015;11(4):282-9.

Questions 24-26
A 23-year-old primigravida in 32nd week of pregnancy is shifted to hospital with the seizures. She is administered with injection lorazepam 4 mg, but she continues to have convulsions. She is intubated for airway protection, and monitor shows a blood pressure of 200/100 and SpO$_2$ of 91% on room air.

Q.24. Which of the following is the least appropriate of the management in the above clinical condition?
   a. Stabilization of blood pressure
   b. Prevention of further seizure activity

c. Safe delivery of the fetus
d. To do magnetic resonance imaging (MRI) of brain to confirm diagnosis.

Ans. d

Q.25. **Which of the following is false about the neuroimaging in this patient?**
a. CT highly sensitive for subarachnoid blood, large masses, and early stroke evaluation.
b. The fetal radiation exposure during cerebral CT imaging with shielding is minimal (-10 mrads).
c. MRI has the advantage of being magnetic based, and therefore having no radiation exposure.
d. The use of MRI contrast (gadolinium) is considered safe in pregnancy.

Ans. d

Q.26. **The first-line intravenous (IV) drug for blood pressure control in this patient is:**
a. Hydralazine
b. Labetalol
c. Esmolol
d. Nitroprusside

Ans. b

Explanation (Q.24–26): Any seizure episode should be treated as eclampsia till the definitive diagnosis is made. After initial management of airway, breathing and circulation, prevention of further seizure episodes should be the priority. This should be followed by the differential diagnosis and safe delivery of the fetus. Risks and safety of the neuroimaging should be considered. MRI is the safe modality and avoid IV gadolinium as much as possible. Beta blockers are the first choice of management in high blood pressure. Oral or intravenous infusion of labetalol is often used as it has lesser adverse effects. The goal is to control blood pressure without compromising the uteroplacental perfusion and approach depends on the expected time to delivery.

Suggested Reading
1. Feat MJ. Pre-eclampsia and eclampsia in critical care. In: Bryden D, Temple A (Eds). Case Studies in Adult Intensive Care Medicine. Cambridge: Cambridge University Press; 2017. pp. 232-8.
2. Wiles R, Hankinson B, Benbow E, Sharp A. Making decisions about radiological imaging in pregnancy. BMJ. 2022;377:e070486.

Q.27. **A 35-year-old diabetic, is in follow-up with gynecologist and physician, presents at 33 weeks gestation with malaise, vomiting, and Kussmaul breathing. Vital signs are blood pressure 140/70 mm Hg, heart rate 110 beats/minute, respiratory rate 25 breaths/minute, and temperature 37°C. Which of the following is false in the statement?**
a. Pregnancy constitutes a state of insulin resistance.
b. Intravascular volume repletion, electrolyte correction, and insulin injection form the mainstay of the treatment.

c. Sodium bicarbonate can cause right shift of oxyhemoglobin dissociation curve.
d. Pregnancy is risk factor for euglycemic ketoacidosis.

Ans. c

Explanation: Pregnancy is a state of relative insulin deficiency with a tendency for ketosis. These two factors decrease the threshold for diabetic ketoacidosis. The consumption of glucose by the fetus results in relative reduction in blood glucose level in the maternal serum. This predisposes the patient to euglycemic ketoacidosis. Fluid resuscitation, electrolyte correction and followed by the insulin infusion remain the sequence of the treatment in diabetic ketoacidosis (DKA). Sodium bicarbonate increases the oxygen dissociation curve to the left.

Suggested Reading
1. Sibai BM, Viteri OA. Diabetic ketoacidosis in pregnancy. Obstet Gynecol. 2014;123(1):167-78.
2. Witcher PM, Graves CR. Role of insulin in normal metabolism. In: Troiano NH, Witcher PM, Baird S (Eds). AWHONN's High-Risk and Critical Care Obstetrics. Netherlands: Wolters Kluwer; 2018.

Questions 28–29
A 38-year-old G5P4 with a twin pregnancy presents to the obstetric emergency assessment at 9th month of gestation with dyspnea and bilateral lower limb swelling. She has no complaints related to obstetrics. On examination, she is in tachypnea, hypoxemia requiring high flow of oxygen, high blood pressure, and cold peripheries. The bedside thoracic ultrasound shows pulmonary edema with diastolic dysfunction. She is conscious and had told that she has not suffered from any chronic disease prior to this pregnancy. A clinical diagnosis of heart failure was made by the multidisciplinary team and patient is shifted to MICU for further management.

Q.28. What is the most likely diagnosis in this patient?
   a. Peripartum cardiomyopathy
   b. Dilated cardiomyopathy
   c. Hypertrophic cardiomyopathy
   d. Ebstein's anomaly

Ans. a

Q.29. Which of the following is true about her further management?
   a. Noninvasive ventilation is an absolute contraindication in this patient.
   b. Ramipril can be administered for hypertension.
   c. Heparin is indicated for DVT prophylaxis and anticoagulation.
   d. Aldosterone antagonists can be considered for diuresis.

Ans. c

Explanation (Q.28–29): Peripartum cardiomyopathy is characterized by echocardiographic evidence of left ventricular dysfunction with dilated cardiomyopathy. It is typically seen between the last month of pregnancy and 5 months postpartum. Multiparity, elderly mother and preeclampsia are the common risk factors. Usually the preexisting cardiac conditions are manifested in the first two trimester of pregnancy. The management of peripartum cardiomyopathy (PPCM) is use of hydralazines, nitrates, beta blockers. Anticoagulation is indicated for deep venous thrombosis prophylaxis.

Suggested Reading
1. Austine O, Henry AO. Cardiovascular diseases in pregnancy. In: Okonofua F, Balogun JA, Odunsi K, Chilaka VN (Eds). Contemporary Obstetrics and Gynecology for Developing Countries. Cham: Springer. 2021. pp. 269-80.
2. Simcox LE, Ormesher L, Tower C, Greer IA. Pulmonary thrombo-embolism in pregnancy: diagnosis and management. Breathe. 2015;11(4):282-9.

The 27-week pregnant patient is admitted in ICU with the consumption of 100 tablets of unknown name 2 hours back. She is conscious, oriented, with stable oxygenation and hemodynamics.

Q.30. Which of the following is false in further management of this patient?
   a. Gastric lavage is contraindicated as she is at high risk of aspiration.
   b. Gastric lavage is indicated but is of little use as she is presented after 1 hour.
   c. If this is paracetamol tablets, N-acetyl cysteine should be administered to avoid liver injury.
   d. If this is iron tablets deferoxamine can be administered.

Ans. b

Explanation: The pregnancy is characterized by delayed gastric emptying. Hence the oral activated charcoal can be tried beyond 1 hour of toxin ingestion up to 4 hours. The line of management will be similar to toxin ingestion like any other adults.

Suggested Reading
1. Cumpston KL, Erickson TB, Leikin JB. Poisoning in pregnancy. In: Critical Care Toxicology: Diagnosis and Management of the Critically Poisoned Patient. Philadelphia: Elsevier Mosby. 2005. p. 134.

CHAPTER

End of Life/Transplant

Nishant Agrawal, Jignesh Shah

Q.1. Which of the following should be used as a first line of treatment for the management of acute rejection of a renal allograft?
  a. Cyclosporin
  b. Plasmapheresis
  c. 500 mg intravenous (IV) methylprednisolone
  d. Antithymocyte globulin

Ans. c

Explanation: Cell-mediated acute rejection typically manifests within the first 6 months following renal transplantation. Acute T cell-mediated rejection and acute antibody-mediated rejection are the two types of acute rejection recognized histologically.

Suggested Reading
  1. Burton SA, Amir N, Asbury A, Lange A, Hardinger KL. Treatment of antibody-mediated rejection in renal transplant patients: a clinical practice survey. Clin Transplant. 2015;29(2):118-23.

Q.2. Following a renal transplant, delayed graft function is described as:
  a. Dialysis is necessary within 7 days of transplantation.
  b. Even after transplantation, the serum creatinine level failed to drop.
  c. A week of urine output of <0.5 mL/kg.
  d. Proteinuria >1 g/day

Ans. a

Explanation: Most frequently, it is described as requiring dialysis within 7 days of the transplant. Following renal transplantation, it is characterized by acute tubular necrosis.

Suggested Reading
  1. Siedlecki A, Irish W, Brennan DC. Delayed graft function following kidney transplant. Int J Transplant. 2011;11(11):2279-96.

Q.3. A total of 5 hours after receiving a kidney transplant from a live donor, a 65-year-old man is complaining of abdominal discomfort. Despite a 1:1 replacement of fluids, the nurse caring for him notices that the urinary catheter has not drained any urine in the last 2 hours (1 mL of crystalloid being transfused for every milliliter (mL) of

urine output in the previous hour). The catheter not being obstructed is eliminated. What among the following is most likely to be the cause?
   a. Rupture of the urinary bladder
   b. Thrombosis of the renal arteries
   c. Postoperative bleeding
   d. Extremely rapid rejection

Ans. b

Explanation: Usually leading to graft loss, renal artery thrombosis is a severe post-transplant complication. Multiple renal arteries, hypercoagulable state, and hypotension are the risk factors.

Suggested Reading
1. Humar A, Matas AJ. After-kidney transplant surgical complications. Semin Dial. 2005;18(6):505-10.

Q.4. Which of the following is true about the idea of "respect for autonomy"?
   a. A credible threat can be used to coerce a patient into receiving treatment.
   b. A patient may be convinced to undergo treatment using a strong argument.
   c. The duty of physicians is to "do whatever the patient wants".
   d. There is no way that a doctor can be held responsible for injuries that result from not providing treatment if a patient refuses a treatment.

Ans. b

Explanation: The patients must be fully informed of the risks, advantages, and alternative treatment options, according to the autonomy concept. The act of persuading someone by making persuasive arguments can be a part of the informational process about various treatment options.

Suggested Reading
1. Waisel DB, Truog RD. Conscientious consent. Anesthesiology. 1997;87(4):968978.

Q.5. A 62-year-old man who was admitted to the intensive care unit (ICU) needs noninvasive ventilation (NIV) support because his breathing is working harder than it should. The results of a thorough evaluation of the CT scan point to lung cancer that has spread to the liver. Prior to disclosing results of imaging to the patient, the patient's wife requests to speak with you privately. She states that her husband does not wish to know anything regarding his condition. What is the most suitable course of action?
   a. Determine the basis for the wife's assertion that her husband is reluctant to discuss his diagnosis.
   b. Inquire about the patient's preferences for learning about imaging results, likely diagnoses, and treatment plans.
   c. Determine the patient's decision-making capacity in more detail.
   d. Involve the ethics committee in the assessment of the patient's decision-making capacity.

Ans. b

Explanation: Patient autonomy includes the power to choose which treatments he/she will and will not accept. In order to exercise autonomy, a patient must be given the freedom to choose his/her own medical treatment, armed with sufficient information and free from outside pressure. Making a family member a healthcare proxy is a decision that must be made by the patient alone, with the understanding that additional medical information may be withheld from them. In this case, a conversation with the patient would need to take place first.

Suggested Reading

1. Entwistle VA, Carter SM, Cribb A, McCaffery K. Supporting patient autonomy: the significance of relationships between clinicians and patients. J Gen Intern Med. 2010;25(7):741-5.

Q.6. A 78-year-old man who has 1.5 mg/dL of serum bilirubin and slightly elevated liver function tests is admitted. Temperature is 37.1°C, and serum amylase and lipase levels are normal. His magnetic resonance cholangiopancreatography revealed that he had choledocholithiasis [magnetic resonance cholangiopancreatography (MRCP)]. Which of the following discussions with the patient when getting his consent for an endoscopic retrograde cholangiopancreatography (ERCP) is the least appropriate?

a. The diagnosis of choledocholithiasis and need for additional procedures after ERCP.
b. Propose and explain ERCP and alternative treatment options.
c. The contact information of family members not present.
d. The risks of refusing treatment.

Ans. c

Explanation: A doctor's duty to provide care is both legally and morally mandated.

A patient should receive adequate information about medical procedures so that he/she can process it and make the best decision possible. As part of informed consent followings are notables:

1. Justification for the action and its goal, as well as any potential need for additional actions
2. Procedure explanation
3. Additional options
4. Procedure risks and advantages
5. Pitfalls of forgoing treatment
   Unless the doctor determines that the patient does not have.

Family members or a healthcare proxy do not need to be contacted or present during consent for the procedure if the patient lacks decisional capacity (is intoxicated, delirious, demented, comatose, or is unable to remember/understand what is being said) or has been found to be legally incompetent.

Suggested Reading

1. Entwistle VA, Carter SM, Cribb A, McCaffery K. Supporting patient autonomy: the significance of relationships between clinicians and patients. J Gen Intern Med. 2010; 25(7):741-5.

Q.7. Which of the following is the correct order for highest to lowest priority of surrogate decision-makers for an incompetent adult patient?
   a. Individual appointed by patient, spouse, adult child, parent, adult sibling
   b. Individual appointed by patient, spouse, parent, adult child, adult sibling
   c. Individual appointed by patient, spouse, adult sibling, adult child, parent
   d. Individual appointed by patient, spouse, parent, adult sibling, adult child

Ans. a

Explanation: The following hierarchy is used for surrogate decision-makers when an adult patient is determined to be incapacitated:
1. A person the patient appointed
2. Spouse
3. Older juvenile
4. Parent
5. The older sibling

In the event that a patient has a living will, the surrogate decision:

The decision-maker should refer to this document when making medical decisions for the patient. By making decisions that the incompetent person would make if he/she was competent, the surrogate should also apply the substituted judgment principle.

Suggested Reading
1. Buchanan AE, Brock DW. Deciding for Others: The Ethics of Surrogate Decision Making. New York: Cambridge University Press; 1989.

Q.8. A 65-year-old male presents with a left middle cerebral artery stroke. On arrival patient was intubated in view of low Glasgow Coma Scale (GCS). His wife is his durable power of attorney for healthcare decisions. She notes that he did not want to end up, "connected to machines to keep him alive," and his living will state: "I do not want aggressive measures to extend my life." The neurointerventional team feels that his prognosis is likely good with an endovascular revascularization procedure, but the wife is hesitant to consent to this procedure. What is the most appropriate next step?
   a. Explore the patient's wishes with regard to medical care with his wife.
   b. Consult the hospital ethics committee.
   c. Proceed with the procedure without his wife's consent because it is likely lifesaving, any delay may make his outcome worse.
   d. Consult other members of the family and seek their consent for the procedure.

Ans. a

Explanation: Due to his inability to make medical treatment decisions, this patient deteriorated mental state. The principle of substituted judgment should be applied because of how ambiguous his living will is regarding his wishes. A surrogate decision-maker is required by this principle to make choices for the patient based on their comprehension of the patient's beliefs and values. In this case, the patient's wife, who is his durable power of attorney, is acting as his legal surrogate decision-maker and has the final say on all medical decisions. It is appropriate to talk to her about the treatment, get her informed consent, and then further investigate her objections if she declines.

Suggested Reading
1. Bernat JL. Ethical Concerns in Neurology, 3rd edition. Philadelphia: Lippincott Williams and Wilkins; 2008. pp. 81-110.

Q.9. Bioethical principles fundamental to critical care practice include all except:
   a. Autonomy
   b. Beneficence
   c. Quality of care
   d. Distributive justice
   e. Nonmaleficence

Ans. c

Explanation: The term "autonomy" refers to the right of the informed patient to choose how he/she will be treated. Beneficence refers to acting in a way that is (or is believed to be) best for the patient.

Distributive justice states that a patient in a similar situation should receive a similar level of care.

Nonmaleficence refers to doing no harm and not placing an unnecessary or unjustifiable burden on the patient.

Suggested Reading
1. Mani RK, Amin P, Chawla R, Divatia JV, Kapadia F, Khilnani P, et al. Guidelines for end-of-life and palliative care in Indian intensive care units' ISCCM consensus Ethical Position Statement. Indian J Crit Care Med. 2012;16(3):166-81.

Q.10. The fundamentals of bioethical principles which impart that patients with the same condition admitted to the hospital should receive similar treatment and care. Which of the following terms correlates to the same?
   a. Beneficence
   b. Quality of care
   c. Distributive justice
   d. Nonmaleficence

Ans. c

Explanation: In order to be benevolent, one must act in the patient's best interest and highest good. Distributive justice states that a patient in a comparable situation should get the same level of care. Nonmaleficence refers to not inflicting harm or unnecessary restrictions or placing an unreasonable burden on the patient.

Suggested Reading
1. Mani RK, Amin P, Chawla R, Divatia JV, Kapadia F, Khilnani P, et al. Guidelines for end-of-life and palliative care in Indian intensive care units' ISCCM consensus Ethical Position Statement. Indian J Crit Care Med. 2012;16(3):166-81.

Q.11. The Health Insurance Portability and Accountability Act (HIPAA) privacy rule permits healthcare providers to disclose protected healthcare information concerning a patient with major depression, who has capacity and requests that his or her family not be contacted in which of the following situations?
  a. When the family member is the healthcare proxy.
  b. When the healthcare provider perceives a serious patient safety concern.
  c. When the family member is the spouse or next of kin.
  d. When the healthcare provider does not agree with the patient's healthcare decisions.
  e. When the healthcare provider believes that the patient's medical decisions are being influenced by his/her mental illness.

Ans. b

Explanation: A patient with a mental illness may have his/her protected health information disclosed under the HIPAA in a few very limited circumstances. The patient retains the right to make his/her own healthcare decisions if he/she is found to be competent. If the healthcare provider believes there is a "serious and imminent threat to the health or safety of the patient or others and the family members are in a position to lessen the threat," HIPAA permits the disclosure of protected healthcare information about a patient with a mental illness.

Suggested Reading
  1. HHS.GOV. U.S. Office for Civil Rights of the Department of Health and Human Services. Information sharing and the HIPAA Privacy Rule. [online] Available from https://www.hhs.gov/sites/default/files/hipaa-privacy-rule-and-sharinginfo-related-to-mental-health.pdf [Last accessed June, 2023].

Q.12. "The Indian Law Commission" published a draught bill on "medical treatment of terminally ill patients (for the protection of patients and medical practitioners)" in 2006. Which of the following statements does not stand true according to the draught?
  a. Euthanasia and physician-assisted suicide remain criminal offences, but are clearly distinct from withholding and withdrawal of life support.
  b. Adult patients' right to self-determination and right to refuse treatment are binding on doctors if based on informed choice.
  c. Applying invasive therapies contrary to patient's will is legally permitted in case of emergencies.
  d. Refusal to accept medical treatment does not amount to "attempt to commit suicide" and endorsement of forgoing life-sustaining treatment (FLST) by the physician does not constitute "abetment of suicide".
  e. Withholding and withdrawal are viewed as an "omission to struggle" on the part of the physician that will not be unlawful unless there is a breach of duty toward the patient.

Ans. c

Explanation: It is battery or, in some cases, culpable homicide to administer invasive therapies against a patient's wishes.

Suggested Reading
1. Government of India's Law Commission. Report 196. Medical care for patients who are near death (for the protection of patients and Medical practitioners). [online] Available from http://lawcommissionofindia.nic.in/reports/rep196.pdf [Last accessed June, 2023].

Q.13. The available evidence suggests that the impact of ICU-based palliative care includes all the following except:
a. Decrease ICU and hospital length of stay
b. Decrease healthcare cost
c. Improve communication with patient
d. Increase in-hospital mortality

Ans. d

Explanation: Interprofessional assistance is provided for both in the ICU's palliative care program providing care for patients and their families in the spiritual, physical, and emotional spheres of serious illness. Contrary to hospice care, palliative care is not based on prognosis and is frequently provided in conjunction with life-prolonging care. ICU-based palliative care interventions are still being studied in an effort to define outcomes and measure their effectiveness. Palliative care interventions are thought to significantly shorten hospital and ICU stays and lower healthcare costs, according to a number of meta-analyses and systematic reviews of the impact of ICU-based palliative care on a variety of outcomes. Although some studies point to a decline in in-hospital mortality, other studies find no difference. But there is no proof that using palliative care interventions causes mortality to rise.

Suggested Reading
1. Aslakson RA, Curtis JR, Nelson JE. Palliative care's evolving role in the intensive care unit. Crit Care Med. 2014;42:2418-28.

Q.14. Single best response among the following concerns to the principles of medical ethics and consent:
a. Respect for a patient's autonomy means that an operation cannot be performed if a patient who has capacity refuses, even if it is deemed in the patient's best interest by the medical team.
b. Oral consent is never considered as explicit consent.
c. Nonmaleficence retains primacy over autonomy as shown by blood and marrow donation.
d. In order to obtain informed consent the patient must be informed of all conceivable risks and benefits of the treatment.
e. Consent is needed from the next of kin to perform a procedure on an adult patient who lacks capacity.

Ans. a

Explanation: In terms of ethics, respect for autonomy, beneficence, nonmaleficence, and justice are the four fundamental tenets. We can make our own decisions based on deliberation if we have autonomy, which is defined as "deliberate self-rule." The moral responsibility to respect another person's autonomy exists insofar as doing so is consistent with respecting the autonomy of all parties who may be affected. The goal of beneficence and nonmaleficence, which can be thought of together, is to produce a net benefit over harm. Autonomy continues to take precedence over nonmaleficence in the case of bone marrow and blood donation. Justice is the moral duty to act so that competing claims are fairly adjudicated. Explicit consent is consent that has been verbally or in writing expressed. When patients are informed that their information will be disclosed, along with why and how much, and that they have the right to object, but they choose not to, implied consent can be assumed.

While the sharing of information between a doctor and patient is essential for informed consent, it should be respected as much as possible if a patient prefers to remain anonymous regarding his/her condition or course of treatment. The treating medical professional may approve a procedure when it is thought to be in the patient's best interests when it is being considered for a patient who lacks capacity. Getting the patient's next of kin's consent is a good idea, but it is not required by law.

Suggested Reading
1. Gillon R. Medical ethics: four guiding principles plus scope-consciousness. BMJ. 1994;309(6948):184-8.

Q.15. Regarding the ethical and legal aspects of organ donation after cardiac death and after brainstem death, which of the following statements is false:
   a. Once the decision for organ donation in a brainstem dead patient has been made, management should move from a "patient-focused approach" to an "organ management approach".
   b. Regarding donation after cardiac death, it is ethically acceptable to delay the process of withdrawal in the donor until the donor process is in place.
   c. Verbal expression of a wish to donate organs expressed before death is a valid form of consent for organ retrieval after death.
   d. The family does not have legal authority to refuse organ donation if the dead patient previously consented to this.
   e. Patients must be at least 16 years of age to register on the Organ Donor Register.

Ans. e

Explanation: The insertion of new invasive monitoring (if indicated) is frequently thought to be appropriate because once a diagnosis of brainstem death is made; the patient is legally dead and the focus of management shifts from a patient-focused approach to an organ management approach. The patient in the potential heart-beating donor is still alive, and best interests are used to manage his/her care. It is in the patient's best interests to take into account all the variables influencing his/her interests. According to Department of Health guidance, delaying treatment withdrawal "may be considered to be in the best interests of someone who wanted to be a donor if this facilitates donation and does not cause the person harm or distress, or place them at significant risk of experiencing harm or distress." The Human Tissue Act of 2004 acknowledges that the desire to donate may have been expressed in a variety of ways, including verbally, in writing, on a donor card, or through the NHS Organ Donor Register (ODR). All of these methods are recognized as equally valid forms of consent under the Act. There is no legal authority for the family to disregard a person's known wishes. However, if the person's wishes are unknown, the designated representative and then the family gain the power of decision-making. The ODR does not have an age restriction for self-registration. Parents are presumed to have registered children under the age of 12 at the time of registration, while individuals aged 12 and older are presumed to have self-registered.

Suggested Reading
1. Gordon JK, McKinlay J. The management of the heart-beating donor and physiological changes following brain stem death. Contin Educ Anaesth Crit Care Pain. 2012;12(5):225-9.

Q.16. **The following principles are true regarding the end of life care of intensive care patients, which of the following statements holds true:**
   a. Any management plan specifying limits of invasive interventions must be reviewed daily.
   b. Unanimity amongst the medical and nursing team is necessary before withdrawal of life-sustaining treatment can take place.
   c. The healthcare professional responsible for making the decision about the extent of treatment in a patient lacking capacity should consult with those close to the patient to help reach a decision.
   d. Should be appointed an independent mental capacity advocate (IMCA); they assume the responsibility of making the final decision about withdrawal.
   e. A legally binding advance care plan which includes requests for specific treatments must be honored by the treating medical team.

Ans. c

Explanation: Most ICU patients lack the mental capacity to participate in discussions about delaying or stopping treatment. There should be a specific management plan in place when patients are admitted to the ICU that specifies the extent, if any, of invasive interventions. This plan needs to be reviewed and updated frequently, though not necessarily daily. Following discussion with other nurses and doctors on the medical team, the decision to withdraw or withhold is typically made. Unanimity is ideal but might not be possible. The consultant-in-charge of the ICU has the final say and is responsible for that decision, but it is crucial that the family's or the patient's close friends' opinions be taken into consideration.

The doctor must speak with their employing or contracting organization about appointing an IMCA, as required by the Mental Capacity Act, 2005, if there is no legal proxy, close relative, or other person who is willing or able to support or represent the patient and the decision involves serious medical treatment. While it has the power to gather information about the patient and represent his/her interests in the decision-making process, the IMCA is not allowed to act as the patient's decision-maker. It is advisable to have conversations with patients about their course of treatment and care as they near the end of their lives in order to ensure timely access to safe, effective care, and continuity in its delivery to meet the patient's needs. Patients' wishes for their medical care can be recorded in an advance care plan. This can include in-advance treatment refusals (which are legally binding) and requests for particular treatments, but the consultant-in-charge of the patient ultimately decides whether to provide these treatments.

Suggested Reading
1. Intensive Care Society Standards Committee. For adults who need intensive care, there are guidelines for treatment restrictions. London, UK: ICS; 2003.
2. The General Medical Council. Decision-making best practices for treatment and care in the final stages of life. London, UK: GMC; 2010.

Q.17. Regarding the logistics of organ donation:
a. Functional warm ischemic time begins with the onset of asystole.
b. Cold ischemic time is the time from initiation of cold preservation until the restoration of warm circulation after transplant.
c. Age >80 years is a contraindication to organ donation.
d. A donation after cardiac death (DCD) patient is always suitable for heart donation.
e. Noradrenaline is the first-line agent for the management of fluid resistant hypotension in the brainstem-dead donor.

Ans. b

Explanation: Functional warm ischemia time starts when there is insufficient oxygenation or perfusion of the organ, which is defined by a systolic arterial pressure 50 mm Hg, oxygen saturation 70% or both, such as during treatment withdrawal or cardiac standstill, and it lasts until the start of cold perfusion. From the start of cold perfusion until warm circulation is restored after transplantation, there is a cold ischemic period.

Although there are age recommendations for specific organs, there is no longer a maximum or minimum age for potential donors. From donors who are undergoing donation after cardiac death, kidneys, liver, pancreas, lungs, and tissue are all suitable for transplantation. The only source of hearts for transplantation is donation following brain death. In most brain-dead donors, hypotension will develop as a result of relative hypovolemia, which is aggravated by a decrease in systemic vascular resistance. Titration of crystalloid or colloid infusions is necessary to reach euvolemia. Early re-establishment of vascular tone promotes hemodynamic stability and lowers the danger of administering too much fluid.

When fluid therapy fails to relieve hypotension, vasopressin is thought of as the first-line treatment. It improves vascular tone, manages diabetes insipidus, reduces the need for catecholamines, and has a lower propensity than noradrenaline to result in metabolic acidosis or pulmonary hypertension. Dopamine is the preferred agent in some facilities, so when implementing such therapies, it is crucial to be aware of local regulations.

Suggested Reading
1. Dunne K, Doherty P. Donation following circulatory death. Contin Educ Anaesth Crit Care Pain 2011;11(3):82-6.
2. Gordon JK, McKinlay J. Physiological alterations following brain stem death and the care of the heart-beating donor. Contin Educ Anaesth Crit Care Pain. 2012;12(5):225-9.

Q.18. Regarding the potential organ donor patient which of the following statements is true:
  a. Warm ischemic time is reduced in DCD cases, compared to donation after brainstem death (DBD).
  b. DCD patients cannot donate lungs.
  c. Controlled DCD patients are Maastricht category I and II.
  d. Organ retrieval should be commenced immediately following the onset of asystole in DCD donors.
  e. A nurse with a specialist role in organ donation is an appropriate person to make the initial approach to the family.

Ans. e

Explanation: Donation after cardiac death is the process of removing a patient from care with the goal of retrieving his/her organs as soon as death has been officially confirmed. In comparison to donation following brainstem death, the warm ischemic time—during which there is insufficient oxygenation or perfusion to the organs—is thus prolonged. A certain amount of warm ischemia time is unavoidable in DCD patients. Warm ischemia time is defined as the interval between the onset of asystole and cold perfusion of the organs. Functional warm ischemia time, which is defined as starting when the donor's systolic arterial pressure is <50 mm Hg or SpO_2 is <70%, and ending with cold perfusion of the organs, is a more helpful concept.

The lungs are a good organ for DCD because they can tolerate being without blood flow as long as they are still inflated with oxygen. Even though the procedure is still new, it is becoming more popular. The modified Maastricht classification system divides potential DCD patients into five categories, of which IV is cardiac arrest in a brainstem-dead donor and III is awaiting cardiac arrest. All of the patients in other groups have uncontrolled DCD.

According to guidelines, confirmation of death should occur after 5 minutes of ongoing cardiorespiratory arrest. After the death has been officially declared, there should be another 5 minutes of grace before organ retrieval begins. Prior to making any attempts at retrieval, this 10-minute "hands off" period—which is collectively known as such—ensures irreversible brainstem death in addition to cardiac death.

Suggested Reading
1. Kootstra G, Daemen JHC, Oomen APA. Categories of non-heart-beating donors. Transpl Proc. 1995;27:2893-4.
2. Vincent A, Logan L. Consent for organ donation. Br J Anaesth. 2012;108(Suppl 1):i80-7.

Q.19. A 24-year-old male with traumatic brain injury has been declared brainstem dead on your ICU this morning. He was on the organ donor register and his family has been consulted. They, in agreement with the medical team, are keen to proceed to donation after brainstem death. While awaiting the transplant team he becomes cardiovascularly unstable with a blood pressure of 90/30 mm Hg [mean arterial pressure (MAP) 50 mm Hg]. He has crystalloid fluid running through a peripheral IV line and is currently 3L positive on cumulative balance. He has no central access. Which course of action is ideal to take next?
  a. He should start receiving a peripheral metaraminol infusion.
  b. To hasten surgery, get in touch with the transplant team.
  c. Stop mechanical ventilation and abandon your plans for organ donation.
  d. He should be given low-dose vasopressin after placing a central venous catheter.
  e. Give the patient another 500 mL bolus of a 4.5% human albumin solution.

Ans. d

Explanation: This patient's brain injury cannot be repaired. Your responsibility now is to ensure a respectful passing in accordance with his wishes. This situation allows for interventions like central venous catheter placement and the start of cardiovascular support to maximize the chances of a successful outcome for the donated organs and their recipients. Acting ethically in the "best interests" of the patient can be reasonably interpreted as ensuring his wish to donate organs is carried out.

Despite being an option, peripheral metaraminol is not advised as a first-line treatment due to the possibility of bradyarrhythmias. An untimely surgical procedure is more likely to have a negative effect on either the donor or the recipients. To measure central venous pressure (CVP) and administer medications, it is advised to place a central line; low-dose vasopressin is the vasopressor of choice in this situation. Because low vasopressin levels are linked to brainstem death, it is possible to consider that this medication will return "normal physiological tone." As needed, noradrenaline can also be used.

While maintaining normovolemia is crucial, it has been shown that avoiding excessive fluid administration greatly increases the proportion of transplantable lungs in this cohort.

Suggested Reading
  1. McKeown DW, Bonser RS, Kellum JA. Management of the heartbeat-inducing brain-dead organ donor. Br J Anaesth. 2012;108(Suppl 1):i96-i107.
  2. ODT Clinical. Donor management guidelines for brain-stem dead donors. [online] Available from http://www.odt.nhs.uk/donation/deceased-donation/donor-optimisation/resources/ [Last accessed June, 2023].

Q.20. True among the following statements regarding acute graft versus host disease (AGVHD):
  a. Rarely do the skin, liver, or gut get involved.
  b. B lymphocyte donors attack the host's tissues.
  c. First-line therapies include infliximab or mycophenolate mofetil.

d. The prevention of AGVHD frequently employs calcineurin inhibitors.
e. The mortality rate for AGVHD associated with transfusions is <45%.

Ans. d

Explanation: The skin, liver, and gut are frequently affected by AGVHD, a side effect of allogeneic hematopoietic stem cell transplantation (HSCT). A maculopapular rash typically begins on the palms and soles, but it can begin on any area of the skin before spreading. Toxic epidermal necrolysis can manifest itself in severe forms. There may be severe diarrhea. Liver involvement is frequently signaled by jaundice and cholestasis.

T-cells from the donor blood, bone marrow, and stem cells attack the host's tissues and cause AGVHD.

Although first-line treatment for AGVHD steroids may only be 50% effective in some patients, extracorporeal photopheresis, T cell immunosuppression (cyclosporine, tacrolimus), anti-TNF antibodies (infliximab, etanercept), mTOR inhibitors (sirolimus), mycophenolate mofetil, and IL-2 receptor antibodies are among the second-line treatments for AGVHD [mycophenolate mofetil (MMF)].

Acute graft versus host disease prophylaxis frequently involves the use of calcineurin inhibitors (ciclosporin/tacrolimus).

A nearly 100% mortality rate is linked to transfusion-associated graft versus host disease (TA-GVHD).

Suggested Reading
1. Clevenger B, Kelleher A. Hazards of blood transfusion in adults and children. Contin Educ Anaesth Crit Care Pain. 2014;14(3):112-8.

Q.21. All of the following are true with regard to liver transplantation for acute liver failure (ALF):
a. The first 3 months following surgery are when most transplant-related deaths happen.
b. A donor graft from a donor without an identical ABO donor carries a higher risk of death for the recipient.
c. Patients with ALF receive 20% of liver transplant surgeries.
d. Impaired graft function that occurs early after surgery is poorly tolerated.
e. ALF patients outlive patients with chronic liver failure after the first year following transplantation.

Ans. c

Explanation: At 1 year and 5 years after liver transplantation for ALF, the survival rates are 79% and 72%, respectively. Most fatalities happen within the first 3 months following surgery.

Acute liver failure patients who are older and who receive partial or older grafts have a higher risk of death after liver transplantation. Additionally, it is higher in patients who have had a donor graft from a donor who does not have the same ABO blood group as them.

Less than 10% of liver transplants are done on patients with ALF. Survival rates after liver transplantation for ALF are consistently lower than those seen after elective liver transplantation for chronic liver disease, making perioperative management of the procedure difficult.

Impaired graft function in the early postoperative period is poorly tolerated and increases the risk of sepsis and intracranial hypertension.

Compared to patients with chronic liver failure, ALF patients have a higher initial mortality rate after liver transplantation. However, after the first year, this trend reverses, and patients with ALF have better long-term survival.

Suggested Reading
1. Bernal W, Wendon J. Acute liver failure. New Engl J Med. 2014;369(26):2525-34.
2. Wang DW, Yin YM, Yao YM. Advances in the management of acute liver failure. World J Gastroenterol. 2013;19(41): 7069-77.

Q.22. All the following statements are true with regard to liver transplantation, but:
  a. For patients with acute liver failure, the 12-month survival rate is about 65%.
  b. At 1 year, there is a 12% mortality rate among patients waiting for liver transplants.
  c. Donation after circulatory death donors is the ones who undergo the majority of liver retrievals.
  d. Venovenous bypass is not necessary when using the surgical technique that preserves the vena cava.
  e. Perioperative thromboelastography could detect elevated LY30 and LY60.

Ans. c

Explanation: A liver transplant for acute liver failure results in a 65% 1-year survival rate. As a result of chronic liver failure transplantation, this is less.

Data from April 2010 to March 2011 reveals that 12% of patients on the transplant waiting list had passed away or been removed from the list after 1 year due to clinical deterioration.

By using the Maastricht classification, DCD donors can be categorized.

Currently, only controlled donors can be used to harvest liver and lungs for transplant (category III-IV).

The "piggyback technique" refers to this. Hemodynamic stability and the avoidance of venovenous bypass are benefits of this procedure.

In some recipients of liver transplants, the fibrinolytic system may become activated during the anhepatic and postreperfusion phases. A thromboelastogram's LY30 and LY60 measurements of the percentage decrease in amplitude at 30 and 60 minutes after the clot's maximum amplitude provide an indication of the degree of fibrinolysis.

Suggested Reading
1. Bersten AD, Soni N. Oh's Intensive Care Manual, 6th edition. Butterworth Heinemann: Elsevier; 2009. p. 1292.
2. Ridley S, Bonner S, Bray K, Falvey S, Mackay J, Manara A, et al. UK guidance for non-heart-beating donation. Br J Anaesth. 2005;95(5):592-5.

Q.23. Following liver transplantation, which of the following is true?
a. Rejection is the only factor in graft dysfunction.
b. An appropriate management strategy for an episode of acute rejection at an incremental dose is pulsed methylprednisolone.
c. After solid organ transplantation, cytomegalovirus (CMV) infection is the most prevalent opportunistic infection.
d. In the postoperative period, immunosuppression should be treated with steroids or a calcineurin inhibitor.
e. There are no indicators of readmission following critical care discharge.

Ans. c

Explanation: Graft dysfunction can be brought on by a number of factors, such as primary nonfunction (a type of reperfusion injury), rejection, preservation injury, vascular and biliary complications, drug-induced dysfunction, infection, and the recurrence of chronic illness.

A typical methylprednisolone regimen would be 1 g/day for 3 days, then a tapering of the dose.

A total of 23–85% of patients who undergo orthotopic liver transplantation will contract cytomegalovirus (CMV) infection in the absence of antiviral prophylaxis. The preferred medication for CMV disease is still ganciclovir.

The traditional cornerstone of immunosuppressive therapy following liver transplantation consists of calcineurin inhibitors (ciclosporin, tacrolimus), especially in the early stages. Drugs like azathioprine or MMF may be added over time after transplantation to allow for dose reduction of steroids and calcineurin inhibitors. The immunosuppressive regimen after a liver transplant may also include other medications such as antilymphocyte antibodies (ALA), monoclonal antibodies (basiliximab), and/or sirolimus.

A total of 20% of liver transplant recipients need to be readmitted to intensive care. Patient survival and graft function are both negatively correlated with readmission. The following factors increase the risk of readmission to intensive care—abnormal predischarge chest X-ray, high central venous pressure, tachypnea, advancing patient age, abnormal pretransplant synthetic function, abnormal bilirubin, significant intraoperative blood product requirement, and renal dysfunction. Cardiorespiratory failure brought on by infection and fluid overload is the most typical reason for readmission. Other significant reasons for readmission include biliary anastomotic leaks, graft dysfunction, severe sepsis, bleeding, and other surgical complications.

Suggested Reading
1. Bersten AD, Soni N. Oh's Intensive Care Manual, 6th edition. Butterworth Heinemann: Elsevier; 2009. p. 1292.

Q.24. Which of the following statements about consent and privacy is true?
a. Without their prior written consent, treatment cannot be administered to patients in critical care.

b. Competent intensive care patients have the right to reject care that might be in their best interests, even if doing so might lead to their demise.
c. For an adult who lacks mental capacity, an enduring power of solicitor may make medical decisions.
d. The use of anonymized patient data for quality improvement purposes requires the consent of each individual patient.
e. Information disclosure to third parties is not thought to require the consent of each patient individually.

Ans. b

Explanation: Treatment that is lifesaving or in the patient's best interests can be given without a patient's consent in cases where they are unable to give it.

Any competent adult is allowed to reject medical advice and refuse treatment.

Enduring powers of solicitor can make decisions for a patient's financial affairs, but not for his/her medical care.

Individual patient consent is not required for the analysis of anonymized data for internal quality control procedures.

If a patient's information is to be disclosed to a third party, only with that patient's consent should that information be disclosed.

Suggested Reading
1. British Medical Association. Advanced claims regarding medical treatment: the working party's 1995 report. London: BMA, 1995.
2. British Medical Association. Health information confidentiality and disclosure: working party report for 1999. London: BMA; 1999.
3. British Medical Association. Report of the consent working party: incorporating consent tool kit. London: BMA; 2001.

Q.25. The following is accurate regarding calcineurin inhibitors:
a. Tacrolimus has a good oral bioavailability.
b. Avoid having B cells produce cytokines or multiply.
c. Tacrolimus prevents IL-2 from being produced.
d. Do not negatively impact renal functions.

Ans. c

Explanation: By attaching to the intracellular immunophilins cyclophilin and FKBP-12, calcineurin inhibitors inhibit the production of IL-2 by T cells. Tacrolimus has a very lipophilic structure and a poor, inconsistent bioavailability; the oral dose is nearly three times that of intravenous. Chronic nephrotoxicity is the most significant adverse effect, often resulting in dose reduction.

Suggested Reading
1. Irwin RS, Rippe JM. Intensive Care Medicine, 6th edition. Philadelphia: Lippincott Williams and Wilkins; 2007.

Q.26. Which of the following claims regarding allograft rejection is accurate?
 a. Without immunosuppression, transplant rejection between unrelated donors and recipients varies greatly in terms of timing and ferocity.
 b. Cells or antibodies may play a role in allograft rejection.
 c. Th2 cells are believed to be the culprit behind allograft rejection.
 d. The main reason clinical organ transplants fail is acute cellular rejection.
 e. An allograft cannot be rejected by a person who has "tolerance."

Ans. b

Explanation: In the absence of immunosuppression, allografts from randomly chosen donors are always rejected, and the rate of rejection is high compared to the rate at which most immune responses develop. Antidonor antibodies can lead to very serious types of rejection, such as hyperacute and acute vascular rejection, even though allograft rejection in naive recipients is primarily mediated by cells. The development of chronic rejection, currently the most common reason for graft loss, may be influenced by antidonor antibodies or cellular reactions. Recent research has shown that helper T cells can differentiate in one of the two ways. Allograft rejection and delayed-type hypersensitivity are linked to the Th1 pathway, which results in the release of interferon-gamma and other cytokines. The Th2 pathway is connected to the release of IL-10 and IL-4 and may actually suppress alloimmune reactions. Thus, the maturation of Th2 responses may aid in tolerance. Tolerance is extremely specific, just like allograft rejection. An individual who is tolerant to one antigen or one person can still mount an immune response against other antigens and other people.

Suggested Reading
 1. Irwin RS, Rippe JM. Intensive Care Medicine, 6th edition. Philadelphia: Lippincott Williams and Wilkins; 2007.

Q.27. All things except—can result in post-transplantation hypertension.
 a. Rejection
 b. Nephrotoxicity from cyclosporine
 c. Hypertension reactive
 d. Artery stenosis following renal transplant [renal tubular acidosis (RTAS)]
 e. Disease that returns to the allograft.

Ans. c

Explanation: Hypertension may be caused by acute or chronic rejection. The former results in acute fluid retention and inflammatory cell plugging of peritubular capillaries; as a result of endothelial proliferation and the destruction of small vessels, this may progress to intimal swelling, medial necrosis, and eventually ischemia. Chronic rejection, which is thought to be related to long-term humoral injury, causes intimal hyperplasia, which destroys capillaries. Because of the vasoconstrictive effects of cyclosporine, hypertension may develop as a result of renin-angiotensin system activation. In 4–12% of recipients of renal allografts, hypertension is caused by RTAS. Percutaneous angioplasty works well in treating it. RTAS may be diagnosed through a careful evaluation of angiotensin-converting enzyme inhibitors. Significant hypertension may develop in recipients of renal allografts due to recurrent illness such as membranoproliferative glomerulonephritis and focal glomerular sclerosis.

Suggested Reading
1. Luke RG. Pathophysiology and treatment of posttransplant hypertension. J Am Soc Nephrol. 1991;(2 Suppl 1):S37-44.

Q.28. The recipient of a cadaver kidney allograft is still on dialysis and oliguric 1 week after the transplant. A larger perigraft fluid collection is seen on ultrasound. Your following management step entails:
   a. No more research is necessary (since perigraft collections are fairly common after renal transplantation).
   b. A fibrosis-inducing agent is injected after the perigraft fluid collection is aspirated to eliminate the dead space.
   c. Angiography to identify the location of the bleeding in the renal allograft.
   d. The collection of perigraft fluid being aspirated for chemical analysis.

Ans. d

Explanation: The most frequent source of urine leakage is the ureteroneocystostomy or ischemic ureter, which typically occurs early after transplantation. Before leakage from the wound is seen, there are clinical signs such as pain, swelling, and a decline in renal function. It would be easier to distinguish between lymphocele and urinoma by aspirating the perigraft fluid collection for blood urea nitrogen (BUN) and creatinine chemical analysis. When compared to lymphocele values, which are comparable to blood values, the BUN and creatinine concentrations in urinoma are several orders of magnitude higher.

Suggested Reading
1. Pollak R, Veremis SA, Maddux MS, Mozes MF. The natural history of and therapy for perirenal fluid collections following renal transplantation. J Urol. 1988;140(4):716-20.

Q.29. All of the statements are true, except for the one that refers to hepatic artery thrombosis after liver transplantation.
   a. Children are more likely than adult patients to experience hepatic artery thrombosis after liver transplantation.
   b. Several weeks after transplant, arteriosclerosis usually causes thrombosis of the hepatic artery.
   c. If retransplantation cannot be done within 36–72 hours after the initial transplant, thrombosis of the hepatic artery is a serious complication that can be fatal.
   d. Multiple intrahepatic bile duct strictures and/or hepatic abscesses may result from the hepatic artery narrowing or late thrombosis.
   e. After liver transplantation, thrombosis of the portal vein occurs more frequently than hepatic artery thrombosis.

Ans. b

Explanation: One of the worst initial side effects of liver transplantation is still thrombosis of the hepatic artery. Children experience this complication three to five times more frequently than adults do. Technical error is the main reason for this complication, but in some cases the hypercoagulable state may also be a significant factor. If a transplant cannot be done within 36–72 hours after an early hepatic artery thrombosis, the patient will die from rapid liver failure. The majority of these patients need retransplantation, even though thrombolytic therapy administered via percutaneous or surgical access can be effective. Multiple intrahepatic bile duct strictures and/or hepatic abscesses may result from the hepatic artery narrowing or late thrombosis. This complication frequently necessitates retransplantation as well. A less common side effect is portal vein thrombosis. When it develops early, it can be fatal, but if it takes place after a few months, it can be well tolerated. Shunt surgery is frequently effective in treating portal hypertension brought on by late portal vein thrombosis.

Suggested Reading
1. Silva MA, Jambulingam PS, Gunson BK, Mayer D, Buckels JA, Mirza DF, et al. Hepatic artery thrombosis following orthotopic liver transplantation: a 10-year experience from a single centre in the United Kingdom. Liver Transpl. 2006;12(1):146-51.

Q.30. Which of the following treatments is currently preferred for heart-lung transplant patients?
a. Right ventricular function is largely unaffected by primary pulmonary hypertension.
b. A patient with end-stage lung disease and cystic fibrosis was found to have a confirmed cardiomyopathy.
c. CF and end-stage pulmonary failure with healthy heart function.
d. A defect in the atrial septum causes Eisenmenger's syndrome.
e. Emphysematous end-stage lung disease.

Ans. b

Explanation: Only those with advanced heart and lung diseases should now undergo heart-lung transplants. The best course of treatment for a patient with primary pulmonary hypertension and moderately well-preserved right ventricular function is a single or bilateral lung transplant. Combination heart-lung transplantation would be a better course of treatment for someone who has end-stage heart and lung disease or who has complex congenital heart disease and Eisenmenger's syndrome. Eisenmenger's syndrome patients with relatively simple congenital defects (e.g., atrial septal defect, ventricular septal defect) respond best to concurrent congenital defect correction and single or bilateral lung transplantation. Similar to this, an individual with end-stage emphysema who has normal heart function can benefit greatly from a single or bilateral lung transplant, saving the donor heart for a patient who actually has heart failure.

Suggested Reading
1. De Geest S, Dobbels F, Fluri C, Paris W, Troosters T. Adherence to the therapeutic regimen in heart, lung, and heart-lung transplant recipients. J Cardiovasc Nurs. 2005;20(5 Suppl):S88-98.

CHAPTER 19

Oncology/Hematology

Shilpushp Jagannath Bhosale, Atul Prabhakar Kulkarni

Q.1. A 44-year-old male is recently diagnosed with acute myeloid leukemia (AML). He had a chemoport placed for chemotherapy administration and he received induction chemotherapy regimen with cytarabine and daunorubicin. He was placed on neutropenic precautions, started on appropriate antimicrobial prophylaxis. Seven days after the completion of his induction chemotherapy he spiked a fever of 38.8°C (101.8°F) and complained of chills and nausea. His temperature is 38.8°C, pulse (P) 105 bpm, respiration rate (RR) 16 breaths/minute, blood pressure (BP) 112/78 mm Hg, and SpO_2 98%. Absolute neutrophilic count (ANC) is 1,500 cells/mL. Which of the following is correct in terms of further care for this patient?
a. Administer paracetamol and suggest to observe at home.
b. Patient is considered low risk of infection since ANC count is normal.
c. The patient is a case of febrile neutropenia (FN) and needs strict observation.
d. Does not fit in FN criteria since ANC count is normal.

Ans. c

Explanation: Febrile neutropenia is considered an emergency. In neutropenic patients infectious etiology cannot be determined and most of the times labeled as a fever of unknown origin (FUO). Neutropenic fever is defined as a single oral temperature greater than or equal to 101°F (38.3°C) or a temperature greater than or equal to 100.4°F (38°C) for at least an hour, with an absolute ANC of <1,500 cells/µL or expected to fall over next 48 hours.

Severe febrile neutropenia is defined as the ANC <500/µL, or ANC is expected to decrease below 500 cells/µL in the next 24–48 hours.
- ANC = WBC (cells/µL) × percent (PMNs + bands)/100

Suggested Reading
1. Rivera-Salgado D, Valverde-Muñoz K, Ávila-Agüero ML. [Febrile neutropenia in cancer patients: management in the emergency room]. Rev Chilena Infectol. 2018;35(1):62-71.
2. Villafuerte-Gutierrez P, Villalon L, Losa JE, Henriquez-Camacho C. Treatment of febrile neutropenia and prophylaxis in hematologic malignancies: a critical review and update. Adv Hematol. 2014;2014:986938.

Q.2. A 44-year-old male, a known case of AML status postchemotherapy (cytarabine and daunorubicin), presented to ED 1 week after the completion of his induction chemotherapy with fever, chills, and pain in abdomen. The ANC count is 1,000 cells/mL. On examination his temperature is 38.8°C, P 135 bpm, RR 26/minute, BP 90/70 mm Hg, and SpO_2 98%. Which of the following is correct in terms of further care for this patient?
   a. Start oral ciprofloxacin 500–750 mg orally every 12 hours.
   b. Ciprofloxacin 500–750 mg orally every 12 hours and amoxicillin/clavulanate 500 mg.
   c. Start oral ciprofloxacin 500–750 mg orally every 12 hours plus vancomycin 500 ng 8 hourly.
   d. Meropenem standard—1–2 g intravenous (IV) every 8 hours.

Ans. d

Explanation: This is a high-risk febrile neutropenia patient and intravenous antibiotic therapy should be given within 1 hour after triage and monitored aggressively. The Infectious Disease Society of America (IDSA) recommends monotherapy with antipseudomonal beta-lactam agents such as cefepime, carbapenems, or piperacillin/tazobactam.

The usual recommended dosages are as follows:
- *Cefepime or ceftazidime:* 2 g IV every 8 hours or
- *Piperacillin/tazobactam:* 4.5 g IV every 6–8 hours or
- Antipseudomonal carbapenems:
  - *Imipenem-cilastatin:* 500 mg IV every 6 hours
  - *Meropenem standard:* 1–2 g IV every 8 hours

Ciprofloxacin 500–750 mg orally every 12 hours and amoxicillin/clavulanate 500 mg orally every 8 hours can be used only in low-risk patients in the outpatient setting; if a low risk hemodynamically stable patient remains febrile for 48–72 hours, he will be considered high risk and will need hospital admission for intense monitoring. Clindamycin can be used for those with penicillin allergies.

Vancomycin is not recommended for initial therapy but should be considered if suspecting catheter-related infection, skin or soft tissue infections, pneumonia, or hemodynamic instability.

If patients do not respond to treatments, coverage should be expanded to include resistant species such as:
- Methicillin-resistant *Staphylococcus aureus*—vancomycin, linezolid, and daptomycin
- Vancomycin-resistant *Enterococci*—linezolid and daptomycin
- Extended-spectrum beta-lactamase producing organisms—carbapenems
- *Klebsiella pneumoniae*—carbapenems, polymyxin, colistin, or tigecycline

Suggested Reading
   1. Randy A. Taplitz, et al. Journal of Clinical Oncology. 36, no. 30 (October 20, 2018) 3043-54.

Q.3. A 44-year-old male is recently diagnosed with AML. He had a chemoport placed for chemotherapy administration and he received induction chemotherapy regimen with cytarabine and daunorubicin. Seven days after the completion of his induction chemotherapy he presented to the ED with history of (H/O) fever of 38.8°C (101.8°F) for 2 days, chills, and nausea. On examination in emergency department (ED), he is conscious; his temperature is 38.8°C, P 105 bpm, RR 26 breaths/minute, BP 100/78 mm Hg, and SpO_2 98%. His ANC is 1,500 cells/mL. He was on oral ciprofloxacin 500–750 mg orally every 12 hours for 3 days. Which of the following is correct in terms of further care for this patient?
a. Change to empirical antimicrobial therapy and discharge home.
b. Continue oral prophylaxis and advice to observe at home.
c. Change to IV ciprofloxacin and observe in ED.
d. Needs urgent admission as high risk FN.

Ans. d

Explanation: Multinational Association for Supportive Care in Cancer (MASCC) score is most commonly used to identify if patient needs an inpatient treatment.

An MASCC score of 21 or more identified low-risk patients (eligible for outpatient care) with a positive pressure ventilation (PPV) of 91%, a specificity of 68%, and a sensitivity of 71%.

Limitations of MASCC: Several important factors are not considered such as newer neutropenia cutoff, hypotension, type of cancer, chemotherapy, performance status, laboratory markers, and complications such as acute kidney injury, electrolyte disturbances, and surrogates of invasive infection. MASCC score has only been validated to identify low-risk patients, and any threshold score of <21 does not adequately distinguish high-risk patients. A very low level (<15) demonstrates a high rate of complications.

Suggested Reading
1. Klastersky J, Paesmans M, Rubenstein EB, Boyer M, Elting L, Feld R, et al. The multinational association for supportive care in cancer risk index: a multinational scoring system for identifying low-risk febrile neutropenic cancer patients. J Clin Oncol. 2000;18:3038-51.
2. Wijeratne DT, Wright K, Gyawali B. Risk-stratifying treatment strategies for febrile neutropenia—tools, tools everywhere, and not a single one that works? JCO Oncol Pract. 2021;17(11):651-4.

Q.4. A 44-year-old male, a known case of AML status postchemotherapy (cytarabine and daunorubicin), presented to ED 1 week after the completion of his induction chemotherapy with fever, cough, chills, and pain in abdomen for 3 days. The ANC count is 1,000 cells/mL. On examination his temperature is 38.8°C, P 135 bpm, RR 26/minute, BP 90/70 mm Hg, and SpO_2 98%. The chest X-ray is normal. Which is the best way evaluating this patient's febrile neutropenia?
a. Consider bronchoscopy.
b. Consider computed tomography (CT) of the chest, abdomen, and pelvis.

c. Chest X-ray should be enough for diagnosis.
d. Consider echocardiography.

Ans. b

Explanation: Patients with neutropenia may not have an inflammatory response and hence chest radiography may not be diagnosed early. Those who have normal chest radiographic findings should undergo CT of the chest when they have persistent fever and has suspicion of infection. More than 50% of neutropenic patients with normal chest radiographic findings have evidence of pneumonia on CT. chest CT help identify invasive pulmonary infection, commonly mold infections. CT of the abdomen and pelvis can identify typhlitis, intra-abdominal abscesses, neutropenic colitis, cholecystitis, or appendicitis. Echocardiography should be considered in neutropenic febrile patients when clinical suspicion for endocarditis exists but would not be the most appropriate next step in the evaluation of fever in this patient. Bronchoscopy is used to obtain a microbiologic diagnosis in patients with identified pulmonary infiltrates.

Suggested Reading
1. Heussel CP, Kauczor HU, Heussel GE. Pneumonia in febrile neutropenic patients and in bone marrow and blood stem-cell transplant recipients: use of high-resolution computed tomography. J Clin Oncol. 1999;17(3):796-805.
2. Maschmeyer G. Pneumonia in febrile neutropenic patients: radiologic diagnosis. Curr Opin Oncol. 2001;13(4):229-35.

Q.5. **A 55-year-old male diagnosed case of diffuse large B-cell lymphoma (DLBCL) stage IVB shifted to ICU with fever and septic shock status post two cycles of R-CHOP (rituximab, cyclophosphamide, doxorubicin, vincristine, and prednisone) chemotherapy. He had a history of neutropenic sepsis 2 months back for which he was treated with cefepime for 2 weeks. He is currently on trimethoprim-sulfamethoxazole prophylaxis. On examination: He is conscious febrile, his temperature is 39.1°C, swelling and tenderness at the peripherally inserted central catheter (PICC) entry site, investigations—hemoglobin 7 g/dL, leukocyte count 0.5×10^9/L, platelet count 10×10^9/L, and lever function test (LFT) renal function test (RFT) normal. Which of the following is correct in terms of further care for this patient?**
a. Convert to therapeutic septran and remove the PICC.
b. Continue gram-negative coverage.
c. Consider gram-positive.
d. Consider gram-negative and gram-positive and remove the PICC.

Ans. d

Explanation: In the past gram-negative bacilli were the most commonly identified pathogens in patients with neutropenic fever and hematologic malignancies. Since the suspected source is the PICC line, most common pathogens would be gram-positive organisms that historically account for 60–70% of bloodstream infections in patients with neutropenic fever. The most common gram-positive organisms are *Staphylococcus aureus*, *Staphylococcus* epidermidis, and *Streptococci* species. High risk factors for these infections are long-term indwelling central venous catheters, use of empirical antibiotics targeted to cover gram-negative organisms. Anaerobic, atypical, and acid-fast bacteria are not the most commonly identified organisms.

Suggested Reading
1. Kanamaru A, Tatsumi Y. Microbiological data for patients with febrile neutropenia. Clin Infect Dis. 2004;39(Suppl 1):S7-S10.

Q.6. A 44-year-old male, a known case of AML status day 14 postinduction chemotherapy (cytarabine and daunorubicin), was admitted to the ICU with febrile neutropenia and septic shock. The ANC count remains low 100 cells/mL. He has intermittent fever spikes, temperature 39°C, P 125 bpm, RR 26/minute, BP 90/70 mm Hg, and SpO_2 98% on room air. He received 7 days of meropenem 2 g IV every 8 hours and vancomycin 500 mg 8 hourly for 2 weeks. His cultures are negative but he continues to have fever spikes and continues to remain on noradrenaline 0.01 µg/kg/minute. Which of the following is correct in terms of further care for this patient?
a. Continue same antibiotics for 2 weeks and review.
b. Consider antifungal therapy.
c. Consider changing the antibiotics depending on the hospital antibiogram.
d. Consider deescalating antibiotics as fever is due to leukemia.

Ans. b

Explanation: Appropriate antibiotics may be continued until the ANC is ≥500 cells/mm, or when the infection is cleared with the resolution of all signs and symptoms of documented infection. If the patients remain neutropenic after the appropriate treatment course is completed, oral fluoroquinolone prophylaxis can be resumed until marrow recovers.

Invasive fungal infection (IFI) is major cause of mortality (>30%) among FN patients after chemotherapy or hematopoietic stem cell transplantation.

Empiric antifungal coverage is advised in high-risk patients with persistent fever after 4–7 days of broad-spectrum antibacterial regimen and suspicion of fungal infection.

Diagnosis of IFI is categorized as proven, probable or possible. Proven IFI is defined as demonstration of fungal elements in infected tissue for most conditions irrespective of host factors or clinical features. Cases of probable IFIs require a host factor, clinical features, and mycological evidence. Possible IFIs include cases with appropriate host factors and sufficient clinical evidence but no mycological support. The most commonly identified fungal species associated with IFI are *Candida* species, *Aspergillus*, *Cryptococcus*, and *Pneumocystis*.

Suggested Reading
1. Chen K, Wang Q, Pleasants RA, Ge L, Liu W, Peng K, et al. Empiric treatment against invasive fungal diseases in febrile neutropenic patients: a systematic review and network meta-analysis. BMC Infect Dis. 2017 Feb 20;17(1):159.

2. Patterson TF, Thompson GR 3rd, Denning DW, Fishman JA, Hadley S, Herbrecht R, et al. Practice Guidelines for the Diagnosis and Management of Aspergillosis: 2016 Update by the Infectious Diseases Society of America. Clin Infect Dis. 2016;63:e1-60

Q.7. A 55-year-old male diagnosed case of diffuse large B-cell lymphoma (DLBCL) stage IVB shifted to ICU with fever, nausea, and septic shock, status post R-CHOP (rituximab, cyclophosphamide, doxorubicin, vincristine, and prednisone) chemotherapy. He is on cefepime and vancomycin for 1 week and currently on granulocyte colony-stimulating factor (GCSF) for prolonged neutropenia and on trimethoprim-sulfamethoxazole prophylaxis. On examination—He is conscious febrile, temperature 39.1°C. Investigations—hemoglobin 7 g/dL, leukocyte count 0.5×10^9/L, platelet count 10×10^9/L, and LFT RFT normal. Which of the following is true regarding this patient? Patient is high risk of invasive fungal disease because of:
a. White blood cell growth-stimulating factors.
b. Prolonged neutropenia and antibiotic use.
c. Presence of an indwelling intravascular catheter.
d. Degree of neutropenia.

Ans. b

Explanation: Invasive fungal disease has also been associated with prolonged neutropenia, usually regarded as >7 days in duration. The duration and magnitude of neutropenia are the most important risk factors for development of invasive mold infection. Invasive fungal disease has also been associated with prolonged antibiotic use. Growth-stimulating factors have shown to reduce the incidence of neutropenic fever and the need for hospitalization however the use of growth-stimulating factors has not been associated with an increase in invasive fungal disease.

Suggested Reading
1. Smith TJ, Khatcheressian J, Lyman GH. 2006 Update of recommendations for the use of white blood cell growth factors: an evidence-based clinical practice guideline. J Clin Oncol. 2006;24(19):3187-3205.

Q.8. A 55-year-old male diagnosed case of diffuse large B-cell lymphoma stage (DLBCL) IVB status post R-CHOP (rituximab, cyclophosphamide, doxorubicin, vincristine, and prednisone) chemotherapy. Day 8 in the ICU still has fever spikes, and on norepinephrine 0.2 μg/kg/min. He is on cefepime, vancomycin, and fluconazole for 1 week. Ultrasound showed multiple hypodense lesions in the liver on spleen and was diagnosed to have hepatosplenic candidiasis. Investigations—hemoglobin 7 g/dL leukocyte count 0.5×10^9/L, platelet count 10×10^9/L, and LFT RFT normal. Which of the following is true regarding this patient?
a. Continue fluconazole for 2 weeks and reassess.
b. Suspicion of hepatosplenic candidiasis, change fluconazole to echinocandins.
c. Wait for the blood culture report.
d. Ultrasound-guided aspiration of the liver lesion and decide according to the tissue culture.

Ans. b

Explanation: The findings on USG are consistent with the hepatosplenic candidiasis. It is not uncommon for disseminated candidacies to cause persistent fevers for weeks despite appropriate treatment. However since persistent shock and fever is a concern for treatment failure and should warrant escalation of antifungal treatment to echinocandins.

Suggested Reading
1. Kanda Y, Yamamoto R, Chizuka A. Prophylactic action of oral fluconazole against fungal infection in neutropenic patients: a meta-analysis of 16 randomized, controlled trials. Cancer. 2000;89(7):1611-25.

Q.9. A 55-year-old male diagnosed case of diffuse large B-cell lymphoma stage (DLBCL) IVB status post R-CHOP (rituximab, cyclophosphamide, doxorubicin, vincristine, and prednisone) chemotherapy. Day 8 in the ICU still he has fever spikes, and on norepinephrine 0.2 µg/kg/min. He is on cefepime and vancomycin for 1 week and on fluconazole prophylaxis. Ultrasound showed hepatosplenic candidiasis and USG aspiration culture showed Candida (C.) non-albicans. Which of the following is true regarding this patient?
a. Continue therapeutic fluconazole for 2 weeks.
b. Wait for blood culture for further plan.
c. Change fluconazole to echinocandins.
d. Reassess with USG aspiration for efficacy of treatment.

Ans. c

Explanation: Fluconazole has no intrinsic activity against mucormycosis/Rhizopus, Aspergillus, and Fusarium species or against Candida (C.) krusei.

In patients who are on fluconazole prophylaxis there is higher incidence of colonization with fluconazole-resistant fungi and this should be considered to guide therapy in patients receiving fluconazole prophylaxis.

Also if the patient has persistent fever in the setting of appropriate antifungal therapy, treatment failure due to resistant strain of Candida should be suspected.

Suggested Reading
1. Kontoyiannis DP, Luna MA, Samuels BI, Bodey GP. Hepatosplenic candidiasis: a manifestation of chronic disseminated candidiasis. Infect Dis Clin North Am. 2000;14(3):721-39.

Q.10. A 65-year-old male patient, a known case of extensive stage small cell lung cancer (SCLC), received six cycles of chemotherapy with cisplatin and etoposide, was brought to the emergency department with one episode of generalized tonic-clonic convulsions (GTC). On examination the patient is disoriented and did not recognize his family members and relatives. Vitals were stable. Investigations—CBC normal, serum bilirubin (43 µmol/L) and liver enzymes (alanine aminotransferase 145 U/L, aspartate aminotransferase 107 U/L), as well as increased levels of alkaline phosphatase (460 U/L) and lactate dehydrogenase (798 U/L). Sodium level of is 104 mmol/L. Serum levels of potassium, glucose, creatinine, urea, and ammonia were normal. What is the correct statement?
a. Spurious value of sodium and needs to be repeated.
b. No drug history to cause hyponatremia.

c. Needs urgent CT evaluation.
d. Treat hyponatremia urgently.

Ans. d

Explanation: Hyponatremia in the cancer patient is usually caused by the syndrome of inappropriate antidiuretic hormone (SIADH), which develops more frequently with SCLC than with other malignancies such as breast, head, and neck, etc.

Syndrome of inappropriate antidiuretic hormone may be driven by production of arginine vasopressin (AVP) by tumors or by effects of anticancer medications on AVP production or action.

Cisplatin stimulates AVP secretion to cause SIADH, but uniquely can also directly damage renal tubules to interfere with sodium reabsorption and may lead to hyponatremia via salt wasting nephropathy.

Hyponatremia is generally a negative prognostic factor in patients with non-small cell lung cancer.

Suggested Reading
1. Hamdi T, Latta S, Jallad B, Kheir F, Alhosaini MN, Patel A. Cisplatin-induced renal salt wasting syndrome. South Med J. 2010;103:793-99.
2. Lassen U, Osterlind K, Hansen M, Dombernowsky P, Bergman B, Hansen HH. Long-term survival in small-cell lung cancer: posttreatment characteristics in patients surviving 5 to 18+ years—an analysis of 1,714 consecutive patients. J Clin Oncol. 1995;13:1215-20.
3. Ray P, Quantin X, Grenier J, Pujol JL. Predictive factors of tumor response and prognostic factors of survival during lung cancer chemotherapy. Cancer Detect Prev. 1998;22:293-304.

Q.11. A 65-year-old male patient, a known case of extensive stage SCLC, received six cycles of chemotherapy with cisplatin and etoposide was brought to the emergency department with one episode of GTC. On examination, the patient has altered sensorium, vitals were stable. CT scan done just before shifting to ICU reveals no stroke or metastasis. Investigations—CBC normal, serum bilirubin 4 mg/dL, AST 140 U/L, ALT 120 U/L, alkaline phosphatase 540 U/L, LDH 878 U/L, serum Na 104 mmol/L, serum osmolality 208 mOsm/L, urine sodium, and osmolality were consistent with SIADH. Serum levels of potassium, glucose, creatinine, urea, and ammonia were normal. What is the correct way to treat symptomatic hyponatremia?
a. Restrict water to 1.5L/day and give extra salt in diet.
b. Normal saline infusion 100 mL/hour and repeat serum sodium after 4 hours.
c. 3% saline infused at a rate of 0.5-2 mL/kg/hour until symptoms resolve.
d. 3% NS at 100 mL/hour for 4 hours.

Ans. c

Explanation: Severe hyponatremia with neurological symptoms such as seizures, coma typically occurs when the sodium level falls below 120 mEq/L, but can occur at <125 mEq/L.

Severe symptomatic hyponatremia must be corrected promptly because it can lead to cerebral edema, irreversible neurologic damage, respiratory arrest, brainstem herniation, and death. The rate of sodium correction should be 6–12 mEq/L in the first 24 hours and 18 mEq/L or less in 48 hours.

An increase of 4–6 mEq/L is usually sufficient to reduce symptoms of acute hyponatremia.

Suggested Reading
1. Braun MM, Barstow CH, Pyzocha NJ. Diagnosis and management of sodium disorders: hyponatremia and hypernatremia. Am Fam Physician. 2015;91(5):299-307.

Q.12. A 65-year-old male patient, a known case of SCLC status post six cycles of chemotherapy with cisplatin and etoposide, was brought to the emergency department with altered sensorium and one episode of GTCs secondary to SIADH-induced hyponatremia. His CT scan was unremarkable. He received 3% NS (0.5–2 mL/kg/hour), his serum sodium level improved from 104 mmol/L to 112 mmol/L. On examination, he is conscious, oriented, afebrile, and systemic examination is unremarkable. Other investigations are CBC normal, serum bilirubin 4 mg/dL, AST 140 U/L, ALT 120 U/L, alkaline phosphatase 540 U/L, and LDH 878 U/L. Which is not correct regarding:
a. Tolvaptan is routinely recommended for hyponatremia correction.
b. Loop diuretics may be needed in patients with concurrent symptomatic hyponatremia and volume overload.
c. Fluid restriction should be limited to 500 mL less than the daily urinary volume.
d. Volume status can be difficult to determine and hence a trial of intravenous fluids can be given.

Ans. a

Explanation: Vaptans are vasopressin-receptor antagonists approved for the treatment of hospitalized patients with severe hypervolemic and euvolemic hyponatremia. Studies have shown that tolvaptan is associated with reduction in cardiovascular morbidity and mortality patients with hyponatremia and heart failure.

However tolvaptan should not be used in patients with hepatic impairment because they may worsen liver function. The European Society of Endocrinology guidelines in fact recommend against the routine use of vaptans due to lack of reduction in overall mortality rates and risk of rapid overcorrection.

Suggested Reading
1. Dahl E, Gluud LL, Kimer N, Krag A. Meta-analysis: the safety and efficacy of vaptans (tolvaptan, satavaptan and lixivaptan) in cirrhosis with ascites or hyponatraemia. Aliment Pharmacol Ther. 2012;36(7):619-26.
2. Spasovski G, Vanholder R, Allolio B, Annane D, Ball S, Bichet D, et al.; Hyponatraemia Guideline Development Group. Clinical practice guideline on diagnosis and treatment of hyponatraemia. Eur J Endocrinol. 2014;170(3):G1-G47.

Q.13. A 51-year-old male with newly diagnosed, poorly differentiated cholangiocarcinoma with hepatic and pulmonary metastases presented to ICU with right upper quadrant abdominal pain, cough, and weakness. Empiric vancomycin, cefepime,

and levofloxacin were started. X-ray chest showed multiple bilateral pulmonary nodules, right basilar effusion, and consolidation. On examination, laboratory findings—Hb 7, WBC 53,500/mm^3, platelet 180,000/mm^3, BUN 55, Cr 2, Na 138, K 6, Cl 96, Ca 9.4, PO$_4$ 4.6, UA 10.2, alkaline phosphatase 1640, serum glutamic-oxaloacetic transaminase (SGOT) 480, and serum glutamate pyruvate transaminase (SGPT) 460. What is appropriate for this patient?
a. Spontaneous TLS (STLS)
b. TLS ruled out since its cholangiocarcinoma and phosphate is normal.
c. Repeat uric acid.
d. Needs bone marrow to confirm other malignancy.

Ans. a

Explanation: Tumor lysis syndrome (TLS) is a complication that is more commonly associated with hematologic malignancy such as acute lymphocytic leukemia and Burkitt lymphoma upon initiation of chemotherapy.

Tumor lysis syndrome can occur rarely in some solid tumors, including small cell lung cancer, breast cancer, colorectal cancer, neuroblastoma, ovarian cancer, and hepatocellular carcinoma. It is relatively rare for tumor lysis to occur spontaneously in solid tumors.

It is also known that hyperphosphatemia and hypocalcemia is less likely in STLS as compared to chemotherapy-induced TLS, due to the continued phosphate uptake into rapidly dividing tumor cells that would have been destroyed in typical TLS.

Given its uncommon occurrence and vague clinical picture, STLS may very likely be underdiagnosed, and a high degree of clinical suspicion is needed to ensure prompt intervention to change clinical outcomes.

Suggested Reading
1. Ali AM, Barbaryan A, Zdunek T, Khan M, Voore P, Mirrakhimov AE. Spontaneous tumor lysis syndrome in a patient with cholangiocarcinoma. J Gastrointest Oncol. 2014;5(2):E46-9.

Q.14. A 18-year-old male presented with 3 days' history of fever breathlessness, malaise, bone pain, and cervical lymphadenopathy. Chest radiography revealed a small mediastinal mass, and an electrocardiogram was normal. Laboratory findings—Hb 6, WBC 84,600/mm^3 with circulating blasts, Na 133 mmol/L, K 5.9 mmol/L, HCO$_3$ 16 mmol/L, Cr 1.0 mg/dL, PO$_4$ 8.5 mg/dL, Ca 6.7 mg/dL, UA 4.3 mg/dL, and LDH 4233 IU/L.
a. Does not have TLS since UA is not elevated.
b. Not TLS since not yet diagnosed to have cancer.
c. Does not have TLS since yet to be treated.
d. TLS

Ans. d

Explanation: The above patient's clinical and laboratory findings are consistent with diagnosis of TLS.

According to the current classification system of Cairo and Bishop, the tumor lysis syndrome can be classified as laboratory or clinical.

Laboratory tumor lysis syndrome requires that two or more of the following metabolic abnormalities occur within 3 days before or up to 7 days after the initiation of therapy—hyperuricemia, hyperkalemia, hyperphosphatemia, and hypocalcemia.

Clinical tumor lysis syndrome is present when laboratory tumor lysis syndrome is accompanied by an increased creatinine level, seizures, cardiac dysrhythmia, or death.

The modified Howard definition of LTLS is ≥2 of the following metabolic abnormalities occurring simultaneously within 3 days prior to and up to 7 days after treatment initiation—hyperuricemia (>8.0 mg/dL), hyperkalemia (>6.0 mmol/L), hyperphosphatemia (>4.5 mg/dL), and hypocalcemia (corrected Ca <7.0 mg/dL, ionized Ca <1.12 mg/dL). The modified Howard definition for CTLS is the same as laboratory-defined TLS, and is accompanied by elevated creatinine level, seizures, cardiac dysrhythmia, or death.

Suggested Reading
1. Cairo MS, Bishop M. Tumour lysis syndrome: new therapeutic strategies and classification. Br J Haematol. 2004;127:3-11.
2. Howard SC, Jones DP, Pui CH. The tumor lysis syndrome. N Engl J Med. 2011;364:1844-54.

Q.15. A 18-year-male diagnosed case of T-cell acute lymphoblastic leukemia presented with history of fever breathlessness, malaise, bone pain, and cervical lymphadenopathy. Chest radiography revealed a small mediastinal mass, and an electrocardiogram was normal. Laboratory findings—Hb 6, WBC 84,600/mm^3, Na 133 mmol/L, K 5.9 mmol/L, HCO$_3$ 16 mmol/L, Cr 1.0 mg/dL, PO$_4$ 8.5 mg/dL, Ca 6.7 mg/dL, UA 14.3 mg/dL, and LDH 4233 IU/L. The patient is started on hydration and allopurinol. What is the true regarding use of rasburicase?
a. Not required when allopurinol is already initiated.
b. Hydration is enough to reduce the uric acid levels.
c. Rasburicase is superior to allopurinol to reduce the incidence of nephropathy.
d. Rasburicase is safe in presence of G6PD deficiency.

Ans. c

Explanation: Rasburicase is a recombinant form of urate oxidase, an enzyme responsible for the breakdown of UA into soluble allantoin. Rasburicase rapidly lowers UA levels, usually within 4 hours of administration. It also provides better control of UA compared to allopurinol.

Rasburicase should not be administered in patients with glucose-6-phosphate dehydrogenase (G6PD) deficiency due to the risk of hemolysis. Rasburicase breaks down UA and results in the production of hydrogen peroxide. In patients with G6PD deficiency, it may result in an increased risk of hemolytic anemia and methemoglobinemia.

Suggested Reading
1. Goldman SC, Holcenberg JS, Finklestein JZ, Hutchinson R, Kreissman S, Johnson FL, et al. A randomized comparison between rasburicase and allopurinol in children with lymphoma or leukemia at high risk for tumor lysis. Blood. 2001;97(10):2998-3003.
2. Ibrahim U, Saqib A, Mohammad F, Atallah JP, Odaimi M. Rasburicase-induced methemoglobinemia: The eyes do not see what the mind does not know. J Oncol Pharm Pract. 2018;24(4):309-13.

Q.16. A 18-year-old male diagnosed case of T-cell acute lymphoblastic leukemia presented with TLS to the ICU. Laboratory findings—Hb 6, WBC 84,600/mm^3, Na 133 mmol/L, K 5.9 mmol/L, HCO$_3$ 16 mmol/L, Cr 1.0 mg/dL, PO$_4$ 8.5 mg/dL, Ca 6.7 mg/dL, UA 14.3 mg/dL, and LDH 4233 IU/L. He was started on intravenous fluids 3 L/m^2, rasburicase (0.15 mg/kg), and 800 mg of aluminum hydroxide. What is true regarding further management?
  a. Urinary alkalinization is the effective in treatment of renal failure.
  b. Urinary alkalinizing the urine may prevent calcium phosphate deposition in kidney.
  c. Urinary alkalization can prevent xanthine nephropathy.
  d. Urinary alkalinization is no longer routinely recommended.

Ans. d

Explanation: Urinary alkalinization was considered for prevention of TLS as increasing the urine pH, UA remains ionized and more soluble and less likely to precipitate in the renal tubules thus decreasing the incidence of UA nephropathy.

However, alkalinizing the urine facilitates calcium phosphate precipitation and deposition in the kidneys in patients with severe hyperphosphatemia.

Urinary alkalization can in fact cause a xanthine nephropathy by decreasing the solubility of xanthine, a precursor of UA.

Thus urinary alkalinization is no longer routinely recommended because it may be associated with metabolic acidosis and calcium phosphate precipitation.

Suggested Reading
1. Davidson MB, Thakkar S, Hix JK, Bhandarkar ND, Wong A, Schreiber MJ. Pathophysiology, clinical consequences, and treatment of tumor lysis syndrome. Am J Med. 2004;116(8):546-54.
2. Wilson FP, Berns JS. Onco-nephrology: tumor lysis syndrome. Clin J Am Soc Nephrol. 2012;7(10):1730-9.

Q.17. A 18-year-old male diagnosed case of T-cell acute lymphoblastic leukemia presented with TLS to the ICU. Laboratory findings—Hb 6, WBC 84,600/mm^3, Na 133 mmol/L, K 5.9 mmol/L, HCO$_3$ 16 mmol/L, Cr 1.0 mg/dL, PO$_4$ 8.5 mg/dL, Ca 6.7 mg/dL, UA 14.3 mg/dL, and LDH 4233 IU/L. He was started on intravenous fluids 3 L/m^2, rasburicase (0.15 mg/kg), and 800 mg of aluminum hydroxide and oral sodium polystyrene sulfonate however he developed oliguria, hyperphosphatemia (11.2 mg/dL) and creatinine 2 mg/dL and started to develop broad complex tachyarrythmias on ECG which was managed by glucose insulin drip. What is the true regarding further management?
  a. Continue IV fluids with loop diuretics.
  b. Continue GI drip.
  c. Start NaHCO$_3$ infusion.
  d. Consider urgent continuous renal replacement therapy (CRRT).

Ans. d

Explanation: Hyperkalemia in TLS is most dangerous as it can cause sudden death due to cardiac dysrhythmia. Glucose plus insulin, beta-agonists, and calcium gluconate are used as temporary measures while awaiting hemodialysis.

Administration of excessive calcium increases the risk of calcium phosphate crystallization, particularly if the product is >60 mg^2/dL^2.

The thresholds for renal-replacement therapy are lower in patients with the tumor lysis syndrome as compared to other causes of acute kidney injury.

Continuous renal replacement therapy modalities such as continuous venovenous hemofiltration, continuous venovenous hemodialysis, or continuous venovenous hemodiafiltration are preferred over conventional hemodialysis since it can allow the use of larger pore size filters facilitating more rapid clearance of molecules.

Suggested Reading
1. Gutzwiller JP, Schneditz D, Huber AR, Schindler C, Gutzwiller F, Zehnder CE. Estimating phosphate removal in haemodialysis: an additional tool to quantify dialysis dose. Nephrol Dial Transplant. 2002;17(6):1037-44.

Q.18. A 22-year-male newly diagnosed to have acute myeloid leukemia presented to the ICU with headache, pain in abdomen, and blurring of vision. Emergent CT head done just before shifting to ICU was unremarkable. On examination his chest was clear with normal heart sounds, abdomen examination revealed gross hepatosplenomegaly. While getting evaluated in the ICU he developed priapism for which urology consult was sorted. His laboratory findings revealed—Hb 6, WBC 520 × 10^9/L, uric acid 8.5 mg/dL. Rest investigations—electrolytes, liver function tests, coagulation indices, and the level of amylase and lipase were normal. What is the most appropriate in terms of further management?
   a. Start hydroxyurea, allopurinol and intravenous fluids.
   b. Start low dose chemotherapy.
   c. Consider leukopheresis.
   d. Start chemotherapy with monitoring of TLS.

Ans. c

Explanation: Hyperleukocytosis syndrome can present with headache, dizziness, altered mental status and pulmonary insufficiency due large numbers of circulating blasts (monocytic, myelocytic or myelomonocytic cell lines which are considered the "stickiest") causing leukostasis, vascular occlusion, and perivascular leukemic infiltration.

The huge cell load can cause severe inflammatory response due release of lysosomal contents and can initiate the coagulation cascade causing catastrophic microvascular coagulation.

Leukopheresis can be considered in such group of patients for rapid reversal of leukostasis-mediated symptoms. Evidences suggest that patients presenting with neurological, respiratory or renal complications had higher early mortality rates than those without such complications despite similar initial leukocyte counts and comparable leukoreductions. This lack of correlation between the degree of leukoreduction and early mortality has discouraged the use of leukoreduction as routine modality of care.

Suggested Reading
1. Bunin NJ, Kunkel K, Callihan TR. Cytoreductive procedures in the early management in cases of leukemia and hyperleukocytosis in children. Med Pediatr Oncol. 1987;15:232-5.
2. Porcu P, Danielson CF, Orazi A, Heerema NA, Gabig TG, McCarthy LJ. Therapeutic leukapheresis in hyperleucocytic leukaemias: lack of correlation between degree of cytoreduction and early mortality rate. Br J Haematol. 1997;98:433-6.

Q.19. A 81-year-old woman recently diagnosed with multiple myeloma was admitted with altered sensorium to the ICU. She had history of constipation for 4 days. On examination, she was irritable and stuporous, dehydrated, and pale. Vitals were stable GCS – E2V2M4, no neck rigidity, Babinski's sign negative, and pupils reacted normally. Laboratory findings—Hb 9.2 g/dL, WBC 4.5 × 10^9/L, Ca 18.1 mEq/L, PO_4 5.2 mg/dL, serum Na 123 mEq/L, BUN 96 mg/dL, and Cr 2.6 mg/dL. What is the most appropriate in terms of further management?
a. Parathyroid hormone and vitamin D_3 to diagnose hypercalcemia of malignancy (HCM).
b. Parathyroid hormone-related protein (PTHrP) to diagnose HCM.
c. Consider intravenous saline, furosemide, calcitonin and zoledronic acid infusion and consider hemodialysis.
d. Continue intravenous saline, furosemide, calcitonin zoledronic acid infusion, and discuss goals of care with the oncologist.

Ans. d

Explanation: Hypercalcemia of malignancy occurs in 10–30% of patients with cancer. HCM is often considered as a sign of advanced cancer. HCM can be graded as mild, moderate, and severe depending on the serum calcium concentrations (10.5–11.9, 12–13.4, and ≥13.5 mg/dL respectively)

Pathogenesis of HCM can be:
1. Humoral HCM mediated by PTHrP (commonly seen in squamous cell carcinoma and renal cell carcinoma).
2. HCM secondary to osteolysis of bone due to metastasis or direct involvement (metastatic carcinoma breast, multiple myeloma, and leukemia).
3. Ectopic production of calcitriol by malignancy (lymphomas and ovarian tumors) and ectopic production of PTH.

Suggested Reading
1. Ralston SH, Gallacher SJ, Patel U, Campbell J, Boyle IT. Cancer-associated hypercalcemia: morbidity and mortality. Ann Intern Med. 1990;112:499-504.
2. Stewart AF. Hypercalcemia associated with cancer. N Engl J Med. 2005;352:373-9.

Q.20. A 22-year-old male presented to the ICU with cough and breathlessness NYHA III which was worse in supine position. There was no history of fever, chest pain, and cyanosis or wheezing. On examination afebrile, HR 140 bpm regular, BP 110/80 mm Hg, RR 28/minute, SpO_2 95% on room air. His jugular venous pulse (JVP) is elevated. Heart sounds were diminished, while lung auscultation showed a

reduced right side air entry. Laboratory findings—Hb 7.5, WBC 15 × 10⁹/L, ABG pH of 7.45, PO$_2$ 60 mm Hg, PCO$_2$ 30 mm Hg, chest X-ray (CXR)—enlarged mediastinum suggesting anterior mediastinal mass and a significant right-sided pleural effusion. What is next most appropriate step?
  a. Advice urgent CT chest to evaluate the disease status.
  b. Urgent bedside echo.
  c. Tissue biopsy to confirm diagnosis.
  d. Oncology consult for chemotherapy.

Ans. b

Explanation: Anterior mediastinal tumors can cause cardiac tamponade due to direct mass effect and should not be dismissed in the presence of a pericardial effusion.

Cardiac tamponade may be the first or predominant symptom of some pathologies.

Echo can confirm the diagnosis and also guide emergent subxyphoid pericardiotomy which can be lifesaving.

Suggested Reading
  1. Perek B, Tomaszewska I, Stefaniak S, Katynska I, Jemielity M. Cardiac tamponade - unusual clinical manifestation of undiagnosed malignant neoplasm Neoplasma. 2016;63(4):601-6.

Q.21. A 37-year-old male presented to the emergency department with the chief complaint of neck swelling for a week and a half, a dry cough that worsened with exertion and was relieved by rest. Vital signs—conscious, heart rate 82 beats/minute, blood pressure 137/79 mm Hg, and temperature 36.0°C, pupils equal, chest on auscultation is clear, heart sounds normal, regular with no murmur. *Laboratory findings*—Hb 7.5, WBC 15 × 10⁹/L, platelet count 392 × 10⁹/L, sodium 140 mmol/L, potassium 4.7 mmol/L, chloride 102 mmol/L, bicarbonate 27 mmol/L, blood urea nitrogen 7 mmol/L, and creatinine 88.4 µmol/L, and ECG normal. CT scan—large lobulated mass on the right upper chest invading the mediastinum measuring 8 cm × 6 cm × 8 cm with compressed superior vena cava (SVC) and dilated azygos vein. What is the appropriate management?
  a. Dexamethasone 4 mg every 6 hours
  b. Radiotherapy
  c. Thrombolysis and anticoagulation
  d. Endovascular dilation and stenting of the SVC

Ans. d

Explanation: Superior vena cava syndrome is a clinical diagnosis and X-ray, computed tomography (CT), and venography are used only for confirmation.

Thrombolysis and anticoagulation may be indicated in SVC thrombus is found on venography. Fibrinolytic therapy with urokinase and endovascular catheter-directed (intraclot) thrombolytic infusion therapy are currently being used.

However in cases of SVC syndrome due to mediastinal tumor-related compressions, percutaneous stent placement is a simple, safe, and effective technique to rapidly relieve SVC syndrome symptoms.

Suggested Reading
1. Higdon ML, Higdon JA. Treatment of oncologic emergencies. Am Fam Physician. 2006;74:1873-80.
2. Nunnelee JD. Superior vena cava syndrome. J Vasc Nurs. 2007;25:2-5.

Q.22. A 75-year-old female, a known hypertensive, diagnosed case of diffuse large B-cell lymphoma. Her 2D Echo showed a left ventricular ejection fraction (LVEF) of 70%. She received six cycles chemotherapy R-CHOP (rituximab, cyclophosphamide, doxorubicin hydrochloride vincristine, and prednisone) protocol. A total cumulative dose of doxorubicin (550 mg/m^2) rituximab (7.7 g/m^2), cyclophosphamide (8.4 g/m^2), vincristine (12 mg/m^2), and prednisone (3 g/m^2) was administered. She completed her last cycle 6 months back. Presently she was admitted with exertional dyspnea, orthopnea, and decreased effort capacity. No previous history of chest pain or angina was noted. On examination—conscious, afebrile, HR 110/minute regular, BP 100/70 mm Hg, bilateral pretibial edema, tachycardia, chest—bilateral crackles, normal heart sounds, CXR—increased bronchovascular markings with bilateral pleural effusion, ECG—sinus, tachycardia, no ST-T changes, high sensitivity troponin I of 110 pg/mL, BNP of 847.2 pg/mL. 2D Echo showed—global hypokinesia, no wall motion abnormalities, moderate to severe aortic regurgitation, LVEF 35%. What is the most appropriate for this patient?
a. Consider a cardiac MRI to diagnose.
b. Consider coronary angiography to rule out CAD.
c. Diagnosis is consistent with anthracycline cardiomyopathy.
d. Consider endocardial biopsy for the diagnosis.

Ans. c

Explanation: Chemotherapy-induced cardio toxicity is described as type I or type II depending on the type of injury. Type I cardiotoxicity is irreversible as it leads to cardiomyocyte death by necrosis or apoptosis. Type II cardiotoxicity is caused by cardiomyocyte dysfunction and, as such, may be reversible. Anthracycline cardiotoxicity is considered as type I as it occurs by oxidative stress, inhibiting topoisomerase 2β and the resulting activation of cell death pathways and inhibition of mitochondrial biogenesis. However, recent studies seem to suggest that cardiomyopathy is mostly reversible if detected early and treated promptly. Genetic factors such as hereditary hemochromatosis, C282Y HFE gene mutation are recognized as risk factors to increased anthracycline cardiotoxicity.

Suggested Reading
1. Cardinale D, Iacopo F, Cipolla CM. Cardiotoxicity of anthracyclines. Front Cardiovasc Med. 2020;7:26.
2. Henriksen PA. Anthracycline cardiotoxicity: an update on mechanisms, monitoring and prevention. Heart. 2018;104(12):971-7.

Q.23. A 35-year-old male admitted with acute chest pain after receiving chemotherapy. He is known case of testicular germ cell tumor. He was receiving third cycle of BOP regimen. There is no significant past medical history. On examination, conscious,

afebrile, HR 126 bpm, BP 160/90 mm Hg, auscultation, bilateral crepts present with S_3 gallop. 12-lead ECG—ST segment depression with T inversion in anterolateral leads. 2D Echo—anterolateral wall hypokinesia, LVEF 35%. Troponin T test was positive. What is the most appropriate?
a. Unlikely to have AMI since no risk factors.
b. Possibility of coronary spasm due to cisplatin.
c. CAG is the not necessary for the diagnosis.
d. Cardiac MRI is the diagnostic test.

Ans. b

Explanation: Cisplatin-induced coronary thrombosis or spasm occurs due to direct action on myocytes or production of reactive oxygen species that induce oxidative stress and cause coronary spasm or thrombus formation.

Direct cardiotoxicity has also been suggested due to oxidative stress on the cardiac cells with lipid peroxidation causing physical injury and functional damage.

Cisplatin can also alter potassium and magnesium levels within and outside the cells predisposing to arrhythmias. Direct action on sodium channels has also been suggested to cause arrhythmias.

Suggested Reading
1. Nuver J, Smit AJ, van der Meer J, van den Berg MP, van der Graaf WT, Meinardi MT, et al. Acute chemotherapy-induced cardiovascular changes in patients with testicular cancer. J Clin Oncol. 2005;23(36):9130-7.
2. Raja W, Mir MH, Dar I, Banday MA, Ahmad I. Cisplatin induced paroxysmal supraventricular tachycardia. Indian J Med Paediatr Oncol. 2013;34(4):330-2.

Q.24. A 18-year-old male patient diagnosed as high-grade osteosarcoma of the right tibia. Before chemotherapy all his investigations were normal. He received IV methotrexate (12 g/m^2). Day after the chemotherapy he developed altered sensorium and hypotension and was shifted to ICU. He was intubated and mechanically ventilated and started on noradrenaline 0.03 µg/kg/min. Injection meropenem and Vancomycin started. Cr 3 mg/dL and hyperkaliemia up to 6.1 mmol/L. AST 10,121 U/L, ALT 6,510 U/L, Bilirubin 4 g%, INR 3.28. What is most appropriate step regarding methotrexate toxicity?
a. Urine alkalinization is a not recommended during MTX infusion.
b. Leucovorin should be administered before methotrexate infusion.
c. Plasma methotrexate monitoring is an unreliable indicator specifically of nephrotoxicity.
d. Leucovorin, glucarpidase, cholestyramine and N-acetylcysteine should be administered considering methotrexate toxicity.

Ans. d

Explanation: The patient is suspected to have acute renal failure secondary to methotrexate toxicity. He should receive leucovorin 100 mg/m^2 QDS for the competitive inhibition of the activity of methotrexate, glucarpidase (50 U/kg) to eliminate methotrexate faster, cholestyramine to decrease enterohepatic circulation and N-acetylcysteine to reduce the oxidative damage on the liver. Hyperhydration 4,500 mL/m^2/24 hours with sodium bicarbonate should be used to maintain urine alkalinization. In refractory metabolic acidosis and hyperkalemia, hemodialysis was initiated along with liver organ support and liver dialysis.

Suggested Reading
1. Aumente D, Buelga DS, Lukas JC, Gomez P, Torres A, García MJ. Population pharmacokinetics of high-dose methotrexate in children with acute lymphoblastic leukaemia. Clin Pharmacokinet. 2006;45(12):1227-38.
2. Saland JM, Leavey PJ, Bash RO, Hansch E, Arbus GS, Quigley R. Effective removal of methotrexate by high-flux hemodialysis. Pediatr Nephrol. 2002;17(10):825-9.
3. Widemann BC, Adamson PC. Understanding and managing methotrexate nephrotoxicity. Oncologist. 2006;11(6):694-703.

Q.25. A 50-year-old female known case of phleomorphic sarcoma, she received ifosfamide (2 g/m^2/day), epirubicin (50 mg/m^2), and cisplatin (80 mg/m^2). On day 4 of chemotherapy the patient presented to ICU with altered sensorium and myoclonic jerks. Laboratory findings—Hb 9.2 g/dL, WBC 12,700/mm^3, LDH 238 IU, blood sugar, and LFT/RFT normal. CNS examination—Drowsy, arousal, GCS E3 M5 V2, no neck rigidity, no neurodeficit pupils B/L sluggish with diffuse myoclonus. CT brain was unremarkable. Injection ceftriaxone and vancomycin was started. What is the most appropriate for management of this patient?
a. MRI is diagnostic of ifosfamide neurotoxicity.
b. CT scan is diagnostic.
c. CSF is necessary for diagnosis.
d. Clinically ifosfamide toxicity and administer methylene blue

Ans. d

Explanation: Patient should be started on intravenous hydration (3000 mL/day) and methylene blue 50 mg every 4 hours.

Ifosfamide-induced encephalopathy is a clinical diagnosis, with a variable onset after ifosfamide (2–140 hours). Methylene blue has shown to be effective in symptom resolution. Methylene blue serves as electron acceptor and preventing chloroethylamine from inhibiting flavoprotein and thus improves mitochondrial function. Methylene blue inhibits extrahepatic monoamine oxidases, prevents dehydrogenation of aldehydes and formation of chloroacetaldehyde.

Thiamine has been tried in ifosfamide-induced encephalopathy with variable results.

Suggested Reading
1. Kataria PS, Kendre PP, Patel AA. Ifosfamide-induced encephalopathy precipitated by aprepitant: a rarely manifested side effect of drug interaction. J Pharmacol Pharmacother. 2017;8(1):38-40.
2. Richards A, Marshall H, McQuary A. Evaluation of methylene blue, thiamine, and/or albumin in the prevention of ifosfamide-related neurotoxicity. J Oncol Pharm Pract. 2011;17(4):372-80.

Q.26. A 55-year-old male known case of carcinoma prostrate was found unresponsive and was shifted to the ED. Past medical history of COPD, DM and IHD. On examination—GCS 3/15, HR 120/minute, RR 20/minute shallow, BP 110/70 mm Hg, SpO$_2$ 85% on O$_2$ by mask, ABG pH 7.2/PCO$_2$ 22/PO$_2$ 57/HCO$_3$ 30. The decision is made to intubate. What is the best method to assess airway?

a. LEMON score
b. 3-3-2 rule
c. Wilson score
d. MACOCHA score

Ans. d

Explanation: The MACOCHA score is a predictive score of difficult intubation in the ICU that has been externally validated.

The MACOCHA score allows identification of patients at risk of difficult intubation.

The main predictors of difficult intubation are classified according to:
- Patient factors (Mallampati score III or IV, obstructive apnea syndrome, reduced mobility of cervical spine, limited mouth opening)
- Operator factor (nonanesthesiologist)
- Pathology factors (coma, severe hypoxia)
- A score of 3 or greater was indicative of difficult intubation.

	Points
Factors related to patient:	
• **M**allampati Score III or IV	5
• Obstructive Sleep **A**pnea Syndrome	2
• Reduced Mobility of **C**ervical Spine	1
• Limited Mouth **O**pening <3 cm	1
Factors related to pathology:	
• **C**oma	1
• Severe **H**ypoxemia (<80%)	1
Factor related to operator:	
• Non-**A**nesthesiologist	1
Total	**12**

M. Mallampati score III or IV
A. Apnea syndrome (obstructive)
C. Cervical spine limitation
O. Opening mouth <3 cm
C. Coma
H. Hypoxia
A. Anesthesiologist non-trained

Coded from 0 to 12
0 = easy
12 = very difficult

Source: De Jong A, Molinari N, Terzi N, Mongardon N, Arnal JM, Guitton C, et al. Early identification of patients at risk for difficult intubation in the intensive care unit: development and validation of the MACOCHA score in a multicenter cohort study. Am J Respir Crit Care Med. 2013;187(8):832-9.

Suggested Reading
1. De Jong A, Molinari N, Terzi N, Mongardon N, Arnal JM, Guitton C, et al. Early identification of patients at risk for difficult intubation in the intensive care unit: development and validation of the MACOCHA score in a multicenter cohort study. Am J Respir Crit Care Med. 2013;187(8):832-9.

Q.27. A 58-year-old woman came to an ED with history of palpitation dizziness and headache. She had no chest pain, dyspnea, fever, seizures, or gastrointestinal (GI) symptoms. History of hypertension—5 mg amlodipine. On examination—Conscious, afebrile, HR 70/minute regular, RR 20/minute, BP 190/90 mm Hg, temperature 36.4°C, SpO$_2$ 98%. Troponin I 0.30 ng/mL, CK-MB 41 IU/L, NT-pro BNP 5,138.77 pg/mL. Rest investigations were within normal limits. Electrocardiograph (ECG)—ST-segment depression in V2-V6. Echocardiography revealed a hypertrophic ventricular wall with an ejection fraction of 60%. Coronary CT angiography (CTA) suggested mild stenosis of the left anterior descending branch. Chest CT and cerebral CT were normal. CT abdomen showed 5 cm × 4 cm tumor of the left adrenal gland. What is true regarding this patient?
a. CT scam 4 fludeoxyglucose positron emission tomography CT is diagnostic of pheochromocytoma.
b. Blood norepinephrine, epinephrine, and dopamine most sensitive MRI diagnostic of pheochromocytoma.
c. VMA, metanephrines, and catecholamines in a 24-h urine or plasma is diagnostic.

Ans. b

Explanation: Pheochromocytomas and paragangliomas (PPGLs) are rare neuroendocrine chromaffin tumors that maybe secretory and produce catecholamines.

About 80–85% of PPGLs come from the adrenal medulla (pheochromocytoma), whereas about 15–20% of PPGLs come from the sympathetic or parasympathetic paravertebral ganglia (paragangliomas).

The effects of catecholamines on different organs depend on their blood concentration and the types of adrenergic receptors in the organs causing highly variable clinical symptoms and signs.

The most common symptoms are headaches, sweating, heart palpitations, and hypertension while serious potential cardiovascular complications include arrhythmia, hypotension, myocardial ischemia, shock, aortic dissection, cardiomyopathy, and peripheral ischemia.

PPGLs may express neuroendocrine markers such as chromogranin A and synaptophysin which helps distinguish them from other neuroendocrine tumors.

Suggested Reading
1. Carrasquillo JA, Chen CC, Jha A, Ling A, Lin FI, Pryma DA, et al. Imaging of pheochromocytoma and paraganglioma. J Nucl Med. 2021;62:1033-42.
2. Gunawardane PTK, Grossman A. Phaeochromocytoma and paraganglioma. Adv Exp Med Biol. 2017;956:239-59.

Q.28. A 22-year-old female came to an ED with history of palpitation dizziness and headache. She had no chest pain, dyspnea, fever, seizures, or GI symptoms. On examination—Conscious, afebrile, HR 70/minute regular, RR 20/minute, BP 190/90 mm Hg, temperature 36.4°C, SpO$_2$ 98%. ECG and ECHO were normal. Abdominal MRI showed a retroperitoneal tumor and diagnosis of pheochromocytoma was made. 24-hour urine test—secretion of norepinephrine significantly increased. What is true regarding this patient?
   a. Somatostatin receptor scintigraphy is necessary to confirm sites of secretion.
   b. Consider emergent surgery.
   c. Start phenoxybenzamine and take for surgery urgently.
   d. Malignancy can be confirmed if metanephrines are elevated.

Ans. a

Explanation: Pheochromocytomas arising outside the adrenal gland is called paraglioma, which is mostly seen in thoracic and abdominal sympathetic nerves. The retroperitoneal paraganglioma accounts for over 50% of all paragangliomas and the functional paraganglioma 15–24%.

Malignancy can be confirmed only if there is a definite diffuse infiltration of surrounding organs/tissues or distant metastasis.

Somatostatin receptor scintigraphy and DOTA scan can help localize secretory metastatic paraganglioma and should be considered before resecting adrenal tumor.

Suggested Reading
1. Ezzat Abdel-Aziz T, Prete F, Conway G, Gaze M, Bomanji J, Bouloux P, et al. Phaeochromocytomas and paragangliomas: A difference in disease behaviour and clinical outcomes. J Surg Oncol. 2015;112(5):486-91.
2. Thompson LD. Pheochromocytoma of the Adrenal gland Scaled Score (PASS) to separate benign from malignant neoplasms: a clinicopathologic and immunophenotypic study of 100 cases. Am J Surg Pathol. 2002;26:551-66.

Q.29. A 70-year-old male presented with sudden onset of seizures. He had a history of headache, nausea, and visual disturbance for week before. On examination—GCS E3M5V2, HR 50, BP 190/90 mm Hg, SpO$_2$ 98% on room air, neurological examination left UL/LL power 3/5. pupils B/L, sluggish RTL, and no neck rigidity. Magnetic resonance imaging (MRI) showed a right temporal lobe tumor suggestive of glioblastoma multiforme (GBM) and an acute ischemic stroke at the posterior limb of the internal capsule. The acute ischemic stroke was identified at the tumor invasion site. The angiographic study showed that the MCA was occluded. What is the next best approach?
   a. IV thrombolysis
   b. Catheter-directed thrombolysis
   c. Emergent surgery
   d. Urgent chemotherapy

Ans. c

Explanation: Due to the clinical emergency secondary to the tumor, emergent surgery should be considered to relieve and educe ICP. The mechanisms of acute ischemic stroke in GBM may be secondary to mechanical compression, arterial dissection or tumor infiltration to the vascular wall.

Ischemic strokes are commonly seen even after surgery possibly due to radiation vasculopathy, chemotherapy, and cerebral inflammation.

Suggested Reading
1. Farkas A, Schlakman B, Khan M, Joyner D. Glioblastoma presenting with acute middle cerebral artery territory infarct. J. Stroke Cerebrovasc Dis. 2018;27(7):e113-e114.
2. Omuro A, DeAngelis LM. Glioblastoma and other malignant gliomas: a clinical review. JAMA. 2013;310(17):1842-50.

Q.30. A 18-year-old male with lymphoma underwent autologous bone marrow transplant (BMT) after high-dose chemotherapy (etoposide, carboplatin, and cyclophosphamide). He was engrafted on day 19 after transplantation. He developed hemolytic anemia on day 90 and presented to ICU with cough, hemoptysis, and respiratory distress. Chest computed tomography showed diffuse pulmonary hemorrhage and bilateral pleural effusions. On examination—Conscious, afebrile, HR 120/minute, BP 150/90 mm Hg, SpO$_2$ 92% on O$_2$ mask Laboratory findings—Hb 7, WBC 2.3 × 10^9/L, platelets 30 k, urea 70 mg/dL, Cr 2.1. Fragmented red blood cells and elevated LDH levels consistent with hemolytic anemia, negative direct and indirect Coombs tests, normal ADAMTS13 levels. Urine examination—proteinuria and hematuria. What is true regarding this patient?
a. GVHD
b. C5b-9 levels to confirm diagnose TA-TMA
c. Dialysis
d. Plasma exchange

Ans. b

Explanation: According to the clinical presentation, the laboratory findings, and based on the diagnostic criteria of Jodele et al. this patient can be diagnosed to have systemic transplant associated thrombotic microangiopathy (TA-TMA). TA-TMA is characterized by microangiopathic hemolytic anemia, consumptive thrombocytopenia, and organ damage due to microcirculatory failure.

C5b-9 and CH50 levels need to be sent to decide the use of eculizumab. Eculizumab is a humanized monoclonal antibody to complement protein C5 that can prevent tissue damage by inhibiting the formation of C5b-9.

Plasma exchange is effective in acquired thrombotic thrombocytopenic purpura, in which ADAMTS13 activity is severely reduced.

High proteinuria and high C5b-9 levels, as in this case, are poor prognostic factors for TA-TMA.

Suggested Reading
1. Jodele S, Dandoy CE, Lane A, Laskin BL, Teusink-Cross A, Myers KC, et al. Complement blockade for TA-TMA: lessons learned from a large pediatric cohort treated with eculizumab. Blood. 2020;135:1049-57.
2. Jodele S, Laskin BL, Dandoy CE, Myers KC, El-Bietar J, Davies SM, et al. A new paradigm: diagnosis and management of HSCT-associated thrombotic microangiopathy as multi-system endothelial injury. Blood Rev. 2015;29:191-204.

CHAPTER 20

Thromboembolism

Kushal Rajeev Kalvit

Q.1. A 20-year-old female suffering from acute lymphoblastic leukemia (ALL) was started on induction chemotherapy which included vincristine, daunorubicin, prednisone, and asparaginase. One week after the therapy, patient had acute-onset dyspnea and was diagnosed to have submassive pulmonary embolism (PE). Her platelet count was 90,000/mm^3 and her international normalized ratio (INR) was 1.5. Which of the following statements is true regarding anticoagulation in asparaginase-associated thrombosis?
  a. Heparins (UFH or LMWH) are contraindicated in asparaginase therapy-associated PE due to very low antithrombin levels.
  b. Therapeutic dose of enoxaparin should be given for 3–6 months only if the platelet count is >100,000/mm^3 and after FFP transfusion.
  c. There is no change in the prevention and management strategy of PE in asparaginase-associated thrombosis.
  d. Start therapeutic dose of enoxaparin and continue for 6 months along with short-term antithrombin concentrate in the initial stabilization phase.

Ans. d

Explanation: Asparaginase therapy leads to a hypercoagulable state as it reduces the levels of anticoagulants such as antithrombin, protein C, and S. The maximum reduction occurs within 10 days of therapy. Hence, it is advisable to monitor serum antithrombin levels on a weekly basis after initiation of therapy. Antithrombin concentrate needs to be given for levels below 50–60% and a target of 80–120% needs to be achieved to prevent venous thromboembolism (VTE). Moreover, it is now recommended to start daily low-molecular-weight heparin (LMWH) prophylaxis for all patients receiving asparaginase and continue it throughout the induction phase. There is no role of prophylactic fresh frozen plasma (FFP) transfusion to prevent VTE. Once thrombosis has occurred, therapeutic dose of LMWH has to be started with monitoring of anti-Xa levels as the efficacy is unpredictable due to low antithrombin levels. LMWH has to be continued for minimum 6 months with extended therapy based on individual case. In case of a major thrombotic event such as central PE or cerebral venous thrombosis, concurrent antithrombin administration is recommended till the patient improves clinically. Asparaginase therapy has to be withheld during the acute thrombotic event and may be restarted with caution after at least 4 weeks. Direct oral anticoagulants (DOAC) may be alternative if the platelet count is >50,000/mm^3.

Suggested Reading

1. Zwicker JI, Wang TF, DeAngelo DJ, Lauw MN, Connors JM, Falanga A, et al. The prevention and management of asparaginase-related venous thromboembolism in adults: Guidance from the SSC on Hemostasis and Malignancy of the ISTH. J Thromb Haemost. 2020;18(2):278-84.

Q.2. A 50-year-old male was being treated in the intensive care unit (ICU) for ascending cholangitis with septic shock. He was receiving thromboprophylaxis with enoxaparin 40 mg OD. One week later, he developed an acute drop in platelet count from 3.2 to 1.4 lakh/mm^3 without any bleeding manifestations. Routine ultrasound screening of lower limbs revealed proximal deep vein thrombosis (DVT) in left femoral vein. A provisional diagnosis of heparin-induced thrombocytopenia with thrombosis (HITT) was considered. Which of the following statements is true regarding management of HITT?

a. Convert prophylactic dose of enoxaparin to therapeutic dose.
b. Stop enoxaparin, transfuse platelets, and start warfarin.
c. Stop enoxaparin, do not transfuse platelets and start bivalirudin.
d. Stop enoxaparin and start oral rivaroxaban.

Ans. c

Explanation: Heparin-induced thrombocytopenia (HIT) is a prothrombotic phenomenon that occurs during or after heparin therapy [either unfractionated heparin (UFH) or LMWH]. It is caused by antibodies formed against the complex of heparin-platelet factor 4. It leads to thrombocytopenia as these platelet complexes get destroyed by IgG antibodies. 30–50% cases are associated with thrombosis formation (HITT) which may be venous or arterial. Diagnosis of HIT is suspected by the 4T score and confirmed by an immunoassay (IgG) and/or functional (serotonin release) assay. Once HITT is suspected, all heparin anticoagulants need to be stopped immediately. A nonheparin anticoagulant needs to be started for thromboprophylaxis such as argatroban, bivalirudin, fondaparinux, or a DOAC. Bivalirudin and argatroban are the preferred agents for critically ill patients at high risk of bleeding, while DOAC and fondaparinux are used in clinically stable patients with a low bleeding risk. Administration of vitamin K antagonist (VKA) like warfarin is not recommended unless the platelet count is >1.5 lakh/mm^3. There is no role of platelet transfusion. Platelet count recovers within 7 days in 90% of cases. Patients who have recovered from HIT should receive nonheparin anticoagulant if need arises in future.

Suggested Reading

1. Cuker A, Arepally GM, Chong BH, Cines DB, Greinacher A, Gruel Y, et al. American Society of Hematology 2018 guidelines for management of venous thromboembolism: heparin-induced thrombocytopenia. Blood Adv. 2018;2(22):3360-92.

Q.3. A 30-year-old, 32-week pregnant female was diagnosed with proximal femoral vein thrombosis (DVT) in left lower limb. She was hemodynamically stable, had a normal platelet count and coagulation parameters. Which statement is true regarding the management of the same?

a. Start prophylactic dose LMWH, continue in the intrapartum and the postpartum period.
b. Start therapeutic dose LMWH, withhold before delivery and switch to oral DOAC in the postpartum period.
c. Start therapeutic dose UFH in addition to catheter-directed thrombolysis and discontinue heparin after delivery.
d. Start therapeutic dose LMWH, withhold before delivery and continue the same dose in postpartum period.

Ans. d

Explanation: All pregnant females with acute venous thromboembolism (VTE) should be treated with therapeutic dose anticoagulation in which LMWH is preferred over UFH. There is no role of monitoring of anti-Factor Xa level or the use of catheter-directed thrombolysis in these patients. Therapeutic dose of LMWH should be withheld prior to scheduled delivery and then restarted in the postpartum period. The anticoagulant in the postpartum breastfeeding woman could be LMWH, UFH, warfarin, acenocoumarol, fondaparinux, or danaparoid. DOACs are not recommended in the breastfeeding period due to lack of safety data.

Suggested Reading
1. Bates SM, Rajasekhar A, Middeldorp S, McLintock C, Rodger MA, James AH, et al. American Society of Hematology 2018 guidelines for management of venous thromboembolism: venous thromboembolism in the context of pregnancy. Blood Adv. 2018;2(22):3317-59.

Q.4. A 50-year-old male was admitted with acute onset of chest pain and dyspnea. He landed at the airport after a long-haul flight few hours back. He has diabetes mellitus for 10 years and is on metformin along with aspirin for cardiovascular disease risk reduction. He was diagnosed with DVT/PE and had right ventricular (RV) dysfunction on echocardiography. He had normal vital signs except for sinus tachycardia and had no risk factor for DVT/PE. It was decided to anticoagulate him with dabigatran. Which of the following is correct regarding the treatment?
a. Thrombolyse with streptokinase, start anticoagulation with dabigatran, continue aspirin as usual, and continue dabigatran for 3-6 months.
b. Start anticoagulation with enoxaparin for 5-10 days and then start dabigatran; stop aspirin and continue dabigatran lifelong.
c. Start anticoagulation with dabigatran directly for 6 months; continue aspirin thereafter.
d. Anticoagulate with enoxaparin bridged with warfarin for 3-6 months as dabigatran cannot be given in this case.

Ans. b

Explanation: Systemic thrombolysis along with anticoagulation is indicated if any patient with DVT/PE develops hemodynamic compromise. DVT/PE with evidence of RV dysfunction without hypotension (submassive PE) requires only anticoagulation and does not need thrombolysis. DOACs are preferred over VKA for anticoagulation due to better pharmacodynamic and pharmacokinetic profile. There is no recommendation for one DOAC over another. Initial bridging with UFH or LMWH is indicated if anticoagulation is being done with VKA (warfarin), dabigatran, or edoxaban. Bridging with UFH/LMWH is not indicated for rivaroxaban and apixaban. The duration for anticoagulation is usually 3–6 months but has to be continued lifelong in case of either an unprovoked DVT/PE or due to a chronic risk factor. During the period of anticoagulation, it is recommended to stop aspirin if it was being taken for cardiovascular risk reduction [not applicable for recent myocardial infarction (MI) or coronary interventions].

Suggested Reading
1. Ortel TL, Neumann I, Ageno W, Beyth R, Clark NP, Cuker A, et al. American Society of Hematology 2020 guidelines for management of venous thromboembolism: treatment of deep vein thrombosis and pulmonary embolism. Blood Adv. 2020;4(19):4693-738.

Q.5. A 55-year-old male underwent Whipple's procedure for pancreatic cancer. He had no known comorbidities. Which of the following statements is wrong regarding postoperative thromboprophylaxis?
   a. Thromboprophylaxis with enoxaparin can be started after 12 hours if there is no surgical bleeding risk.
   b. Thromboprophylaxis with enoxaparin along with intermittent pneumatic compression (IPC) is preferred over enoxaparin alone.
   c. In case of high-surgical bleeding risk, mechanical thromboprophylaxis with IPC is better than graduated compression stocking (GCS).
   d. Mechanical thromboprophylaxis with GCS alone is sufficient in this case.

Ans. d

Explanation: For any major general, gynecological, cardiac, vascular, or orthopedic surgery, pharmacological thromboprophylaxis should be started in the immediate postoperative period if there is no surgical high risk of bleeding. LMWH is the preferred agent in case of major general or gynecological surgery while DOAC is preferred for total hip arthroplasty and total knee arthroplasty. LMWH or UFH can be used for cardiovascular surgery patients. The timing of initiation can be early (within 12 hours) or late (after 12 hours). It has to be continued for at least 3 weeks. Pharmacological thromboprophylaxis is not recommended after laparoscopic cholecystectomy, laparoscopic prostatectomy, transurethral resection of prostate (TURP), and neurosurgical procedures. In case pharmacological thromboprophylaxis cannot be given, mechanical thromboprophylaxis is indicated in all patients. Mechanical prophylaxis is done by use of intermittent pneumatic compression devices. The combination of LMWH with IPC is better than either of them alone. Use of graduated compression stockings (GCS) only is not recommended in the postoperative period. There is no role of inferior vena cava (IVC) filters for thromboprophylaxis.

Suggested Reading
1. Anderson DR, Morgano GP, Bennett C, Dentali F, Francis CW, Garcia DA, et al. American Society of Hematology 2019 guidelines for management of venous thromboembolism: prevention of venous thromboembolism in surgical hospitalized patients. Blood Adv. 2019;3(23):3898-944.

Q.6. A 30-year-old male was admitted with shortness of breath that started 2 hours back. He did not have any other complaints. His heart rate (HR) was 90 beats/min, blood pressure (BP) was 130/80 mm Hg, and respiratory rate (RR) was 24 breaths/min. He has recovered from a femur fracture 1 month back for which his limb was immobilized for 2 weeks. Which of the following is the correct statement regarding diagnosis of VTE in this case?
   a. A single positive D-dimer test (>500 µg/L) is sufficient to diagnose VTE in this scenario.
   b. A D-dimer test should be done; if D-dimer is negative, a CT pulmonary angiogram should be done.
   c. CT pulmonary angiogram should be done directly without the need for D-dimer testing.
   d. A D-dimer test should be done; if positive, diagnosis of VTE should be confirmed by a CTPA scan.

Ans. d

Explanation: D-dimer testing strategy is preferred when the pretest probability of DVT/PE is low or intermediate. An age-adjusted cut-off value should be used instead of an arbitrary cut-off. A negative D-dimer test rules out VTE and does not need any additional testing. A positive D-dimer test should be followed by either a computed tomography pulmonary angiogram (CTPA) or a VQ scan to confirm VTE. A negative CTPA or VQ scan rules out PE. In case the pretest probability of VTE is high, direct CTPA is advised to diagnose/rule out VTE. Validated prediction scores such as Geneva score, pulmonary embolism rule out criteria (PERC), or Wells criteria can be used in outpatients to decide about the testing strategy.

Suggested Reading
1. Lim W, Le Gal G, Bates SM, Righini M, Haramati LB, Lang E, et al. American Society of Hematology 2018 guidelines for management of venous thromboembolism: diagnosis of venous thromboembolism. Blood Adv. 2018;2(22):3226-56.

Q.7. A 60-year-old female was diagnosed with DVT/PE and was started on LMWH anticoagulation. She was then transitioned to rivaroxaban for 1 month. However, patient cannot afford DOAC and wants a cheaper alternative. A decision was made to start warfarin. Which of the following statements is correct regarding transitioning of anticoagulants?
   a. DOACs can be stopped anytime and warfarin has to be started from the next day.
   b. DOAC needs to be overlapped with warfarin till the INR is in the therapeutic range, then DOAC will be stopped.

c. DOAC needs to be stopped followed by initiation of LMWH and bridging with warfarin for 5 days.
d. DOAC to be stopped only if the DOAC-specific anti-Xa level is in the recommended range, then switch to warfarin next day.

Ans. b

Explanation: Initiation of warfarin in a patient already on DOAC needs overlapping the two drugs with measurement of INR serially. DOAC can be stopped only when the INR is in the therapeutic range of 2-3. There is no need of LMWH or UFH bridging in this case. Routine testing for DOAC-specific assays is not recommended currently. While converting from warfarin to dabigatran, rivaroxaban, or apixaban, start DOAC once the INR is <2. If DOAC is to be started after an initial LMWH/UFH therapy, the DOAC can be given whenever the next dose of heparin is due. One DOAC to another DOAC can be easily converted by giving the new DOAC at the scheduled next dose of the previous drug.

Suggested Reading
1. Chen A, Stecker E, A Warden B. Direct oral anticoagulant use: A practical guide to common clinical challenges. J Am Heart Assoc. 2020;9(13):e017559.
2. Witt DM, Nieuwlaat R, Clark NP, Ansell J, Holbrook A, Skov J, et al. American Society of Hematology 2018 guidelines for management of venous thromboembolism: optimal management of anticoagulation therapy. Blood Adv. 2018;2(22):3257-91.

Q.8. A 36-year-old female with acute myeloid leukemia (AML) is undergoing induction chemotherapy. She is diagnosed to have an acute symptomatic DVT in left proximal femoral vein without PE. Her blood tests show hemoglobin (Hb) of 7.5 g/dL, white blood cell (WBC) of 400/mm^3, platelet count of 30,000/mm^3, and INR of 1.1. Which of the following statements is correct regarding her treatment?
a. Start therapeutic dose anticoagulation with enoxaparin and transfuse platelets.
b. Do not start heparin; insert a retrievable IVC filter in this case till the bone marrow recovers.
c. There is no role of heparin or IVC filter; treat with bed rest and catheter-directed thrombolysis.
d. Start prophylactic dose enoxaparin and explain the risk of subsequent PE to the patient.

Ans. a

Explanation: In patients with cancer-associated thrombosis (CAT) and platelet count >50,000/mm^3, therapeutic dose anticoagulation is recommended for proximal DVT/PE. If the platelet count is <50,000/mm^3, platelet transfusion is to be done to maintain the platelet count >40,000–50,000/mm^3 along with therapeutic anticoagulation. In case of distal DVT or subsegmental PE and platelet <50,000/mm^3, prophylactic dose of LMWH is recommended till the platelet count becomes >50,000/mm^3. If the platelet count falls below 25,000/mm^3, anticoagulation should be discontinued.

Suggested Reading
1. Samuelson Bannow BT, Lee A, Khorana AA, Zwicker JI, Noble S, Ay C, et al. Management of cancer-associated thrombosis in patients with thrombocytopenia: guidance from the SSC of the ISTH. J Thromb Haemost. 2018;16(6):1246-9.

Q.9. A 31-year-old male was admitted with swelling of the right upper extremity for 5 days. He is a case of non-Hodgkin's lymphoma and is receiving chemotherapy for the same. A PICC (peripherally inserted central catheter) was inserted in the right upper limb 3 weeks back. Doppler USG shows DVT in the right axillary vein extending into right subclavian vein. There is no evidence of RV dysfunction on 2D Echo. The nurse says that the catheter is working well after flushing and the patient is due for his next cycle 2 days later. Which statement is correct from the following?
   a. Remove the PICC, insert new catheter in left upper limb, and start therapeutic enoxaparin.
   b. Continue using the same PICC and start therapeutic dose enoxaparin.
   c. Shift the patient to IR for clot-directed thrombolysis and then continue therapeutic dose enoxaparin.
   d. Start prophylactic dose enoxaparin only as upper extremity DVT is not harmful.

Ans. b

Explanation: There is no role of routine administration of heparin flushes or prophylactic enoxaparin in patients with indwelling catheters to prevent DVT. It is recommended to start therapeutic dose of LMWH without removal of catheter if the catheter is functioning and is needed for later use. If the catheter is blocked or infected, it is recommended to remove the catheter and resume therapeutic anticoagulation. In case anticoagulation cannot be administered due to bleeding risk, it is advised to remove the catheter without anticoagulation. Clot-directed thrombolysis is recommended only for refractory thrombosis not resolving with anticoagulation alone. Upper extremity DVT can also lead to PE, which requires systemic thrombolysis.

Suggested Reading
1. Zwicker JI, Connolly G, Carrier M, Kamphuisen PW, Lee AY. Catheter-associated deep vein thrombosis of the upper extremity in cancer patients: guidance from the SSC of the ISTH. J Thromb Haemost. 2014;12(5):796-800.

Q.10. A 60-year-old male was admitted to the hospital with fever and abdominal pain. He was a known case of decompensated cirrhosis of liver and had ascites with pedal edema. He was diagnosed to have spontaneous bacterial peritonitis. His blood investigations showed Hb of 8 g/dL, WBC of 13,400/mm^3, platelet count of 80,000/mm^3, INR of 2.2, creatinine of 1.7 mg/dL, and blood urea nitrogen (BUN) of 38 mg/dL. Which of the following statements is correct regarding thromboprophylaxis in this case?
   a. Unfractionated heparin should be started 5,000 U BD as the patient has renal dysfunction.
   b. Anticoagulation should not be given and only mechanical thromboprophylaxis should be started.

c. Correct platelet and INR by FFP and platelet transfusion and then start thromboprophylaxis.
d. Start dose-adjusted enoxaparin without platelet or INR correction.

Ans. d

Explanation: International Society on Thrombosis and Haemostasis (ISTH) guidelines recommend against the use of thrombocytopenia and/or prolongation of PT/INR as absolute contraindications for thromboprophylaxis in patients with cirrhosis of liver. For hospitalized patients with cirrhosis, the use of anticoagulant thromboprophylaxis should be followed as for general critically ill patients and the use of LMWH or fondaparinux over UFH is suggested. In patients with renal impairment, use of dose-adjusted LMWH over UFH is recommended. For critically ill unstable patients (particularly with acute on chronic liver failure), thromboprophylaxis should be considered on a case-by-case basis.

Suggested Reading
1. Roberts LN, Hernandez-Gea V, Magnusson M, Stanworth S, Thachil J, Tripodi A, et al. Thromboprophylaxis for venous thromboembolism prevention in hospitalized patients with cirrhosis: Guidance from the SSC of the ISTH. J Thromb Haemost. 2022;20(10):2237-45.

Q.11. **A 35-year-old female was admitted with seizures and was diagnosed to have cerebral venous sinus thrombosis (CVST). She is a known case of antiphospholipid antibody (APLA) syndrome and is currently on warfarin therapy and is compliant with it. No other precipitating factor could be identified for CVST. Her last INR was 2.4. Which of the following statements is wrong regarding further anticoagulant management?**
a. The dose of warfarin should be increased to a target INR of 3–4.
b. Current dose and INR target should be continued with addition of aspirin.
c. Warfarin therapy should be stopped and enoxaparin should be started for a long duration.
d. Warfarin therapy should be stopped and DOAC (rivaroxaban) should be started.

Ans. d

Explanation: Most of the patients with APLA should take low-dose aspirin (LDA) for primary thromboprophylaxis. In case of a first episode of venous thrombosis, therapy with VKA is recommended with a target INR of 2–3. The duration of anticoagulation should be lifelong for an unprovoked episode or 3–6 months for a provoked episode. If the patient develops recurrent thrombosis despite good adherence to warfarin and achievement of target INR, the therapy can either be changed to LMWH or addition of LDA or increase in the dose of warfarin with a target INR of 3–4 can be done. DOAC is not recommended in APLA due to high risk of recurrent thrombosis. DOAC may be considered in cases where VKA is contraindicated or INR cannot be achieved despite high doses. In case of a first unprovoked arterial thrombosis, therapy with VKA is recommended with a target INR of 2–3 or 3–4 depending on the bleeding risk of the individual.

Suggested Reading
1. Tektonidou MG, Andreoli L, Limper M, Amoura Z, Cervera R, Costedoat-Chalumeau N, et al. EULAR recommendations for the management of antiphospholipid syndrome in adults. Ann Rheum Dis. 2019;78(10):1296-304.

Q.12. Which of the following statements is wrong with respect to the risk of thromboembolism among combined hormonal contraceptive (CHC) users?
   a. CHC containing >50 µg of ethinylestradiol (EE) has a higher risk of venous thromboembolism (VTE) as compared to lower doses.
   b. CHC containing <35 µg of ethinylestradiol (EE) has a lower risk of VTE as compared to higher doses.
   c. Levonorgestrel-containing CHC has a lower risk of VTE as compared to drospirenone-containing CHC.
   d. Contraceptive patch-containing CHC does not carry a higher risk of VTE as compared to oral contraceptives.

Ans. b

Explanation: Use of combined hormonal contraceptives containing an estrogen and a progesterone preparation increases the risk of VTE as compared to nonusers. It has been seen that CHC with >50 µg EE carries a higher risk of VTE as compared to <50 µg EE. However, there is no evidence that dose <35 µg provides any additional benefit (lower risk of VTE) as compared to CHC with >35 µg EE. As far as progesterone is concerned, CHC with levonorgestrel or norethindrone has a lower risk of VTE as compared to those containing drospirenone or third-generation progestins. There is insufficient evidence to show that contraceptive patches or rings carry a different risk of VTE as compared to oral contraceptives. Even in the setting of CHC use, other risk factors such as hypertension, obesity, tobacco use, and hereditary thrombophilia increase the risk of VTE further.

Suggested Reading
1. Practice Committee of the American Society for Reproductive Medicine. Electronic address: ASRM@asrm.org; Practice Committee of the American Society for Reproductive Medicine. Combined hormonal contraception and the risk of venous thromboembolism: a guideline. Fertil Steril. 2017;107(1):43-51.

Q.13. Which of the following statements is correct with respect to testing for hereditary thrombophilia in a 30-year-old male presenting with an unprovoked symptomatic deep vein thrombosis (DVT)?
   a. Testing for hereditary thrombophilia is recommended in unprovoked symptomatic DVT cases.
   b. Factor V Leiden mutation and prothrombin gene mutation assay should be performed only after 3 months of anticoagulation therapy to avoid false-positive results.
   c. Testing of phenotypic activated protein C resistance ratio (APC-R) can be performed at any time point during the thrombosis episode and/or anticoagulation.

d. Antithrombin III deficiency testing should be performed only after 3 months of anticoagulation and in the absence of heparin therapy.

Ans. d

Explanation: Hereditary thrombophilia consists of conditions such as Factor V Leiden mutation, prothrombin gene mutation, protein C deficiency, protein S deficiency, and antithrombin III deficiency. Acquired thrombophilia is APLA syndrome, myeloproliferative neoplasms, paroxysmal nocturnal hemoglobinuria (PNH), etc. Routine testing for these conditions is not recommended to predict the risk of thrombosis or the evaluation for any provoked or unprovoked VTE episode. This is because the identification of a thrombophilia does not alter the therapy or the duration of therapy. Identification of hereditary thrombophilia by testing of clotting factor concentrations should not be done as they are unreliable predictors. Testing for hereditary thrombophilia is not recommended even for arterial thrombosis or venous thrombosis at unusual sites. If at all testing is to be performed, only the genetic assays for Factor V Leiden or prothrombin gene mutation can be done at any time point since they are not affected by clotting process. On the contrary, testing for protein C, protein S, antithrombin III, or APC-R should be done only after 3 months of anticoagulation. Protein C, protein S, and antithrombin III can be falsely low in case of sepsis, disseminated intravascular coagulation (DIC), nephrotic syndrome, and liver failure. Heparin use lowers the levels of antithrombin III by binding to it, while increases the levels of protein C and S.

Suggested Reading
1. Arachchillage DJ, Mackillop L, Chandratheva A, Motawani J, MacCallum P, Laffan M. Thrombophilia testing: A British Society for Haematology guideline. Br J Haematol. 2022;198(3):443-58.

Q.14. Which of the following statements is wrong with respect to antithrombin in venous thromboembolism?
a. Antithrombin III level testing is not recommended for patients with first unprovoked DVT.
b. The target concentration for antithrombin after initiating antithrombin concentrate therapy is 80-120%.
c. Heparin therapy leads to falsely elevated levels of antithrombin III.
d. DOAC therapy leads to falsely elevated levels of antithrombin III.

Ans. c

Explanation: Heparin binds to antithrombin in vivo and enhances its natural activity as an anticoagulant. Antithrombin is the major endogenous anticoagulant that inhibits thrombin and activated factor X (Factor Xa). Binding of heparin to antithrombin leads to reduced levels of antithrombin. On the contrary, use of DOAC such as rivaroxaban and apixaban may falsely elevate the levels of antithrombin III. Laboratory testing of antithrombin is based on either thrombin-based assay or the activated factor X-based assay. Owing to the inhibition of factor X by DOAC, it leads to interference in the measurement of antithrombin via the factor X-based assay. This leads to falsely elevated levels and can label someone with antithrombin deficiency as "normal".

Suggested Reading
1. Ząbczyk M, Natorska J, Kopytek M, Malinowski KP, Undas A. The effect of direct oral anticoagulants on antithrombin activity testing is abolished by DOAC-stop in venous thromboembolism patients. Arch Pathol Lab Med. 2021;145(1):99-104.

Q.15. A 55-year-old female was suspected of developing heparin-induced thrombocytopenia and thrombosis (HITT) based on a 4T score of 6. Her enoxaparin thromboprophylaxis was stopped and bivalirudin was started. An HIT antibody assay was reported as 1.6 OD. Which of the following is true regarding diagnostic tests for HITT?
  a. A 4T score of 3 warrants testing for HIT antibody by ELISA.
  b. HIT antibody assay of >2 OD confirms the presence of HITT and does not need further testing.
  c. HIT antibody assay 1.6 OD with a 4 T score of 6 requires additional testing with serotonin release assay for confirmation.
  d. Heparin should be stopped only after the results of HIT antibody assay.

Ans. b

Explanation:
When HITT is suspected in a case, the 4T score is calculated based on severity of thrombocytopenia, timing of start of heparin, presence of thrombosis, and other causes for thrombocytopenia. A score of 3 or less is low risk, 4–5 is intermediate risk, while 6–8 is high risk for HITT. An intermediate- or high-risk score warrants further testing with HIT antibody ELISA assay *and* stopping all heparin therapy. A score of 3 or less makes HITT unlikely. HIT antibody assay is reported as optical density (OD) units. An OD >1.5 with a score of 6–8 *or* OD >2 confirms HITT and does not need further testing. However, an OD between 0.6 and 2.0 *or* 0.6 and 1.5 with 4T score of 6–8 warrants further testing by serotonin release assay (SRA). A positive SRA confirms HITT and vice versa. An OD of <0.6 rules out HITT.

Suggested Reading
1. Cuker A, Arepally GM, Chong BH, Cines DB, Greinacher A, Gruel Y, et al. American Society of Hematology 2018 guidelines for management of venous thromboembolism: heparin-induced thrombocytopenia. Blood Adv. 2018;2(22):3360-92.

Q.16. A 27-year-old 24 weeks' pregnant female was admitted to the ICU for pneumonia with acute hypoxemic respiratory failure. High-flow nasal oxygenation and antibiotics were started. Her mother has a history of recurrent deep vein thrombosis (DVT) and was tested positive for protein S deficiency. Which of the following statements is correct with respect to thromboprophylaxis in this case?
  a. Thromboprophylaxis with enoxaparin is required only for the current ICU stay.
  b. Thromboprophylaxis will be required for the ICU stay and entire antepartum period.

c. Thromboprophylaxis will be required for the ICU stay, antepartum period, and the postpartum period.
d. Thromboprophylaxis will be required only during this ICU stay and the postpartum period.

Ans. d

Explanation: All hereditary thrombophilias do not require primary and/or secondary thromboprophylaxis. Thromboprophylaxis during the ICU stay is a must for all patients. The decision to administer thromboprophylaxis during the antenatal and/or postnatal period depends on the specific type of hereditary thrombophilia, genotype, and the presence of a positive family history for VTE.

	Antepartum prophylaxis	*Postpartum prophylaxis*
FVL or PGM heterozygous	No	No
FVL homozygous	Yes	Yes
PGM homozygous	Only if positive FH	Yes
FVL and PGM compound heterozygosity	Yes	Yes
Protein C or S deficiency	No	Only if positive FH
Antithrombin deficiency	Only if positive FH	Only if positive FH

(FH: family history; FVL: factor V Leiden mutation; PGM: prothrombin gene mutation)

Suggested Reading
1. Langer AL, Connell NT. (2022). Update on pregnancy-associated venous thromboembolism. [online] Available from https://www.sciencedirect.com/science/article/pii/S2666572722000116?via%3Dihub. [Last accessed June, 2023]

Q.17. Which of the following statements is true regarding radiological imaging for VTE in pregnancy?
   a. CTPA delivers higher radiation dose to the fetus as compared to V/Q scan.
   b. Magnetic resonance (MR) venography to visualize iliac vein thrombosis is done without gadolinium contrast in pregnancy.
   c. If available in the hospital, an abnormal V/Q scan can accurately diagnose PE in all the cases.
   d. V/Q scan delivers higher radiation dose to the breast tissue of the mother.

Ans. b

Explanation: Both CTPA and V/Q scans are highly sensitive and specific to diagnose pulmonary embolism in all cases including pregnant females. However, CTPA delivers a higher radiation dose to the mother and especially to the breast tissue as compared to V/Q scan. On the contrary, CTPA delivers a lower radiation dose to the fetus as compared to V/Q scan. The exposure can be further lowered by applying an abdominal shield on the mother. A normal chest X-ray is a prerequisite to conduct a V/Q scan. A normal V/Q scan rules out PE. However, an abnormal V/Q scan (perfusion defect) can diagnose PE only in the presence of a normal chest X-ray. Moreover, CTPA is more beneficial if mechanical thrombectomy is being planned and anatomical details of vessels and clot are required. DVT in pregnancy is diagnosed as usual with compression ultrasonography (CUS). MR venography is an excellent alternative if CUS is equivocal or not feasible due to extensive edema or the clinical suspicion is high despite a negative CUS. MR venography can visualize the iliac vasculature too but gadolinium cannot be used as it crosses the placenta and is associated with stillbirths.

Suggested Reading
1. Langer AL, Connell NT. (2022). Update on pregnancy-associated venous thromboembolism. [online] Available from https://www.sciencedirect.com/science/article/pii/S2666572722000116?via%3Dihub. [Last accessed June, 2023]
2. Tromeur C, van der Pol LM, Le Roux PY, Ende-Verhaar Y, Salaun PY, Leroyer C, et al. Computed tomography pulmonary angiography *versus* ventilation-perfusion lung scanning for diagnosing pulmonary embolism during pregnancy: a systematic review and meta-analysis. Haematologica. 2019;104(1):176-88.

Q.18. Which of the following surgeries does not warrant pharmacological thromboprophylaxis in the postoperative period?
a. Laparoscopic total gastrectomy
b. Laparoscopic abdominopelvic resection (APR)
c. Laparoscopic total nephrectomy
d. Laparoscopic cholecystectomy

Ans. d

Explanation: For any major general, gynecological, cardiac, vascular, or orthopedic surgery, pharmacological thromboprophylaxis should be started in the immediate postoperative period if there is no surgical high risk of bleeding. LMWH is the preferred agent in case of major general or gynecological surgery while DOAC is preferred for total hip arthroplasty and total knee arthroplasty. LMWH or UFH can be used for cardiovascular surgery patients. The timing of initiation can be early (within 12 hours) or late (after 12 hours). It has to be continued for at least 3 weeks. Pharmacological thromboprophylaxis is not recommended after laparoscopic cholecystectomy, laparoscopic prostatectomy, TURP, and neurosurgical procedures.

Suggested Reading
1. Anderson DR, Morgano GP, Bennett C, Dentali F, Francis CW, Garcia DA, et al. American Society of Hematology 2019 guidelines for management of venous thromboembolism: prevention of venous thromboembolism in surgical hospitalized patients. Blood Adv. 2019;3(23):3898-944.

Q.19. Which of the following echocardiographic abnormalities is not suggestive of pulmonary embolism?
a. Decreased peak systolic velocity of tricuspid annulus (S' < 9.5 cm/s)
b. Increased tricuspid annular plane systolic excursion (TAPSE > 16 mm)
c. Acceleration time of pulmonary blood ejection < 60 ms
d. Peak systolic pressure gradient at the tricuspid valve < 60 mm Hg

Ans. b

Explanation: The echocardiographic manifestations suggestive of pulmonary embolism are:
- Decreased peak systolic velocity of tricuspid annulus (S' < 9.5 cm/s)
- Decreased tricuspid annular plane systolic excursion (TAPSE < 16 mm)
- Acceleration time of pulmonary blood ejection < 60 ms with midsystolic notch + peak systolic pressure gradient at the tricuspid valve < 60 mm Hg (60/60 sign)
- Enlarged right ventricle with basal RV/LV ratio > 1.0
- Flattened interventricular septum with D-shaped left ventricle
- Distended IVC with diminished inspiratory collapsibility
- McConnell's sign
- Mobile thrombus in the right heart chambers

Suggested Reading

1. Konstantinides SV, Meyer G, Becattini C, Bueno H, Geersing GJ, Harjola VP, et al.; ESC Scientific Document Group. 2019 ESC Guidelines for the diagnosis and management of acute pulmonary embolism developed in collaboration with the European Respiratory Society (ERS). Eur Heart J. 2020;41(4):543-603.

Q.20. A 50-year-old female came to the emergency department with acute-onset dyspnea and hypotension. She was diagnosed to have pulmonary embolism after CTPA scan. While being treated in the emergency department, she suffered a cardiac arrest with pulseless electrical activity (PEA) rhythm. Which of the following statements is correct in this scenario?
a. Epinephrine should be avoided during CPR in this case.
b. Thrombolysis with streptokinase is ineffective once cardiac arrest occurs in a case of PE.
c. CPR should be continued for at least 60-90 minutes after administration of streptokinase.
d. VV-ECMO should be immediately started during CPR.

Ans. c

Explanation: Cardiac arrest in PE commonly presents as PEA. The initial resuscitation should be as per the American Heart Association (AHA) Advanced Cardiac Life Support (ACLS) guidelines, i.e., high-quality chest compressions along with epinephrine 1 mg every 3-5 minutes. Perform echocardiography during ongoing cardiopulmonary resuscitation (CPR) to support the diagnosis. Administer systemic thrombolytic drug in a cardiac arrest situation due to suspected PE. Once thrombolysis is done, CPR should be continued for at least 60-90 minutes before termination. When conventional CPR fails to revive the patient, extracorporeal CPR should be considered. The efficacy of venoarterial extracorporeal membrane oxygenation (VA-ECMO) as a stand-alone modality is controversial and is usually combined with surgical embolectomy or percutaneous mechanical thrombectomy. There is no role of VV-ECMO in cardiac arrest due to PE.

Suggested Reading

1. Konstantinides SV, Meyer G, Becattini C, Bueno H, Geersing GJ, Harjola VP, et al.; ESC Scientific Document Group. 2019 ESC Guidelines for the diagnosis and management of

acute pulmonary embolism developed in collaboration with the European Respiratory Society (ERS). Eur Heart J. 2020;41(4):543-603.
2. Lott C, Truhlář A, Alfonzo A, Barelli A, González-Salvado V, Hinkelbein J, et al.; ERC Special Circumstances Writing Group Collaborators. European Resuscitation Council Guidelines 2021: Cardiac arrest in special circumstances. Resuscitation. 2021;161:152-219.

Q.21. Which of the following is a strong predisposing factor for venous thromboembolism?
a. Fracture of lower limb
b. Pregnancy
c. Prolonged air travel
d. Varicose veins

Ans. a

Explanation: Weak risk factors (OR < 2) for VTE are varicose veins, pregnancy, prolonged car or air travel, obesity, bed rest > 3 days, increasing age, diabetes mellitus, and hypertension. Strong risk factors (OR > 10) for VTE are fracture of lower limb, hip or knee replacement, major trauma, previous VTE, spinal cord injury, recent MI, and recent hospitalization for heart failure and/or atrial fibrillation.

Suggested Reading
1. Anderson FA Jr, Spencer FA. Risk factors for venous thromboembolism. Circulation. 2003;107(23 Suppl 1):I9-16.
2. Rogers MA, Levine DA, Blumberg N, Flanders SA, Chopra V, Langa KM. Triggers of hospitalization for venous thromboembolism. Circulation. 2012;125(17):2092-9.

Q.22. A 45-year-old male with pulmonary embolism was hemodynamically stable and was being treated with heparin anticoagulation. His 2D Echo showed RV dysfunction with a normal LV. His troponin I test results were normal. His simplified PESI (pulmonary embolism severity index) score is 2. Which of the following severity categories of PE does this patient belong?
a. High risk
b. Intermediate-high risk
c. Intermediate-low risk
d. Low risk

Ans. c

Explanation: Risk stratification of PE is based on hemodynamic stability, presence of RV dysfunction, troponin I test results, and simplified PESI score. Any patient with hemodynamic stability is considered as "high-risk" with an increased 30-day mortality risk. A patient who is hemodynamically stable with a simplified PESI score of 0, negative troponin I, and normal RV function is considered as "low-risk". Presence of RV dysfunction and/or positive troponin results places a patient in the intermediate-risk category.

Suggested Reading
1. Konstantinides SV, Meyer G, Becattini C, Bueno H, Geersing GJ, Harjola VP, et al.; ESC Scientific Document Group. 2019 ESC Guidelines for the diagnosis and management of acute pulmonary embolism developed in collaboration with the European Respiratory Society (ERS). Eur Heart J. 2020;41(4):543-603.

Q.23. A 50-year-old female came to the emergency department with acute-onset dyspnea and hypotension. She was diagnosed to have pulmonary embolism after CTPA scan. While being treated in the emergency department, she suffered a cardiac

arrest with PEA rhythm. Which of the following is the correct accelerated dose for thrombolysis in this scenario?
   a. Urokinase 4,400 IU/kg over 10 minutes followed by 4,400 IU/kg/h for 12 hours.
   b. Recombinant tissue plasminogen activator (rtPA) 100 mg over 2 hours
   c. Streptokinase 250,000 IU over 30 minutes followed by 100,000 IU/hour over 12–24 hours
   d. Streptokinase 1.5 million units over 2 hours

Ans. d

Explanation: The doses mentioned in the options A, B, and C are the approved doses for thrombolysis in PE. However, in case of cardiac arrest, accelerated regimens need to be given due to the emergent situation. Streptokinase 1.5 million IU over 2 hours, rtPA 0.6 mg/kg over 15 minutes, and urokinase 3 million IU over 2 hours are the accelerated regimens of each drug to be given in cardiac arrest situations.

Suggested Reading
1. Konstantinides SV, Meyer G, Becattini C, Bueno H, Geersing GJ, Harjola VP, et al.; ESC Scientific Document Group. 2019 ESC Guidelines for the diagnosis and management of acute pulmonary embolism developed in collaboration with the European Respiratory Society (ERS). Eur Heart J. 2020;41(4):543-603.

Q.24. Which of the following risk factors present during an episode of PE predisposes a patient for the development of chronic thromboembolic pulmonary hypertension (CTEPH)?
   a. Thrombophilic disorders
   b. Myeloproliferative disorders (MPS)
   c. Inflammatory bowel disease (IBD)
   d. All of the above

Ans. d

Explanation: Certain conditions that are present at the time of PE or diagnosed in the 3–6 months of follow-up predispose a patient for the development of CTEPH. These include ventriculoatrial shunts, infected chronic IV lines or pacemakers, history of splenectomy, IBD, MPS, thrombophilic disorders, chronic osteomyelitis, hypothyroidism, and non-O blood group.

Suggested Reading
1. Konstantinides SV, Meyer G, Becattini C, Bueno H, Geersing GJ, Harjola VP, et al.; ESC Scientific Document Group. 2019 ESC Guidelines for the diagnosis and management of acute pulmonary embolism developed in collaboration with the European Respiratory Society (ERS). Eur Heart J. 2020;41(4):543-603.

Q.25. Which of the following findings is not essential for the diagnosis of CTEPH?
   a. Completion of 3 months of anticoagulation after the episode of PE.
   b. Left heart catheterization demonstrating pulmonary capillary wedge pressure (PCWP) > 15 mm Hg.
   c. Right heart catheterization demonstrating mean pulmonary artery pressure (PAP) > 25 mm Hg.
   d. V/Q lung scan showing mismatched perfusion defect.

Ans. b

Explanation: The diagnosis of CTEPH is based on findings obtained after at least 3 months of effective anticoagulation, to distinguish this condition from acute PE. The diagnosis requires a mean PAP of >25 mm Hg along with a pulmonary arterial wedge pressure of <15 mm Hg, documented at right heart catheterization in a patient with mismatched perfusion defects on V/Q lung scan. Specific diagnostic signs for CTEPH on multidetector CT angiography or conventional pulmonary cineangiography include ring-like stenoses, webs, slits, and chronic total occlusions.

Suggested Reading
1. Konstantinides SV, Meyer G, Becattini C, Bueno H, Geersing GJ, Harjola VP, et al.; ESC Scientific Document Group. 2019 ESC Guidelines for the diagnosis and management of acute pulmonary embolism developed in collaboration with the European Respiratory Society (ERS). Eur Heart J. 2020;41(4):543-603.

Q.26. Which of the following statements regarding placement of an IVC filter in VTE is true?
   a. IVC filter should be placed in all patients with a large proximal femoral vein thrombus and PE.
   b. A patient undergoing therapeutic anticoagulation for DVT beyond the acute phase should be posted for IVC filter placement if contraindication to anticoagulation develops.
   c. A patient undergoing therapeutic anticoagulation for acute DVT should be posted for IVC filter placement if contraindication to anticoagulation develops.
   d. IVC filter should be placed upfront if a patient develops recurrent VTE with ongoing anticoagulation.

Ans. c

Explanation: IVC filter should not be routinely inserted in all patients with acute VTE. It is indicated only if a patient with acute VTE develops a contraindication to anticoagulation. It is not indicated if a patient has completed the initial acute phase of anticoagulation and develops a contraindication in the extended phase. If a patient develops recurrent VTE despite anticoagulation, the primary focus is to optimize the drug, dose, route, and frequency of the anticoagulant used and to choose IVC filter only if there are no modifiable factors.

Suggested Reading
1. Kaufman JA, Barnes GD, Chaer RA, Cuschieri J, Eberhardt RT, Johnson MS, et al. Society of Interventional Radiology Clinical Practice Guideline for Inferior Vena Cava Filters in the Treatment of Patients with Venous Thromboembolic Disease: Developed in collaboration with the American College of Cardiology, American College of Chest Physicians, American College of Surgeons Committee on Trauma, American Heart Association, Society for Vascular Surgery, and Society for Vascular Medicine. J Vasc Interv Radiol. 2020;31(10):1529-44.

Q.27. Which of the following tests is not very useful for monitoring the efficacy of dabigatran?
   a. Activated partial thromboplastin time
   b. Thrombin time

c. Ecarin clotting time
d. Mass spectrometry

Ans. a

Explanation: Prothrombin time (PT) and activated partial thromboplastin time (aPTT) can be used as first-line tests to provide a qualitative assessment of rivaroxaban and dabigatran, respectively. Direct thrombin inhibitors tend to disproportionately prolong the aPTT rather than PT, while direct factor Xa inhibitors prolong the PT to a greater extent than the aPTT. However, because of their limited sensitivities, PT and aPTT are not suitable for quantification of the anticoagulant effect. There is a poor correlation between plasma concentrations of DOACs and PT/APTT prolongation. Mass spectrometry, when calibrated with each drug individually, to be measured, is considered the gold-standard method for quantification of DOAC level. More rapid methods including dilute thrombin time (dTT), ecarin methods, and chromogenic anti-Xa assays are potentially suitable means to measure DOACs.

Suggested Reading
1. McRae HL, Militello L, Refaai MA. Updates in Anticoagulation Therapy Monitoring. Biomedicines. 2021;9(3):262.

Q.28. Which of the following is not an absolute contraindication to systemic thrombolysis in a case of pulmonary embolism?
a. Major surgery in the previous 3 weeks
b. Active peptic ulcer
c. Central nervous system (CNS) neoplasm
d. Ischemic stroke in the previous 6 months

Ans. b

Explanation: Absolute contraindications for systemic thrombolysis are major trauma, surgery or head injury in the last 3 weeks, ischemic stroke in the last 6 months, history of hemorrhagic stroke or stroke of unknown origin, CNS neoplasm, bleeding diathesis, and active bleeding. Relative contraindications for the same are oral anticoagulation, active peptic ulcer, noncompressible puncture sites, pregnancy, advanced liver disease, infective endocarditis, and TIA (transient ischemic attack) in the previous 6 months.

Suggested Reading
1. Konstantinides SV, Meyer G, Becattini C, Bueno H, Geersing GJ, Harjola VP, et al.; ESC Scientific Document Group. 2019 ESC Guidelines for the diagnosis and management of acute pulmonary embolism developed in collaboration with the European Respiratory Society (ERS). Eur Heart J. 2020;41(4):543-603.

Q.29. Which of the following is *not* an indication for catheter-directed thrombectomy in PE?
a. High-risk PE with absolute contraindication to systemic thrombolysis
b. Intermediate-high risk category at-risk of clinical deterioration with absolute contraindication to thrombolysis
c. High-risk category PE with failed thrombolysis
d. None of the above

Ans. d

Explanation: Percutaneous embolectomy is reserved for selected patients with contraindications to thrombolysis and/or failure of thrombolysis, when surgical embolectomy is not available, and if the interventional equipment and expertise are available. Indications of catheter-directed thrombectomy are:
- Intermediate-high risk PE with risk for clinical deterioration with absolute or relative contraindications to thrombolysis
- High-risk PE with absolute contraindications to thrombolysis
- After failed systemic thrombolysis
- Thrombus-in-transit in the right atrium or right ventricle

Suggested Reading
1. Rivera-Lebron B, McDaniel M, Ahrar K, Alrifai A, Dudzinski DM, Fanola C, et al.; PERT Consortium. Diagnosis, Treatment and Follow Up of Acute Pulmonary Embolism: Consensus Practice from the PERT Consortium. Clin Appl Thromb Hemost. 2019;25:1076029619853037.

Q.30. Which of the following are indications for surgical embolectomy in PE?
a. High-risk PE with failed thrombolysis
b. Right heart thrombi with large thrombus burden
c. Thrombus in-transit across a patent foramen ovale
d. All of the above

Ans. d

Explanation:
Indications for surgical pulmonary embolectomy are as follows:
- High-risk PE, with contraindications to, or failure of thrombolysis.
- Intermediate-high risk PE, with contraindications to, or failure of thrombolysis, with risk for clinical deterioration.
- Right-heart thrombi, especially with large thromboembolic burden.
- Thrombus-in-transit across a patent foramen ovale (PFO).

Suggested Reading
1. Rivera-Lebron B, McDaniel M, Ahrar K, Alrifai A, Dudzinski DM, Fanola C, et al.; PERT Consortium. Diagnosis, treatment and follow up of acute pulmonary embolism: Consensus Practice from the PERT Consortium. Clin Appl Thromb Hemost. 2019;25:1076029619853037.

CHAPTER 21

Postoperative Care

Suhail Sarwar Siddiqui, Arshad Ayub, Anuja Pandit

Q.1. A 62-year-old male patient underwent right-sided intrapericardial pneumonectomy for carcinoma of right lung. In the surgical intensive care unit (ICU), 3 hours after the surgery, he acutely develops tachycardia, profound hypotension, and shock. Central venous pressure (CVP) rises, and cyanosis develops that does not respond to oxygen administration. Chest radiograph is suggestive of mediastinal shift to the right. Identify the *wrong* statement:
   a. Cardiac herniation could be the cause of this clinical scenario and should be ruled out immediately
   b. In case of cardiac herniation, medical management is the choice.
   c. Pulmonary thromboembolism is an important differential in this case.
   d. Cardiac herniation may present as arrhythmias.

Ans. b

Explanation: Acute cardiac herniation is a rare but well-documented complication of pneumonectomy, which may occur when the pericardium is incompletely closed or the closure breaks down. Lobar resection with pericardial opening or other chest tumor resections involving the pericardium or trauma can be complicated by cardiac herniation. Typically, it happens immediately or within 24 hours following the surgery and is linked to a mortality rate of >50%.

The clinical manifestation of cardiac herniation following right pneumonectomy is brought on by impairment of venous return to the heart, which is accompanied by an increase in CVP, tachycardia, extreme hypotension, and shock. Acute superior vena cava syndrome develops as a result of the heart's torsion. In contrast, there is less cardiac rotation when the herniation happens after a left-sided pneumonectomy, yet the margin of the pericardium compresses the myocardium. This could result in myocardial ischemia, the emergence of arrhythmias, and obstruction of the ventricular outflow tract. After chest closure, cardiac herniation happens as a result of the pressure differential between the two hemithoraces. The heart could be forced out through a pericardial defect as a result of this pressure difference, such as when suction is applied to the intercostal drain on the operated side or during noninvasive positive pressure ventilation (NIPPV) applied to ventilate the remaining lung. A patient who has a cardiac herniation should undergo emergent surgery.

A high index of suspicion based on the clinical situation along with radiological investigations helps to arrive at the diagnosis. On the plain chest radiograph, the heart may seem to shift toward the operative side and appear as a little bulge at the site of the pericardial defect (snow cone sign) in cases with partial or imminent herniation. Right-sided cardiac herniation is typically obvious; on chest radiographs, the herniated heart's shadow can be clearly seen in the open right pleural space and is pathognomonic. The remaining pericardial sac is thus empty and might be outlined by air. The symptoms of left-sided herniation can include a mediastinal shift to the left, an irregular cardiac contour, and a bulging left heart border. In situations where a diagnosis is questionable, bedside echocardiogram may be useful. The acuteness and severity of the clinical setting typically impedes a computed tomography (CT) scan which would have comparable findings.

Massive intrathoracic bleeding, pulmonary embolism, or mediastinal shift as a result of poor chest drain care should all be considered in the differential diagnosis.

Suggested Reading

1. Baisi A, Cioffi U, Nosotti M, De Simone M, Rosso L, Santambrogio L. Intrapericardial left pneumonectomy after induction chemotherapy: the risk of cardiac herniation. J Thorac Cardiovasc Surg. 2002;123(6):1206-7.
2. Brady MB, Brogdon BG. Cardiac herniation and volvulus: radiographic findings. Radiology. 1986;161(3):657-8.
3. Gurney JW, Arnold S, Goodman LR. Impending cardiac herniation: the snow cone sign. Radiology. 1986;161(3):653-5.
4. Mehanna MJ, Israel GM, Katigbak M, Rubinowitz AN. Cardiac herniation after right pneumonectomy: case report and review of the literature. J Thorac Imaging. 2007;22(3): 280-2.
5. Rippey JCR, Rao S, Fatovich D. Blunt traumatic rupture of the pericardium with cardiac herniation. CJEM. 2004;6(2):126-9.
6. Sugarbaker DJ, Jaklitsch MT, Bueno R, Richards W, Lukanich J, Mentzer SJ, et al. Prevention, early detection, and management of complications after 328 consecutive extrapleural pneumonectomies. J Thorac Cardiovasc Surg. 2004;128(1):138-46.
7. Trentin C, Veronesi G, Tosoni A, Bellomi M. Cardiac herniation after pneumonectomy: report of 2 cases. Radiol Med. 2003;105(3):230-3.

Q.2. **A 35-year-old gentleman with carcinoma thyroid underwent thyroidectomy with radical neck dissection. He denies any other significant medical history. Review of symptoms reveals orthopnea and dysphagia with a recent change in voice. At the conclusion of a complicated 4-hour resection, the patient is extubated and brought to the recovery room. One hour after extubation, the patient complains of dyspnea with stridorous respiration. Initial steps include all of the following, *except*:**

a. Intravenous administration of calcium
b. Nebulized racemic epinephrine
c. Inspection of the surgical site
d. Direct laryngoscopy

Ans. a

Explanation: Examination of the neck is typically the first step since it could identify a potentially fatal and treatable cause of airway obstruction like a compressing hematoma. Open chords on direct visualization by laryngoscopy may indicate recurrent laryngeal nerve injury as a cause of the dyspnea. Despite the possibility of hypocalcemia as a result of parathyroid gland removal, signs, and symptoms often appear considerably later in the perioperative course (24-96 hours) and are therefore unlikely to be a cause of dyspnea in the postanesthesia care unit (PACU). When stridor develops following extubation, racemic epinephrine is frequently administered via inhalation for management of laryngeal edema.

Other causes of dyspnea after thyroidectomy could include tracheomalacia, which will present immediately on extubation. While unilateral recurrent laryngeal nerve palsy may present as breathlessness, bilateral palsy can result in airway obstruction necessitating reintubation.

Suggested Reading
1. Christou N, Mathonnet M. Complications after total thyroidectomy. J Visc Surg. 2013;150(4):249-56.

Q.3. **A 58-year-old male, a diagnosed case of carcinoma colon, known diabetic since 10 years, postneoadjuvant chemotherapy (NACT) underwent cytoreductive surgery (CRS) and hyperthermic intraperitoneal chemotherapy (HIPEC). He received intraperitoneal instillation of cisplatin during HIPEC. He was extubated and shifted to ICU for postoperative monitoring and care.**
Which of the following medications should be used with caution in this patient?
 a. Opioids
 b. Nonsteroidal anti-inflammatory drugs (NSAIDs)
 c. Sodium thiosulfate
 d. Antibiotics

Ans. b

Explanation: Perioperative acute kidney injury (AKI) has high morbidity and mortality. In a retrospective study done by Cata et al. in patients undergoing CRS with HIPEC, a number of probable processes that could account for the AKI were observed. The primary mediators of AKI, according to the authors, are ischemia-reperfusion injury owing to periods of arterial hypotension, fluid redistribution, the direct effects of nephrotoxic medications, and inflammation.

Mitomycin-c and platinum-based chemotherapeutic agents such as cisplatin and oxaliplatin administered during HIPEC are also nephrotoxic. Also, age, the use of pregabalin, placement of ureteral stents, and major blood loss are independent risk factors of AKI.

Many institutions start a bolus of sodium thiosulfate 20 minutes before the commencement of HIPEC and continue a drip of the same drug for the following 12 hours in an effort to lessen the side effects of AKI after HIPEC due to cisplatin. This medication significantly reduced AKI in this situation and aids in preventing drug precipitation within the kidney. Since patients undergoing HIPEC are at high risk of developing renal dysfunction; nephrotoxic drugs such as NSAIDs are avoided in the perioperative period.

Suggested Reading
1. Cata JP, Zavala AM, Van Meter A, Williams UU, Soliz J, Hernandez M, et al. Identification of risk factors associated with postoperative acute kidney injury after cytoreductive surgery with hyperthermic intraperitoneal chemotherapy: a retrospective study. Int J Hyperthermia. 2018;34(5):538-44.
2. Hübner M, Kusamura S, Villeneuve L, Al-Niaimi A, Alyami M, Balonov K, et al. Guidelines for Perioperative Care in Cytoreductive Surgery (CRS) with or without hyperthermic IntraPEritoneal chemotherapy (HIPEC): Enhanced Recovery After Surgery (ERAS®) Society Recommendations-Part II: Postoperative management and special considerations. Eur J Surg Oncol J Eur Soc Surg Oncol Br Assoc Surg Oncol. 2020;46(12):2311-23.
3. Kurreck A, Gronau F, Alberto Vilchez ME, Abels W, Enghard P, Brandl A, et al. Sodium Thiosulfate Reduces Acute Kidney Injury in Patients Undergoing Cytoreductive Surgery Plus Hyperthermic Intraperitoneal Chemotherapy with Cisplatin: A Single-Center Observational Study. Ann Surg Oncol. 2022;29(1):152-62.

Q.4. **A 45-year-old female patient who underwent robotic nephroureterectomy with standard modified flank positioning developed postoperative pain and weakness of the dependent thigh. Serum creatine phosphokinase (CPK) values peaked 22,000 U/L (normal range 0–170 U/L) with urine that was positive for myoglobin and negative for significant microscopic hematuria. Which of the following statements is *false* regarding this condition?**
   a. It is a known but rare complication following prolonged robotic pelvic/renal surgery.
   b. Mannitol diuresis is the treatment of choice.
   c. Can be prevented by vigilance during patient positioning and an emphasis on proper cushioning
   d. Most commonly seen in the gluteal area

Ans. b

Explanation: Following laparoscopic or robotic renal surgery, rhabdomyolysis has been described as a rare complication affecting the dependent lower extremity, most frequently the gluteal region, and has been associated with risk factors like a high body mass index (BMI), an extended operating time, lateral decubitus positioning, and Trendelenburg position. Extra caution was advised while positioning to ensure adequate gluteal cushioning. Acute kidney injury (AKI) is the most frequent complication reported in literature to be linked to rhabdomyolysis, and a protracted hospital course required some sort of renal replacement therapy. Preventive measures generally concentrated on being watchful when positioning patients, emphasizing appropriate cushioning and pressure relief for the gluteal area, and adequate hydration in patients with suspected rhabdomyolysis.

When identified, treatment of postoperative rhabdomyolysis should be initiated immediately and without delay. Aggressive intravenous fluid hydration titrated to a urine output of roughly 3 mL/kg/hour is the cornerstone of therapy. Myoglobin-induced renal vasoconstriction is hypothesized to be prevented by alkalinization, which also inhibits reactive oxygen species and reduces protein-myoglobin complex precipitation within renal tubules. Mannitol diuresis is still controversial. Also, care must be taken to administer the diuretic only after sufficient fluid resuscitation has been completed.

Suggested Reading
1. Deras P, Amraoui J, Boutin C, Laporte S, Ripart J. Rhabdomyolysis and compartment syndrome of two forearms after robotic assisted prolonged surgery. Ann Fr Anesth Reanim. 2010;29:301-3.
2. Galyon SW, Richards KA, Pettus JA, Bodin SG. Three-limb compartment syndrome and rhabdomyolysis after robotic cystoprostatectomy. J Clin Anesth. 2011;23:75-8.
3. Mattei A, Di Pierro GB, Rafeld V, Konrad C, Beutler J, Danuser H. Positioning injury, rhabdomyolysis, and serum creatine kinase-concentration course in patients undergoing robot-assisted radical prostatectomy and extended pelvic lymph node dissection. J Endourol. 2013;27:45-51.
4. Terry RS, Gerke T, Mason JB, Sorensen MD, Joseph JP, Dahm P, et al. Postoperative rhabdomyolysis following robotic renal and adrenal surgery: a cautionary tale of compounding risk factors. J Robot Surg. 2015;9:195-200.

Q.5. A 35-year-old male with carcinoma gingivobuccal sulcus underwent hemi-mandibulectomy and reconstructive surgery. Preoperatively, he had a history of using fentanyl transdermal patch of 100 μg/hour for management of his cancer pain for the past 2 months. Which of the following is *true* regarding analgesia for this patient?
 a. Fentanyl patch should be removed intraoperatively.
 b. Nalbuphine can be used as an alternative analgesic.
 c. All opioids need to be discontinued.
 d. Only epidural analgesia is analgesic modality of choice.

Ans. a

Explanation: If the patient has been using a fentanyl patch, it should be removed. Skin temperature affects fentanyl transdermal absorption, and forced air warming devices placed over the patches could result in unexpectedly high uptake or overdose. Moreover, fentanyl distribution may be impacted by intraoperative fluid changes. Fentanyl patches should be removed as a result during surgery. To reduce the risk of withdrawal symptoms, transcutaneous fentanyl patches are replaced postoperatively or a similar "basal" narcotic is given in the early postoperative period.

In chronic opioid users, withdrawal symptoms might start anywhere between 6 and 18 hours following cessation. Even those experiencing a strong analgesic response from neuraxial or regional anesthetic blockade will need to take an opioid medication on a regular basis for maintenance. Opioid agonists having high binding affinity for the mu opioid receptor such as hydromorphone, fentanyl, and sufentanil are frequently favored for such individuals. Chronic opioid users should not be administered opioid agonist-antagonists like nalbuphine since they might precipitate withdrawal. While effective as a supplemental pain reliever, epidural anesthetic alone can cause withdrawal if oral or intravenous opioids are not additionally administered.

Opioids must be taken consistently to avoid withdrawal, but a multimodal therapeutic regimen may also include acetaminophen, nonsteroidal anti-inflammatory medicines, gabapentin, and pregabalin. In the perioperative period, ketamine has been used to reduce the amount of narcotics required and to decrease hyperalgesia.

Suggested Reading
1. Greene D. Total necrosis of the intranasal structures and soft palate as a result of nasal inhalation of crushed OxyContin. Ear Nose Throat J. 2005;84(8):512, 514, 516.
2. Griffith CC, Raval JS, Nichols L. Intravascular talcosis due to intravenous drug use is an underrecognized cause of pulmonary hypertension. Pulm Med. 2012;2012:617531.
3. Preston KL, Bigelow GE, Liebson IA. Antagonist effects of nalbuphine in opioid-dependent human volunteers. J Pharmacol Exp Ther. 1989;248(3):929-37.
4. Richebe P, Beaulieu P. Perioperative pain management in the patient treated with opioids: continuing professional development. Can J Anaesth. 2009;56(12):969-81.

Q.6. **A 32-year-old lady with grade 1 obesity and hypertension underwent total abdominal hysterectomy with bilateral salpingo-oophorectomy for ovarian malignancy. Which of the following statement is *incorrectly* related to postoperative deep venous thrombosis (DVT) prophylaxis?**
   a. Aspirin should never be considered as the sole anticoagulant for DVT prophylaxis.
   b. Neuraxial increase vasodilation in the lower limb and decreases the risk of DVT
   c. DVT pharmacotherapy should not be started immediately postsurgery.
   d. Mechanical thromboprophylaxis is usually recommended during the early postoperative period.

Ans. b

Explanation: Neuraxial or epidural catheter reduces the risk of DVT by 30–50%.

In immediate postoperative period, mechanical thromboprophylaxis should be started till the risk of bleeding decreases followed by pharmacotherapy after 6–12 hours as the female's obesity and HTN increase the risk of postoperative DVT.

Suggested Reading
1. Geerts WH, Bergqvist D, Pineo GF, Heit JA, Samama CM, Lassen MR, et al. Prevention of venous thromboembolism: American College of Chest Physicians Evidence-Based Clinical Practice Guidelines (8th Edition). Chest. 2008;133(6 Suppl):381S-453S.

Q.7. **In continuation of the above question, which of the following is *correct* for routine DVT scanning of the postoperative patient?**
   a. Contrast venography is a highly sensitive and specific DVT screening tool.
   b. Ultrasound techniques are highly reliable in diagnosing calf vein thrombosis.
   c. Duplex ultrasonography is the standard for routine DVT screening of patients.
   d. D-dimer has a high positive predictive value for DVT.

Ans. c

Explanation: Contrast venography is highly sensitive; however, venography is invasive, 20–40% of venograms are considered nondiagnostic, and the clinical relevance of small thrombi is uncertain. Ultrasound screening is noninvasive and has high sensitivity

90–95% and specificity but is unreliable in diagnosing calf vein thrombosis. Dimer has high negative predictive value.

Suggested Reading
1. Geerts WH, Pineo GF, Heit JA, Bergqvist D, Lassen MR, Colwell CW, et al. Prevention of venous thromboembolism: the Seventh ACCP Conference on Antithrombotic and Thrombolytic Therapy. Chest. 2004;126(3 Suppl):338S-400S.
2. Tovey C, Wyatt S. Diagnosis, investigation, and management of deep vein thrombosis. BMJ. 2003;326(7400):1180-4.

Q.8. A 30-year-old gentleman suffered blunt trauma abdomen during a road traffic accident and underwent exploratory laparotomy with splenectomy. Identify the *incorrect* statement regarding the case:
a. This patient will be at higher risk of infections with encapsulated organisms, e.g., pneumococci, meningococci, and *Haemophilus influenzae*.
b. Conjugated vaccines are preferred over polysaccharide vaccines for vaccination against pneumococci, meningococci, and *Haemophilus influenzae* in this case.
c. In this case ideally the vaccination against pneumococci, meningococci, and *Haemophilus influenzae* should be done on postoperative day 1.
d. *Babesia* and *Capnocytophaga canimorsus* infections are also common in these patients.

Ans. c

Explanation: The spleen is a lymphoid organ that plays an important role in both innate and acquired immunity. Its role is particularly crucial for the elimination of encapsulated bacteria, the clearance of intraerythrocytic parasites, and for potentiating the immune response to vaccines against polysaccharide antigens. Due to decreased response to encapsulated bacteria, the principal bacteria involved in postsplenectomy sepsis are primarily *Streptococcus pneumoniae* (50–70%), and *Neisseria meningitidis* and *Haemophilus influenzae* B (15–25% each), although the epidemiology of postsplenectomy infection has not been reassessed since the advent of vaccines against pneumococcus, meningococcus, and *Haemophilus*. There is also an increased risk of serious infection due to *Capnocytophaga canimorsus* after animal bites, *Bordetella holmesii*, *Ehrlichia* species and intraerythrocytic parasites such as *Babesia* after tick bites, and *Plasmodium* species in malaria-endemic areas.

When elective splenectomy is planned, it is preferable to administer the vaccine at least 2 weeks before surgery to ensure better immunogenicity. For emergency splenectomy or when vaccines were not administered beforehand, it is recommended that the immunization should be administered at least 2 weeks after surgery because the vaccine response is lower in the first 2 weeks after splenectomy. However, when patients are discharged early from the hospital, the risk of nonvaccination or loss to follow-up after splenectomy may encourage the administration of immunizations before that time.

Since asplenia causes an impaired immune response to polysaccharide antigens, conjugate vaccines must be used. Conjugate vaccines consist of polysaccharide antigens covalently bonded to bacterial protein antigens resulting in improved antigenicity and a more-prolonged immune response. T-cell-independent polysaccharide antigens are poorly immunogenic in such individuals. Recently developed pneumococcal conjugate vaccines (PCV, initially marketed as a 7-valent vaccine, now replaced with PCV13/PCV10—Prevenar 13/Synflorix) contain capsular polysaccharides from the 10 or 13 most common serotypes that cause disease, covalently linked to a nontoxic carrier protein.

Suggested Reading
1. Buzelé R, Barbier L, Sauvanet A, Fantin B. Medical complications following splenectomy. J Visc Surg. 2016;153(4):277-86.
2. Kuchar E, Miśkiewicz K, Karlikowska M. A review of guidance on immunization in persons with defective or deficient splenic function. Br J Haematol. 2015;171(5):683-94.

Q.9. Which of the following is *incorrect* regarding blood picture presentation of the above patient?
a. Howell Jolly bodies present
b. Thrombocytopenia
c. Pappenheimer bodies present
d. Raised total leukocyte counts

Ans. b

Explanation: Spleen plays the role of a phagocytic filter, allowing the culling and destruction of senescent erythrocytes and platelets and the selective elimination of intracytoplasmic elements (pitting). This "cleansing" of red blood cells (RBCs) also allows the clearance of intraerythrocyte pathogens such as *Plasmodium* and *Babesia*. With the loss of this culling function, the postsplenectomy patient often develops transient thrombocytosis (600–800,000/mm^3). Elevated counts of polymorphonuclear leukocytes (PMNs) also typical occur early after splenectomy and an elevated white blood cell (WBC) count > 15,000/mm^3 may lead to the erroneous suspicion of an infectious complication. The failure to remove intraerythrocytic nuclear fragments (pitting) results in the typical finding of Howell-Jolly bodies on review of blood smear or by simple phase-contrasted microscopy (basophilic stippling of RBCs).

The following may be observed in the laboratory results of individuals with hyposplenism: mild thrombocytosis and leukocytosis, the presence of Howell-Jolly bodies (nuclear remnants), Heinz and Pappenheimer bodies in erythrocytes, increased number of misshapen erythrocytes (target cells and irregular contracted cells), and erythrocytes with reduced deformability.

Suggested Reading
1. Buzelé R, Barbier L, Sauvanet A, Fantin B. Medical complications following splenectomy. J Visc Surg. 2016;153(4):277-86.
2. Kuchar E, Miśkiewicz K, Karlikowska M. A review of guidance on immunization in persons with defective or deficient splenic function. Br J Haematol. 2015;171(5):683-94.

Q.10. **A 85-year-old patient underwent total knee replacement under combined spinal epidural anesthesia and shifted to postoperative care with an epidural infusion of ropivacaine with fentanyl. Which of the following statement is *not true* related to postoperative complications of the patient?**
   a. Urinary retention is the most common complication of neuraxial opioid in males and a urinary catheter should be ensured.
   b. Emergence delirium is quite common with geriatric patients operated under general anesthesia.
   c. Nausea vomiting is more common with neuraxial opioids and an antiemetic should be added.
   d. None of the above

Ans. c

Explanation: Although nausea and vomiting is overall most common complication but urinary retention is more common with neuraxial opioids in old-aged males.

Suggested Reading
1. Shafer SL, Rathmell JP, Flood P. Stoelting's Pharmacology and Physiology in anesthetic Practice, 5th edition. Philadelphia: Wolters Kluwer Health; 2015.

Q.11. **A 62-year-old male patient was taken up for robotic cystoprostatectomy. The surgery went on for 8 hours in steep Trendelenburg position. In the recovery room, the patient was noted to have inspiratory stridor with SpO_2 of 92% on O_2 mask. The SpO_2 rose to 98% following administration of nebulized epinephrine. Which of the following is the *most likely* cause of the symptoms?**
   a. Airway edema
   b. Vocal cord paralysis
   c. Arytenoids subluxation
   d. Laryngospasm

Ans. a

Explanation: Around 12.5% of patients who underwent robotic surgery in a prolonged Trendelenburg posture were observed to develop head and neck edema. Such edema has been known to be severe enough to postpone extubation and rarely can be severe enough to require reintubation. Prolonged steep Trendelenburg positioning is thought to frequently result in chemosis and conjunctival edema, with no apparent clinical impact. Yet, there is evidence between the development of higher upper airway resistance and the occurrence of chemosis. As a result, the degree of chemosis has been employed as a potential airway edema warning indication.

The reduction in venous outflow from the head brought on by pneumoperitoneum during prolonged, deep Trendelenburg positioning contributes to upper airway edema. It may present as swollen and dull, edematous tongues, snoring, noisy inspiration with signs of accessory respiratory muscle use when patients are extubated. By obstructing the lymphatic and venous drainage of the tongue, endotracheal cuff pressure at the base of the mouth can both produce and worsen tongue edema. Reintubation was the most often reported consequence from airway edema followed by delayed extubation and ventilator support in patients whose edema was identified prior to extubation.

Treatment for airway edema apart from delayed extubation and mechanical ventilation included head up position, continuous positive airway pressure (CPAP), a nasopharyngeal airway, and a combination of head-up extubation at the end of the case followed by diuretics.

Suggested Reading
1. Maerz DA, Beck LN, Sim AJ, Gainsburg DM, et al. Complications of robotic-assisted laparoscopic surgery distant from the surgical site. Br J Anaesth. 2017;118(4):492-503.
2. Oksar M, Akbulut Z, Ocal H, Balbay MD, Kanbak O. Anesthetic considerations for robotic cystectomy: a prospective study. Braz J Anesthesiol. 2014;64:109-15.
3. Phong SV, Koh LK. Anaesthesia for robotic-assisted radical prostatectomy: considerations for laparoscopy in the Trendelenburg position. Anaesth Intensive Care. 2007;35:281-5.

Q.12. A 22-year-old male with a maxillary Ewing's sarcoma was operated for tumor asportation and reconstruction with free fibula flap. Which of the following is *false* regarding his postoperative care in compliance with enhanced recovery after surgery (ERAS) protocol?
   a. Free flap monitoring should be performed at least hourly for the first 24 hours postoperatively.
   b. Opioid-sparing, multimodal analgesia, utilizing NSAIDs, cyclooxygenase (COX) inhibitors, and paracetamol are preferred for postoperative analgesia.
   c. Urinary catheters should be removed as soon as the patient is able to void, ideally less than 24 hours after completion of surgery.
   d. ERAS strongly recommends the use of near-infrared spectroscopy for flap monitoring

Ans. d

Explanation: Frequent monitoring of free flaps in the acute postoperative period is important. There is general agreement that early flap monitoring following surgery should be frequent, reducing with time as the risk of flap problems reduces. Free flap monitoring is strongly advised by the ERAS Society to be carried out at least hourly for the first 24 hours following surgery, then continued throughout the remainder of the patient's stay with intensity dropping off gradually. The ERAS Society further strongly advises that the monitoring strategy should at the very least include a clinical examination by personnel knowledgeable on free flap monitoring; alternative monitoring methods may also be taken into consideration.

Other ERAS recommendations for postoperative care of free flap surgeries are:
- Routine ICU admission to facilitate an immediate postoperative period of deep sedation and artificial respiration is not necessary. A subset of low-risk uncomplicated patients may be treated safely after recovery from anesthesia in a high-dependency unit or specialist ward, provided adequate skilled nursing and medical coverage are provided.
- Opioid-sparing, multimodal analgesia, utilizing NSAIDs, COX inhibitors, and paracetamol are preferred for patients undergoing head and neck cancer surgery.

Patient-controlled analgesia can be considered if multimodal analgesia approaches are insufficient. No recommendation can be made on the role of additional nerve blocks.
- Free flap monitoring should be performed at least hourly for the first 24 hours postoperatively. Monitoring should be continued for the duration of the patient's stay with tapering of intensity after the first 24 hours. Method of monitoring should include, at a minimum, clinical examination by staff experienced with free flap monitoring. Adjunct monitoring techniques should be considered.
- Early mobilization, within the first 24 hours of surgery is recommended for patients undergoing major head and neck cancer surgery.
- Urinary catheters should be removed as soon as the patient is able to void, ideally less than 24 hours after completion of surgery.

Suggested Reading
1. Dort JC, Farwell DG, Findlay M, Huber GF, Kerr P, Shea-Budgell MA, et al. Optimal Perioperative Care in Major Head and Neck Cancer Surgery With Free Flap Reconstruction: A Consensus Review and Recommendations From the Enhanced Recovery After Surgery Society. JAMA Otolaryngol Head Neck Surg. 2017;143(3):292-303.

Q.13. During a postoperative check on a 53-year-old patient who underwent a total thyroidectomy 2 days prior, you notice that he is stridorous and is complaining of muscle cramps. The best treatment for this symptom is:
   a. Administration of calcium gluconate
   b. Opening the neck wound
   c. Reintubation for airway protection
   d. Administration of sodium bicarbonate

Ans. a

Explanation: One possible side effect of thyroid surgery is hypoparathyroidism, which develops when the parathyroid gland is unintentionally removed. Low blood calcium levels can cause cramping, weakness, tetany, laryngospasm, and stridor by interfering with normal muscular contraction and nerve conduction. Symptoms of hypocalcemia range from mild (e.g., paresthesias around the lips, mouth, hands, and feet) or moderate (e.g., muscle twitches or frank cramps) to severe (e.g., trismus or tetany).

Asymptomatic patients may or may not require calcium supplementation, but all patients with symptomatic hypocalcemia require oral calcium and some may need to be managed with extraintravenous calcium or calcitriol.

Following thyroid surgery, calcium supplementation is often administered orally as calcium carbonate, with a daily dose of 1,250–2,500 mg divided into 2–4 doses. The starting dose is modified and gradually tapered off depending on symptoms and/or calcium levels. Sometimes patients with persistently low calcium levels and symptoms despite oral treatment need intravenous calcium. Peripheral intravenous infusion sites should be closely watched in these individuals because calcium solution infiltration can cause soft tissue damage. When hypocalcemic symptoms disappear and serum calcium levels reach 7.8 mg/dL, patients can be discharged on oral calcium supplements. Measurement of serum magnesium should also be prompted by persistent hypocalcemia with replacement if necessary.

Patients with very low or undetectable parathyroid hormone (PTH) levels may also require 1,25-dihydroxyvitamin D (calcitriol), which is necessary for proper calcium absorption. As calcitriol can take up to 48 hours to achieve maximal effect, patients should continue to be monitored for both hypocalcemia and any potential resulting hypercalcemia.

Muscle cramps are not likely to be caused by a neck hematoma, despite the fact that compression can impair the airway. Difficulty caused by bilateral vocal cord paralysis is immediately noticeable after extubation, and reintubation would be necessary to create a patent airway. By lowering ionized calcium levels, sodium bicarbonate would result in a metabolic alkalosis and perhaps exacerbate hypocalcemia symptoms.

Suggested Reading
1. Bellantone R, Lombardi CP, Raffaelli M, Boscherini M, Alesina PF, De Crea C, et al. Is routine supplementation therapy (calcium and vitamin D) useful after total thyroidectomy? Surgery. 2002;132(6):1109-12; discussion 1112-3.
2. Ritter K, Elfenbein D, Schneider DF, Chen H, Sippel RS. Hypoparathyroidism after total thyroidectomy: incidence and resolution. J Surg Res. 2015;197(2):348-53.

Q.14. A 26-year-old gentleman with malignant bowel obstruction underwent laparotomy and end colostomy. He had been unable to eat for last 2 weeks and was on total parenteral nutrition (TPN) for several days. After the surgery, he was extubated in the operating room. However, 15 minutes after arriving to PACU he is unable to maintain adequate ventilation and oxygenation. On examination, profound global weakness was present with absent deep tendon reflexes. The specific electrolyte abnormality that should be evaluated is:
a. Magnesium
b. Phosphate
c. Sodium
d. Glucose

Ans. b

Explanation: It is crucial to guarantee that the patient receiving total parenteral feeding has normal serum phosphate levels since hypophosphatemia has been linked to abrupt respiratory failure brought on by significant areflexive muscular weakness. Sodium and magnesium do not present with respiratory failure and areflexia. TPN causes hyperglycemia.

Hypophosphatemia can occur when there are increased losses, decreased intake, or cellular shifts of phosphate. Cellular changes can result in hypophosphatemia when glucose or TPN is given to malnourished patients. Phosphate moves to the intracellular compartment as a result of an increase in insulin. High-energy phosphate bonds are also formed as a result of the enhanced anabolism, further depleting the phosphate levels.

The severity and persistence of low plasma phosphate levels determine the clinical signs and symptoms of hypophosphatemia. Individuals with mild hypophosphatemia (1.5-2.5 mg/dL) typically exhibit no symptoms. Patients with severe hypophosphatemia

(1.5 mg/dL) may experience symptoms related to muscular dysfunction, metabolic encephalopathy, bone pain, or symptoms secondary to muscle dysfunction (decreased strength, rhabdomyolysis, cardiomyopathy, and respiratory failure). Hematologic abnormalities can also be seen in hypophosphatemic patients [hemolysis secondary to decreased 2,3-DGP and adenosine triphosphate (ATP) levels, leukocyte dysfunction, and thrombocytopenia].

Management: It is crucial to remember that serum phosphate levels do not always correspond to total body stores when selecting how to treat hypophosphatemia. The presence of low, normal, or high total stores might result in hypophosphatemia. When there is a deficiency in the body stores of phosphorus, clinically significant hypophosphatemia can develop.

Phosphorus can be replaced orally or parenterally. Orally, it is considered safer. Phosphate-containing salts, such as sodium phosphate or potassium phosphate, and dairy products, such as milk, which has 1 mg of phosphorus per milliliter, are used as oral treatments. Moderate hypophosphatemia may usually be corrected orally with 60 mmol of phosphate per day given in 3-4 separate doses of the preferred formulation over the course of 7-10 days. Patients taking oral salt supplements could experience diarrhea, which can be prevented by giving divided doses.

Parenteral therapy is often only used in cases of severe hypophosphatemia or when oral medications are not tolerated or effective. Potassium and sodium phosphate are components in intravenous formulations. In cases of severe hypophosphatemia without obvious clinical symptoms, a typical regimen is 2.5 mg/kg body weight of phosphate administered over 6 hours, while in cases of hypophosphatemic emergency, 5.0 mg/kg body weight administered over 6 hours. Side effects of phosphate replacement are possible. Patients should be continuously monitored for hypernatremia, hyperkalemia, hyperphosphatemia, and volume overload when phosphate-containing salts are used. Also, it is crucial to keep an eye on the calcium phosphate product when receiving parenteral repletion. Overaggressive repletion can cause hypocalcemia and metastatic calcium deposition.

In addition to lowering the phosphorus levels in the plasma, the underlying causes of hypophosphatemia must be found and addressed.

Suggested Reading
1. Mushlin SB, Greene HL. Decision Making in Medicine: An algorithmic approach. Philadelphia, PA: Elsevier Health Sciences; 2009.

Q.15. A 60-year-old male patient presented with history of fever, vomiting, and abdominal pain for 5 days to emergency room. On examination, he was tachycardic, tachypnic, febrile, in circulatory shock with distended and rigid abdomen. X-ray abdomen showed gas under diaphragm. Patient was explored and two small bowel perforations of 1 cm diameter were found 25 cm prior to ileocecal junction. Peritoneal lavage with small bowel resection of involved segment and end-to-end anastomosis was done and patient improved and shifted to ward on postoperative day 5. On postoperative day 10, patient again became febrile, tachypnic, tachycardic, and in

circulatory shock. The abdomen was distended and resonant to percussion. A few abdominal sutures were opened and there was feculent material coming out of the suture line and signs of fistula development were present. Daily fistula output was around 800–1,000 mL. A diagnosis of postoperative enterocutaneous (EC) fistula was made. Identify the *incorrect* statement related to this case:
a. The patient is having a high output EC fistula.
b. EC fistula of ileum is less likely to resolve spontaneously and requires surgical closure.
c. A surgical etiology of EC fistula portends grave prognosis
d. A transferrin level <200 mg/dL is a poor prognostic indicator.

Ans. c

Explanation: There are several ways in which ECF has been classified, including by output, etiology, and source. Most often, a high-output ECF is characterized as one with >500 mL/24 hours, low output <200 mL/24 hours, and a moderate output fistula between 200 and 500 mL/24 hours. While the great majority of ECFs are iatrogenic (75–85%), between 15 and 25% occur spontaneously. Fistulas arising from the esophagus, duodenal stump after gastric resection, pancreaticobiliary tract, and jejunum are more likely to close without operative intervention. Additionally, those with long tracts and small enteric wall defects are associated with higher spontaneous closure rates. In contrast, those associated with the stomach, the lateral wall of the duodenum, the ligament of Treitz, and the ileum are more likely to require surgical correction. Surgical etiology of EC fistula, absence of sepsis, low-medium output EC fistula, and transferrin >200 mg/dL are indicators of good prognosis.

Suggested Reading
1. Gribovskaja-Rupp I, Melton GB. Enterocutaneous Fistula: Proven Strategies and Updates. Clin Colon Rectal Surg. 2016;29(2):130-7.
2. Haack CI, Galloway JR, Srinivasan J. Enterocutaneous Fistulas: A Look at Causes and Management. Curr Surg Rep. 2014;2(10):71.

Q.16. A 26-year-old gentleman presented to ICU with severe traumatic brain injury following a motor vehicular accident. During ICU management, tracheostomy was performed on day 2 of ICU admission; patient was successfully weaned and discharged home with tracheostomy on day 10. On day 4 of discharge, patient presented with bleeding from tracheostomy. The ICU resident calls ENT resident suspecting it to be tracheo-innominate artery (TIA) fistula. Which of the following statement is *wrong* regarding the case?
a. TIA fistula is a common complication of tracheostomy.
b. TIA fistula is associated with very high mortality rate (>80%).
c. Nearly three-fourths of the cases of TIA fistula present within first 3 weeks of tracheostomy
d. Mucosal ischemic necrosis and tracheostomy at lower than third tracheal cartilage are common predisposing factors for TIA fistula.

Ans. a

Explanation: Tracheo-innominate artery fistula (TIF) as described by Weisman is rare, but the most dramatic and adrenaline-producing complication of tracheostomy. Jones et al., who analyzed 137 reported cases in the literature including 10 of their own, reported that this life-threatening complication of tracheostomy is seen in approximately one in every 150 cases with a mortality of 92.7% (127/137). Although it is underlined that this incidence should have fallen with the application of "*low-pressure, soft-cuffed*" cannulas and endotracheal tubes, TIF can also be formed by "*non-cuffed*" cannulas. Since the mechanism of injury leading to TIF is pressure necrosis, it is of vital importance to be aware of the predisposing factors and to take preventive measures. After this catastrophic and almost always fatal complication, only patients who can be treated with emergency surgery tend to survive. Therefore, in any patient with tracheostomy, a high index of suspicion should be maintained, and important therapeutic steps must be taken in every suspected case.

A more frequent mechanism is mucosal ischemic necrosis caused by the pressure of the inflated cuff. Sometimes, especially when the tracheostomy is performed lower than the second to third tracheal ring, arterial erosion can be caused by direct pressure from the curved portion of the cannula.

Hemorrhage occurring 3 days to 6 weeks after tracheostomy should be thought of as a result of TIF until proven otherwise. Other causes of catastrophic pulmonary hemorrhage include pulmonary artery flotation, catheter-induced arterial rupture, thoracic aneurysm rupture, and less common vascular fistula (carotid artery and inferior thyroid). It is likely that the majority will occur in the critical care unit as 70% of all delayed hemorrhages occur during the first 3 weeks. A sentinel bleed is reported in >50% of patients who then develop massive delayed hemorrhage.

Suggested Reading
1. Grant CA, Dempsey G, Harrison J, Jones T. Tracheo-innominate artery fistula after percutaneous tracheostomy: three case reports and a clinical review. Br J Anaesth. 2006;96(1):127-31.
2. Jones JW, Reynolds M, Hewitt RL, Drapanas T. Tracheo-innominate artery erosion: Successful surgical management of a devastating complication. Ann Surg. 1976;184:194-204.
3. Weissman BW. Tracheo-innominate artery fistula. Laryngoscope. 1974;84:205-9.
4. Yaliniz H, Tokcan A, Ulus T. Tracheo-innominate artery fistula: two cases. Ulus Travma Acil Cerrahi Derg. 2009;15(5):505-8.

Q.17. **A 35-year-old male patient with morbid obesity, mild obstructive sleep apnea (OSA), and type 1 diabetes mellitus (DM) was admitted for bariatric surgery. He underwent laparoscopic sleeve gastrectomy. The patient was induced with fentanyl 2 µg/kg, propofol induction dose, and the trachea was intubated after a loading dose of atracurium. Anesthesia was maintained with sevoflurane and a mixture of 50% oxygen and air. The surgery lasted for 3 hours, two doses of fentanyl were repeated at the interval of 1 hour, and a single dose of muscle relaxant was repeated 1 hour before the end of the surgery. A total dose of reversal was given, and the patient was extubated after ensuring an awake, cooperative, and sustained hand grip of 5 seconds. The patient was shifted to the postoperative care unit. Soon, the**

SpO$_2$ **of the patient dropped; which of the following statements might be correct for the cause of desaturation?**
a. Airway obstruction can be ruled out in an awake, cooperative patient at extubation.
b. Respiratory depression can be ruled out as there was sustained head lift and hand grip.
c. Since the patient was not using CPAP earlier, it is unnecessary in postoperative period.
d. None of the above

Ans. d

Explanation: Respiratory complications and airway obstruction are the leading cause of postoperative adverse outcomes in obese patients. Airway obstruction in the postoperative period is because by two reasons—(1) fall of the tongue onto the posterior pharyngeal wall and (2) loss of pharynx muscular tone. The stimulation associated with tracheal extubation may keep the patient awake and airway open during extubation and transport to the PACU. Only after the patient calmly rests in the PACU does upper airway obstruction become evident.

Also, clinical parameters at extubation of the patient have low sensitivity and specificity and do not rule out the risk of hypoventilation, atelectasis, and airway collapse in the postoperative area.

The hypercapnic ventilatory response is depressed in obese patients, even with subanesthetic effects in the postoperative period leading to an increased risk of hypoxemia and desaturation. CPAP and noninvasive ventilation (NIV) is thus considered first-line treatment in patients with postoperative acute respiratory failure due to atelectasis or pneumonia.

Suggested Reading
1. Chiumello D, Chevallard G, Gregoretti C. Non-invasive ventilation in postoperative patients: a systematic review. Intensive Care Med. 2011;37:918-29.
2. Ferreyra GP, Baussano I, Squadrone V, Richiardi L, Marchiaro G, Del Sorbo L, et al. Continuous positive airway pressure for treatment of respiratory complications after abdominal surgery: a systematic review and meta-analysis. Ann Surg. 2008;247:617-26.
3. Isono S, Warner DS, Warner MA. Obstructive Sleep Apnea of Obese Adults: Pathophysiology and Perioperative Airway Management. Anesthesiology. 2009;110:908-21.

Q.18. **In the above-mentioned patient, the attending clinician in the recovery area rushed to the patient and noted that the patient was deeply sedated and was not breathing. As he tapped the patient for a response, he became awake and started breathing again. While the clinician observed the patient, he noted chest rise and respiratory rate was adequate but the patient started snoring again and went into apnea soon. Which of the following interventions is the most appropriate for the patient?**
a. A nasopharyngeal airway will open the airway.
b. A dose of naloxone should be given to restore neural response to hypoxemia.

c. There is a loss of neural response to apnea and hypoxemia, thus, patients need to be on invasive ventilation.
d. None of the above

Ans. d

Explanation: This is a case of postoperative airway obstruction and OSA augmented by the effects of anesthesia. Postoperative airway obstruction is more common in obese patients for two reasons—(1) fall of the tongue onto the posterior pharyngeal wall and loss of tone of muscles of the pharynx. This is followed by hypoxemia, desaturation, and should lead to a neural response of awakening and thus opening the airway. This response might be suppressed in obese patients who are overtly sensitive to anesthetics effects.

Though restoration of the neural response might be desirable, the opening of the airway is the primary treatment. A nasopharyngeal airway might prevent the fall of the tongue; it does not help with pharyngeal tone. A CPAP, when applied above a critical pressure opens the complete airway, decreases the work of breathing, and even helps with atelectasis and decreases the risk of pneumonia.

Suggested Reading
1. Hodgson LE, Murphy PB, Hart N. Respiratory management of the obese patient undergoing surgery. J Thorac Dis. 2015;7(5):943-52.
2. Spicuzza L, Caruso D, Di Maria G. Obstructive sleep apnoea syndrome and its management. Ther Adv Chronic Dis. 2015;6(5):273-85.

Q.19. In the above-mentioned case residual neuromuscular blockade (NMB) was considered as one of the cause of the decreased pharyngeal tone and airway obstruction of the patient. Which of the following is correct about the residual neuromuscular blockade in this patient?
a. Incidence of the residual blockade is as high as 40%.
b. Sustained head lift or palmar grasp should be sufficient to rule out residual effects.
c. Sugammadex will lead to complete reversal of this patient.
d. Supplemental dose of neostigmine can be given to the patient.

Ans. a

Explanation: The incidence of residual neuromuscular blockade has been found to be as high as 20-40%. This can be especially prolonged in obese patients with hypercarbia and can always be considered a cause of hypoventilation or collapsed airway. A train-of-four (TOF) reading of >0.9 is considered an adequate reversal. Clinical parameters have shown wide variability, with senstivity as low as 18-19%. Sugammadex is a modified γ-cyclodextrin that selectively binds amino steroid NMB and completely reverses it. However, our patient was given atracurium which is a nonamino steroid. Although, we can give an additional dose of neostigmine, but if there is already complete inhibition of acetylcholinesterase, giving further neostigmine will not serve any useful purpose.

Suggested Reading
1. Brull SJ, Murphy GS. Residual neuromuscular block: lessons unlearned. Part 2: Methods to reduce the risk of residual weakness. Anesth Analg. 2011;111:129-40.
2. Murphy GS, Brull SJ. Residual neuromuscular block: lessons learned. Part 1: definitions, incidence, and adverse physiologic effects of residual neuromuscular block. Anesth Analg. 2010;111:120-8.

Q.20. A 30-year-old male was brought to the trauma center as a suspected case of the blunt trauma patient with *fast* positive. The patient was hemodynamically unstable. The patient was intubated and resuscitated with blood and fluids. The patient did not respond to fluids and thus was posted for emergency laparotomy. The patient underwent general anesthesia with fentanyl 100 µg and muscle relaxant. Surgery started with a midline incision from the xiphoid to pubic symphysis. A mesenteric bleed was located, hemostasis was achieved, and primary closure was done. Intraoperative anesthesia and analgesia were maintained with morphine 4.5 mg, repeated doses of fentanyl 100 µg, and intermittent muscle relaxants. Norepinephrine was started for a while and soon was not needed after hemostasis. Intraoperative, a total of two units of packed RBC, RDP, FPP, and 1.5 L of Ringer's lactate were transfused. Surgery lasted for 3 hours following which the trachea was extubated and shifted to intensive care. Soon the SpO$_2$ of the patient dropped to 78% on 6 L oxygen therapy. On bedside, evaluation and mean arterial pressure was normal with slight tachycardia but with dyspnea. An arterial blood gas analysis was done, a diagnosis of respiratory failure was made, and he was soon intubated, which of the following is not true to the definition of postoperative respiratory failure?
   a. Postoperative PaO$_2$ <8 kPa (60 mm Hg) on room air
   b. *PaO$_2$*: FiO$_2$ ratio <40 kPa (300 mm Hg)
   c. No evidence of cardiac failure or fluid overload
   d. Patient needing oxygen therapy

Ans. c

Explanation: European Perioperative Clinical Outcome definitions for postoperative respiratory failure is—Postoperative PaO$_2$ <8 kPa (60 mm Hg) on room air, a PaO$_2$: FiO$_2$ ratio <40 kPa (300 mm Hg), or arterial oxyhemoglobin saturation measured with pulse oximetry <90% and requiring oxygen therapy. So, fluid overload and pulmonary edema is one of the etiologies of postoperative pulmonary complications (PPCs).

Suggested Reading
1. Gropper MA, Eriksson LI, Fleisher LA, Wiener-Kronish JP, Cohen NH, Leslie K. Miller's Anesthesia, 9th edition. Philadelphia: Elsevier Health Sciences; 2019.
2. Jammer I, Wickbold N, Sander M, Smith A, Schultz MJ, Pelosi P, et al. Standards for definitions and use of outcome measures for clinical effectiveness research in perioperative medicine: European Perioperative Clinical Outcome (EPCO) definitions: a statement from the ESA-ESICM joint taskforce on perioperative outcome measures. Eur J Anaesthesiol. 2015;32:88-105.

Q.21. What could not be the possible cause of respiratory failure in the above-mentioned patient?
a. Type 4 respiratory failure
b. Type 3 respiratory failure
c. Type 2 respiratory failure
d. Type 1 respiratory failure

Ans. a

Explanation: European Society of Anaesthesiologists has given a list of etiologies that can lead to or be included in the spectrum of postoperative respiratory failure.
- Atelectasis—resulting in postoperative hypoxemia (most typical complication)
- Alveolar hypoventilation (residual effects of muscle relaxants, opioids, etc.)
- Pneumonia and bronchitis
- Bronchospasm
- Exacerbation of previous lung disease
- Pulmonary collapse due to mucus plugging of the airways
- Respiratory failure with ventilatory support >48 hours
- Acute lung injury (ALI) including aspiration pneumonitis, transfusion-related ALI (TRALI), and acute respiratory distress syndrome (ARDS)
- Pulmonary embolism
- Obstructive pulmonary edema

Respiratory failure is of 4 types:
- *Type 1 (hypoxia without hypercarbia)*: It is due to V/Q mismatch, decreased diffusion capacity, and venous admixture. Postoperative pneumonia, chronic obstructive pulmonary disease (COPD), pulmonary edema, embolism, etc. can lead to type 1 respiratory failure.
- *Type 2 (hypoxia with hypercarbia)*: Due to hypoventilation, peripheral or central causes, it can be the cause of central respiratory depression because of the effect of opioids, inhalational, etc., and decreased respiratory efforts due to residual neuromuscular blockade, or splinting action of pain due to upper abdominal surgery.
- Type 3 is also called postoperative respiratory failure due to atelectasis, common in emergency abdominal surgery lasting >2 hours.
- Type 4 respiratory failure, also known as shock failure. It is due to shock leading to fatigue and failure of respiratory muscles.

Suggested Reading
1. Gropper MA, Eriksson LI, Fleisher LA, Wiener-Kronish JP, Cohen NH, Leslie K. Miller's Anesthesia, 9th edition. Philadelphia: Elsevier Health Sciences; 2019.
2. Jammer I, Wickbold N, Sander M, Smith A, Schultz MJ, Pelosi P, et al. Standards for definitions and use of outcome measures for clinical effectiveness research in perioperative medicine: European Perioperative Clinical Outcome (EPCO) definitions: a statement from the ESA-ESICM joint taskforce on perioperative outcome measures. Eur J Anaesthesiol. 2015;32:88-105.

Q.22. Which of the following statements about managing and preventing postoperative pulmonary complications (PPCs) is incorrect for the above-mentioned patient with abdominal surgery?
a. Supplemental oxygen can treat hypoxemia due to alveolar hypoventilation.
b. High intraoperative positive end-expiratory pressure (PEEP) is recommended to correct postoperative atelectasis and pneumonia.
c. Intraoperative lung-protective ventilation with low tidal volume is beneficial to prevent postoperative pneumonia.
d. Nasogastric tube (NGT) can be removed to prevent aspiration and PPC.

Ans. b

Explanation: Arterial hypoxemia due to hypoventilation and hypercarbia can treated with increasing FiO_2 (oxygen therapy) and partial pressure of alveolar oxygen.

$$PAO_2 = FiO_2 (Patm + Pvapour) - PaCO_2/RQ$$

Ventilation strategies for preventing/managing atelectasis and pneumonia: Various studies and meta-analysis showed reduced PPC incidence with low tidal volumes and recruitment maneuvers. However, regarding PEEP, there is low-quality evidence in favor of moderate PEEP, a large RCT PROVHILO trial has shown no benefit rather hemodynamic instability with the use of high PEEP.

Various studies and a meta-analysis have shown that patients undergoing abdominal surgery are 5-8 times more likely to have a PPC if an NGT is used in the perioperative period. A NGT decreases the swallowing reflex, risk increases the risk of upper respiratory secretions, and infection going down lower respiratory tract and also keeps the lower esophageal sphincter open thus increasing the risk aspiration as well.

Suggested Reading
1. Cheatham ML, Chapman WC, Key SP, Sawyers JL. A meta-analysis of selective versus routine nasogastric decompression after elective laparotomy. Ann Surg. 1995;221:469-76; discussion 476-8.
2. Futier E, Constantin JM, Paugam-Burtz C, Pascal J, Eurin M, Neuschwander A, et al. IMPROVE Study Group: a trial of intraoperative low-tidal-volume ventilation in abdominal surgery. N Engl J Med. 2013;369:428-37.
3. Hemmes SN, Serpa Neto A, Schultz MJ. Intraoperative ventilatory strategies to prevent postoperative pulmonary complications: a meta-analysis. Curr Opin Anesthesiol. 2013;26:126-33.
4. PROVE Network Investigators for the Clinical Trial Network of the European Society of Anaesthesiology; Hemmes SN, Gama de Abreu M, Pelosi P, Schultz MJ. High versus low positive end-expiratory pressure during general anaesthesia for open abdominal surgery (PROVHILO trial): a multicentre randomised controlled trial. Lancet. 2014;384:495-503.
5. Serpa Neto A, Hemmes SN, Barbas CS, Beiderlinden M, Biehl M, Binnekade JM, et al. Protective versus conventional ventilation for surgery: A systematic review and individual patient data meta-analysis. Anesthesiology. 2015;123:66-78.

Q.23. A 65-year-old male patient presented to the emergency with signs and symptoms suggestive of peritonitis. Upon further investigation, the patient was diagnosed with perforation peritonitis, and sepsis with shock. The patient is a known case of uncontrolled DM on insulin and is a known smoker. The patient did not have any history suggestive of cardiac or cerebral events. The patient was operated under general anesthesia. The shock was managed with intraoperative fluids and vasopressors. Postoperatively the patient was shifted to PACU, where the patient's blood pressure further crashed. A bedside Echo revealed anterolateral wall hypokinesia; which of the following statements is *true* to the management of the patient?

a. Bowel perforation is an intermediate-risk surgery.
b. Revised cardiac risk index (RCRI) score for this patient reveals an increased risk of major adverse cardiac events (MACEs)
c. Routine postoperative ECG is recommended to diagnose such events.
d. Routine troponin is recommended to diagnose such events.

Ans. d

Explanation:

Revised cardiac risk index:

Clinical parameter	RCRI point
Elevated-risk surgery Intraperitoneal, intrathoracic, suprainguinal vascular	1
History of ischemic heart disease	1
History of congestive heart failure	1
History of cerebrovascular disease	1
Preoperative treatment with insulin	1
Preoperative creatinine >2 mg/dL/176.8 µmol/L	1

Low risk-0 (0.4%), moderate risk 1–2 (0.9–6.6%), high risk >2 (>11%)

According to American Heart Association (AHA) recommendations, all abdominal surgeries including bowel perforations are high-risk. RCRI is an assessment risk score to evaluate the risk score of perioperative MACE. Our patient does have two risk factors, i.e., (1) high-risk surgery and (2) DM on insulin. However, RCRI is not valid for emergencies and thus inappropriate for risk assessment. Myocardial ischemia after noncardiac surgery (MINS) is often not associated with clinical signs and symptoms or even ECG changes. AHA therefore recommends routine troponin for every patient undergoing vascular or high-risk surgery.

Suggested Reading

1. Fleisher LA, Fleischmann KE, Auerbach AD, Barnason SA, Beckman JA, Bozkurt B, et al. 2014 ACC/AHA guideline on perioperative cardiovascular evaluation and management of patients undergoing noncardiac surgery: executive summary: a report of the American College of Cardiology/American Heart Association Task Force on Practice Guidelines. Circulation. 2014;130(24):2215-45.
2. Lee TH, Marcantonio ER, Mangione CM, Thomas EJ, Polanczyk CA, Cook EF, et al. Derivation and prospective validation of a simple index for prediction of cardiac risk of major noncardiac surgery. Circulation. 1999;100(10):1043-9.

Q.24. In continuation of the above question, an investigation of serum markers revealed elevated troponin levels with normal ECG findings. What should be the correct approach for diagnosing and managing the case?
   a. Elevated troponin levels could be because of sepsis and is insignificant.
   b. Normal ECG rules out the diagnosis of ischemia
   c. Troponin levels are a prognostic marker of myocardial ischemia.
   d. Fibrinolysis must be considered as the event is acute and severe.

Ans. c

Explanation: Myocardial ischemia after noncardiac surgery (MINS) is defined as elevated postoperative troponin levels without any clinical symptoms or any changes in the ECG. Elevated troponin levels and serial elevations are a highly sensitive marker and are associated with poor outcome and 30-day mortality rate. Troponins are elevated in sepsis but the serial troponin should be followed to establish the diagnosis.

In the postoperative period, fibrinolysis or percutaneous coronary intervention (PCI) should be considered for acute and severe cases. However, since these patients just had surgery, there are conflicting goals in terms of postoperative bleeding versus coronary blood flow.

Suggested Reading
   1. Gropper MA, Eriksson LI, Fleisher LA, Wiener-Kronish JP, Cohen NH, Leslie K. Miller's Anesthesia, 9th edition. Philadelphia: Elsevier Health Sciences; 2019.

Q.25. A 26-year-old female, gravida 1, para 1 at 39 weeks' gestation was admitted to the hospital for termination of pregnancy. She is a known case of mitral stenosis with atrial fibrillation. Her first trimester antenatal Echo showed severe mitral stenosis with a dilated left atrium, mild tricuspid regurgitation, and normal biventricular function. She reported to the antenatal care (ANC) clinic in her second trimester and was started on furosemide 20 mg 12 hourly, tablet warfarin for anticoagulation, and metoprolol for controlling ventricular rate. She was planned for elective cesarean section. Warfarin was replaced with bridge therapy of unfractionated heparin, which was stopped 12 hours before surgery. The cesarean section was conducted under spinal anesthesia. The surgery was uneventful, and she was sent to the postoperative care unit. On postoperative day 1, a sudden fall in blood pressure to 70/25 mm Hg. Uncontrolled atrial fibrillation with an effective heart rate of 158 was noted on the ECG monitor. Heparin was not yet started due to the risk of postpartum hemorrhage. Which of the following is the treatment of choice for the patient?
   a. Treatment with β-blocker will control the rate and improve hemodynamic.
   b. Digoxin is the treatment of choice.
   c. Cardioversion is the treatment of choice.
   d. Perform transesophageal echocardiogram (TEE) before cardioversion to rule out left atrial (LA) clot

Ans. c

Explanation: AHA gives following recommendation for prevention of thromboembolism and cardioversion in AF.

Class I:

- For patients with AF or atrial flutter of 48 hours' duration or longer, or when the duration of AF is unknown, anticoagulation with warfarin [international normalized ratio (INR) 2.0-3.0] is recommended for at least 3 weeks before and 4 weeks after cardioversion.
- For patients with AF or atrial flutter of >48 hours or unknown duration requiring immediate cardioversion for hemodynamic instability, anticoagulation should be initiated as soon as possible and continued for at least 4 weeks after cardioversion unless contraindicated.

Class IIa: For patients with AF or atrial flutter of 48 hours duration or longer or of unknown duration who have not been anticoagulated for the preceding 3 weeks, it is reasonable to perform TEE before cardioversion and proceed with cardioversion if no LA thrombus is identified, including in the left atrial appendage (LAA), provided that anticoagulation is achieved before TEE and maintained after cardioversion for at least 4 weeks.

So, in case of emergency or where the patient was on anticoagulation just 2 days back, cardioversion is the intervention of choice.

Suggested Reading

1. January CT, Wann LS, Alpert JS, Calkins H, Cigarroa JE, Cleveland JC Jr, et al. 2014 AHA/ACC/HRS guideline for managing patients with atrial fibrillation: a report of the American College of Cardiology/American Heart Association Task Force on practice guidelines and the Heart Rhythm Society. Circulation. 2014;130(23):e199-267.
2. Writing Group Members; January CT, Wann LS, Calkins H, Chen LY, Cigarroa JE, et al. 2019 AHA/ACC/HRS focused update of the 2014 AHA/ACC/HRS guideline for the management of patients with atrial fibrillation: A Report of the American College of Cardiology/American Heart Association Task Force on Clinical Practice Guidelines and the Heart Rhythm Society. Heart Rhythm. 2019;16(8):e66-e93.

Q.26. A 29-year-old male presented to the trauma center with a stab injury to abdomen, and shock. The trachea was intubated, and the patient was resuscitated with fluids, blood, and blood components. The shock was unresponsive and patient shifted for surgery. The patient was operated on, a grade 2 liver injury was noted, hemostasis was achieved, and primary closure was done without an abdominal drain. Intraoperative, further fluids, and blood and components were transfused. The patient was shifted to the ICU due to a significant fluid shift and the need for postoperative ventilation. In the ICU, 6 hours after shifting, airway pressures increased with hypotension and tachycardia. On palpation, the abdomen was not tense, which of the following should help make the correct diagnosis and management?
 a. Absence of abdominal distension should rule out abdominal compartment syndrome (ACS).
 b. Bedside CT is needed to diagnose ACS.

c. A fluid challenge can be diagnostic as well as therapeutic.
d. Point of care ultrasound can help make diagnosis.

Ans. d

Explanation: A postoperative patient with shock features should suggest a provisional diagnosis of ACS, hemorrhage, or sepsis with ARDS or pulmonary thromboembolism. However, the trauma patient with major abdominal surgery of liver injury, without drains and major fluid shift, and increased airway pressures should raise suspicion of ACS.

A tense abdomen should be a unique pathognomonic feature helping in the diagnosis. However, recent data suggest that some of the adverse effects of elevated abdominal pressure manifest before the development of a distended abdomen. CT helps to confirm the diagnosis but is never a gold standard or necessary to make a diagnosis. A bedside ultrasound can be used to assess inferior vena cava (IVC) compression, cardiac filling pressures and functions, and help to differentiate diagnosis. Ultrasound is however neither specific not sensitive of ACS.

Suggested Reading
1. Cheatham ML, Malbrain ML, Kirkpatrick A, Sugrue M, Parr M, De Waele J, et al. Results from the International Conference of Experts on Intra-Abdominal Hypertension and Abdominal Compartment Syndrome. II. Recommendations. Intensive Care Med. 2007;33(6):951-62.
2. Malbrain ML, Cheatham ML, Kirkpatrick A, Sugrue M, Parr M, De Waele J, et al. Results from the International Conference of Experts on Intra-Abdominal Hypertension and Abdominal Compartment Syndrome. I. Definitions. Intensive Care Med. 2006;32(11): 1722-32.

Q.27. A provisional diagnosis of ACS was made in the above-mentioned patient. What is the next course of action for the patient?
a. Urinary bladder pressure measurement is gold standard for the ACS.
b. A diuretic must be added for the management of secondary ACS.
c. Surgical intervention is the intervention of choice.
d. None of the above

Ans. a

Explanation: Primary ACS is the most common after both blunt and penetrating trauma. This risk is higher in patients with liver trauma or combined abdominopelvic injury and in those who have undergone abdominal packing for bleeding or primary fascial closure after laparotomy. Secondary ACS occurs because of bowel edema or ascites formation following an extensive volume fluid resuscitation and visceral reperfusion injury.

As mentioned, the patient is a case of both primary and secondary ACS with shock and respiratory failure. While surgical intervention is the intervention of choice for primary ACS, medical therapy includes sedation, neuromuscular blockade, evacuating intraluminal contents, paracentesis of ascites or hemoperitoneum, percutaneous drainage, and cautious fluid resuscitation. Diuretics are used in case of fluid overload. They are not the first choice of treatment in patient with shock or organ failure.

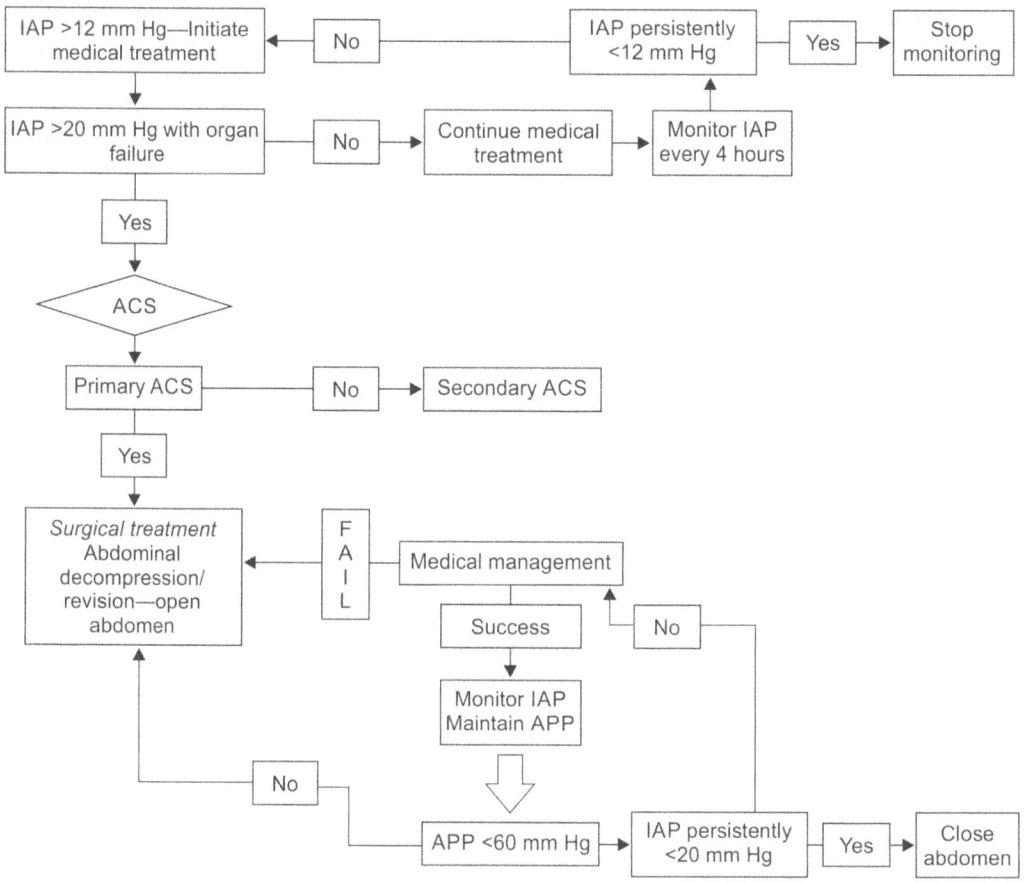

Suggested Reading
1. Cheatham ML, Malbrain ML, Kirkpatrick A, Sugrue M, Parr M, De Waele J, et al. Results from the international conference of experts on intra-abdominal hypertension and abdominal compartment syndrome. II. Recommendations. Intensive Care Med. 2007;33(6):951-62.
2. Malbrain ML, Cheatham ML, Kirkpatrick A, Sugrue M, Parr M, De Waele J, et al. Results from the international conference of experts on intra-abdominal hypertension and Abdominal compartment syndrome. I. Definitions. Intensive Care Med. 2006;32(11): 1722-32.

Q.28. A 48-year-old male patient with a known case of triple vessel disease presented to the outpatient department. His echocardiography report showed an anterolateral wall hypokinesia with an ejection fraction of 35% and no valvular abnormalities. The patient was started on β-blockers and spironolactone by a previous cardiologist. He was NYHA class 2 and could climb one flight of stairs. An on-pump coronary artery

bypass grafting (CABG) from right internal mammary artery and saphenous vein graft was performed. The patient was shifted to intensive care in the postoperative period. The patient soon went into shock. A provisional diagnosis of hemorrhagic shock was considered; which of the following statements is true for the shock?
a. Class III shock is associated with a urine output of approximately 10 mL/hour.
b. Pulse pressure is decreased in class I shock.
c. Class III shock is a loss of approximately 25% of the blood volume.
d. Pulmonary capillary wedge pressure (PCWP) is increased in hemorrhagic shock.

Ans. a

Explanation: *There are four stages/class of hemorrhagic shock:*

	Class of hemorrhagic shock			
	I	II	III	IV
Blood loss (mL)	Up to 750	750–1,500	1,500-2,000	>2,000
Blood loss (% blood volume)	Up to 15	15–30	30–40	>40
Pulse rate (per minute)	<100	100–120	120–140	>140
Blood pressure	Normal	Normal	Decreased	Decreased
Pulse pressure (mm Hg)	Normal or increased	Decreased	Decreased	Decreased
Respiratory rate (per minute)	14–20	20–30	30–40	>35
Urine output (mL/hour)	>30	20–30	5–15	Negligible
Central nervous system/mental status	Slightly anxious	Mildly anxious	Anxious, confused	Confused, lethargic

Suggested Reading
1. American College of Surgeons Committee on Trauma. ATLS: advanced trauma life support for doctors: student course manual (8th edition). Chicago, IL: American College of Surgeons; 2008.
2. Guly HR, Bouamra O, Little R, Dark P, Coats T, Driscoll P, et al. Testing the validity of the ATLS classification of hypovolaemic shock. Resuscitation. 2010;81(9):1142-7.

Q.29. In the above patient, after assessing the chest drain, patient chest X-rays, bedside ultrasound, ACT, and thromboelastogram, a diagnosis of hemorrhagic shock was ruled out. Assessing cardiac pressures led to a provisional diagnosis of hypovolemic/vasodilatory shock. Which of the following is *incorrect* for vasodilatory/hypovolemic shock of the patient?
a. Vasodilatory shock is refractory to fluids and β-agonists.
b. Most of the patients reach recovery with fluid overload
c. Hypothermia can lead to vasodilatory shock.
d. Methylene blue may be used to treat shock.

Ans. c

Explanation: Cardiopulmonary bypass (CPB) typically results in fluid sequestration into the interstitial compartment. Fluid shifts into or out of the interstitial and intracellular compartments can be anticipated in the hours following surgery. Most CPB patients reach the recovery area with excess body fluids that need to be mobilized. A healthy patient with good renal and cardiac function diurese this fluid over the next few days without assistance.

Hypothermia further complicates fluid management. It leads to vasoconstriction rather than dilation, shivering, increased myocardial oxygen demand, and decreased cardiac output.

Hypotension in the postbypass period can be due to the following reasons:
- *Cardiac*: Ventricular dysfunction, arrhythmias, tamponade, and bleeding.
- *Vascular*: Hypotension due to vasodilation—8% of cardiac surgery patient experience refractory vasodilatory shock after bypass. These patients do not respond to either traditional vasopressors or volume expansion. An intravenous bolus of methylene blue or vasopressin may be useful and has been shown to benefit in this patient population.

Suggested Reading
1. Hensley FA, Martin DE, Gravlee GP (Eds). A Practical Approach to Cardiac Anesthesia, 5th edition. Philadelphia, PA: Lippincott, Williams and Wilkins; 2013.

Q.30. A 60-year-old patient was operated on for CABG for left main artery disease with right internal mammary artery. Postcardiopulmonary bypass patient complained of right-sided weakness of the upper limb. Which is not the common cause of neurological complications with CPB in the above-mentioned patient?
a. Cerebral ischemia
b. Intracranial hemorrhage
c. Encephalopathy
d. Peripheral nerve injury

Ans. b

Explanation: It is estimated that between 6 and 28% of patients experience some perioperative neurological injury. Between 0.8 and 5.2% of individuals undergoing CABG surgery have clinically evident stroke postoperatively. Neurological complications can be divided into three groups: (1) Focal ischemic injury (Stroke-MC), (2) neurocognitive dysfunction (diffuse encephalopathy), and (3) peripheral nerve injury (e.g., brachial plexus injury due to sternal retraction, especially due to mammary artery dissection).

Clinical picture may vary widely from subtle changes in personality or behavior to fatal central nervous system (CNS) damage as presented in the table here.

Complication	*Incidence*
Fatal brain injury	0.3%
Nonfatal diffuse encephalopathy	
Depressed conscious level	3%
Behavioral changes	1%

Contd...

Contd...

Complication	Incidence
Intellectual/cognitive dysfunction	30–79%
Seizures	
Choreoathetosis	0.3%
Ophthalmological	
Visual field defects	25%
Reduced visual acuity	4.5%
Focal brain injury (stroke)	2–5%
Primitive reflexes	39%
Spinal cord injury	0–0.1%
Peripheral nerve injury	
Brachial plexopathy	7%
Other peripheral neuropathy	6%

Suggested Reading

1. Arrowsmith JE, Grocott HP, Reves JG, Newman MF. Central nervous system complications of cardiac surgery. Br J Anaesth. 2000;84(3):378-93.
2. Hensley FA, Martin DE, Gravlee GP (Eds). A Practical Approach to Cardiac Anesthesia, 5th edition. Philadelphia, PA: Lippincott, Williams and Wilkins; 2013.

CHAPTER

Sepsis and Antimicrobial Stewardship

Natesh Prabu R, Carol D'Silva, Dipali A Taggarsi

Q.1. A 60-year-old male patient was admitted with renal stones and hydrouretero-nephrosis with septic shock. On examination, he was drowsy, but he was responding to verbal commands, blood pressure—100/64 mm Hg, heart rate—112 bpm, and respiratory rate—22 bpm. His laboratory values are as follows, hemoglobin—8.2 g/dL, white blood counts—4,100 cells/mm³, platelets—76,000 cells/µL, serum creatinine—2.1 mg/dL, serum bilirubin—2.8 g/dL, INR—1.6, and serum sodium—134 mmol/L. Choose the correct response.
   a. The patient is having disseminated intravascular coagulation (DIC) needing aggressive blood products and anticoagulation.
   b. Disseminated intravascular coagulation is common in patients with sepsis and the key to the diagnosis is evidence of at least one vessel thrombosis and overt bleeding simultaneously.
   c. The diagnosis of sepsis-induced coagulopathy (SIC) is based on the SOFA score along with platelet count and the INR.
   d. Antithrombin and heparin are avoided in patients with sepsis-induced coagulopathy.

Ans. c

Explanation: Disseminated intravascular coagulation is defined by scientific subcommittee (SSC) on DIC of the International Society on Thrombosis and Haemostasis (ISTH DIC-SSC) as "an acquired syndrome characterized by the intravascular activation of coagulation with loss of localization arising from different causes. It can originate from and cause damage to the microvasculature, which if sufficiently severe, can produce organ dysfunction." Recently, ISTH DIC-SSC proposed a simpler definition for sepsis-induced coagulopathy that depends only on Sepsis-3 definition [Sepsis-3—infection with organ dysfunction—Sequential Organ Failure Assessment (SOFA) score platelet count, and the international normalized ratio (INR)]. SIC is diagnosed when the score is >4. Antithrombin, thrombomodulin, and heparin are potential treatment strategies that are tried in patients with SIC/DIC.

Suggested Reading
  1. Iba T, Levi M, Levy JH. Sepsis-induced coagulopathy and disseminated intravascular coagulation. Semin Thromb Hemost. 2020;46(1):89-95.

Q.2. Choose the true statement regarding septic cardiomyopathy.
  a. Patients with septic cardiomyopathy will have predominant left ventricular systolic dysfunction which is reversible.
  b. Patients with hyperkinetic profiles will respond well to fluid administration and have better outcomes compared to hypokinetic profiles.
  c. The predominant mechanism proposed is the altered sensitivity of adrenergic receptors in the myocardium.
  d. Patients with septic cardiomyopathy with poor ejection fraction will have low intraventricular pressures.

Ans. d

Explanation: Patients with septic cardiomyopathy commonly present with left ventricular systolic dysfunction but it is known to cause biventricular dysfunction and it can involve diastolic function as well. The common profile is hypokinetic with a low ejection fraction. The patients with hyperkinetic profiles had poor outcomes since it may be an indicator of poor vasomotor tone and the ventricle may be contracting against less resistance. The mechanism of injury proposed was coronary artery involvement, altered adrenergic receptors, direct myocardial injury, etc., but later the evidence is more in favor of cytokine-related injury. The common feature of septic cardiomyopathy is low intraventricular pressures, varied spectrum, and severity of biventricular involvement. It is reversible usually within a week after clinical improvement.

Suggested Reading
  1. L'Heureux M, Sternberg M, Brath L, Turlington J, Kashiouris MG. Sepsis-Induced Cardiomyopathy: a Comprehensive Review. Curr Cardiol Rep. 2020;22(5):35.
  2. Vieillard-Baron A. Septic cardiomyopathy. Ann Intensive Care. 2011;1(1):6.

Q.3. All are true regarding Pk/Pd alterations in patients with septic shock, except.
  a. The volume of distribution (Vd) is increased for hydrophilic drugs in patients with septic shock.
  b. In patients with septic shock, oral absorption may be affected due to sepsis-related gastrointestinal dysfunction and shock.
  c. Lipophilic drugs do not need a dose change despite alteration in Vd during septic shock and critical illness.
  d. Hydrophilic antibiotics require a normal loading and maintenance dose in patients with septic shock with normal renal function.

Ans. d

Explanation: The patients with septic shock will have increased Vd due to capillary leak, fluid infusion, and low albumin concentration and this will increase Vd of hydrophilic drugs, e.g., beta-lactams, carbapenems, and aminoglycosides. So due to increased Vd, hydrophilic drugs may need higher loading and maintenance doses. The Vd is not affected for lipophilic drugs; the dose adjustment is needed only when there are abnormal renal and hepatic functions. Oral absorption is usually not affected unless there is associated gastrointestinal dysfunction or unstable shock.

Suggested Reading
1. Póvoa P, Moniz P, Pereira JG, Coelho L. Optimizing antimicrobial drug dosing in critically ill patients. Microorganisms. 2021;9(7):1401.

Q.4. A 30-year-old male is admitted to ICU with right leg necrotizing fasciitis, septic shock, and multiorgan dysfunction. Choose the appropriate choice regarding the choice of antimicrobials.
   a. Aggressive surgery after optimal antibiotics and hemodynamic stabilization is the key to a good outcome.
   b. Beta-lactams and carbapenems are preferred choices due to less volume of distribution, better intracellular penetration, and rapid administration.
   c. Choose broad-spectrum antibiotics that attain high blood levels and stay in the vascular compartment.
   d. Clindamycin may have added advantage of toxin neutralization in case of toxic shock syndromes.

Ans. d

Explanation: Necrotizing fasciitis is a rapidly spreading infection of soft tissues, commonly polymicrobial requires emergency surgery and appropriate antibiotics (gram-positive, gram-negative, and anaerobic with good tissue penetration) that are administered rapidly as soon as possible. Clindamycin is commonly added in such cases due to its broad-spectrum activity, and good tissue penetration and it can neutralize toxins, particularly in case of toxic shock syndromes. The patients with septic shock will have altered volume of distribution (Vd) due to capillary leak, fluid infusion, and low albumin concentration and this will increase Vd of hydrophilic drugs, e.g., beta-lactams, carbapenems, aminoglycosides, etc. So due to increased Vd, hydrophilic drugs may need higher loading and maintenance doses. It is logical to give longer infusion times for drugs that are time-dependent, but this may take time to complete, and action may not be quick. So, it is suggested to give a bolus of these drugs as the first dose.

Suggested Reading
1. BMJ Best Practice. (2022). Necrotising fasciitis. [online] Available from: https://bestpractice.bmj.com/topics/en-gb/3000241 [Last accessed June, 2023].

Q.5. Choose the false statement regarding augmented renal clearance in patients with septic shock.
   a. Commonly seen in patients with polytrauma and septic shock.
   b. Augmented renal clearance affects the hydrophilic drugs that need higher dosages in patients with septic shock.
   c. High cardiac output with high renal blood flow and low systemic vascular resistance contributes to ARC in patients with septic shock.
   d. It is diagnosed with increased urine output with normal serum creatinine with normal kidneys in ultrasonography.

Ans. d

Explanation: Augmented renal clearance (ARC) is diagnosed when there is a >10% increase in glomerular filtration rate (GFR) or GFR > 130–150 mL/min, but there is no standard definition. Ideally, we should measure the GFR either using serum creatinine or 24 hours of urine creatinine clearance to find the increase in GFR. But, more commonly for ease the urinary creatinine clearance that is measured 8th hourly is used to diagnose increased GFR. ARC happens when there is increased renal blood flow which is due to high cardiac output and low systemic vascular resistance in patients with sepsis. Due to increased GFR, hydrophilic drugs are excreted more needing higher maintenance dosages. So, to avoid less dosing, the dose of hydrophilic drugs should be increased, though there are no guides available for appropriate dosing. ARC scoring system and ARC in trauma intensive care (ARCTIC) score are proposed scoring system to find high-risk patients.

Suggested Reading
1. Chen IH, Nicolau DP. Augmented renal clearance and how to augment antibiotic dosing. Antibiotics (Basel). 2020;9(7):393.

Q.6. Choose the false statement regarding sepsis-associated encephalopathy.
   a. Sepsis-associated encephalopathy (SAE) occurs due to bacteremia and small vessel ischemia leading to microvascular damage which is reversible.
   b. The prevalence is more when there are more organ failures and bacteremia.
   c. The diagnosis is made by exclusion.
   d. Inflammation, ischemia, and disruption of blood-brain barrier are proposed mechanism.

Ans. a

Explanation: The brain plays a vital role in maintaining homeostasis of immune response by fine-tuning neuroendocrine systems like the sympathetic and parasympathetic nervous system and hypothalamic-pituitary-adrenal (HPA) axis, which help in immunomodulation. SAE happens when there is intractable immune-related neuroinflammation. Overtime, this may lead to persistent brain injury leading to cognitive impairment, peripheral nervous system involvement, and uncertain neurological recovery. Both immunosuppression and hyperactivity are possible due to neuromodulatory mechanisms. It may lead to a vicious cycle of inflammation, brain dysfunction, and further immune modulation. SAE can be diagnosed when there is an extracranial focus of sepsis with brain dysfunction. Common manifestations are altered consciousness, delirium, seizures, involuntary movements, focal deficits, and comatose state. Later, it may lead to cognitive impairment, dementia, anxiety, post-traumatic stress, etc. It is usually a diagnosis of exclusion, close differential diagnoses are neuroinfection, thrombotic thrombocytopenic purpura, hemolytic uremic syndrome, and antiphospholipid syndrome.

Suggested Reading
1. Chung HY, Wickel J, Brunkhorst FM, Geis C. Sepsis-Associated Encephalopathy: From Delirium to Dementia? J Clin Med. 2020;9(3):703.

2. Huang Y, Chen R, Jiang L, Li S, Xue Y. Basic research and clinical progress of sepsis-associated encephalopathy. J Intensive Med. 2021;1(2): 90-5.
3. Mazeraud A, Righy C, Bouchereau E, Benghanem S, Augusto Bozza F, Sharshar T. Septic-Associated Encephalopathy: a Comprehensive Review. Neurotherapeutics. 2020;17:392-403.

Q.7. In patients with sepsis-induced respiratory failure, it is better to use all the strategies given below, except:
 a. Use low oxygen targets rather than high oxygen targets in critically ill patients with sepsis.
 b. It is desirable to use high-flow nasal cannula (HFNC) rather noninvasive ventilation (NIV) in patients with sepsis-induced respiratory failure.
 c. It is good to use intermittent boluses of muscle relaxants rather than infusion.
 d. In patients with sepsis without acute respiratory distress syndrome (ARDS), it is suggested to use low tidal volume (TD) ventilation rather than normal tidal volume.

Ans. a

Explanation: It is good to use HFNC rather than NIV as the first choice in patients with sepsis and respiratory failure. Prolonged infusion of muscle relaxants may increase the risk of critical illness polymyopathy, so better to avoid and if required better to use intermittent bolus muscle relaxants. For all patients with sepsis, it is suggested to use low TV (sepsis with or without ARDS), and target plateau pressure (Pplat) 30 mm Hg. The evidence is more in favor of usual oxygen targets, especially in patients with septic shock and low oxygen targets are still not proven superior, pending more evidence.

Suggested Reading
1. Evans L, Rhodes A, Alhazzani W, Antonelli M, Coopersmith CM, French C, et al. Surviving sepsis campaign: international guidelines for management of sepsis and septic shock 2021. Intensive Care Med. 2021;47:1181-247.

Q.8. Choose the true statement regarding the management of patients with sepsis.
 a. Quick SOFA (qSOFA) is a good screening tool to identify sepsis early.
 b. Clinical evaluation along with procalcitonin is useful to start antimicrobials in patients with sepsis.
 c. It is better to use more than one antimicrobial with gram-negative coverage in high-risk patients with suspected sepsis with multidrug-resistant organisms.
 d. Beta-lactam antibiotics are effective when given as prolonged infusion and initial loading bolus dose is not required to rapidly achieve the desired concentration.

Ans. c

Explanation: Administration of a loading dose of antibiotic before prolonged infusion is essential to avoid delays in achieving effective beta-lactam concentrations. For adults with sepsis or septic shock, it is suggested using a prolonged infusion of beta-lactams for maintenance (after an initial bolus) over a conventional bolus infusion. Procalcitonin should be used to initiate the antimicrobials but rather can be used as a guide to stop antimicrobials. It is suggested to use more than one gram-negative cover antimicrobials when you suspect multidrug-resistant organisms.

Suggested Reading
1. Evans L, Rhodes A, Alhazzani W, Antonelli M, Coopersmith CM, French C, et al. Surviving sepsis campaign: international guidelines for management of sepsis and septic shock 2021. Intensive Care Med. 2021;47:1181-247.

Q.9. Choose the correct statement regarding drug resistance of antimicrobials.
a. Extremely drug resistance (XDR) is defined as when the microbes are resistant to all antimicrobials agents in a given class of antimicrobials.
b. Difficult-to-treat resistance is defined as when the microbe is resistant to all agents in beta-lactams, carbapenems, and fluoroquinolones.
c. Drug synergy is not useful when the microbe is resistant to individual agents.
d. Multidrug resistance is defined as when the microbe is not susceptible to one or more agents in all antimicrobial classes.

Ans. b

Explanation: Drug resistance is defined as the acquired nonsusceptibility of microbes to previous susceptible antimicrobials. Drug resistance is defined when the microbe is *nonsusceptible* to:
- ≥1 agent in ≥3 antimicrobial categories as MDR
- ≥1 agent in all but ≤2 categories as XDR
- All antimicrobial agents listed as PDR
- Difficult-to-treat resistance (DTR) as a treatment-limiting resistance to all first-line agents including all beta-lactams, carbapenems, and fluoroquinolones.

When there is a synergy, the combination of drugs will be active against the bacteria when it is resistant to individual agents, e.g., combination of ceftazidime-avibactam and aztreonam has synergistic action pseudomonas.

Suggested Reading
1. Kadri SS, Adjemian J, Lai YL, Spaulding AB, Ricotta E, Prevots DR, et al.; National Institutes of Health Antimicrobial Resistance Outcomes Research Initiative (NIH-ARORI). Difficult-to-Treat Resistance in Gram-negative Bacteremia at 173 US Hospitals: Retrospective Cohort Analysis of Prevalence, Predictors, and Outcome of Resistance to All First-line Agents. Clin Infect Dis. 2018;67(12):1803-14.
2. Magiorakos AP, Srinivasan A, Carey RB, Carmeli Y, Falagas ME, Giske CG, et al. Multidrug-resistant, extensively drug-resistant and pandrug-resistant bacteria: an international expert proposal for interim standard definitions for acquired resistance. Clin Microbiol Infect. 2012;18(3):268-81.

Q.10. A 32-year-old female was admitted to the hospital with a pelvic fracture after polytrauma. She was shifted to ICU after 10 days of hospital stay with urosepsis, septic shock, and breathlessness. She was empirically started on injection meropenem 1 g 8th hourly and injection vancomycin 1 g 12th hourly. She improved after 72 hours of ICU care, but she remained afebrile, off vasopressors. The urine culture grew extended spectrum beta-lactamase (ESBL) *Escherichia coli* sensitivity to amikacin, gentamycin, meropenem, and colistin. Choose the appropriate intervention.
a. Procalcitonin levels should be sent to help in the de-escalation of antibiotic therapy.
b. Antibiotics should be changed to amikacin and stop vancomycin.

c. Continue meropenem as the patient is clinically responding and stop vancomycin.
d. De-escalate to amikacin but continue vancomycin pending other cultures.

Ans. b

Explanation: The antibiotics should be de-escalated whenever there is clinical improvement and culture reports are available to narrow the spectrum. Switching to a narrow spectrum, reducing the number of antibiotics, and stopping when it is not necessarily important. Procalcitonin values are not needed to de-escalate. It is important to consider whether the drug can penetrate the tissue of interest and less adverse effects before choosing from the list of narrow-spectrum drugs available.

Suggested Reading
1. De Waele JJ, Schouten J, Beovic B, , Tabah A, Leone M. Antimicrobial de-escalation as part of antimicrobial stewardship in intensive care: no simple answers to simple questions—a viewpoint of experts. Intensive Care Med . 2020;46(2):236-44. https://doi.org/10.1007/s00134-019-05871-z

Q.11. Which of the following statements is true?
1. Newborns have higher baseline levels of procalcitonin.
2. Procalcitonin levels do not change with dialysis.
3. Normal levels of procalcitonin rule out the presence of bacterial infection.
4. Procalcitonin levels peak faster than C-reactive protein (CRP) levels in response to bacterial infection.

a. 1, 2, and 3
b. 1 and 3
c. 2 and 4
d. 1 and 4

Ans. d

Explanation: Newborns have a higher baseline level of procalcitonin at birth. Procalcitonin levels reduce with dialysis by 21–83%. Procalcitonin levels can be normal when the infection is localized such as empyema or infective endocarditis. Procalcitonin levels peak at 24 hours whereas CRP levels peak at 36–50 hours.

Suggested Reading
1. Samsudin I, Vasikaran SD. Clinical utility and measurement of procalcitonin. Clin Biochem Rev. 2017;38(2):59-68.

Q.12. As per Surviving Sepsis Campaign Guidelines 2021, which of the following is not part of the 1-hour bundle?
a. Measure lactate level/remeasure lactate if initial value >2 mmol/L.
b. Administer broad-spectrum antibiotics.
c. Secure central venous access for administration of vasopressors.
d. Rapid administration of crystalloid 30 mL/kg in case of hypotension or lactate ≥4.

Ans. c

Explanation: Securing central venous access is not part of the 1-hour bundle. Vasopressors can be initiated within the first hour through a peripheral cannula proximal to the antecubital vein if the mean arterial pressure (MAP) target of 65 mm Hg has not been achieved with initial fluid resuscitation.

Suggested Reading
1. Lehman KD. Update: Surviving sepsis campaign recommends hour-1 bundle use. Nurse Pract. 2019;44(4):10.

Q.13. A 66-year-old female, diabetic and hypertensive for 30 years, presented to a primary care hospital with a 3-day history of fever followed by a 2-day history of multiple episodes of loose stools and 1-day history of decreased urine output and altered sensorium. On examination in emergency room (ER), she was found to have temperature 101°F, heart rate (HR): 132 beats/min, blood pressure (BP): 94/56 mm Hg, and respiratory rate (RR): 32 breaths/min which was rapid and shallow, oxygen saturation (SpO_2): 90% on room air, peripheries were warm, Glasgow coma scale (GCS): E2V3M4. Abdominal examination revealed tenderness over the left flank. Catheterization revealed no urine output. How can fluids be titrated during initial resuscitation in this patient based on clinical parameters in the absence of point-of-care ultrasound or blood gas analysis?
   a. An initial bolus of 30 mL/kg is sufficient as the patient appears to be in septic shock.
   b. Urine output can serve as a good guide to titrate resuscitation. Fluid boluses of 500 mL can be given till urine output of at least 0.5 mL/kg is achieved.
   c. Targeting heart rate < 100 beats/min and MAP of 65 mm Hg can serve as a guide for initial fluid resuscitation.
   d. After an initial bolus of 20–30 mL/kg, resuscitation can be guided using smaller fluid boluses, by a combination of clinical parameters like skin mottling score, and capillary refill time (CRT) for initial stabilization.

Ans. d

Explanation: In the absence of more advanced equipment, skin mottling scores, skin temperature gradients, and capillary refill time can be used to titrate fluids. Urine output may not be reliable in the presence of acute kidney injury and acute tubular necrosis or preexisting kidney disease. Heart rate may be affected by multiple factors and no targets have been described.

Suggested Reading
1. Evans L, Rhodes A, Alhazzani W, Antonelli M, Coopersmith CM, French C, et al. Surviving sepsis campaign: international guidelines for management of sepsis and septic shock 2021. Intensive Care Med. 2021;47(11):1181-247.
2. Misango D, Pattnaik R, Baker T, Dünser MW, Dondorp AM, Schultz MJ, et al. Haemodynamic assessment and support in sepsis and septic shock in resource-limited settings. Trans R Soc Trop Med Hyg. 2017;111(11):483-9.

Q.14. Which of the following is true with respect to vasopressors/inotropes in septic shock?
   a. Dopamine is an effective vasopressor used in septic shock.
   b. Vasopressin should be initiated after norepinephrine levels exceed 0.25–0.5 µg/kg/min.
   c. Levosimendan is recommended in the presence of sepsis-induced cardiac dysfunction.
   d. Terlipressin can be used as part of second-line treatment in septic shock.

Ans. b

Explanation: As per Surviving Sepsis Campaign Guidelines 2021, vasopressin can be added instead of escalating the dose of norepinephrine if MAP attained is inadequate. Neither terlipressin nor dobutamine is second-line therapy. Levosimendan is not recommended in the treatment of septic shock.

Suggested Reading
1. Evans L, Rhodes A, Alhazzani W, Antonelli M, Coopersmith CM, French C, et al. Surviving sepsis campaign: international guidelines for management of sepsis and septic shock 2021. Intensive Care Med. 2021;47(11):1181-247.

Q.15. A 45-year-old male presented with a 4-day history of fever, a 2-day history of rash over the chest, and 1-day history of excess fatigue. At presentation, he was found to have HR: 122 beats/min, BP: 80 systolic mm Hg, RR: 24 breaths/min, and SpO_2: 98% on room air. Peripheries were warm and CRT >4 seconds. Arterial blood gas (ABG) done showed pH 7.22, partial pressure of carbon dioxide (pCO_2): 34 mm Hg, HCO_3: 17.7 mmol/L, and Lac: 7.5 mmol/L. An initial bolus of 30 mL/kg was given and noradrenaline was started at 0.1 µg/kg/min. Broad-spectrum antibiotics were given after sending a blood culture. After 2 hours, his HR: 126 beats/min, invasive blood pressure, MAP: 66 mm Hg on noradrenaline at 0.12 µg/kg/min, and lactates: 6. He developed worsening breathing difficulty and saturation reduced to 86% requiring oxygen at 5 L/min via face mask. Ultrasound showed bilateral B lines with irregular pleura in axillary and infra-axillary areas. The anterior lung still showed an A profile. ECHO done showed hypercontractile left ventricle. What will your next step be?
a. Initiation of NIV and 40 mg IV frusemide to treat the pulmonary edema.
b. As lactates are persistently high, 30 mL/kg of fluid bolus should be repeated and lactates should be checked again after 2 hours.
c. Initiation of advanced hemodynamic monitoring
d. Initiation of IV steroid, thiamine, and high-dose vitamin C

Ans. c

Explanation: This patient has persistently high lactates despite initial fluids. However, a drop in oxygen saturation and the development of B lines with irregular pleura may indicate that he is developing extrapulmonary ARDS. Invasive cardiac output monitoring is useful in such patients as it helps to assess fluid responsiveness and titrate fluids using parameters like extravascular lung water, thus limiting over-resuscitation. Apart from this, an ongoing attempt at source control is imperative. NIV and frusemide form the mainstay of treatment in cardiogenic pulmonary edema, and not in noncardiogenic pulmonary edema, as is the case in this scenario. A second bolus of 30 mL/kg may be detrimental to the patient as it appears the patient is already beginning to develop hypoxia due to ARDS. There is no evidence supporting the use of steroid, thiamine, and vitamin C.

Suggested Reading
1. Evans L, Rhodes A, Alhazzani W, Antonelli M, Coopersmith CM, French C, et al. Surviving sepsis campaign: international guidelines for management of sepsis and septic shock 2021. Intensive Care Med. 2021;47(11):1181-247.

Q.16. **Which of the following pharmacologic agents is recommended in septic shock?**
   a. Hydrocortisone with fludrocortisone
   b. Intravenous immunoglobulin (IVIG)
   c. Hydrocortisone alone
   d. Ulinastatin

Ans. c

Explanation: Hydrocortisone has been recommended for the treatment of septic shock if norepinephrine/epinephrine are at > 0.25 µg/kg/min for at least 4 hours. Other forms of immunomodulation have not been recommended in septic shock. Fludrocortisone is not routinely used although previous studies have used it along with hydrocortisone.

Suggested Reading
   1. Evans L, Rhodes A, Alhazzani W, Antonelli M, Coopersmith CM, French C, et al. Surviving sepsis campaign: international guidelines for management of sepsis and septic shock 2021. Intensive Care Med. 2021;47(11):1181-247.

Q.17. **A 38-year-old female, with no comorbidities, presented with right lower limb cellulitis following trauma to right foot 3 days back. She was drowsy, tachycardic, and hypotensive. Her serum lactate 4.5 mmol/L and central venous oxygen saturation ($ScVO_2$) was 76%. Lactate levels remained around 4 mmol/L and the $ScVO_2$ level was 77% after fluid therapy after 4 hours and she continued to require noradrenaline at 0.2 µg/kg/min. What could this signify?**
   a. Sepsis-related mitochondrial dysfunction resulting in cytopathic dysoxia
   b. Improvement in tissue perfusion since the time of admission
   c. The presence of anemic dysoxia indicates the need for blood transfusion.
   d. The patient is suffering from cardiogenic shock and not septic shock.

Ans. a

Explanation: Mitochondrial dysfunction results in cytopathic hypoxia due to decreased oxygen extraction at the tissue level. The oxygen utilization is affected at the mitochondrial level, so $ScVO_2$ either normal or high may not guide to monitor the therapy. Only when the $ScVO_2$ is low, it serves as a marker of tissue hypoxia. Lactates can be high in patients with sepsis and mitochondrial dysfunction.

Suggested Reading
   1. Ltaief Z, Schneider AG, Liaudet L. Pathophysiology and clinical implications of the veno-arterial PCO_2 gap. Crit Care. 2021;25(1):318.

Q.18. **A 40-year male patient was admitted with community-acquired pneumonia, septic shock, and multiorgan failure. He is mechanically ventilated with fraction of inspired oxygen (FiO_2) of 50% and positive end-expiratory pressure of 8 cmH$_2$O. He had received 1.5 L of fluids from admission and his heart rate is 114 beats/min, invasive mean arterial pressure is 68 mm Hg, noradrenaline is 0.3 µg/kg/min, and**

serum lactate is 2.8 mmol/L. In the scenario given previously, what would be the next step to guide patient management?
a. Repeat fluid bolus and then reassess lactate after 2 hours.
b. Measurement of Pv-aCO_2 gap to determine the status of tissue perfusion.
c. Measure central venous pressure (CVP) to guide further fluid requirement and achieve target CVP 12 cmH_2O.
d. Use of colloids for resuscitation as the shock is persistent.

Ans. b

Explanation: Measurement of ScVO_2 and Pv-aCO_2 gap is a part of the basic hemodynamic assessment in a patient with circulatory failure. The high pCO_2 gap indicates that the improvement in cardiac output will be beneficial and is a marker of tissue perfusion. CVP target is not routinely used nowadays and it is recommended not to use CVP as a target of fluid resuscitation. Crystalloids are always preferred over colloids except in special situations, albumin can be administered in patients with septic shock.

Suggested Reading
1. Evans L, Rhodes A, Alhazzani W, Antonelli M, Coopersmith CM, French C, et al. Surviving sepsis campaign: international guidelines for management of sepsis and septic shock 2021. Intensive Care Med. 2021;47(11):1181-247.
2. Ltaief Z, Schneider AG, Liaudet L. Pathophysiology and clinical implications of the venoarterial PCO_2 gap. Crit Care. 2021;25(1):318.

Q.19. With regard to recommendations made by the Surviving Sepsis Guidelines regarding antibiotic therapy in sepsis, which of the following is not true?
a. In patients with septic shock, antibiotics should be given for at least a duration of 2–3 weeks.
b. Reassessment for antibiotic de-escalation is recommended to be done every 48–72 hours.
c. CRP can serve as an appropriate marker to stop antibiotic therapy.
d. Daily reassessment for antibiotic de-escalation has been suggested.

Ans. d

Explanation: It has been suggested that shorter duration of antibiotics is preferable over a longer duration once adequate source control has been achieved. Procalcitonin and clinical examination can aid in de-escalation and stopping therapy. Daily reassessment for de-escalation has been suggested.

Suggested Reading
1. Evans L, Rhodes A, Alhazzani W, Antonelli M, Coopersmith CM, French C, et al. Surviving sepsis campaign: international guidelines for management of sepsis and septic shock 2021. Intensive Care Med. 2021;47(11):1181-247.

Q.20. A 45-year-old patient, a known diabetic, presented with left-sided pyelonephritis with obstructive left hydroureteronephrosis. The patient was started on broad-spectrum antibiotics and left DJ stenting was done. Postprocedure patient was shifted to ICU with temperature 100°F, HR: 140/min, BP: 90/50 mm Hg on noradrenaline at 0.05 µg/kg/min, and SpO_2: 96% with the patient on volume control

mode, FiO$_2$: 50%, PEEP: 8 cmH$_2$O, RR: 26 breaths/min, tidal volume: 420 mL, ABG: pH 7.25, PaCO$_2$: 28 mm Hg, PaO$_2$: 85 mm Hg, HCO$_3$: 12 mEq/L, lactate: 4 mmol/L, serum creatinine: 2.2 mg/dL, and CRP: 42 mg/L. Patient has been producing 5 mL/h of urine for last 12 hours. What is the next best course of actions?
   a. Initiate RRT in form of CVVHDF or SLED
   b. Start bicarbonate infusion to treat acidosis
   c. Initiate polymyxin B hemoperfusion to treat cytokine storm
   d. Initiate IVIG to counter sepsis and cytokine storm

Ans. a

Explanation: As the patient's urine output has been <0.5 mL/kg/h for >6 hours in the presence of severe metabolic acidosis, initiation of RRT is indicated. Bicarbonate therapy is not indicated for pH > 7.2. Polymyxin B hemoperfusion and IVIG have not shown any mortality benefit and are presently not recommended as part of sepsis management.

Suggested Reading
   1. Evans L, Rhodes A, Alhazzani W, Antonelli M, Coopersmith CM, French C, et al. Surviving sepsis campaign: international guidelines for management of sepsis and septic shock 2021. Intensive Care Med. 2021;47(11):1181-247.
   2. Hellman T, Uusalo P, Järvisalo MJ. Renal replacement techniques in septic shock. Int J Mol Sci. 2021;22(19):10238.

Q.21. The concept of "antibiotic timeout" is best described by which statement?
   a. De-escalation of antibiotics
   b. Reassessing the need for continuation of empirical antibiotics after a duration of 48–72 hours postcommencement
   c. Discontinuation of antibiotics after a fixed period of time
   d. Choosing the best frequency of dosing of antibiotics based on pharmacokinetic parameters.

Ans. b

Explanation: An antibiotic timeout is a provider-led reassessment of the continuing need and choice of antibiotics when the clinical picture is clearer and more diagnostic information, especially results of cultures and rapid diagnostics, is available. Antibiotic timeouts are different from prospective audits and feedback because the providers, not the stewardship team, are doing the reviews.

Suggested Reading
   1. Centers for Disease Control and Prevention. (2021). Core elements of hospital antibiotic stewardship programs. [online] Available from: https://www.cdc.gov/antibiotic-use/core-elements/hospital.html [Last accessed June, 2023].

Q.22. The AWaRe classification of antimicrobials as per World Health Organization (WHO) classifies them on the basis of:
   a. Cost in each country
   b. Levels of antimicrobial resistance

c. Mechanism of action
d. Antibiotic consumption across countries

Ans. b

Explanation: The AWaRe classification of antibiotics was developed in 2017 by the WHO Expert Committee on Selection and Use of Essential Medicines as a tool to support antibiotic stewardship efforts at local, national, and global levels. Antibiotics are classified into three groups: (1) access, (2) watch, and (3) reserve, taking into account the impact of different antibiotics and antibiotic classes on antimicrobial resistance, to emphasize the importance of their appropriate use.

Suggested Reading
1. WHO. (2021). 2021 AWaRe classification. [online] Available from: https://www.who.int/publications/i/item/2021-aware-classification [Last accessed June, 2023].

Q.23. Which of the following is true about colistin?
a. Preferred over polymyxin B for urinary tract infections
b. Belongs to the "Watch" category of antimicrobials as per WHO AWaRe classification
c. Bacteriostatic antibiotic
d. Active against gram-negative and anaerobic infections

Ans. a

Explanation: Colistin (polymyxin E) or polymyxin B are antibiotics used to treat multidrug-resistant (MDR) gram-negative bacteria (GNB), particularly *Escherichia coli*, *Klebsiella pneumoniae, Pseudomonas aeruginosa,* and *Acinetobacter baumannii*. It has no activity against gram-positive and anaerobic organisms. It is classified under the reserve category of antibiotics as per the WHO AwaRe classification. It is bactericidal in high concentrations. The colistin gets converted to the active form in urine and hence has high urinary concentrations compared to polymyxin-B.

Suggested Reading
1. Ahmed MAEG, Zhong LL, Shen C, Yang Y, Doi Y, Tian GB. Colistin and its role in the era of antibiotic resistance: an extended review (2000–2019). Emerg Microbes Infect. 2020;9(1):868-5.
2. Nation RL, Velkov T, Li J. Colistin and polymyxin B: Peas in a pod, or chalk and cheese? Clin Infect Dis. 2014;59(1):88-94.
3. WHO. (2021). 2021 AWaRe classification. [online] Available from: https://www.who.int/publications/i/item/2021-aware-classification [Last accessed June, 2023].

Q.24. A 60-year-old rice farmer, on treatment for psoriasis, is admitted with high-grade fever on and off, upper abdominal pain, and right knee pain, gradually increasing over 14 days. He is admitted to the ICU. He is febrile, hemodynamically stable, and appears confused. Blood culture is sent and the initial Gram stain report suggests the presence of a gram-negative bacillus with bipolar staining and a characteristic "safety pin" appearance. His course in the ICU is complicated by acute kidney injury and septic shock. What is the treatment of choice?

a. Penicillins
b. Amikacin
c. Meropenem
d. Linezolid

Ans. c

Explanation: Clinical diagnosis of melioidosis, caused by the gram-negative organism *Burkholderia pseudomallei*, which exhibits a bipolar staining giving a classical safety pin appearance on Gram staining.

Melioidosis is transmitted to humans through direct skin contact with contaminated soil or water. The patient in question is a farmer, with history of psoriasis which made him likely to have breaks in skin barrier.

Melioidosis can be categorized as an acute or localized infection, acute pulmonary infection, acute bloodstream infection, or disseminated infection. Subclinical infections are also possible. Disseminated melioidosis presents with abscess formation in various organs of the body, and may be associated with sepsis. Organs involved include the liver, lung, spleen, and prostate; involvement of joints, bones, viscera, lymph nodes, skin, or brain may also occur. Disseminated infection is seen in acute or chronic melioidosis. Signs and symptoms, in addition to fever, include weight loss, stomach or chest pain, muscle or joint pain, and headache or seizure. The treatment of choice includes ceftazidime or meropenem IV for 2 weeks followed by treatment with cotrimoxazole [trimethoprim/sulfamethoxazole (TMP SMZ)] for at least 3 months.

Suggested Reading
1. Wiersinga W, Virk H, Torres A, Currie BJ, Peacock SJ, Dance DAB, et al. Melioidosis. Nat Rev Dis Primers. 2018;4:17107.

Q.25. All the following antimicrobials exhibit concentration-dependent (Cmax/MIC) pharmacokinetics, except:
a. Colistin
b. Linezolid
c. Fluoroquinolones
d. Aminoglycosides

Ans. b

Explanation: Linezolid follows time-dependent pharmacokinetics. For antibiotics that are time-dependent in their effect, the concentration should at least be above the MIC for >50% of the time. The optimal target for Cmax-dependent antibiotics is usually recommended to be 8–10 times above the minimum inhibitory concentration (MIC) (Cmax/MIC = 8–10).

Suggested Reading
1. Roger C, Roberts JA, Muller L. Clinical pharmacokinetics and pharmacodynamics of oxazolidinones. Clin Pharmacokinet. 2018;57:559-75.

Q.26. Choose the correct statement regarding minimum inhibitory concentrations (MIC) and clinical breakpoints.
a. Both MIC and breakpoint concentrations are determined by Clinical and Laboratory Standards Institute (CLSI) or European Committee on Antimicrobial Susceptibility Testing (EUCAST).

b. An organism is considered susceptible to an antibiotic if the MIC is less than the breakpoint concentration.
c. Breakpoints vary from patient to patient for the same organisms and type of sample.
d. MIC is defined as the chosen concentration of an antibiotic which defines whether bacteria are susceptible or resistant to an antibiotic.

Ans. b

Explanation: MIC is the lowest concentration of an antibacterial agent expressed in mg/L (μg/mL) which, under strictly controlled in vitro conditions, completely prevents visible growth of the test strain of an organism.

Minimal inhibitory concentration (MIC) defines in vitro levels of susceptibility or resistance of specific bacterial strains to applied antibiotic. MIC are usually determined by both dilution and disk diffusion (Kirby–Bauer testing) methods.

Breakpoints is defined as the chosen concentration of an antibiotic which defines whether bacteria are susceptible or resistant to an antibiotic.

Clinical breakpoints are currently set and published primarily by two organizations in the world: The European EUCAST (European Committee on Antimicrobial Susceptibility Testing) and the American CLSI (Clinical and Laboratory Standards Institute), and partly by the FDA (Food and Drug Administration).

Clinical breakpoints are standardized for a specific organism and each antibiotic tested for that organism, not for an individual patient.

A MIC less than the determined clinical breakpoint for that organism is reported susceptible, while a MIC higher than the breakpoint is reported as resistant.

Suggested Reading
1. Kowalska-Krochmal B, Dudek-Wicher R. The minimum inhibitory concentration of antibiotics: Methods, interpretation, clinical relevance. Pathogens. 2021;10(2):165.

Q.27. All the following are important interventions used by antimicrobial stewards to optimize antimicrobial use, except:
a. Prospective audit and feedback
b. Preauthorization
c. Following facility-specific treatment guidelines
d. Identifying the ideal duration for all antimicrobials

Ans. d

Explanation: Prospective audit and feedback (sometimes called postprescription review) and preauthorization are the two most effective antibiotic stewardship interventions in hospitals.

Prospective audit and feedback is an external review of antibiotic therapy by an expert in antibiotic use, accompanied by suggestions to optimize use, at some point after the agent has been prescribed.

Preauthorization requires prescribers to gain approval prior to the use of certain antibiotics. This can help to optimize initial empiric therapy because it allows for expert input on antibiotic selection and dosing, which can be lifesaving in serious infections, like sepsis. It can also prevent unnecessary initiation of antibiotics. Facility-specific treatment guidelines are also considered a priority because they can greatly enhance the effectiveness of both prospective audit and feedback and preauthorization by establishing clear recommendations for optimal antibiotic use at the hospital. These guidelines can optimize antibiotic selection and duration, particularly for common indications for antibiotic use such as community-acquired pneumonia, urinary tract infection, intra-abdominal infection, skin and soft tissue infection, and surgical prophylaxis.

While an optimal duration of antimicrobials is 5–7 days, however, the duration can vary depending on various factors such as host factors, nature of pathogen, site of infection, etc.

Suggested Reading
1. Centers for Disease Control and Prevention. (2021). Core Elements of Hospital Antibiotic Stewardship Programs. [online] Available from: https://www.cdc.gov/antibiotic-use/core-elements/hospital.html [Last accessed June, 2023].

Q.28. Which of the following does not define de-escalation of antimicrobials?
a. Switching from empirical broad spectrum to narrow-spectrum antimicrobials once culture report is available.
b. Change broad spectrum to narrow-spectrum antibiotic if patient is improving clinically and cultures are negative.
c. Changing from intravenous to oral preparations.
d. Reducing one antimicrobial if many empirical broad-spectrum antimicrobials were initiated.

Ans. c

Explanation: Changing from IV to oral preparations is called an oral switch and does not indicate de-escalation of the antibiotic.

Suggested Reading
1. Cyriac JM, James E. Switch over from intravenous to oral therapy: a concise overview. J Pharmacol Pharmacother. 2014;5(2):83-7.
2. Masterton RG. Antibiotic de-escalation. Crit Care Clin. 2011;27(1):149-62.

Q.29. Choose the correct statement with respect to the pharmacokinetics of antimicrobials.
a. Beta-lactams should be given dosed once a day for the best action.
b. Augmented renal clearance is typically seen in patients with chronic kidney disease patients.
c. Therapeutic drug monitoring is needed for patients on vancomycin treatment.
d. Linezolid has poor oral bioavailability.

Ans. c

Explanation: Beta-lactams follow time-dependent pharmacokinetics. Hence, they are dosed more frequently and given as prolonged infusions to maintain the free plasma concentration above the minimum inhibitory concentration levels. Linezolid has an excellent oral bioavailability.

Augmented renal clearance (ARC) is the pathologic phenomenon wherein the kidneys display increased filtering activity beyond that expected under normal physiological conditions of renal function. Patients in this state have a creatinine clearance of > 130 mL/min/1.73 m^2.

Suggested Reading
1. He N, Su S, Ye Z, Du G, He B, Li D, et al. Evidence-based guideline for therapeutic drug monitoring of vancomycin: 2020 Update by the Division of Therapeutic Drug Monitoring, Chinese Pharmacological Society. Clin Infect Dis. 2020;71(Suppl 4):S363-S371.
2. Luo Y, Wang Y, Ma Y, Wang P, Zhong J, Chu Y. Augmented renal clearance: What have we known and what will we do? Front Pharmacol. 2021;12:723731.

Q.30 **Choose the most correct statement regarding *Clostridium difficile* (*C. difficile*) diarrhea.**
a. Fidaxomicin is recommended as first-line treatment for first episode of nonsevere *C. difficile* infections (CDI).
b. The recommended dose of oral vancomycin in 500 mg BD for 10–14 days.
c. There is no role of fecal microbiota transplantation for refractory *C. difficile* infection.
d. Intravenous vancomycin is the treatment of choice for severe *C. difficile* infections.

Ans. a

Explanation: As per the recent Infectious Diseases Society of America and Society for Healthcare Epidemiology of America (IDSA/SHEA) update, fidaxomicin has been recommended as first-line treatment for initial episode of nonsevere CDI. Oral vancomycin is given in a dose of 125 mg QID.

Oral vancomycin plus intravenous metrogyl is recommended for treatment of severe CDI.

Fetal microbiota transplant is recommended for recurrent episodes of CDI, refractory to medical treatment.

Suggested Reading
1. Johnson S, Lavergne V, Skinner AM, Gonzales-Luna AJ, Garey KW, Kelly CP, et al. Clinical Practice Guideline by the Infectious Diseases Society of America (IDSA) and Society for Healthcare Epidemiology of America (SHEA): 2021 Focused Update Guidelines on Management of Clostridioides difficile Infection in Adults. Clin Infect Dis. 2021;73(5):e1029-44.

CHAPTER 23

Neuromonitoring

Vasudha Singhal

Q.1. Intracranial pressure (ICP) monitoring is indicated in all of the following scenarios of traumatic brain injury, except:
   a. Glasgow coma scale (GCS) <8
   b. Computed tomography (CT) head showing bilateral frontotemporal contusions
   c. Male patient with a normal CT with bilateral motor posturing
   d. A 42-year-old comatose patient with a normal CT with systolic blood pressure (BP) <90 mm Hg

Ans. c

Explanation: As per the brain trauma foundation guidelines for the management of severe traumatic brain injury (level II recommendations), ICP monitoring is indicated in patients with a GCS <8 with an abnormal CT head, and if a normal CT head—with at least two of these: Age >40 years, unilateral or bilateral posturing, or systolic BP <90 mm Hg.

Suggested Reading
   1. Brain Trauma Foundation; American Association of Neurological Surgeons; Congress of Neurological Surgeons; Joint Section on Neurotrauma and Critical Care, AANS/CNS; Bratton SL, Chestnut RM, Ghajar J, McConnell Hammond FF, Harris OA, Hartl R, et al. Guidelines for the management of severe traumatic brain injury. VI. Indications for intracranial pressure monitoring. J Neurotrauma. 2007;24 (Suppl 1):S37-44.

Q.2. In the Fourth Edition of the Brain Trauma Foundation (BTF) guidelines for the management of severe traumatic brain injury (TBI), the ICP threshold for treatment has been described as:
   a. 22 mm Hg
   b. 20 mm Hg
   c. 25 mm Hg
   d. 16 mm Hg

Ans. a

Explanation: As per the latest BTF guidelines, it is recommended to treat ICP values >22 mm Hg, as studies have shown that values above this level best predict an increased mortality and morbidity (level IIb evidence). Furthermore, the guidelines say that management decisions should be based on a combination of ICP values, and clinical and imaging findings.

Suggested Reading
1. Carney N, Totten AM, O'reilly C, Ullman JS, Hawryluk GWJ, Bell MJ, et al. Guidelines for the management of severe traumatic brain injury. Neurosurgery. 2017;80(1):6-15.
2. Sorrentino E, Diedler J, Kasprowicz M, Budohoski KP, Haubrich C, Smielewski P, et al. Critical thresholds for cerebrovascular reactivity after traumatic brain injury. Neurocrit Care. 2012;16(2):258-66

Q.3. All of the following are cerebral blood flow (CBF) monitoring techniques, except:
a. Positron emission tomography (PET)
b. Thermal diffusion flowmetry
c. CT angiography
d. Transcranial Doppler

Ans. c

Explanation: Thermal diffusion flowmetry is considered the gold standard technique to measure the cerebral blood flow. It provides continuous and invasive bedside monitoring of local CBF, though the findings may be sensitive to ambient light and temperature. PET is a minimally invasive technique to measure the regional CBF, but is expensive and hence used as a research tool only, rather than a clinical tool. Transcranial Doppler (TCD) is a noninvasive technique that can be used to measure the cerebral blood flow at the patient's bedside. It, however, provides only a relative index of CBF.

Computed tomography perfusion (CTP), and not CT angiography, is the modality to estimate the cerebral blood flow, most commonly used in acute ischemic stroke, where CTP is a part of the imaging protocol to assess for the eligibility for endovascular thrombectomy, using the ratio of the ischemic core and penumbra.

Suggested Reading
1. Fantini S, Sassaroli A, Tgavalekos KT, Kornbluth J. Cerebral blood flow and autoregulation: current measurement techniques and prospects for noninvasive optical methods. Neurophotonics. 2016;3(3):031411.
2. Yang MT. Multimodal neurocritical monitoring. Biomed J. 2020;43(3):226-30.

Q.4. Which component of the ICP waveform most reliably predicts a poor brain compliance and intracranial hypertension?
a. P1 (percussion wave)
b. P2 (tidal wave)
c. P3 (dicrotic wave)
d. Lundberg C waves

Ans. b

Explanation: The pulse component of the ICP waveform consists of three peaks: (1) P1 (percussion wave) due to arterial pulsation; (2) P2 (tidal wave) representing brain compliance; and (3) P3 (dicrotic wave) owing to aortic valve closure. As the brain compliance decreases with a rising ICP, the amplitude of the ICP waveform increases, and the P2 component rises beyond the P1 and P3 resulting in the rounding of the waveform. Lundberg A waves are pathological waves, also called the plateau waves, where the ICP rises to high levels for a period of 5-10 minutes, and are indicative of a poor prognosis. Lundberg B and C waves may be seen in normal individuals.

Suggested Reading
1. Abraham M, Singhal V. Intracranial pressure monitoring. J Neuroanaesthesiol Crit Care. 2015;2:193-203.

Q.5. Intraventricular catheters are considered the gold standard for ICP monitoring. All of the following may be true for intraventricular ICP monitoring, except:
 a. Intraventricular catheters measure the global ICP.
 b. It allows for therapeutic drainage of CSF in cases of a raised ICP.
 c. Insertion in a young patient with traumatic brain injury is easier.
 d. It can be rezeroed after placement to minimize drift.

Ans. c

Explanation: Intracranial pressure (ICP) and cerebral perfusion pressure (CPP) monitoring are recommended as a part of protocol-driven care in patients who are at a risk of elevated intracranial pressure based on clinical or imaging features. While both parenchymal ICP monitors and intraventricular catheters (also known as external ventricular drainage or EVD) provide reliable and accurate data for ICP measurement, the intraventricular catheter system is considered the gold standard modality. EVD gives the most accurate assessment of global ICP; can be recalibrated after placement to minimize measurement drift; is cost effective; and allows therapeutic CSF drainage in cases of a raised ICP. It may, however, be difficult to insert in young patients with TBI, presenting with slit-like or displaced ventricles due to cerebral edema post injury.

Suggested Reading
1. Brain Trauma Foundation, American Association of Neurological Surgeons, Congress of Neurological Surgeons; Bratton SL, Chestnut RM, Ghajar J, Hammond FFM, Harris OA, Hartl R, et al. Guidelines for the management of severe traumatic brain injury. VII. Intracranial pressure monitoring technology. J Neurotrauma. 2007;24(supplement 1):S45-S54.
2. Le Roux P, Menon DK, Citerio G, Vespa P, Bader MK, Brophy G, et al. The international Multidisciplinary Consensus Conference on Multimodality Monitoring in Neurocritical Care—a list of recommendations and additional conclusions: A statement for healthcare professionals from the Neurocritical Care Society and the European Society of Intensive Care Medicine. Neurocrit Care. 2014;21(Suppl 2):S282-96.

Q.6. All of the following are noninvasive methods of ICP monitoring, except:
 a. Camino's monitor
 b. Pupillometry
 c. Optic nerve sheath diameter (ONSD)
 d. MRI brain

Ans. a

Explanation: Although the intraventricular catheter remains the gold standard for monitoring ICP, several noninvasive modalities can be used in scenarios where invasive monitoring is not feasible (nonavailability of neurosurgeon) or is contraindicated (patients with coagulopathy). Clinical examination and imaging modalities such as CT and MRI brain remain the time-tested noninvasive methods of monitoring a raised ICP. The sonographic optic nerve sheath diameter (measuring the changes in the diameter of the nerve sheath surrounding the optic nerve) and pupillometry (using a handheld infrared device to quantitatively assess pupillary function) detect steady changes in ICP, and are used commonly for screening purposes in patients susceptible to intracranial hypertension.

Camino's monitor is an invasive intraparenchymal ICP monitoring device based on fiberoptic technology.

Suggested Reading
1. Robba C, Bacigaluppi S, Cardim D, Donnelly J, Bertuccio A, Czosnyka M. Noninvasive assessment of intracranial pressure. Acta Neurol Scand. 2016;134(1):4-21.
2. Khan MN, Shallwani H, Khan MU, Shamim MS. Noninvasive monitoring intracranial pressure: a review of available modalities. Surg Neurol Int. 2017;8:51.

Q.7. Which of the following is true regarding the pressure reactivity index (PRx)?
   a. Pressure reactivity measures the correlation between cerebral perfusion pressure and ICP waves.
   b. Pressure reactivity is represented on a scale as a correlation coefficient (from +1.0 to −1.0).
   c. A positive value suggests intact autoregulation whereas a negative PRx value suggests impaired autoregulation.
   d. Mortality has shown to be higher when the PRx value is <0.25.

Ans. b

Explanation: Pressure reactivity index is a tool to monitor the cerebral autoregulation in response to blood pressure changes. It is a secondary index derived from the relative changes in mean arterial pressure (MAP) and intracranial pressure (ICP). It can be determined as a moving correlation coefficient between MAP and ICP, and is represented on a scale from +1.0 to −1.0. It is used as a surrogate marker of cerebrovascular impairment after TBI—a negative PRx value suggests intact autoregulation, whereas a positive value suggests impaired autoregulation. The PRx shows significant deterioration in patients with refractory intracranial hypertension, and a PRx > 0.35 is associated with a high mortality rate (>50%).

Suggested Reading
1. Tasneem N, Samaniego EA, Pieper C, Leira EC, Adams HP, Hasan D, et al. Brain multimodality monitoring: a new tool in neurocritical care of comatose patients. Critical Care Res Prac. 2017;2017:6097265
2. Zweifel C, Lavinio A, Steiner LA, Radolovich D, Smielewski P, Timofeev I, et al. Continuous monitoring of cerebrovascular pressure reactivity in patients with head injury. Neurosurg Focus. 2008;25(4):E2.

Q.8. Hyperventilation should be avoided during the first 24 hours after acute traumatic brain injury, when the cerebral blood flow (CBF) is reduced critically. Controlled

hyperventilation may, however, be used as a lifesaving temporizing measure in severe intracranial hypertension as a tier-II therapy, with the concomitant use of which advanced multimodal monitoring?
  a. Cerebral microdialysis
  b. Quantitative electroencephalogram (qEEG)
  c. Brain tissue oxygenation ($PbtO_2$)
  d. Pupillometry

Ans. c

Explanation: Controlled hyperventilation is effective in reducing ICP, but is associated with a reduction in CBF resulting in serious cerebral and systemic side effects. As such, guidelines suggest that we should maintain normal $PaCO_2$ values in the early phase after TBI, if the ICP is within acceptable limits. Controlled hyperventilation (i.e., $PaCO_2$ around 33–36 mm Hg and never below 30 mm Hg) should be used as a temporary lifesaving intervention in cases of severe intracranial hypertension and imminent herniation, as a tier-II measure after the failure of increased sedation and hyperosmolar therapy, as a bridge toward additional interventions such as a repeat CT and surgery. $PaCO_2$ levels should be adjusted and individualized in each patient using invasive neuromonitoring in the form of jugular venous oxygen saturation ($SjvO_2$) or $PbtO_2$ to monitor oxygen delivery to the injured brain.

Suggested Reading
  1. Carney N, Totten AM, O'reilly C, Ullman JS, Hawryluk GWJ, Bell MJ, et al. Guidelines for the management of severe traumatic brain injury. Neurosurgery. 2017;80(1):6-15.
  2. Gouvea Bogossian E, Peluso L, Creteur J, Taccone FS. Hyperventilation in adult TBI patients: how to approach it? Front Neurol. 2021;11:580859.

Q.9. A 30-year-old male presented to the emergency department (ED) with traumatic brain injury. His CT scan revealed bifrontal contusions. A decision to insert an intraparenchymal ICP monitor was taken. All of the following are true about intraparenchymal ICP monitors, except:
  a. Intraparenchymal monitors are inaccurate as compared to the gold standard intraventricular monitors.
  b. Measure localized pressure and may not be reflective of global intracranial pressures.
  c. Therapeutic CSF drainage is not possible.
  d. May be subject to drift if used for long periods.

Ans. a

Explanation: Intraparenchymal ICP monitors are nonfluid-coupled monitoring devices which may be based on the fiberoptic technology (Camino ICP monitor) or the Strain Gauge Principle (Codman MicroSensor with an implanted microchip transducer). These devices are accurate and a close correlation is seen between the ICP values measured by them and intraventricular monitors. Their recordings are independent of patient positioning, and a repetitive rezeroing is not needed after disconnection for transport, etc. However, they measure only localized pressure around the point of insertion, and may not be reflective of global intracranial pressures. Since the catheters are placed in the brain parenchyma, therapeutic CSF drainage for lowering the ICP is not an option. They may be subject to a gradual drift over a period of time.

Suggested Reading
1. Abraham M, Singhal V. Intracranial pressure monitoring. J Neuroanaesthesiol Crit Care. 2015;2:193-203.
2. Koskinen LO, Olivecrona M. Clinical experience with the intraparenchymal intracranial pressure monitoring Codman Microsensor system. Neurosurgery. 2005;56:693-8.

Q.10. The four components of the Full Outline of UnResponsiveness (FOUR) score used in the clinical monitoring of comatose patients are:
a. Eye response, motor response, brainstem reflexes, respiratory pattern
b. Eye response, motor response, verbal response, brainstem reflexes
c. Eye response, motor response, verbal response, respiratory pattern
d. Eye response, motor response, verbal response, pupillary response

Ans. a

Explanation: The Full Outline of UnResponsiveness (FOUR) score is a simple, easy to use, and comprehensive scale used in the assessment of patients with an altered sensorium. It contains four components, each with a maximal score of 4. It takes into consideration the brainstem reflexes and the respiratory pattern assessment, besides the eye response and motor response that were conventionally measured in the Glasgow coma scale (GCS). The FOUR score has been validated for use in a variety of critical care settings, including the assessment of nonstructural brain injuries and also brain death.

Suggested Reading
1. Iyer VN, Mandrekar JN, Danielson RD, Zubkov AY, Elmer JL, Wijdicks EF. Validity of the FOUR score coma scale in the medical intensive care unit. Mayo Clin Proc. 2009;84(8):694-701.
2. Wijdicks EF, Bamlet WR, Maramattom BV, Manno EM, McClelland RL. Validation of a new coma scale: the FOUR score. Ann Neurol. 2005;58(4):585-93.

Q.11. All are true regarding the Neurological Pupillary Index (NPi) derived from an automated pupillometry assessment, except:
a. Classification of pupil reactivity according to the NPi eliminates ambiguity in clinical pupillary measurements.
b. Pupillary variables such as size, latency, constriction velocity, and dilation velocity are the parameters used to derive the NPi.
c. An NPi score >3 denotes an abnormal pupillary response.
d. The use of NPi from a pupillometer provides a rapid and noninvasive method for the screening and triage of patients with suspected intracranial hypertension.

Ans. c

Explanation: The pupillometer is an infrared handheld, automated device used to analyze the pupillary dynamics over a 3-second-time period. It helps in minimizing the possible interobserver variability in the pupillary evaluation of brain-injured patients, and aids in the detection of brain herniation in its early stages, before pupillary dilatation becomes apparent. The Neurological Pupillary Index (NPi) is derived from pupillary variables such as size, latency, constriction velocity, and dilation velocity, which are standardized to fall on a scale between 0 and 5. An NPi score ≥3 is indicative of a normal pupillary response, whereas a score of <3 denotes an abnormal pupillary light reflex associated with an increased ICP. An NPi difference of >0.7 between the two eyes correlates well with intracranial hypertension. Pupillometry has emerged as a rapid noninvasive screening method of ICP measurement, and may help to guide neuroprotective and neurosurgical interventions in patients with a rising ICP trend.

Suggested Reading
1. Chen JW, Gombart ZJ, Rogers S, Gardiner SK, Cecil S, Bullock RM. Pupillary reactivity as an early indicator of increased intracranial pressure: the introduction of the Neurological Pupil index. Surg Neurol Int. 2011;2:82.
2. Couret D, Boumaza D, Grisotto C, Triglia T, Pellegrini L, Ocquidant P, et al. Reliability of standard pupillometry practice in neurocritical care: an observational, double-blinded study. Crit Care. 2016;20:99.

Q.12. A 45-year-old male patient with traumatic brain injury is admitted to the ICU with right frontotemporal contusions. Besides clinical monitoring and serial CT scans to monitor the brain, the attending intensivist is also performing serial optic nerve sheath diameter (ONSD) assessments using sonography, every 8 hours. Which of the following findings should raise an alarm to the attending intensivist for a neurosurgical consult?
   a. Mean binocular ONSD 4.2 mm
   b. Mean binocular ONSD 3.6 mm
   c. Mean binocular ONSD 5.0 mm
   d. Mean binocular ONSD 6.2 mm

Ans. d

Explanation: The use of ultrasonography (USG) in measuring ONSD is useful in detecting a raised ICP, and has the advantage of being a noninvasive, portable, bedside, and easily repeatable method of ICP measurement, without the risk of radiation exposure. ONSD is measured 3 cm behind the globe in each eye, and a cutoff value of >5 is considered abnormal, indicating an elevated ICP. ONSD shows a linear increment up to 7.5 mm, after which it plateaus off.

Suggested Reading
1. Chen L, Wang L, Hu Y, Jiang HH, Wang YZ, Xing YQ. Ultrasonic measurement of optic nerve sheath diameter: a non-invasive surrogate approach for dynamic, real-time evaluation of intracranial pressure. Br J Ophthalmol. 2019;103:437-41.
2. Shirodkar CG, Rao SM, Mutkule DP, Harde YR, Venkategowda PM, Mahesh MU. Optic nerve sheath diameter as a marker for evaluation and prognostication of intracranial pressure in Indian patients: an observational study. Indian J Crit Care Med. 2014;18(11):728-34.

Q.13. The normal brain tissue oxygenation ($PbtO_2$) levels are:
   a. 23–35 mm Hg
   b. 16–21 mm Hg
   c. 35–50 mm Hg
   d. 8–12 mm Hg

Ans. a

Explanation: The normal PbtO$_2$ as measured by the intraparenchymal oxygen sensors (Licox®) ranges between 23 and 35 mm Hg (though this depends on the probe depth of the PbtO$_2$ sensor, being less in deeper brain regions). PbtO$_2$ values <20 mm Hg are considered abnormal and are associated with cerebral ischemia.

Suggested Reading
1. Pennings FA, Schuurman PR, van den Munckhof P, Bouma GJ. Brain tissue oxygen pressure monitoring in awake patients during functional neurosurgery: the assessment of normal values. J Neurotrauma. 2008;25(10):1173-7.

Q.14. The gold standard technique to measure cerebral oxygenation is:
  a. Intraparenchymal oxygen sensor (Licox®)
  b. Positron emission tomography (PET)
  c. Jugular venous oximetry (SjvO$_2$)
  d. MR spectroscopy

Ans. b

Explanation: Brain tissue oxygenation (PbtO2) is a combination of cerebral arteriovenous oxygen tension difference, cerebral blood flow, and tissue oxygen extraction. Intraparenchymal oxygen sensors (Licox®), inserted in the subcortical white matter, are often used to monitor regional brain tissue oxygen tension. Global brain oxygenation can be measured using SjvO$_2$, and a value of ≤ 55% is recognized as the ischemic threshold requiring intervention. Magnetic resonance spectroscopy (MRS) is noninvasive and measures brain metabolites and biomarkers following acute brain injury. Clinically, the preferred choice for brain oxygenation monitoring is the intraparenchymal PbtO$_2$ monitor (Licox®), but the gold standard technique for measuring cerebral oxygenation is positron emission tomography (PET) using radiolabeled water (^{15}O-water). PET allows the quantitative measurement of CBF, along with a precise information on the cerebral oxygen metabolism and oxygen extraction fraction, thereby giving reliable results about major aspects of cerebral physiology.

Suggested Reading
1. Frontera J, Ziai W, O'Phelan K, Leroux PD, Kirkpatrick PJ, Diringer MN. Regional brain monitoring in the neurocritical care unit. Neurocritical Care. 2015;22:348-59.

Q.15. Which of the following statements about NIRS (near-infrared spectroscopy) monitoring technique is true?
  a. It is a noninvasive monitoring modality that provides real-time information about global cerebral oxygenation and CBF.
  b. It involves placement of optodes over the forehead to measure signals over the temporal lobe and the watershed zone of the middle and posterior cerebral arteries.
  c. The normal range of rSO$_2$ as measured by the NIRS is 35-55%.
  d. It is prone to inaccurate readings in the setting of postoperative pneumocephalus, scalp edema or lacerations, and frontal contusions.

Ans. d

Explanation: Near-infrared spectroscopy (NIRS) is a noninvasive monitoring modality that provides real-time information about regional cerebral oxygenation and CBF. It calculates the concentration of a chromophore (oxygenated hemoglobin in brain injury patients) based upon attenuation of light between the light source and receiver. It involves the placement of optodes over the forehead to measure signals over the frontal lobe gray matter and watershed zone of the anterior and middle cerebral arteries. The normal range of rSO_2 as measured by the NIRS is 55–80%. NIRS requires a close spatial relationship between the cortex and cranium, and is prone to inaccurate readings in the setting of postoperative pneumocephalus, scalp edema or lacerations, and frontal contusions, which are all common in the neurological intensive care unit (ICU). Moreover, it is only sensitive for changes in and around the frontal region where the optodes are placed, and is unable to detect distant ischemic events.

Suggested Reading
1. Mahajan C, Rath GP, Bithal PK. Advances in neuro-monitoring. Anesth Essays Res. 2013;7(3):312-8.
2. Oddo M, Villa F, Citerio G. Brain multimodality monitoring: an update. Curr Opin Crit Care. 2012;18(2):111-8.
3. Wartenberg KE, Schmidt JM, Mayer SA. Multimodality monitoring in neurocritical care. Crit Care Clin. 2007;23(3):507-38.

Q.16. Near-infrared spectroscopy (NIRS) is used to assess cerebral oxygenation in all of the following clinical settings, except:
   a. Coronary artery bypass grafting (CABG)
   b. Arthroscopic elbow surgery
   c. Carotid endarterectomy
   d. Traumatic brain injury

Ans. b

Explanation: Near-infrared spectroscopy is a noninvasive method based on chromophore absorption of infrared light, used for the continuous monitoring of tissue oxygenation in a wide variety of clinical settings. During cardiac surgery such as CABG or carotid endarterectomy, measuring brain tissue oxygenation may help to detect tissue hypoxia during bypass, thereby preventing postoperative complications such as postoperative cognitive dysfunction, stroke, and prolonged hospital stay. NIRS may be used in shoulder arthroscopic procedures performed in the beach-chair position, to detect cerebral desaturation provoked by postural hypotension, head and neck manipulation, or thromboembolic events. In TBI, NIRS is useful in the identification of episodes of impaired cerebral oxygenation, monitoring the cerebrovascular autoregulation, and detection of increased ICP.

Suggested Reading
1. Barud M, Dabrowski W, Siwicka-Gieroba D, Robba C, Bielacz M, Badenes R. Usefulness of Cerebral Oximetry in TBI by NIRS. J Clinl Med. 2021;10(13):2938.
2. Scheeren TW, Schober P, Schwarte LA. Monitoring tissue oxygenation by near infrared spectroscopy (NIRS): Background and current applications. J Clin Monit Comput. 2012;26(4):279-87.

Q.17. Jugular venous oxygen saturation ($SjvO_2$) measures the balance between cerebral oxygen consumption and delivery. Which of the following will lead to a fall in $SjvO_2$ necessitating intervention?
   a. Hypercapnia
   b. Hypothermia
   c. Seizures
   d. Hypertension

Ans. c

Explanation: Jugular venous oxygen saturation is a monitor of global cerebral oxygenation. It reflects the relative balance between the oxygen delivery to the brain and the oxygen consumption by the brain, provided that the arterial hemoglobin saturation and concentration remain stable. Any disturbance that increases cerebral oxygen consumption (e.g., fever, seizures, etc.) or decreases cerebral oxygen delivery (e.g., hypoxia, hypotension, hypocarbia, anemia, and increased ICP) may decrease $SjvO_2$. Normal $SjvO_2$ levels are 60–75%. Desaturation to <50% suggests ischemia, while $SjvO_2$ above 75% indicates hyperemia or infarcted tissue.

Suggested Reading
1. Robertson CS, Gopinath SP, Goodman JC, Contant CF, Valadka AB, Narayan RK. $SjvO_2$ monitoring in head-injured patients. J Neurotrauma. 1995;12(5):891-6.
2. Wartenberg KE, Schmidt JM, Mayer SA. Multimodality monitoring in neurocritical care. Crit Care Clin. 2007;23(3):507-38.

Q.18. Which of the following statements about $SjvO_2$ monitoring is true?
   a. Intraoperative lactate oxygen index (LOI) <0.03 during aneurysm clipping in SAH has been associated with a poor outcome.
   b. The left jugular bulb is mostly cannulated for $SjvO_2$ monitoring.
   c. The rate of aspiration for intermittent sampling of blood for monitoring should be >2 mL/min.
   d. It is of limited value in monitoring patients with infratentorial lesions.

Ans. d

Explanation: Jugular venous oximetry or $SjvO_2$ monitoring is one of the oldest modalities to monitor cerebral oxygenation. It has classically been used to guide hyperventilation or blood pressure targeted management in patients with TBI or other intracranial pathologies. During intracranial aneurysm surgery, $SjvO_2$ monitoring has been used to determine the minimal blood pressure that should be maintained to avoid hypoperfusion, and also to measure lactate oxygen index (LOI) to help in prognostication. LOI is the ratio of venous-arterial difference in lactate/arteriojugular difference in oxygen. Its normal values are <0.03, and an intraoperative value >0.08 during aneurysm clipping surgery is associated with a poor outcome.

With regard to the side of monitoring, most clinicians prefer to cannulate the right jugular venous bulb, as it is usually dominant. While sampling, care must be taken to aspirate the blood at a rate of <2 mL/min in order to avoid extracranial contamination from the facial veins. Since the brainstem and cerebellum contribute very little to the venous outflow from the brain, $SjvO_2$ monitoring may be of a limited value in monitoring patients with infratentorial lesions or injury.

Suggested Reading
1. Artru F, Dailler F, Burel E, Bodonian C, Grousson S, Convert J, et al. Assessment of jugular blood oxygen and lactate indices for detection of cerebral ischemia and prognosis. J Neurosurg Anesthesiol. 2004;16(3):226-31.
2. Bhardwaj A, Bhagat H, Grover VK. Jugular venous oximetry. J Neuroanaesthesiol Crit Care. 2015;2:225-31.

Q.19. Which of the following major vessels in the circle of Willis cannot be insonated through the transtemporal window of the transcranial doppler (TCD)?
   a. Basilar artery
   b. Posterior cerebral artery (PCA)
   c. Anterior cerebral artery (ACA)
   d. Middle cerebral artery (MCA)

Ans. a

Explanation: The transcranial Doppler (TCD) is a noninvasive, bedside technique to monitor the cerebral blood flow velocity in the major vessels of the brain. A 2 MHz ultrasound probe is used to penetrate the skull acoustic windows, namely the transtemporal (above the zygomatic arch between tragus and the lateral eye canthus), suboccipital (gap between the occipital bone and the atlas vertebra), submandibular (through the submandibular area adjacent to the angle of mandible), and the transorbital (through the orbital plate) brain windows. The transtemporal window is the most common window used to insonate the major vessels of the circle of Willis, including the MCA, ACA, PCA, and the terminal ICA (internal carotid artery). Basilar and vertebral arteries are insonated through the suboccipital window. Identification of the cerebral arteries depends on the acoustic window, probe angle, insonation depth, and the blood flow direction (toward or away from the probe).

Suggested Reading
1. Bathala L, Mehndiratta MM, Sharma VK. Transcranial Doppler: technique and common findings (Part 1). Ann Indian Acad Neurol. 2013;16(2):174-9.
2. Nicoletto HA, Burkman MH. Transcranial Doppler series part II: performing a transcranial Doppler. Am J Electroneurodiagnostic Technol. 2009;49(1):14-27.

Q.20. Which of the following is true regarding the Lindegaard ratio (LR)?
   a. It is a ratio between the mean flow velocity of the middle cerebral artery and that of the intracranial internal carotid artery.
   b. Lindegaard ratio helps to distinguish between hyperemia or vasospasm as a cause of increased MCA mean flow velocities.
   c. LR >3 signifies hyperemia.
   d. LR <3 is reflective of vasospasm.

Ans. b

Explanation: The Lindegaard ratio (LR) is calculated from the mean flow velocities of the MCA and extracranial ICA, as measured on the TCD. It is the ratio between the mean flow velocity of the middle cerebral artery (MCA FV_m) and that of the extracranial internal carotid artery (EICA FV_m).

$$LR = MCA\ FV_m / EICA\ FV_m$$

Lindegaard ratio allows differentiation between vasospasm and hyperdynamic circulation as a cause of increased MCA mean flow velocities—LR >3 indicates vasospasm (mild vasospasm 3.0-4.5, moderate vasospasm 4.5-6.0, and severe vasospasm >6.0), whereas LR <3 indicates hyperdynamic circulation or hyperemia (in hyperemia, the FVm of both the MCA and ICA increase, resulting in a LR <3).

Suggested Reading
1. Bonow RH, Young CC, Bass DI, Moore A, Levitt MR. Transcranial Doppler ultrasonography in neurological surgery and neurocritical care. Neurosurg Focus. 2019;47(6):E2.
2. Lindegaard KF, Nornes H, Bakke SJ, Sorteberg W, Nakstad P. Cerebral vasospasm after subarachnoid haemorrhage investigated by means of transcranial Doppler ultrasound. Acta Neurochir Suppl (Wien). 1988;42:81-4.

Q.21. A 52-year-old female is admitted to the ICU with aneurysmal SAH. She undergoes coiling of the left MCA aneurysm on day 2 of her ictus. Her postoperative course was unremarkable and she was recovering well. On day 4 of her admission, she develops a right-sided hemiparesis. A bedside TCD was done to check for the MCA flow velocities on the left side. Which of the following would reflect a severe vasospasm in her left MCA territory?
a. MCA mean flow velocity (FVm) 80 cm/s
b. MCA FVm 150 cm/s
c. MCA FVm 190 cm/s
d. MCA FVm 220 cm/s

Ans. d

Explanation: Transcranial Doppler provides a noninvasive method for measuring the blood flow velocity (indirectly diameter) in the basal cerebral arteries, and therefore is a valuable screening tool in detecting large vessel vasospasm following subarachnoid hemorrhage. The normal mean velocity for the MCA is 62 ± 12 cm/s. Mean velocities of the MCA of 200 cm/s or greater indicate severe spasm and correlate with 50% or greater narrowing on angiogram. FVm <120 cm/s is unlikely to have a clinically significant spasm.

Suggested Reading
1. Mascia L, Fedorko L, ter Brugge K, Filippini C, Pizzio M, Ranieri VM, et al. The accuracy of transcranial Doppler to detect vasospasm in patients with aneurysmal subarachnoid hemorrhage. Intensive Care Med. 2003;29:1088-94.
2. Newell DW, Winn HR. Transcranial Doppler in cerebral vasospasm. Neurosurg Clin N Am. 1990;1(2):319-28.
3. Vora Y, Suarez-Almazor M, Steinke D, Martin M, Findlay JM. Role of transcranial Doppler monitoring in the diagnosis of cerebral vasospasm after subarachnoid hemorrhage. Neurosurgery. 1999;44:1237-48.

Q.22. Which of the following parameters on transcranial Doppler (TCD) best correlates with a rise in intracranial pressure?
a. Mean flow velocity (FVm)
b. Peak flow velocity
c. Lindegaard ratio
d. Pulsatility index

Ans. d

Explanation: Gosling's pulsatility index (PI) can be calculated by taking difference between the systolic and diastolic flow velocity and dividing this difference by the mean flow velocity in the middle cerebral artery. It is a numerical representation of the change in the pulsatile character of the cerebral blood vessel. It is dimensionless and independent of the angle of insonation of the vessel. It has been shown to strongly correlate with ICP in several studies—PI changes approximately 2.4% with each 1 mm Hg change in ICP. The normal PI in the middle cerebral artery (MCA) ranges between 0.6 and 1.0; an MCA PI >2.0 is suggestive of an ICP >20 mm Hg, thereby predicting a poor outcome.

Suggested Reading
1. Bellner J, Romner B, Reinstrup P, Kristiansson KA, Ryding E, Brandt L. Transcranial Doppler sonography pulsatility index (PI) reflects intracranial pressure (ICP). Surg Neurol. 2004;62:45-51.
2. Homburg AM, Jakobsen M, Enevoldsen E. Transcranial Doppler recordings in raised intracranial pressure. Acta Neurol Scand. 1993;87:488-93.
3. Moreno JA, Mesalles E, Gener J, Tomasa A, Ley A, Roca J, et al. Evaluating the outcome of severe head injury with transcranial Doppler ultrasonography. Neurosurg Focus. 2000;8(1):e8.

Q.23. Microembolic signals on TCD are defined by all of the following criteria, except:
 a. High intensity, amplitude >3 dB above background
 b. Typically bidirectional
 c. Transient character
 d. Audible as snaps or chirps

Ans. b

Explanation: Transcranial Doppler is a valuable modality in the evaluation of acute ischemic stroke when assessing for the risk of repeat ischemia due to embolic phenomena. The presence of microembolic signals can be used to stratify the risk for recurrent strokes in the setting of carotid stenosis, blunt cerebrovascular injury, as well as cardiac disease (atrial fibrillation, patent foramen ovale, myocardial infarction, etc.). Microembolic signals (MES) are high-intensity transient signals seen on the TCD, produced when microemboli pass through the insonated vessel. MES are characterized by transient (lasting <300 ms), high intensity (amplitude >3 dB above background), unidirectional blood flow signals occurring randomly in the cardiac cycle, which have a typical "snap" or "chirpy" or "whistling" sound on the audible output. Patients who have detectable MES, especially in larger number, should be considered as high-risk patients for stroke. The presence of microemboli also predicts a higher incidence of postoperative cognitive deficits in surgical patients, especially those who are undergoing carotid endarterectomy and coronary artery bypass grafting.

Suggested Reading
1. Vitt JR, Loper NE, Mainali S. Multimodal and autoregulation monitoring in the neurointensive care unit. Front Neurol. 2023;14:1155986.
2. Vuković-Cvetković V. Microembolus detection by transcranial Doppler sonography: review of the literature. Stroke Res Treat. 2012;2012382361.

Q.24. A 60-year-old male patient suffered from a cardiac arrest, from which he was revived. Post-CPR, targeted temperature management was initiated. After gradual rewarming of the patient, the in-house intensivist performed a bedside TCD in this patient, and the findings suggested a cerebral circulatory arrest. All of the following findings on TCD are suggestive of brain death, except:
  a. Oscillatory flow
  b. Systolic spikes
  c. Diastolic flow reversal
  d. Transient high intensity chirps

Ans. d

Explanation: Transcranial Doppler is the only validated noninvasive ancillary imaging modality used in brain death testing. It is 100% specific and 96% sensitive in the diagnosis of brain death. Oscillating or to-and-fro flow, with antegrade flow during systole and retrograde flow during diastole, is characteristic of cerebral circulatory arrest. This gradually progresses to small systolic spikes with no diastolic flow, a finding that correlates with the cessation of flow in the intracranial vessels on angiography. Transient high-intensity chirps are a hallmark finding in the detection of microembolic signals on the TCD.

Suggested Reading
1. Nicoletto HA, Burkman MH. Transcranial Doppler series part III: Interpretation. Am J Electroneurodiagnostic Technol. 2009;49:244-59.
2. Marda MK, Prabhakar H. Transcranial Doppler. J Neuroanaesthesiol Crit Care. 2015;2:215-20.

Q.25. All of the following methods are used to test cerebral autoregulation with a transcranial Doppler (TCD), except:
  a. Static autoregulation test by infusion phenylephrine
  b. Pressure reactivity index
  c. Transient hyperemic response test
  d. Dynamic autoregulation test by cuff inflation

Ans. b

Explanation: Cerebral autoregulation is a protective mechanism of brain to maintain a relatively constant CBF with respect to changes in CPP between 50 and 150 mm Hg. Static autoregulation is assessed by inducing steady changes in MAP/CPP with phenylephrine infusion and simultaneously measuring the flow velocity (FV); dynamic autoregulation is assessed by inducing continuous changes in MAP/CPP by inflating and deflating thigh cuff. The estimated cerebral vascular resistance (CVRe) is calculated by the formula, CVRe = mean blood pressure/FV. The transient hyperemic response is performed by compressing the common carotid artery for 5–8 seconds and observing the change in the FV after release. A transient increase in the FV occurs due to hyperemia, only when autoregulation is intact. Pressure reactivity index is a secondary index derived from the relative changes in mean arterial pressure (MAP) and intracranial pressure (ICP), not derived from the TCD.

Suggested Reading
1. Marda MK, Prabhakar H. Transcranial Doppler. J Neuroanaesthesiol Crit Care. 2015;2:215-20.

Q.26. **Out of the following cerebral microdialysis metabolites, which is the most reliable marker for anaerobic metabolism and brain ischemia?**
  a. Lactate pyruvate ratio
  b. Glutamate
  c. Lactate
  d. Glycerol

Ans. a

Explanation: Cerebral microdialysis (CMD) is used as a part of multimodal neuromonitoring (with ICP and $PbtO_2$) in order to guide individualized intensive care therapy in comatose patients to prevent secondary brain insults. In clinical practice, the CMD lactate pyruvate (L/P) ratio and glucose are used primarily to guide interventions, as they are the most reliable markers for anaerobic metabolism and brain ischemia. As for reference values, L/P ratio >25 is considered abnormal, while L/P ratio >40 is the critical level above which brain energy crisis is defined. The reference level for CMD glucose is 1 (±0.15) mmol/L. Glutamate is a marker of excitotoxicity, while glycerol is increased with destruction of cell membrane structure and free radical generation. It should, however, be remembered that the CMD biomarkers (generally sampled every hour and analyzed at the bedside) should always be interpreted in the context of the monitor location, type of injury, and the patient's clinical condition.

Suggested Reading
1. Carteron L, Bouzat P, Oddo M. Cerebral microdialysis monitoring to improve individualized neurointensive care therapy: an update of recent clinical data. Front Neurol. 2017;8:601.

Q.27. **A 46-year-old female, admitted to the ICU with subarachnoid hemorrhage (SAH), experiences a fall in the level of consciousness and a right-sided weakness on day 5 of the ictus. The intensivist applies a continuous EEG (cEEG) monitoring to see the underlying pathology, as a part of multimodal monitoring (besides TCD and cerebral oxygenation). Which of the following parameters suggest the presence of a delayed cerebral ischemia as a cause of neurological deterioration in this patient?**
  a. Increasing relative alpha-variability
  b. Depressed delta foci
  c. Alpha/delta ratio (ADR) <50%
  d. No epileptiform discharges

Ans. c

Explanation: Early detection of delayed cerebral ischemia (DCI) in patients of SAH is critical to allow for timely intervention. While clinical examination in awake patients is the most reliable way to detect and diagnose DCI, early detection may be notoriously difficult in comatose patients with poor grade SAH. Multiple advanced monitoring strategies in the form of TCD, cerebral blood flow monitoring, brain oxygenation, cEEG, and cerebral microdialysis have been described. cEEG accurately predicts DCI following SAH, and may help target therapies to patients at highest risk of secondary brain injury. Reductions in the alpha/delta ratio (ADR) or in alpha variability are most sensitive and specific for predicting DCI at a point where it is potentially reversible. Prominent delta foci and late appearing epileptiform discharges may be seen, along with worsening focal slowing.

Suggested Reading
1. Francoeur CL, Mayer SA. Management of delayed cerebral ischemia after subarachnoid hemorrhage. Crit Care. 2016;20:277.
2. Rosenthal ES, Biswal S, Zafar SF, O'Connor KL, Bechek S, Shenoy AV, et al. Continuous electroencephalography predicts delayed cerebral ischemia after subarachnoid hemorrhage: a prospective study of diagnostic accuracy. Ann Neurol. 2018;83(5):958-69.

Q.28. **All of the following are causes of increased cerebral blood flow velocity on TCD examination, except:**
a. Hyperdynamic circulation
b. Vasospasm
c. Sickle cell anemia
d. Intracranial hypertension

Ans. d

Explanation: An increase in the mean flow velocity (FVm) on the TCD is indicative of one of the two conditions—(1) either a decreased vessel diameter (as seen in vasospasm) or (2) an increased blood flow (as is seen in hyperdynamic circulation). In sickle cell anemia, the sickled red blood cells adhere to the vascular endothelium, leading to vascular occlusion and thus a reduced vessel diameter. FVm is therefore increased in this condition. In fact, a FVm of >200 cm/s in asymptomatic children is associated with a greater risk of stroke in sickle cell disease. Decreased FVm can be due to hypotension, decreased CBF, raised intracranial pressure (ICP), or brainstem death.

Suggested Reading
1. Marda MK, Prabhakar H. Transcranial Doppler. J Neuroanaesthesiol Crit Care. 2015;2:215-20.
2. Purkayastha S, Sorond F. Transcranial Doppler ultrasound: technique and application. Semin Neurol. 2012;32(4):411-20.

Q.29. **Quantitative electroencephalography (qEEG) may be a helpful tool in the diagnosis of all of the following medical conditions, except:**
a. Nonconvulsive seizures
b. Acute ischemic stroke
c. Early detection of delayed cerebral ischemia (DCI) in subarachnoid hemorrhage (SAH)
d. Thalamic injury in traumatic brain injury (TBI)

Ans. b

Explanation: Quantitative EEG (qEEG) is beneficial in analyzing raw EEG data of several hours and presenting the data of relevance in a simplified display. It may be helpful in diagnosing nonconvulsive seizures in comatose patients, which generally go unrecognized in the absence of explicit motor movements. Broad repetitive slow waves correlate with the occurrence of vasospasm in SAH—alpha/delta ratio, power, and percent alpha variability on the EEG are utilized for the detection of DCI in SAH. Thalamic injury in TBI patients is associated with an impaired percent alpha variability on qEEG and poor long-term outcomes. qEEG may not help in the diagnosis of acute ischemic stroke per se, and may only be useful if seizures are suspected.

Suggested Reading
1. Citerio G, Oddo M, Taccone FS. Recommendations for the use of Multimodal monitoring in the neurointensive care unit. Curr Opin Crit Care. 2015;21(2):113-9.
2. Stuart RM, Waziri A, Weintraub D, Schmidt MJ, Fernandez L, Helbok R, et al. Intracortical EEG for the detection of vasospasm in patients with poor-grade subarachnoid hemorrhage. Neurocrit Care. 2010;13(3):355-8.

Q.30. A 25-year-old male presented to the emergency department with a history of road traffic accident. His vitals are stable and his presenting GCS is E1V1M4. The NCCT head does not reveal any significant intracranial pathology. He is intubated and shifted to the ICU for further neuromonitoring in the form of Codman® intraparenchymal ICP and Licox® brain tissue oxygenation. The ICP and PbtO$_2$ show a high normal value at the time of insertion (ICP 22 of mm Hg; PbtO$_2$ of 21 mm Hg). Appropriate sedation, ventilation, and hyperosmolar therapy are initiated. On day 2, an MRI brain is performed which reveals a diffuse axonal injury in the brain. On return from the radiology suite, the patient starts to record an ICP of 26 mm Hg and a PbtO$_2$ of 14 mm Hg. What, according to you, is the least important measure in such a scenario?
 a. Increase sedation/analgesia, repeat a bolus of hypertonic saline.
 b. FiO$_2$ may not be increased as a raised PaO$_2$ has no significant effect on the brain oxygenation.
 c. Increase CPP to >70 mm Hg with fluid boluses, inotropes, and vasopressors.
 d. Consider secondary decompressive craniectomy options.

Ans. b

Explanation: The Seattle International Brain Injury Consensus Conference (SIBICC) (2020) came up with a management algorithm for adult patients with severe TBI, who had both ICP and brain oxygenation monitoring in place. In situations where both intracranial hypertension (ICP >22 mm Hg) and brain hypoxia (PbtO$_2$ <20 mm Hg) are present (as in this case), the consensus is to increase the sedation and analgesia to lower ICP and improve ventilation/PbtO$_2$; administer a repeat bolus of hyperosmolar therapy; ventilator management to increase PaO$_2$ as high as 150 mm Hg; increase CPP to >70 mm Hg with fluid boluses, inotropes, and vasopressors (if cerebral autoregulation intact); and consider secondary decompressive craniectomy options to bring down the ICP and improve cerebral oxygenation.

Suggested Reading
1. Chesnut R, Aguilera S, Buki A, Bulger E, Citerio G, Cooper DJ, et al. A management algorithm for adult patients with both brain oxygen and intracranial pressure monitoring: the Seattle International Severe Traumatic Brain Injury Consensus Conference (SIBICC). Intensive Care Med. 2020;46(5):919-29.

CHAPTER 24

Pharmacotherapeutics

Khalid Ismail Khatib

Q.1. The lipid profile of a patient who suffered from acute coronary syndrome is given below. What drug can be used to treat this condition?
- *Serum low-density lipoprotein:* 127 g/dL
- *Serum high-density lipoprotein:* 32 mg/dL
- *Serum triglycerides:* 278 mg/dL

a. Fenofibrate 160 mg
b. Rosuvastatin + fenofibrate
c. Rosuvastatin 10 mg
d. Atorvastatin 80 mg

Ans. d

Explanation: Atorvastatin 80 mg can be used to treat this condition. The first line of therapy in controlling cholesterol in patients with atherosclerotic cardiovascular disease (ASCVD) is starting a high-intensity statin. High-intensity statins include atorvastatin (40–80 mg) and rosuvastatin (20–40 mg).

Statins are competitive inhibitors of HMG-CoA reductase. This leads to a decrease in cholesterol biosynthesis. Statins are also effective in reducing LDL and triglyceride levels.

Other options:
- *Option a:* Fenofibrate reduces lipoprotein levels by interacting with peroxisome proliferator-activated receptor (PPAR-a) and stimulating lipoprotein lipase. They are used as drugs of choice for treating hyperlipoproteinemia and severe hypertriglyceridemia (>1,000 mg/dL).
- *Option b:* The combination of rosuvastatin and fenofibrate was previously used to reduce atherosclerotic cardiovascular disease risk. But recent studies have indicated no change in reduction and hence is not recommended anymore.
- *Option c:* Rosuvastatin 10 mg is a low-intensity statin and is mainly used for primary prevention against atherosclerotic cardiovascular disease.

Suggested Reading
1. Gurgle HE, Blumenthal DK. Drug therapy for dyslipidemias. In: Bruton LL (Ed). Goodman & Gillman's : The Pharmacological Basis of Therapeutics, 13th edition. McGraw Hill Medical Publishers. pp. 605-18.
2. Vale N, Nordmann AJ, Schwartz GG, de Lemos J, Colivicchi F, den Hartog F, et al. Statins for acute coronary syndrome. Cochrane Database Syst Rev. 2011;(6):CD006870.

Q.2. A 34-year-old woman with multisystem organ dysfunction (MODS) is recovering in the high-dependency unit after a stormy 6-week course. Her sedation and analgesia were stopped 24 hours ago (morphine and midazolam) after running continuously for 3 weeks. She is alert, orientated, and breathing spontaneously on oxygen. Over the next 6 hours, she becomes extremely anxious, agitated, and jittery. She subsequently has a grand mal seizure. What is the most likely reason that she has had a seizure?
  a. Cytokine release syndrome
  b. Benzodiazepine withdrawal syndrome
  c. Central nervous system dysfunction
  d. Hypoglycemia

Ans. b

Explanation: Benzodiazepine withdrawal syndrome is more common, occurs more rapidly and is more severe with short-acting agents such as midazolam rather than long-acting drugs such as diazepam. Withdrawal is more commonly associated with grand mal seizures and myoclonic jerks than with petit mal seizures.

The fit should be controlled with diazepam. Small doses of long-acting benzodiazepine which are progressively decreased will avoid the withdrawal syndrome.

Suggested Reading
1. Pétursson H. The benzodiazepine withdrawal syndrome. Addiction 1994;89(11):1455-9.

Q.3. You have admitted a man with severe ulcerative colitis who requires intubation for respiratory failure secondary to pneumonia. He has been treated with oral prednisolone 60 mg/day and you are asked to give him "equivalent intravenous (IV) steroid." What will you prescribe, and how much?
  a. Prednisolone 5 mg
  b. Methylprednisolone 4 mg
  c. Dexamethasone 0.75 mg
  d. Cortisone 25 mg

Ans. c

Explanation: Either hydrocortisone or dexamethasone is appropriate substitutions (prednisolone does not come in an intravenous preparation).

There is less tendency to sodium retention with dexamethasone and it is cheaper. Approximate equivalent doses and duration of action are as follows:

- Cortisone — 25 mg — 8–12 hours
- Hydrocortisone — 20 mg — 8–12 hours
- Prednisolone — 5 mg — 24 hours
- Methylprednisolone — 4 mg — 24 hours
- Dexamethasone — 0.75 mg — 36 hours

Suggested Reading
1. Buttgereit F, Da Silva JAP, Boers M, Burmester G, Cutolo M, Jacobs J, et al. Standardised nomenclature for glucocorticoid dosages and glucocorticoid treatment regimens: current questions and tentative answers in rheumatology. Ann Rheum Dis. 2002;61:718-22.

Q.4. A 23-year-old woman is admitted having taken a tricyclic overdose. She is hypotensive with a pulse rate of 116 beats/min and wide QRS complexes on the electrocardiogram. Her pH is 7.4 and HCO_3 is 12.8 on arterial blood gas (ABG) testing. What can be administered?
   a. 8.4% sodium bicarbonate
   b. Cyclophosphamide
   c. Calcium gluconate 10%
   d. $MgSO_4$ 1 g

Ans. a

Explanation: The toxicity of tricyclic drugs appears to be reduced in the presence of alkalemia. In an observational study of 91 patients with tricyclic overdose, hypotension resolved within 1 hour in 20 of 21 (96%) patients, QRS prolongation corrected in 39 of 49 (80%), and mental state improved in 40 of 85 (47%) following hypertonic sodium bicarbonate infusion. No complications associated with the administration of bicarbonate infusion were observed.

Suggested Reading
1. Hoffman JR, Votey SR, Bayer M, Silver L. Effect of hypertonic sodium bicarbonate in the treatment of moderate-to-severe cyclic antidepressant over-dose. Am J Emerg Med. 1993; 11(4): 336-41.
2. Khalid MM, Waseem M. Tricyclic Antidepressant Toxicity. [Updated 2022 Aug 7]. In: StatPearls [Internet]. Treasure Island (FL): StatPearls Publishing; 2023 Jan. Available from: https://www.ncbi.nlm.nih.gov/books/NBK430931/

Q.5. A patient with significant coronary artery disease has been admitted to ICU for postoperative monitoring following a colectomy. He becomes hypotensive following an epidural bolus. Despite being given fluid rapidly, he remains hypotensive after 5 minutes and is observed to have some ST segment depression on a V5 ECG trace. Choose the correct drug to be administered.
   a. Noradrenaline 0.05–0.1 µg/kg/min
   b. Dobutamine 5–10 µg/kg/min
   c. Milrinone 0.3–0.7 µg/kg/min
   d. Metaraminol 10 µg/kg/min

Ans. d

Explanation: Metaraminol (Aramine) comes as 10 mg in 1 mL. It needs diluting usually to 10 mL (1 mg/mL) and is then given 0.5–1 mL intravenously.

Do not give 10 mg as severe hypertension is likely to occur.

Suggested Reading
1. Grauslyte L, Bolding N, Phull M, Jovaisa T. The Use of Metaraminol as a Vasopressor in Critically Unwell Patients: A Narrative Review and a Survey of UK Practice. J Crit Care Med (Targu Mures). 2022;8(3):193-203.

Q.6. A 62-year-old male, who has been on dabigatran for pulmonary embolism, presented to the hospital with PR bleeding, presumably from diverticular disease of colon. You would like to reverse the anticoagulation due to the severity of bleeding. Which of the following products will reverse the effect of dabigatran?
   a. Aprotinin
   b. Vitamin K
   c. Idarucizumab
   d. Tranexamic acid

Ans. c

Explanation: Idarucizumab is a humanized antibody fragment that reversibly and with high affinity ties up dabigatran.

Suggested Reading
1. Pollack CV, Reilly PA, Eikelboom J, Glund S, Verhamme P, Bernstein RA, et al. Idarucizumab for Dabigatran Reversal. N Engl J Med. 2015;373:511-20.

Q.7 A 67-year-old man is hospitalized with acutely oliguria and hyperkalemia (K^+ 7.2 mEq/L). He has a history of hypertension, cardiac failure, peripheral vascular disease, and gout for which he is on medications. He is currently hypotensive (BP 65/40 mm Hg) and has poor skin turgor. Which of the following is not associated with acute kidney injury?
 a. Lisinopril
 b. Indomethacin
 c. Frusemide
 d. Cilnidipine

Ans. d

Explanation: In patients with poor renal perfusion (and consequently low glomerular filtration pressure) both nonsteroidal anti-inflammatory drugs (NSAIDs) and ACE inhibitors can provoke renal failure. Diuretics can result in intravascular volume depletion, and this compounds poor renal perfusion and the renal effects of the other drugs.

Under normal conditions, NSAIDs have relatively little effect on the kidney because of low renal production of prostaglandins. However, in the presence of renal hypoperfusion in which local synthesis, a vasodilator prostaglandin, is increased to protect the glomerular hemodynamics and to maintain appropriate renal tubular transport of fluid and electrolytes, inhibition of prostaglandin synthesis by NSAIDs can lead to vasoconstrictive acute renal failure. In the face of decreased glomerular filtration pressure, glomerular filtration becomes critically dependent on angiotensin II-mediated efferent vascular tone. Renal artery stenosis or severe depletion of circulating volume (e.g., acute diarrhea or diuretic therapy) predisposes patients treated with angiotensin-converting enzyme (ACE) inhibitors to develop acute renal failure (ARF).

Following withdrawal of either or both drugs, recovery of renal function can be anticipated even when a period of dialysis or hemofiltration is required.

Suggested Reading
1. Morimoto S, Yano Y, Maki K, Iwasaka T. Renal and vascular protective effects of cilnidipine in patients with essential hypertension. J Hypertens. 2007;25(10):2178-83.

Q.8. A 14-year-old boy was brought to the ER with recurrent seizures. His mother informs you that he is receiving isoniazid prophylaxis since 2 months as she was diagnosed with tuberculosis. ABG revealed a high-anion gap metabolic acidosis. What would be the mainstay of treatment?
 a. Benzodiazepines
 b. Barbiturates
 c. Pyridoxine
 d. Thiamine

Ans. c

Explanation: The given clinical scenario is suggestive of isoniazid overdose for which the mainstay of treatment is intravenous pyridoxine. Isoniazid overdose results in decreased pyridoxine availability to neurons. This decreases the levels of gamma-aminobutyric acid (GABA), which in turn lowers the seizure threshold. Benzodiazepines can be used to control seizures.

Prolonged treatment with isoniazid leads to the deficiency of pyridoxine which can lead to peripheral neuropathy and other neurological manifestations such as ataxia, paresthesia, and numbness.

Clinical triad of isoniazid overdose:
- Seizures refractory to treatment with phenytoin and barbiturates
- High anion gap metabolic acidosis (HAGMA) resistant to treatment with sodium bicarbonate
- Coma

Suggested Reading
1. Shannon MW, Lovejoy FH Jr. Isoniazid. In: Haddad LM, Winchester JF (Eds). Clinical Management of Poisoning and Drug Overdose, 2nd Edition. Philadelphia: Saunders, 1990; pp.970-5.

Q.9. A 50-year-old male patient presents with dyspnea, pedal edema, and congestive hepatomegaly. He is diagnosed with congestive heart failure. Which of the following is not prescribed to prevent progression and revert cardiac remodeling?
a. Beta-blocker
b. ACE inhibitor
c. Digoxin
d. Aldosterone antagonist

Ans. c

Explanation: Digoxin has no role in preventing cardiac remodeling. It increases cardiac contractility and is indicated for symptomatic management of congestive heart failure.

Drugs preventing ventricular remodeling:
- ACE inhibitors/angiotensin receptor blockers (ARBs)
- Beta-blockers
- Aldosterone antagonists (spironolactone and eplerenone)

The activation of renin-angiotensin-aldosterone system (RAAS) and the sympathetic nervous system leads to the remodeling and progressive left ventricular (LV) dysfunction. The RAAS activation is prevented by the ACE inhibitors/ARBs and the aldosterone antagonists (spironolactone), while the overactive sympathetic system is inhibited by the beta-blockers.

Suggested Reading
1. Sullebarger JT, D'Ambra PM, Clark LC, Thanikarry L, Fontanet HL. Effect of digoxin on ventricular remodeling and responsiveness of beta-adrenoceptors in chronic volume overload. J Cardiovasc Pharmacol Ther. 1998;3(4):281-90.

Q.10. A 70-year-old man is brought with complaints of severe chest pain. The ECG shows anterolateral-wall myocardial infarction and echocardiography shows an ejection fraction of 38%. Which of the following is the drug of choice for his condition?
a. Dopamine
b. Dobutamine
c. Epinephrine
d. Norepinephrine

Ans. b

Explanation: The given clinical scenario is suggestive of acute congestive heart failure with systolic dysfunction. Dobutamine is administered as it is the beta-adrenergic agonist of choice for managing this condition.

Dobutamine has a well-balanced action with stimulation of cardiac output. It causes less tachycardia than epinephrine and also has an added advantage of a decrease in pulmonary artery wedge pressure.

At doses that result in a positive inotropic effect, the beta-1 action on the myocardium predominates. In the vasculature, the alpha-1 effects are counterbalanced by beta-2 effects. The net result is an increase in stroke volume, augmented by a small decrease in systemic vascular resistance, thereby resulting in a decrease in afterload.

Suggested Reading
1. Macas A, Baksyte G, Pikciunas A, Semetaite A. Dobutamine in acute myocardial infarction: should we use it for reduction of pulmonary hypertension and pulmonary capillary wedge pressure in acute myocardial infarction? Crit Care. 2008;12(Suppl 2);P262.

Q.11. A 45-year-old woman with multiple sclerosis presents with an exacerbation of her symptoms. Which of the following drugs should be prescribed to her for initial management?
a. Glatiramer
b. Methylprednisolone
c. IFN-3-1a
d. Prednisolone

Ans. b

Explanation: Glucocorticoids are used in the clinical management of either first attacks or acute exacerbations.

Intravenous methylprednisolone administration at a dose of 500–1,000 mg/day for 3–5 days, followed by a course of oral prednisolone beginning at a dose of 60–80 mg/day and gradually tapered over 2 weeks is given.

These medications reduce the severity and shorten the duration of attacks. Disease-modifying therapies for relapsing forms of multiple sclerosis are:
- IFN-B-1a
- IFN-B-1b
- Glatiramer acetate
- Natalizumab
- Fingolimod
- Dimethyl fumarate
- Teriflunomide
- Mitoxantrone
- Alemtuzumab

Suggested Reading

1. Myhr KM, Mellgren SI. Corticosteroids in the treatment of multiple sclerosis. Acta Neurol Scand Suppl. 2009;(189):73-80.

Q.12. Which of the following drugs will you prescribe for a patient with an acute attack of neuromyelitis optica?

a. Rituximab
b. Mycophenolate mofetil
c. Glucocorticoids
d. Azathioprine

Ans. c

Explanation: Acute attacks of neuromyelitis optica are managed by high-dose glucocorticoids or plasma exchange. Drugs used for prophylaxis against relapses include:
- Mycophenolate mofetil
- Rituximab
- Glucocorticoids

Suggested Reading

1. Kimbrough DJ, Fujihara K, Jacob A, Lana-Peixoto MA, Leite MI, Levy M, et al; GJCF-CC&BR. Treatment of Neuromyelitis Optica: Review and Recommendations. Mult Scler Relat Disord. 2012;1(4):180-87.

Q.13. A 21-year-old female complains of fever, headache, and vomiting from the past 3 days. She has been living in a hostel for the last 3 weeks and presented in the ICU. On examination, she has neck stiffness and a maculopapular rash was noted over the trunk and extremities. Which of the following is false about the disease she is likely suffering from?

a. Carriers of this disease can be treated with rifampicin
b. It can lead to adrenal hemorrhage
c. Terminal complement deficiency increases the risk of this disease
d. Metronidazole is the drug of choice

Ans. d

Explanation: The clinical features are suggestive of meningococcal meningitis and the drug of choice is a third-generation cephalosporin such as ceftriaxone. Chloramphenicol is used. It is caused by *Neisseria meningitidis*, a gram-negative, oxidase-positive, catalase-positive diplococci. Outbreaks usually occur in mass gatherings such as in army camps or hostel dorms.

The risk of infection is increased in patients with terminal complement deficiency, hypogammaglobulinemia, and hyposplenism.

This is because opsonization by complement is a major mechanism by which the bacteria is cleared from the blood.

Characteristic clinical findings include:
- Maculopapular or purpuric rash
- Shock due to capillary leak
- Bilateral adrenal hemorrhage (Waterhouse-Friderichsen syndrome)

Rifampicin, ciprofloxacin, and cephalosporins can be used to treat carriers.

Suggested Reading
1. Nadel S, Kroll JS. Diagnosis and management of meningococcal disease: the need for centralized care. FEMS Microbiology Reviews. 2007;31:71-83.

Q.14. A 68-year-old male patient presented with multiple fractures. He has been suffering from recurrent infections for the past 6 months. Bone marrow biopsy shows proliferation of plasma cells. What is the treatment of choice in this condition?
   a. Lenalidomide + bortezomib + dexamethasone
   b. Thalidomide + cyclophosphamide
   c. Rituximab + cyclophosphamide
   d. Bortezomib + cyclophosphamide + dexamethasone

Ans. a

Explanation: In the above clinical scenario, the symptoms and bone marrow biopsy are characteristic of multiple myeloma. Lenalidomide + bortezomib + dexamethasone is the treatment of choice in this condition.

This combination achieves close to a 100% response. Hence, it is one of the preferred induction regimens in transplant-eligible multiple myeloma patients.

Other pharmacological agents are used as second-line and have a 90% response.

Suggested Reading
1. Usmani SZ, Hoering A, Cavo M, Miguel JS, Goldschimdt H, Hajek R, et al. Clinical predictors of long-term survival in newly diagnosed transplant eligible multiple myeloma—an IMWG research project. Blood Cancer J. 2018;8(12):123.

Q.15. A patient was brought to the emergency room with dyspnea, cough, and chest pain. His blood pressure was 180/100 mm Hg and SpO$_2$ was 90%. Chest X-ray shows batwing appearance. Echocardiography revealed reduced LV ejection fraction (LVEF). Which of the following will you not use in the management of this patient?
   a. Digoxin
   b. Morphine
   c. Furosemide
   d. Positive pressure ventilation

Ans. a

Explanation: The above X-ray showing bat-wing appearance along with the given symptoms and reduced LVEF is suggestive of acute decompensated heart failure with pulmonary edema. Digoxin has no role in the management of this condition.

The management of acute cardiogenic pulmonary edema consists of:
- Oxygen therapy and positive pressure ventilation
- *Reduction of preload:*
  - *Diuretics:* Furosemide is the diuretic of choice.
  - *Nitrates*: Sublingual nitroglycerin is the first-line therapy. If pulmonary edema persists, IV nitroglycerin is administered.
  - *Morphine:* It is a transient venodilator that reduces preload, thereby reducing dyspnea and anxiety.

- *ACE inhibitors:* They reduce both preload and afterload and are recommended for hypertensive patients.
- *Nesiritide:* It is an IV recombinant B-type natriuretic peptide (BNP) which is a potent vasodilator with diuretic properties.
- *Inotropic and inodilators:*
  - Dopamine and dobutamine inotropic agents
  - Milrinone stimulates myocardial contractility and promotes peripheral vasodilatation.
  - Intra-aortic balloon counterpulsation or LV assist devices are used in cardiogenic shock.

Suggested Reading
1. HFSA Guidelines Heart Failure Society of America (HFSA) practice guidelines. HFSA guidelines for management of patients with heart failure caused by left ventricular systolic dysfunction: pharmacological approaches. J Card Fail. 1999;5:357-82.

Q.16. In a patient with anemia due to chronic renal failure, which of the following is the long-acting derivative of erythropoietin suitable for treatment?
   a. Oprelvekin
   b. Darbepoetin alfa
   c. Dornase alfa
   d. Filgrastim

Ans. b

Explanation: Darbepoetin alpha is the recombinant derivative of erythropoietin that is long-acting and approved for anemia due to chronic renal failure.
- *Option a:* Oprelvekin is an interleukin-11 (IL-11) analog that stimulates megakaryocyte maturation.
- *Option c:* Dornase alfa is a recombinant human DNase 1 that is used in cystic fibrosis to reduce the viscosity of mucosal secretions.
- *Option d:* Filgrastim is a recombinant human G-CSF, indicated in the treatment of severe neutropenia.

Suggested Reading
1. Agarwal AK. Darbepoetin alfa for anemia in chronic kidney disease. Expert Rev Clin Pharmacol. 2008;1(3):369-79.

Q.17. Performing a vagal maneuver in a stable patient with PSVT is first choice of therapy in such patients. Which of the following muscarinic receptors mediate the therapeutic effect of this maneuver?
   a. M1
   b. M2
   c. M3
   d. M4

Ans. b

Explanation: In vagal maneuver, the parasympathetic nervous system mediates activity on the heart via the M2 muscarinic receptor (most predominant subtype).

The receptors in the autonomic nervous system (ANS) are of two types:
1. *Muscarinic:*
   - Five subtypes—(1) M1, (2) M2, (3) M3, (4) M4, and (5) M5

- M1, M3, and M5 are Gq-coupled receptors.
- M2 and M4 are Gi/Go-coupled receptors.
2. *Nicotinic:*
   - Two subtypes:
     a. Nm (neuromuscular junction)
     b. Nn (CNS, ganglion, and adrenal glands)
   - Nicotinic receptors are ion channels.

Suggested Reading
1. Cohn AE, Fraser FR. Paroxysmal tachycardia and the effect of stimulation of the vagus nerves by pressure. Heart. 1913;93-108.

Q.18. A patient with liver cirrhosis in ICU for 15 days develops fever with hypotension. He is to be started on empirical antifungal drugs. Which of the following drugs should be started?
a. Caspofungin
b. Anidulafungin
c. Micafungin
d. Voriconazole

Ans. b

Explanation: A patient with sepsis/septic shock and who needs empirical antifungal drug treatment should be treated with echinocandins. Caspofungin needs dose adjustments in liver impairment and micafungin should not be used when other echinocandins are available. Anidulafungin does not require dose adjustment in patients with liver impairment and can be given safely.

Suggested Reading
1. Blot S, Charles PE. Fungal sepsis in the ICU: are we doing better? Trends in incidence, diagnosis, and outcome. Minerva Anestesiologica. 2013;79(12):1396-1405.

Q.19. A patient with diabetes and chronic obstructive pulmonary disease (COPD) developed postoperative urinary retention. Which of the following drugs can be used for short-term treatment of the condition?
a. Tamsulosin
b. Bethanechol
c. Terazosin
d. Methacholine

Ans. a

Explanation: Tamsulosin is the drug used to relieve the symptoms in cases of postoperative urinary retention in a patient with COPD.
It is also efficacious in the treatment of benign prostatic hyperplasia (BPH) with little effect on blood pressure.
- *Option b:* Bethanechol is the drug of choice to relieve the symptoms in cases of postoperative urinary retention. However, it can cause bronchoconstriction in patients with COPD. Hence, tamsulosin is the best answer here.
- *Option c:* Terazosin is a receptor antagonist, used in the treatment of benign prostatic hyperplasia (BPH).

- *Option d:* Methacholine is a muscarinic agonist but acts specifically on bronchial smooth muscle causing its contraction. It is available as an inhalational agent and is used for the diagnosis of bronchial hyper-reactivity in patients who do not have clinically apparent asthma.

Suggested Reading
1. Wilt TJ, Mac Donald R, Rutks I. Tamsulosin for benign prostatic hyperplasia. Cochrane Database Syst Rev. 2003;(1):CD002081.

Q.20. A patient with heart disease presents to the emergency room with severe vomiting and blurry vision and mentions that he sees a greenish-yellow tinge over all objects. He then develops ventricular arrhythmia. What would be the most appropriate drug for immediate management?
 a. Procainamide
 b. Lignocaine
 c. Atropine
 d. Propranolol

Ans. b

Explanation: The given clinical scenario is suggestive of digoxin toxicity. Xanthopsia, i.e., yellowing of vision is characteristically seen in this condition. Lignocaine (and phenytoin) has the least effect on AV nodal conduction and is the most appropriate drug for the treatment of digoxin-induced arrhythmias.
- *Option a:* Procainamide and other class IA antiarrhythmic agents are not indicated in digoxin toxicity because of their inhibitory effects on AV nodal conduction.
- *Option c:* Atropine is used for atrial bradyarrhythmias associated with digoxin toxicity.
- *Option d:* Propranolol is used for atrial tachyarrhythmias associated with digoxin toxicity.

Suggested Reading
1. Pincus M. Management of digoxin toxicity. Aust Prescr 2016;39(1):18-20.

Q.21. A 46-year-old man, who is a chronic alcoholic, presented with acute dull and boring abdominal pain. His history is significant for ongoing treatment with ART. Serum lipase levels were noted to be grossly elevated. What is the most likely causative drug?
 a. Nevirapine
 b. Didanosine
 c. Emtricitabine
 d. Stavudine

Ans. b

Explanation: Didanosine is the most likely causative drug. The clinical scenario, suggestive of pancreatitis, is a dose-limiting side effect of didanosine and occurs more frequently in alcoholic patients and those with hypertriglyceridemia.
- *Option a:* Nevirapine side-effects include severe liver problems, skin rash, and skin reactions.
- *Option c:* Emtricitabine is contraindicated in pregnancy and young children.
- *Option d:* Stavudine can cause peripheral neuropathy.

Suggested Reading
1. Kirian MA, Higginson RT, Fulco PP. Acute onset of pancreatitis with concomitant use of tenofovir and didanosine. Ann Pharmacother. 2004;38(10):1660-3.

Q.22. A patient with bronchial asthma was treated with regular inhaled corticosteroids. He is now commenced on theophylline as an add-on therapy. By which of the following mechanism does this drug enhance the effect of corticosteroids?
a. Phosphodiesterase inhibition
b. Blockade of adenosine receptors
c. Interleukin-10 release
d. Activation of histone deacetylase

Ans. d

Explanation: Theophylline enhances the effect of corticosteroids by activation of histone deacetylase.

Theophylline activates histone deacetylase 2. The recruitment of histone deacetylase 2 by glucocorticoid receptors (GRs) switches off inflammatory genes. Through this mechanism, theophylline enhances the anti-inflammatory effects of corticosteroids.

Theophylline is a methylxanthine drug used in the management of asthma and chronic obstructive pulmonary disease. Its other mechanisms of action are as follows:
- It inhibits phosphodiesterase nonselectively (PDE3, PDE4, and PDE5) thereby, increasing cellular cyclic adenosine monophosphate (cAMP) and cyclic guanosine monophosphate (cGMP), causing bronchodilation.
- Adenosine causes bronchoconstriction by releasing histamine and leukotrienes. Theophylline antagonizes adenosine receptors causing bronchodilation.
- It increases IL-10 release, which has an anti-inflammatory effect.
- It decreases gene transcription of proinflammatory cytokines.
- It promotes apoptosis of granulocytes, reducing the inflammatory load in the airways.
- Theophylline is mainly metabolized by the enzyme CYP1A2 enzyme. Various drug interactions of theophylline include:
  - Increased clearance (CYP1A2 enzyme induction) by smoking, phenytoin, rifampicin, and phenobarbitone
  - Decreased clearance (CYP1A2 enzyme inhibition) by erythromycin, cimetidine, ciprofloxacin, oral contraceptives, and allopurinol

Important side effects of this drug due to PDE4 antagonism are nausea, vomiting, and gastric discomfort, and those due to adenosine A1 receptor antagonism are diuresis, cardiac arrhythmias, and seizures.

Suggested Reading
1. Barnes PJ. Theophylline. Pharmaceuticals (Basel). 2010;3(3):725-47.

Q.23. A psychiatric patient with a history of bipolar disorder is brought by her relatives. They give a history suggestive of an acute manic episode. She is already on lithium therapy and the serum lithium levels are measured to be 0.2 mEq/L. What steady-state concentration will you be aiming to achieve in this scenario?
a. 1.2–1.6 mEq/L
b. 0.8–1.2 mEq/L
c. 0.5–0.8 mEq/L
d. 0.3–0.5 mEq/L

Ans. b

Explanation: The given clinical vignette showing increased activity, energy, and euphoria with a decreased need for sleep is indicative of an acute manic episode for which a steady-state concentration of 0.8–1.2 mEq/L of lithium has to be achieved for adequate treatment.

Lithium is used in the management of bipolar disorder, and mania, and has anti-suicidal properties. It has a narrow therapeutic index, and blood levels in excess of this may cause symptoms of toxicity. Therapeutic drug monitoring is done by measuring lithium levels 12 hours after the last dose.

Lithium therapy for acute mania:
- Three individual 10-mg/kg doses of a sustained-release preparation administered at 2-hour intervals.
- The sustained-release form is used to minimize GI adverse effects (e.g., nausea and diarrhea).
- Subsequent treatment may then be continued with Li^+ carbonate.

Steady-state concentrations for therapy:
- For maintenance therapy in bipolar disorder—0.5–0.8 mEq/L
- For episodes of acute mania—0.8–1.2 mEq/L
- Toxic levels >1.5 mEq/L

The blood sample for serum lithium estimation is to be collected after a time interval of 10–12 hours from the previous dose of lithium which is used to estimate the steady-state concentration.

Known significant side effects of lithium therapy include:
- Polyuria-polydipsia (nephrogenic diabetes insipidus)
- Hand tremors
- Confusion
- Electrogastrography (EGG) and electroencephalography (EEG) changes

Suggested Reading
1. Volkmann C, Bschor T, Köhler S. Lithium treatment over the lifespan in bipolar disorders. Front Psychiatry. 2020;11:377.

Q.24. Which of the following is true about pegylated-filgrastim?
a. Duration of action is shorter than normal filgrastim.
b. Added advantage is that it can be taken orally.
c. It should not be administered in sickle cell patients.
d. It is not effective in the treatment of severe neutropenia.

Ans. c

Explanation: Patients with sickle cell anemia should not receive pegylated filgrastim as it can trigger a sickle cell crisis.

Filgrastim is a recombinant human G-CSF (granulocyte colony-stimulating factor). The pegylated forms of filgrastim, pegfilgrastim, and lipegfilgrastim are longer-acting forms. It is administered subcutaneously or by slow intravenous infusion only.

Indications of recombinant G-CSF:
- Severe neutropenia after autologous hematopoietic stem cell transplantation
- Severe neutropenia after high-dose cancer chemotherapy
- Severe congenital neutropenias
- Neutropenia of patients with AIDS receiving zidovudine

Filgrastim is the first FDA-approved drug to treat patients with radiation-induced myelosuppression and to increase survival in such patients.

Suggested Reading
1. Kasi PM, Patnaik MM, Peethambaram PP. Safety of pegfilgrastim (neulasta) in patients with sickle cell trait/anemia. Case Rep Hematol. 2013;2013:146938.

Q.25. A pregnant female at 36 weeks gestation presents with palpitations, protrusion of the eyeball, and heat intolerance. On blood investigations, it was found that she had increased T3 and T4 levels and decreased TSH levels. Which of the following should be the next step in the management of this patient?
   a. Methimazole
   b. Thyroidectomy
   c. Propylthiouracil
   d. Radioactive iodine

Ans. a

Explanation: In the given clinical scenario, the most likely diagnosis is thyrotoxicosis. As she is in her third trimester, the drug of choice for the treatment of thyrotoxicosis is methimazole.

Thyrotoxicosis during pregnancy is usually controlled by thionamide drugs, propylthiouracil was preferred previously because it partially inhibits the conversion of T4 to T3 and crosses the placenta less readily than methimazole. However, since it has a higher risk of causing propylthiouracil-associated liver failure in pregnancy, methimazole is prescribed according to guidelines from the second trimester. Methimazole is usually avoided in the first trimester due to methimazole-associated embryopathy.

Other options:
- *Option b:* A subtotal thyroidectomy is done once the hyperthyroidism is medically controlled. It is usually avoided during pregnancy, however, may be done in some cases where it cannot be controlled via medication.
- *Option d:* Radioactive iodine is contraindicated in pregnant women as it may cause fetal thyroid gland destruction.

Suggested Reading
1. Inoue M, Arata N, Koren G, Ito S. Hyperthyroidism during pregnancy. Can Fam Physician. 2009;55(7):701-3.

Q.26. The risk of carbamazepine-induced Stevens–Johnson syndrome is increased in the presence of which of the following genes?
a. HLA-B*1507
b. HLA-B*1502
c. HLA-B*5701
d. HLA-B*2406

Ans. b

Explanation: Human leukocyte antigen (HLA) allele B*1502 is implicated as a marker for carbamazepine-induced Stevens–Johnson syndrome and toxic epidermal necrolysis in Han Chinese, the USFDA recommends genotyping all Asians for the allele.

Note: The HLA-B*1502 allele is seen in high frequency in many Asian populations other than Han Chinese, but there are few data on whether the allele is a marker for this severe outcome in anyone other than Han Chinese.

Suggested Reading
1. Ferrell PB Jr, McLeod HL. Carbamazepine, HLA-B*1502 and risk of Stevens-Johnson syndrome and toxic epidermal necrolysis: US FDA recommendations. Pharmacogenomics. 2008;9(10):1543-6.

Q.27. A new antibiotic developed for the treatment of infections caused by resistant gram-positive cocci has a volume of distribution of 11 L. It is eliminated by first-order kinetics and has a half-life of 10 hours. If given by a continuous infusion, approximately how much time would it require for the drug to achieve a 95% plasma steady-state concentration?
a. 10 hours
b. 20 hours
c. 30 hours
d. 40 hours

Ans. d

Explanation: During continuous infusion of a drug metabolized by first-order kinetics (i.e., a constant fraction of the drug is eliminated per unit time), the steady-state concentration is reached in 4–5 half-lives. Thus, it would take approximately 40 hours, or four times the half-life of 10 hours, for the drug in question to reach approximately 95% steady-state concentration.

Suggested Reading
1. Borowy CS, Ashurst JV. Physiology, Zero and First Order Kinetics. [Updated 2022 Sep 19]. In: StatPearls [Internet]. Treasure Island (FL): StatPearls Publishing; 2023 Jan. Available from: https://www.ncbi.nlm.nih.gov/books/NBK499866/

Q.28. A 40-year-old female with a history of depression and hypertension is brought to the ER after being found obtunded in her apartment. She is hypotensive and bradycardic on physical examination. Intravenous glucagon is administered, and her condition improves. Which of the following intracellular changes is most likely responsible for the improvement in her condition?
a. Increased synaptic release of glutamate
b. Decreased cAMP in vascular smooth muscle
c. Decreased DAG in vascular smooth muscle

d. Increased cAMP in cardiac myocytes
e. Increased IP3 in cardiac myocytes

Ans. d

Explanation: This patient has most likely overdosed on beta-blocker medications. Beta-blocker overdose causes diffuse nonselective blockade of peripheral beta-adrenergic receptors, causing depression of myocardial contractility, bradycardia, and varying degrees of AV block. The result is a low cardiac output state.

Glucagon is the drug of choice for beta-blocker overdose. Glucagon acts on G protein-coupled receptors, increasing intracellular cAMP and thus increasing the release of intracellular calcium during muscle contraction. This increases heart rate and cardiac contractility. Improvements in heart rate and blood pressure may be observed within minutes.

Patients who have overdosed on beta-blockers should be treated with glucagon, which increases heart rate and contractility independent of adrenergic receptors. Glucagon activates G-protein-coupled receptors on cardiac myocytes, causing activation of adenylate cyclase and raising intracellular cAMP. The result is calcium release from intracellular stores and increased sinoatrial node firing.

Suggested Reading
1. Peterson CD, Leeder JS, Sterner S. Glucagon therapy for beta-blocker overdose. Drug Intell Clin Pharm. 1984;18(5):394-8.

Q.29. A patient is brought with altered sensorium and seizures. He is a chronic alcoholic and has developed liver cirrhosis. His lab shows elevated liver enzymes. Which of the following can be used in this condition?
 a. Midazolam
 b. Diazepam
 c. Alprazolam
 d. Oxazepam

Ans. d

Explanation: Oxazepam can be used in patients with elevated transaminases. It is short-acting and so can be used in patients with liver impairment or brain damage.

Oxazepam is an orally available benzodiazepine used to treat anxiety and alcohol withdrawal states. Hepatic oxidation is decreased in persons with liver disease and the elderly. Oxazepam and lorazepam undergo only hepatic glucuronidation.

Other options:
- *Option a:* Midazolam is the benzodiazepine of choice for induction of anesthesia. The onset of anesthesia is within 30–60 seconds. It can also be used to control seizures, but there is no difference in the efficacy of intravenous midazolam and intravenous diazepam.
- *Option b:* Diazepam is a long-acting benzodiazepine. It is metabolized in the liver to active metabolites like nordazepam which are long-acting. Diazepam and its long-acting metabolites can accumulate significantly in elderly patients with liver disease and therefore should not be used in such cases.

- *Option c:* Alprazolam is metabolized by hepatic oxidation which is significantly decreased in liver impairment and elderly patients.

Suggested Reading
1. Scott AK, Khir AS, Steele WH, Hawksworth GM, Petrie JC. Oxazepam pharmacokinetics in patients with epilepsy treated long-term with phenytoin alone or in combination with phenobarbitone. Br J Clin Pharmacol. 1983;16(4):441-4.

Q.30. **A 38-year-old woman presented with chest pain that was unrelated to physical exertion. ECG showed ST-segment elevation. Intracoronary acetylcholine provocation testing revealed a transient spasm of the right coronary artery. What is the drug of choice in this condition?**
a. Dopamine
b. Diltiazem
c. Propranolol
d. Digoxin

Ans. b

Explanation: The above scenario in which rest pain is associated with ST-segment elevation and transient coronary vasospasm is suggestive of Prinzmetal's angina. The drug of choice is a calcium-channel blocker.

Prinzmetal variant angina (PVA) is a clinical syndrome in which chest pain occurs without the usual precipitating factors. It usually results from coronary vasoconstriction (vasospasm) and tends to involve the right coronary artery.

It is a supply ischemia and usually causes transmural ischemia (subendocardial in classic angina pectoris).

It often affects women under 50 years of age. It characteristically occurs in the early morning, awakening patients from sleep, and may be associated with arrhythmias or conduction defects.

The clinical diagnosis of PVA is made by the detection of transient ST-segment elevation with rest pain.

Coronary angiography demonstrates transient coronary spasm which is the diagnostic hallmark of PVA.

Nitrates and calcium-channel blockers both can be used in alleviating symptoms in prinzmetal angina.

However due to the development of nitrate tolerance in some individuals, they are less preferred and calcium-channel blockers such as verapamil and diltiazem are used as first-line agents.

Suggested Reading
1. McMahon MT, McPherson MA, Talbert RL, Greenberg B, Sheaffer SL. Diagnosis and treatment of Prinzmetal's variant angina. Clin Pharm 1982;1(1):34-42.

CHAPTER 25

Physical Disorders (Drowning, Electrocution, Altitude and Depth Related, Temperature Related, and Rhabdomyolysis)

Sunil Karanth, Raghavendra B Goudar

Q.1. A 20-year-old boy was playing near a deep lake. When his friends were engrossed in the game, the boy dived into the deep lake. The splash alerted his friends and he was rescued by his friends. Which of the following statements is the common sequence of pathophysiological process in the body?
   a. Hypoxia secondary to acute respiratory distress syndrome (ARDS) immediately after extracting from the water
   b. Acidosis secondary to hypoxia causing cardiac arrhythmias and cardiac arrest
   c. Instant death due to cerebral anoxia
   d. Most patients suffer anoxia due to laryngospasm

Ans. b

Explanation: Drowning is a process of submersion or immersion in a liquid medium which results in tissue hypoxia and consequent acidosis resulting in cardiac dysrhythmias. Furthermore, the aspirated fluid results in washout of surfactant and consequent ARDS. Hypothermia may be cerebroprotective but predisposes to arrhythmias. The process of ARDS is often later sequelae, while the instantaneous risk of cardiac arrest is due to hypoxia.

Suggested Reading
1. Buzzacott P, Mease A. Pediatric and adolescent injury in aquatic adventure sports. Res Sports Med. 2018;26 (Suppl 1):20-37.
2. Smith R, Ormerod JOM, Sabharwal N, Kipps C. Swimming-induced pulmonary edema: current perspectives. Open Access J Sports Med. 2018;9:131-7.

Q.2. An 18-year-old boy was learning swimming in a training pool. He accidentally swam toward the deep side of the pool and had accidental drowning. He was rescued by the life-guard, who is trained in BLS. On preliminary evaluation, the boy was found to have no pulse and resuscitation commenced by the first responders. As per the AHA criteria which of the following is the correct sequence of BLS by the trained life-guard?
   a. C–A–B
   b. A–B–C
   c. B–A-C
   d. Any of the above

Ans. b

Explanation: The American Heart Association (AHA) recommends compression first strategy for laypeople, providing resuscitation in cardiac arrest after drowning. However, for healthcare professionals and lifeguards, the AHA recommends rescue breaths or ventilation first (A-B-C) before chest compression. The rationale for ventilation first strategy is based on the mechanism of cardiac arrest in drowning being consequent to hypoxia and the belief is that earlier the ventilation is commenced, better are the chances of early reversal of hypoxia leading on to an early likelihood of return of spontaneous circulation (ROSC).

Suggested Reading
1. Dunne C, Morgan P, Bierens J, Olasveengen T, Morley PT, Perkins GD; International Liaison Committee on Resuscitation BLS Life Support Task Force. (2022). CAB or ABC in drowning: systematic review. [online] Available from https://costr.ilcor.org/document/cab-or-abc-in-drowning-bls-856-tf-systematic-review [Last accessed June, 2023].

Q.3. In the presence of trained personnel, drowning results in respiratory arrest, which of the following measures provides the best chance of survival to hospital discharge?
a. Rescue to the shore and provide BLS
b. In-water ventilation
c. C-spine protection
d. None of the above

Ans. b

Explanation: Efforts at providing floatation to victim will take priority. It is very important to ensure the competence and skill of the rescuer in this process. If the drowning process is not interrupted, it will lead to apnea and cardiac arrest. During this short window of opportunity, immediate in-water ventilation (if safe) can be performed and has been found to improve the rate of hospital discharge by three times. If no response occurs after the first few reduce breaths, it would imply the victim has had a cardiac arrest and will need a full CPR.

Suggested Reading
1. Szpilman D, Soares M. In-water resuscitation—is it worthwhile? Resuscitation. 2004;63(1):25-31.
2. Truhlář A, Deakin CD, Soar J, Khalifa GEA, Alfonzo A, Bierens AJL, et al. European Resuscitation Council Guidelines for Resuscitation 2015: Section 4. Cardiac arrest in special circumstances. Resuscitation. 2015;95:148-201.

Q.4. Which of the following terms is not used in current medical literature?
a. Fatal drowning
b. Nonfatal drowning
c. Near drowning
d. All are accepted terminologies

Ans. c

Explanation: If the victim of drowning is rescued and the process of drowning is interrupted, the event is called nonfatal drowning, but if the victim dies, it is called fatal drowning. Terms such as "near drowning", "dry or wet drowning", and "secondary drowning" should not be used.

Suggested Reading
1. Beeck EF van, Branche CM, Szpilman D, Modell JH, Bierens JJLM. A new definition of drowning: towards documentation and prevention of a global public health problem. Bull World Health Organ. 2005;83(11):853-6.

Q.5. The single most important determinant of outcome in patients with drowning is:
a. Duration of submersion
b. Aspiration
c. ARDS
d. Time of receiving medical aid

Ans. a

Explanation: Drowning is graded from 1 to 6 with first 5 grades having 95% chance of discharge without sequelae. Grade 6 is associated with poor outcomes. Evaluation of multiple studies showed that almost solely the single most important factor that determines the outcome in drowning is the duration of submersion.

Duration of submersion	Death or severe neurological impairment
0 to <10 minutes	10%
5 to <10 minutes	56%
10 to <25 minutes	88%
>25 minutes	99.9%

Note in these data how 5 more minutes of submersion in the 5 to >10-minute group increase morality almost six times compared to the 0 to>5-minute group.

Probability of neurologically intact survival to hospital discharge is based on duration of submersion.

Suggested Reading
1. Szpilman D. Near-drowning and drowning classification: a proposal to stratify mortality based on the analysis of 1,831 cases. Chest. 1997;112(3).660-5.

Q.6. Which of the following is not a type of electrical injury?
a. Flash
b. Flame
c. Lightning
d. True
e. Friction

Ans. e

Explanation: Electrical injuries are broadly categorized into four types:
1. *Flash:* Caused by an arc, usually causing superficial burns with no electrical currents passing past the skin.
2. *Flame:* Caused by the arc flash igniting the victims clothing with or without passage of electrical current past the skin.
3. *Lightning:* Short and high-voltage electrical energy passing through the entire body.

4. *True:* The individual becomes part of an electrical circuit with an entry and exit wound.

Friction burns are a type of mechanical injury which is often due to abrasion against a surface. Heat may be a contributing factor for tissue injuries.

Suggested Reading
1. Burnham T, Hilgenhurst G, McCormick ZL. Second-degree skin burn from a radiofrequency grounding pad: a case report and review of risk mitigation strategies. PM R. 2019;11(10):1139-42.
2. Carrano FM, Iezzi L, Melis M, Quaresima S, Gaspari AL, Di Lorenzo N. A surgical instrument cover for the prevention of thermal injuries during laparoscopic operations. J Laparoendosc Adv Surg Tech. 2019;29:30698493.
3. Kim MS, Lee SG, Kim JY, Kang MY. Maculopathy from an accidental exposure to welding arc. BMJ Case Rep. 2019;12(2):bcr-2018-227677.

Q.7. Which of the following statements is false about electrical injuries?
 a. Electrical current implies flow of electrons down a potential gradient.
 b. Resistance levels in the body vary in the tissues depending on the water and electrolyte content.
 c. More the resistance of the tissues, greater is the level of tissue damage.
 d. The extent of burn injuries on the skin predicts the level of damage internally.

Ans. d

Explanation: Tissues offering the highest level of resistance to the flow of current tend to suffer the greatest amount of damage. If the skin resistance is high, it will tend to cause a large amount of dissipation of energy causing extensive skin burns. On the other hand, if the resistance offered by the skin is low, the damage on the skin is limited. Hence, the external damage on the skin may not necessarily show the extent of internal tissue damage as the latter will depend on the resistance offered to the flow of current.

Suggested Reading
1. Daskal Y, Beicker A, Dudkiewicz M, Kessel B. High voltage electric injury: mechanism of injury, clinical features and initial evaluation. Harefuah. 2019;158(1):65-9.

Q.8. A 45-year-old gentleman suffers electrical injuries following contact with a live wire. Which of the following factors does not correlate with the degree of electrical injuries suffered by the individual?
 a. Comorbidities
 b. Type of current
 c. Current strength
 d. Pathway current takes in the body

Ans. a

Explanation: The degree of electrical injury experienced by an individual can be predicted by Kouwenhoven factors include the type of current, current strength, length of time of exposure, body resistance, and the pathway, the current takes in the body in addition to electrical field strength.

Suggested Reading

1. Daskal Y, Beicker A, Dudkiewicz M, Kessel B. High voltage electric injury: mechanism of injury, clinical features and initial evaluation. Harefuah. 2019;158(1):65-9.

Q.9. A 35-year-old gentleman was returning home from his farm on a stormy evening. He saw a sudden flash of light and was thrown off balance. Which of the following injuries proves that the man suffered a lightning strike?

a. Fractures
b. Damage to solid organs
c. Incised wounds
d. Lichtenberg figure

Ans. d

Explanation: Often lightning injuries happen in places which are isolated. The presentations may be highly variable. When diagnosis is unclear, some important clues may point toward lightning injuries at scene. These include unexplained burns, specific sequelae such as Lichtenberg figures, singed hair, torn clothes, molten metal, and tympanic membrane rupture. Fractures and internal organs damage are rare.

Suggested Reading

1. Ruler R, Eikednal T, Looij FO, Tan ECTH. A shocking injury: a clinical review of lightning injuries highlighting pitfalls and a treatment protocol. Injury. 2022;53(10):3070-7

Q.10. Following an electrical injury, which of the following cardiac manifestations is rare?

a. Ventricular fibrillation
b. Delayed arrhythmias
c. Damage to cardiac myocytes
d. Long-term cardiac sequelae

Ans. d

Explanation: Common cardiac complications include ventricular fibrillation (VF) and damage to cardiac myocytes. VF can occur with exposure to voltage as low as 50 120 mA. Due to damage to cardiac myocytes, patients may experience delayed arrhythmias. Electrical injuries resulting in long-term cardiac sequelae, however, are rare.

Suggested Reading

1. Pawlik AM, Lampart A, Stephan FP, Bingisser R, Ummenhofer W, Nickel CH. Outcomes of electrical injuries in the emergency department: a 10-year retrospective study. Eur J Emerg Med. 2016;23(6):448-54.

Q.11. Which of the following syndromes does not classify as a type of altitude illness?

a. Acute mountain sickness
b. High-altitude cerebral edema
c. High-altitude mountain sickness
d. High-altitude decompression sickness

Ans. d

Explanation: The first three answers are part of high-altitude illness, while there is no entity called high-altitude decompression sickness. Caisson's disease or decompression sickness is seen with rapid ascent from depths.

Suggested Reading
1. Medley T, Grocott MP. Acute high-altitude illness: a clinically orientated review. Br J Pain. 2013;7(2):85-94.

Q.12. Which of the following statements is not true about high-altitude sickness?
a. Physical fitness offers protection against acute high-altitude illness.
b. Past history of high-altitude illness increases the propensity of getting the illness.
c. Exercise may exacerbate the high-altitude mountain illness.
d. Dehydration may be associated with high-altitude mountain sickness.

Ans. a

Explanation: There is no evidence to show that physical fitness offers protection against high-altitude sickness. Dehydration is associated with high-altitude illness though not an independent predictor of risk. Past history of illness, exercising, and rapid ascent may be risk factors to precipitate the disease.

Suggested Reading
1. Cumbo TA, Basnyat B, Graham J, Lescano AG, Gambert S. Acute mountain sickness, dehydration, and bicarbonate clearance: preliminary field data from the Nepal Himalaya. Aviat Space Environ Med. 2002;73:898-901.
2. Milledge JS, Beeley JM, Broome J, Luff N, Pelling M, Smith D. Acute mountain sickness susceptibility, fitness and hypoxic ventilatory response. Eur Respir J. 1991;4:1000-3.
3. Richalet JP, Larmignat P, Poitrine E, Letournel M, Canoui-Poitrine F. Physiological risk factors for severe high-altitude illness: a prospective cohort study. Am J Respir Crit Care Med. 2012;185:192-8.
4. Roach RC, Maes D, Sandoval D, Robergs RA, Icenogle M, Hinghofer-Szalkay H, et al. Exercise exacerbates acute mountain sickness at simulated high altitude. J Appl Physiol. 2000;88:581-5.

Q.13. Which of the following symptoms does not form part of the acute mountain sickness?
a. Exertional dyspnea
b. Loose stools and abdominal cramps
c. Insomnia
d. Dizziness

Ans. b

Explanation: The illness usually develops within 4–34 hours of reaching a new altitude. The symptoms include insomnia, headache, dyspnea on exertion, and nausea. Loose stools and abdominal pain are not a part of this syndrome usually. A scoring system called Lake–Louise score is used for the diagnosis of the illness.

Suggested Reading
1. Hupper T, Gieseler U, Angelini C, Hillebrandt D, Milledge J. Emergency field management of acute mountain sickness, high altitude pulmonary oedema, and high-altitude cerebral oedema. Bern, Switzerland: UIAA Medical Commission; 2008.

Q.14. Which of the following is less likely to be differentials to high-altitude mountain sickness for a traveler to a place of high altitude?
a. Hypothermia
b. Hyponatremia
c. Hypoglycemia
d. Hypokalemia

Ans. d

Explanation: The symptoms of acute mountain sickness are very nonspecific. It is very important to identify the disease which is often thought to be due to fatigue sleep deprivation, etc. Some of the other differentials that can be a part of this syndrome in high altitude is hypothermia, hyponatremia (due to excessive water intake) to compensate for dehydration and hypoglycemia.

Suggested Reading
1. Imray C, Wright A, Subudhi A, Roach R. Acute mountain sickness: pathophysiology, prevention, and treatment. Prog Cardiovasc Dis. 2010;52:467-84.

Q.15. Which of the following measures has not demonstrated efficacy in prevention of mountain sickness?
a. Acetazolamide 125 mg, twice daily
b. Sildenafil 50 mg, three times daily
c. Appropriate ascent rate
d. Dexamethasone 4 mg, twice daily

Ans. b

Explanation: Slow ascent remains the best preventive measure for high-altitude mountain sickness and pulmonary edema. Susceptible individuals should not ascend >300 m/day and avoid high-intensity exercise shortly after ascent. Conventionally, nifedipine 20 m slow-release three times a day reduced the risk. Sildenafil was a preventive strategy that has not been found to be useful in a recently concluded randomized controlled trial (RCT). Based on pathophysiological rationale, acetazolamide and dexamethasone have been used for treatment and prophylaxis. Tadalafil twice a day can also be used for the same. However, the use of sildenafil in a recent RCT increased the severity of mountain sickness. Salmeterol has been trialed for prophylaxis as it increases transepithelial sodium channel function. However, the Wilderness Medical Society guidelines recommend using only 60 mg nifedipine modified-release daily (divided in two or three doses) in susceptible individuals. This should be started 1 day prior to ascent and continued for 5 days. Salmeterol, tadalafil, acetazolamide, and dexamethasone are not currently recommended because of the lack of clinical experience and their limited trial data in the wider population.

Suggested Reading
1. Bartsch P, Maggiorini M, Ritter M, Noti C, Vock P, Oelz O. Prevention of high-altitude pulmonary edema by nifedipine. N Engl J Med. 1991;325:1284-9.
2. Bates MG, Thompson AA, Baillie JK, Sutherland AI, Irving JB, Hirani N, et al. Sildenafil citrate for the prevention of high altitude hypoxic pulmonary hypertension: double blind, randomized, placebo-controlled trial. High Alt Med Biol. 2011;12:207-14.
3. Maggiorini M, Brunner-La Rocca HP, Peth S, Fischler M, Böhm T, Bernheim A, et al. Both tadalafil and dexamethasone may reduce the incidence of high-altitude pulmonary edema: A randomized trial. Ann Intern Med. 2006;145:497-506.
4. Sartori C, Allemann Y, Duplain H, Lepori M, Egli M, Lipp E, et al. Salmeterol for the prevention of high-altitude pulmonary edema. N Engl J Med. 2002;346:1631-6.

Q.16. Which of the following is not part of the pathophysiological process in decompression sickness?
   a. Occurs with rapid transit from an area of low ambient pressure to high pressure
   b. Release of inert gas nitrogen from tissues into the blood causing microcirculatory block and vasospasm
   c. Endothelial activation resulting in activation of inflammatory mediators
   d. Gut translocation

Ans. d

Explanation: Inert gases such as nitrogen remain dissolved in the tissues at ambient temperature in a pressurized environment. When there is a rapid change in ambient pressure due to ascent from an area of higher pressure to a zone of lower pressure these inert gases get released into the blood as microbubbles causing blockage of blood flow and vascular spasm. Gas bubbles also result in endothelial damage resulting in activation of the intrinsic clotting cascade with platelet activation and release of inflammatory mediators, consequently causing increased endothelial permeability development of edema, which leads to tissue ischemia.

Suggested Reading
1. Geng M, Zhou L, Liu X, Li P. Hyperbaric oxygen treatment reduced the lung injury of type II decompression sickness. Int J Clin Exp Pathol. 2015;8(2):1797-803.
2. Hall J. The risks of scuba diving: a focus on decompression illness. Hawaii J Med Public Health. 2014;73(11 Suppl 2):13-6.

Q.17. Joint pain is a part of the syndrome of decompression sickness. The most prevalent joint having pain in this syndrome is:
   a. Shoulder joint
   b. Knee joint
   c. Hip joint
   d. Ankle joint

Ans. a

Explanation: Decompression sickness most frequently presents as pain in the shoulders, elbows, knees, and ankles. These joint pains called "the bends" accounts for most cases, with the shoulder being the most prevalent site. Neurological symptoms and skin manifestations are seen in 10–15% of patients. Pulmonary involvement called "the chokes" is rare. In rare instances, bubbles in the venous blood may cause lung damage, spinal cord involvement, and right-to-left shunt can present as an arterial gas embolism.

Suggested Reading
1. Pollock NW, Buteau D. Updates in decompression illness. Emerg Med Clin North Am. 2017;35(2):301-19.

Q.18. The prevalence of neurologic and skin manifestations in decompression sickness is:
   a. 10–15%
   b. 20–25%
   c. 30–35%
   d. 40–45%

Ans. a

Explanation: Decompression sickness most frequently presents as pain in the shoulders, elbows, knees, and ankles. These joint pains called "the bends" account for most cases, with the shoulder being the most prevalent site. Neurological symptoms and skin manifestations are seen in 10–15% of patients. Pulmonary involvement called "the chokes" is rare. In rare instances, bubbles in the venous blood may cause lung damage, spinal cord involvement, and right-to-left shunt can present as an arterial gas embolism.

Suggested Reading
1. Pollock NW, Buteau D. Updates in decompression illness. Emerg Med Clin North Am. 2017;35(2):301-19.

Q.19. Treatment of decompression sickness includes all, except:
a. Hyperbaric oxygen
b. Oxygen with FiO_2 of 100%
c. Aspirin
d. Judicious fluid administration

Ans. c

Explanation: All patients presenting with decompression sickness will need to be commenced on oxygen at fraction of inspired oxygen (FiO_2) of 100% till hyperbaric oxygen (HBO) therapy is available. Presence of neurological, pulmonary, or skin lesions would need HBO therapy even if several days have passed since the development of disease. Other therapies include judicious fluid administration, to minimize dehydration. Unlike previously believed, there is no role of aspirin in these patients. The Trendelenburg position and the left lateral decubitus position (Durant's maneuver) were considered to be beneficial theoretically and may be potentially beneficial if air emboli are suspected. But this position cannot be continued for prolonged hours in view of the risks and concerns of cerebral edema. Management of airway, breathing, and circulation needs to be addressed as in any other critically ill patient. Critically ill patients should receive hyperbaric oxygen therapy and need to be initiated as soon as possible.

Suggested Reading
1. Pollock NW, Buteau D. Updates in decompression illness. Emerg Med Clin North Am. 2017;35(2):301-19.

Q.20. Most patients with decompression sickness will need to be transferred from scene to a facility having availability of HBO. The points of importance to be aware during the air-retrieval include all of the following, except:
a. Air retrieval in pressurized aircraft
b. Full-fledged retrieval team with doctor, nurse, and ACLS equipment on board
c. Helicopter with an altitude above 300 meters to ensure rapid transport
d. Enroute FiO_2 100%

Ans. c

Explanation: Patients needing evacuation to a definitive treatment center by aeromedical transport should fly on pressurized aircraft. If unpressurized aircraft, such as helicopters, are the only means of transport then flight altitude should be limited to 300 m or 1,000 ft if possible.

Suggested Reading
1. Pollock NW, Buteau D. Updates in decompression illness. Emerg Med Clin North Am. 2017;35(2):301-19.

Q.21. The classical description of a "Classic heat stroke" includes all of the following, except:
a. High ambient temperature
b. Elderly person
c. Following exertion
d. Presence of cardiovascular disease

Ans. c

Explanation: There are two types of heat strokes—(1) classic and (2) exertional. Classic heat stroke is seen in elderly people living alone in areas with high-ambient temperatures stereotypically having a cardiovascular disease. On the other exertional heat stroke is caused by excessive heat generation during physical activity. Although it could occur at room temperature, most cases develop with elevated environmental temperatures. Furthermore, the exertional heat stroke is seen in otherwise healthy athletes, military recruits or soldiers, and individuals who work outdoors.

Suggested Reading
1. Carter R 3rd, Cheuvront SN, Williams JO, Kolka MA, Stephenson LA, Sawka MN, et al. Epidemiology of hospitalizations and deaths from heat illness in soldiers. Med Sci Sports Exerc. 2005;37:1338-44.
2. Centers for Disease Control and Prevention (CDC). (2006). Heat-related deaths—United States, 1999-2003. [online] Available from https://www.cdc.gov/mmwr/preview/mmwrhtml/mm5529a2.htm [Last accessed June, 2023].

Q.22. Which of the following is not a feature of neuroleptic malignant syndrome?
a. Adverse effect related to typical antipsychotics
b. Defective *RYR1* gene leading to unregulated calcium influx causing sustained muscular contraction
c. Present as generalized rigidity, restlessness, and immobility with hyperthermia
d. Tends to occur hours to days after initiation of neuroleptic medications

Ans. b

Explanation: Neuroleptic malignant syndrome (NMS) is a severe adverse effect following administration of typical antipsychotics such as haloperidol. The proposed pathogenesis seems to be secondary to blockade of dopamine-D2 or D1 receptors in the corpus striatum and hypothalamus.

RYR1 gene mutation is related to malignant hyperthermia after exposure to inhalational anesthesia and succinylcholine.

Suggested Reading
1. Anglin RE, Rosebush PI, Mazurek MF. Neuroleptic malignant syndrome: a neuroimmunologic hypothesis. CMAJ. 2010;182:8.
2. Gillman PK. Neuroleptic malignant syndrome: mechanisms, interactions, and causality. Mov Disord. 2010;25:1780-90.
3. Strawn JR, Keck PE Jr, Caroff SN. Neuroleptic malignant syndrome. Am J Psychiatry. 2007;164:870-6.
4. Tao M, Li J, Wang X, Tian X. Malignant syndromes: current advances. Expert Opin Drug Saf. 2021;20:1075-85.

Q.23. A 35-year-old lady on treatment for depression with fluoxetine had a fall and suffered a fracture in the right femur. She had intramedullary nailing done and was commenced on tramadol and diclofenac for analgesia. On the third postoperative day, she developed new-onset fever, altered sensorium, with generalized rigidity. Despite antipyretics her fever increased to 104°F and she was transferred to ICU for further care. Her total counts, CRP and procalcitonin were negative and there was no evidence of any infection. What may be the probable diagnosis of this hyperthermic syndrome?
   a. Neuroleptic malignant syndrome
   b. Malignant hyperthermia
   c. Serotonergic syndrome
   d. Heat stroke

Ans. c

Explanation: This is possibly a serotonin syndrome (SS) precipitated by the combination of SSRI with tramadol. SS is caused by supratherapeutic serotonin levels in the synapses of the brain, and it can lead to hyperthermia. This is often caused by a combination of two or more of the following drugs—SSRIs, monoamine oxidase inhibitors (MAOIs), TCAs, venlafaxine, trazodone, tramadol, linezolid, 3,4-methylenedioxymethamphetamine (MDMA), and several other drugs. These agents often share common mechanisms, including the inhibition of serotonin uptake, decreased serotonin metabolism, increased serotonin synthesis, increased serotonin release, activation of serotonergic receptors, and inhibition of cytochrome P450 enzymes. Hyperstimulation of the postsynaptic 5HT2 A receptors is believed to be the possible cause of hyperthermia.

Suggested Reading
1. Boyer EW, Shannon M. The serotonin syndrome. N Engl J Med. 2005;352:1112-20.
2. Foong AL, Grindrod KA, Patel T, Kellar J. Demystifying serotonin syndrome (or serotonin toxicity). Can Fam Physician. 2018;64:720-7.
3. Takeshita J, Litzinger MH. Serotonin syndrome associated with tramadol. Prim Care Companion J Clin Psychiatry. 2009;11:273.

Q.24. Which of the following definitions of temperature is false?
   a. Fever >100.9°F
   b. Hyperpyrexia >106.7°F
   c. Hypothermia <35°C
   d. Low-grade fever defined as 99.1–101°F

Ans. d

Explanation: The American College of Critical Care Medicine and the Infectious Diseases Society of America define fever as a core body temperature of 38.3°C (100.9°F) or higher. When the core body temperature rises above 38.3°C (100.9°F) but remains <41.5°C (106.7°F), it still falls under the classification of fever. Only once it exceeds 41.5°C (106.7°F), it is known as hyperpyrexia. Fever is graded as follows:
- *Low-grade:* 37.3–38.0°C (99.1–100.4°F)
- *Moderate-grade:* 38.1–39.0°C (100.6–102.2°F)
- *High-grade:* 39.1–41°C (102.4–105.8°F)
- *Hyperthermia:* >41°C (105.8°F)

Suggested Reading
1. Islam MA, Kundu S, Alam SS, Hossan T, Kamal MA, Hassan R. Prevalence and characteristics of fever in adult and paediatric patients with coronavirus disease 2019 (COVID-19): a systematic review and meta-analysis of 17515 patients. PLoS One. 2021;16(4):e0249788.
2. Walter EJ, Hanna-Jumma S, Carraretto M, Forni L. The pathophysiological basis and consequences of fever. Crit Care. 2016;20:200.

Q.25. A 35-year-old gentleman was found unresponsiveness on a cold winter night by patrol officers. He was retrieved and brought to the ER. At evaluation, he was noted to be hypotensive with a systolic blood pressure of 90 mm Hg, Glasgow Coma Scale (GCS)—E3M5V2. His body temperature was found to be 32°C. A junior doctor started resuscitation with fluids. But as he was unable to record the saturation he advised to actively warm the peripheries. 15 minutes after the commencement of warming, a further drop in the systolic blood pressure was noted. What is the reason for a drop in blood pressure despite fluid resuscitation?
a. Sepsis
b. Rewarming collapse
c. Cardiogenic shock
d. Hemorrhagic shock

Ans. b

Explanation: When patients present with moderate-to-severe hypothermia, the priority must be to stabilize the core temperature. Overzealous correction of the peripheries my result in cardiovascular collapse due to vasodilatation of the peripheral circulation causing "rewarming collapse".

Suggested Reading
1. Dow J, Giesbrecht GG, Danzl DF, Brugger H, Sagalyn EB, Walpoth B, et al. Wilderness Medical Society Clinical Practice Guidelines for the Out-of-Hospital Evaluation and Treatment of Accidental Hypothermia: 2019 Update. Wilderness Environ Med. 2019;30(4S):S47-S69.
2. Musi ME, Sheets A, Zafren K, Brugger H, Paal P, Hölzl N, et al. Clinical staging of accidental hypothermia: The Revised Swiss System: Recommendation of the International Commission for Mountain Emergency Medicine (ICAR MedCom). Resuscitation. 2021;162:182.

Q.26. A middle-aged gentleman was recently started on a chlorpromazine as an antipsychotic medication. 1 week after commencement, he developed high-grade fever, rigidity, and altered sensorium. On admission to ER and subsequently to

ICU, he was evaluated with all the routine tests and a brain imaging. Radiology was normal. Biochemistry revealed abnormal renal functions and elevated creatinine phosphokinase levels. Despite antibiotics and antipyretics, he continued to have high-grade fever, eventually becoming hyperpyrexic. CSF studies were normal. What is the most likely diagnosis?
a. Bacterial sepsis with multiorgan failure
b. Tropical fever
c. Neuroleptic malignant syndrome
d. Heat stroke

Ans. c

Explanation: Neuroleptic malignant syndrome (NMS) is a rare disorder seen often in the first few hours or days of initiation of first generation or atypical antipsychotics. The syndrome is characterized by hyperpyrexia, rigidity, and tremors. Unless sought for this diagnosis can be used. A thorough history and suspicion of the syndrome are essential. The important clues are hyperpyrexia and rhabdomyolysis.

Suggested Reading
1. Alpers JP, Jones LK Jr. Natural history of exertional rhabdomyolysis: a population-based analysis. Muscle Nerve. 2010;42(4):487-91.

Q.27. In rhabdomyolysis, which of the following statement for creatine phosphokinase (CPK) values is true?
a. CK-BB isoenzyme is elevated.
b. CPK values decline at 30–50% per day if the process causing muscle break down stops.
c. Peak values of CPK occur within 6 hours of injury.
d. Half-life of CPK is 6 hours.

Ans. b

Explanation: Normal laboratory range of CPK is 20–200 IU/L. There are four isoenzymes of which CK-MM is specific to skeletal muscles, CK-MB1 and two specific to cardiac muscles and CK-BB for the brain.

Its half-life is 36 hours. Serum CPK levels begin to rise within 2–12 hours after the injury peaks within 1–5 days. It declines after 3–5 days in the absence of muscle injury.

Suggested Reading
1. Khan FY. Rhabdomyolysis: a review of the literature. Neth J Med. 2009;67(9):272-83.

Q.28. Which of the following laboratory abnormalities is not a part of the process of rhabdomyolysis?
a. Hyperkalemia
b. Hypercalcemia
c. Hyperphosphatemia
d. Elevated LDH

Ans. b

Explanation: Breakdown of tissues causes third spacing of the extracellular fluid into the myocytes. Disruption of the cell membrane results in release of intracellular ions such as potassium and phosphate causing elevation of these two electrolytes. The pathophysiology is also compounded by influx of calcium into the myocytes causing hypocalcemia. So, hypocalcemia may be a common dyselectrolytemia seen in patients with rhabdomyolysis.

Suggested Reading
1. Gabow PA, Kaehny WD, Kelleher SP. The spectrum of rhabdomyolysis. Medicine (Baltimore). 1982;61(3):141-52.

Q.29. Which of the following factors is not a predictor of AKI in patient with rhabdomyolysis?
   a. Hypocalcemia
   b. Serum level of CPK
   c. State of hydration
   d. Increased serum phosphate
   e. All of the above

Ans. e

Explanation: Acute kidney injury (AKI) in patients with rhabdomyolysis can be multifactorial. The possible causes include hypovolemia, drugs, dehydration, hypoperfusion, and pigment-induced distal tubular damage. AKI is the most common complication of rhabdomyolysis. The risk of AKI is less in patients with CPK levels < 20,000 IU/L. Patients with CK levels of >40,000 IU/L have an increased risk of acute kidney injury. The best predictors for developing acute kidney injury appear to be a state of hydration, high initial serum creatine, low serum bicarbonate, low serum calcium, and increased serum phosphate. Hypoalbuminemia and increased BUN have also been associated with the development of acute kidney injury.

Suggested Reading
1. Trof RJ, Di Maggio F, Leemreis J, Groeneveld AB. Biomarkers of acute renal injury and renal failure. Shock. 2006;26(3):245-53.
2. Wakabayashi Y, Kikuno T, Ohwada T, Kikawada R. Rapid fall in blood myoglobin in massive rhabdomyolysis and acute renal failure. Intensive Care Med. 1994;20(2):109-12.

Q.30. In patients with nontraumatic rhabdomyolysis, which of the following treatment strategies is not recommended?
   a. Hydration and fluid resuscitation with nonpotassium-containing crystalloid
   b. Mannitol
   c. Forced alkaline diuresis
   d. Loop diuretics

Ans. b

Explanation: Adequate fluid resuscitation with nonpotassium-based crystalloid remains the crux of the treatment.

Management includes removing the offending agent at the time of diagnosis and titration of IV fluids to maintain a urine output of 200–300 mL/h with serial monitoring of CPK levels daily to document downtrend levels.

Creatine phosphokinase levels of >5,000 IU/L have increased the risk of the development of AKI. Forceful alkaline diuresis can be considered in severe cases where the CPK is >30,000 IU/L in the absence of oliguria, anuria, and acute kidney injury. Mannitol is *not commonly* used in nontraumatic rhabdomyolysis. Its role even in traumatic rhabdomyolysis is controversial, but still used in circumstance wherein AKI is not present.

Loop diuretics can be considered in the setting of volume overload state from aggressive fluid resuscitation. Patients who remain oliguric, anuric even with aggressive fluid resuscitation, developed AKI should be considered for hemodialysis.

Suggested Reading
1. de Meijer AR, Fikkers BG, de Keijzer MH, van Engelen BG, Drenth JP. Serum creatine kinase as predictor of clinical course in rhabdomyolysis: a 5-year intensive care survey. Intensive Care Med. 2003;29(7):1121-5.

CHAPTER 26

High-resolution Computed Tomography and Magnetic Resonance Imaging

Aditya Kumar Bang

Q.1. A 70-year-old man post Ivor Lewis esophagectomy whose postoperative course was complicated by a hospital-acquired pneumonia is now once again in respiratory distress and has a PaO$_2$ of 8.7 kPa on 15 liters via a nonrebreathing bag and is hypotensive and tachycardic with a blood pressure of 85/59 mm Hg and heart rate of 110 beats/min. His comorbidities include a history of hypertension and chronic obstructive pulmonary disease (COPD). This is a midthoracic computed tomography (CT) image following enteral contrast performed after intensive care admission. What does it demonstrate?

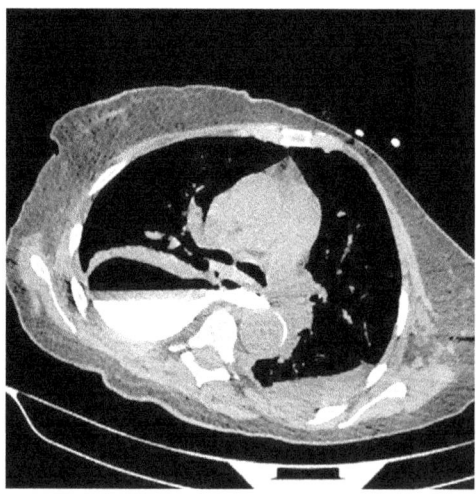

a. Lung abscess
b. Anastomotic leak with underlying consolidation
c. Empyema thoracis
d. None of the above

Ans. b

Explanation: The CT shows bright white enteral contrast leaking from the distal esophagus into a cavity in the right lower part of the thorax. There is noncontrast fluid in the cavity with a clear air–fluid interface. There is some consolidation around the cavity on the right and in the dependent left lung.

Suggested Reading
1. Rakita D, Newatia A, Hines JJ, Siegel DN, Friedman B. Spectrum of CT findings in rupture and impending rupture of abdominal aortic aneurysms. Radiographics. 2007 Mar;27(2):497-507.

Q.2. A 60-year-old man with a history of weight loss and abdominal distension for last 3 months attends the emergency department with acute onset breathlessness. His SpO_2 is 87% on air. This ECG has been done 30 minutes ago.

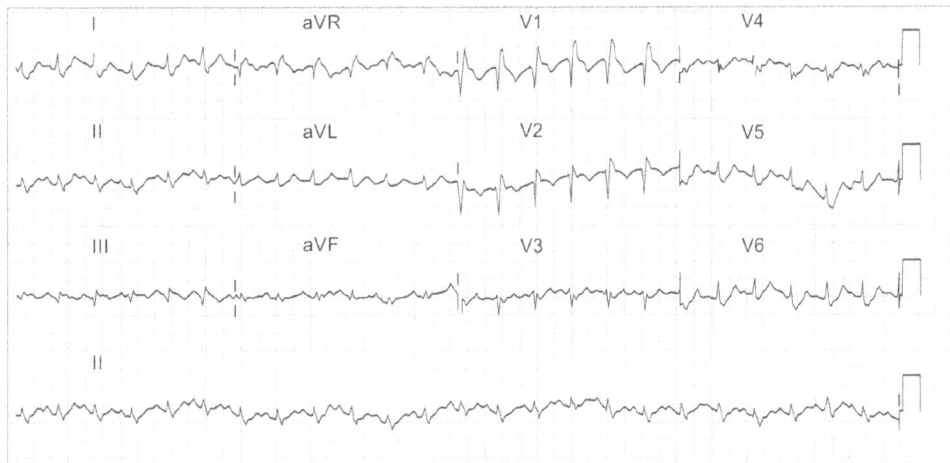

His chest X-ray is unremarkable. Echocardiography shows severe right ventricular (RV) dilatation. His blood pressure is 115/65 mm Hg and there are no signs suggestive of him being in shock. A CT pulmonary angiogram is performed. What is the diagnosis?

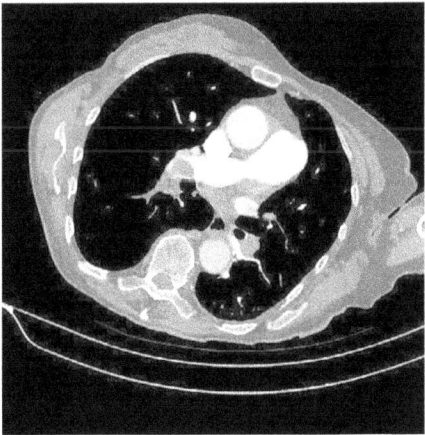

a. Massive pulmonary embolism
b. Low-risk pulmonary embolism
c. Submassive pulmonary embolism
d. None of the above

Ans. c

Explanation: American Heart Association definitions of massive, submassive, and low-risk pulmonary embolism (PE) and associated mortality.

PE classification	Definition	Mortality
Massive	Acute PE with sustained hypotension (90 mm Hg systolic). 15 minutes or requiring inotropic support	25–65% (62)
Submassive	Systolic pressure 90 mm Hg and either: • RV dysfunction (CT, BNP/pro-BNP, and ECG changes) or • Myocardial necrosis (elevated troponins)	3% (20)
Low risk	Absence of hypotension, RV dysfunction, and myocardial necrosis	1% (20)

(BNP: brain natriuretic peptide; CT: computed tomography; ECG: electrocardiography; PE: pulmonary embolism; RV: right ventricular)

Suggested Reading
1. Sista AK, Kuo WT, Schiebler M, Madoff DC. Stratification, imaging, and management of acute massive and submassive pulmonary embolism. Radiology. 2017;284(1):5-24.

Q.3. A 65-year-old man is admitted to the intensive care unit with history of drowsiness and altered behavior. The only significant history is that of regular alcohol intake for more than a decade. A CT brain scan performed on admission was reported as normal. The results of the cerebrospinal fluid (CSF) below:

	CSF sample	Normal range
Color	Clear	Clear
WBC (per mm^3)	250	<5
Differential	Lymphocytes	
CSF plasma:glucose ratio	69%	66% (approximately)
Protein g/L	0.84	<0.45

His MRI scan shows the following. What is the diagnosis?

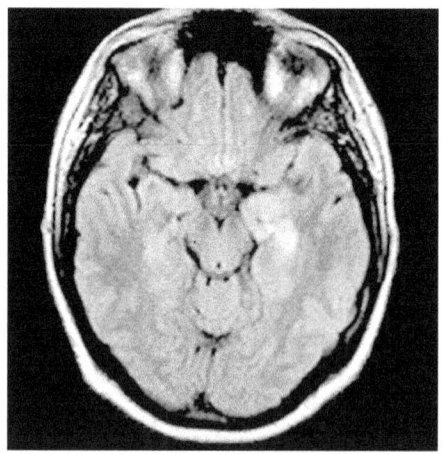

a. CMV encephalitis
b. Japanese encephalitis
c. Herpes simplex encephalitis
d. VZV encephalitis

Ans. c

Explanation: Classical findings of herpes simplex virus (HSV) encephalitis on the magnetic resonance imaging (MRI) are the appearance manifests of bilateral asymmetrical involvement of the limbic system, inferolateral frontal lobes, and medial temporal lobes. MRI fluid-attenuated inversion recovery (FLAIR) image here demonstrates a hyperintense signal in bilateral medial temporal lobe, predominantly involving the left hippocampus.

Suggested Reading
1. Granerod J, Davies NWS, Mukonoweshuro W, Mehta A, Das K, Lim M, et al; UK Public Health England Aetiology of Encephalitis Study Group. Neuroimaging in encephalitis: analysis of imaging findings and interobserver agreement. Clin Radiol. 2016;71(10):1050-8.

Q.4. A 70-year-old man with a history of hypertension and long-term smoking has presented to the emergency department with acute-onset back pain and signs of impaired perfusion. He gives history of similar episodes of intermittent back pain resolving spontaneously. A computed tomography (CT) scan is performed, which shows the following:

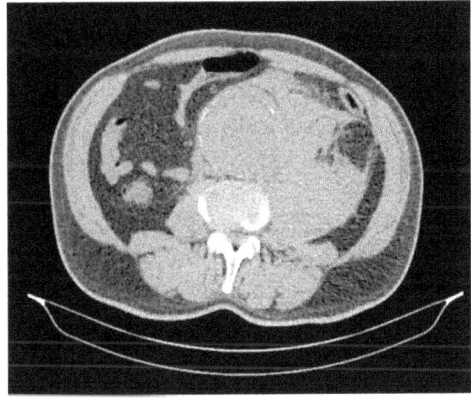

What is the diagnosis and name the sign seen on the CT scan?
a. Unruptured aortic aneurysm
b. Ruptured aortic aneurysm showing hyperattenuation crescent sign
c. Ruptured aortic aneurysm showing draped aorta sign
d. Swirl sign

Ans. b

Explanation: Hyperattenuation crescent sign is an area of increased attenuation within the aortic aneurysmal mural thrombus, can be demonstrated on plain CT images. This is caused by the insinuation of fresh blood into the mural thrombus and aortic wall.

Suggested Reading
1. Rakita D, Newatia A, Hines JJ, Siegel DN, Friedman B. Spectrum of CT findings in rupture and impending rupture of abdominal aortic aneurysms. Radiographics. 2007;27(2):497-507.

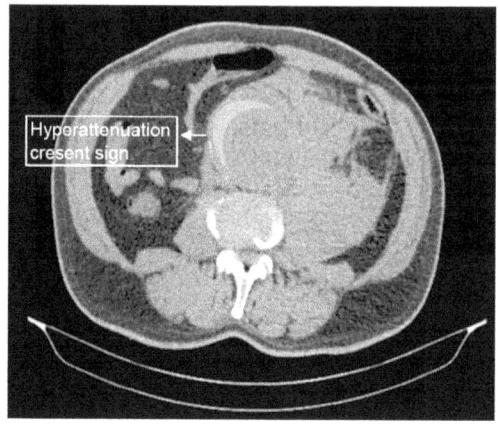

Q.5. A 66-year-old, known case of COPD, female patient recently admitted and treated for severe COVID-19 disease gets admitted on 15th day of her discharge with complaints of progressive dyspnea. Age-adjusted point-of-care brain natriuretic peptide (BNP) and D-dimer are reported to be within normal limits. On examination, patients room air saturation is 82% and auscultation reveals diffuse rhonchi with decreased air entry bilaterally. Patient is started on oxygen therapy with long-acting beta-2 agonist (LABA), steroids, and appropriate intravenous (IV) antibiotics. Sputum for Gram staining and AFB staining and culture sensitivity are sent. Gram stain and acid-fast bacillus (AFB) stain are reported as negative. Patient remains symptomatic after 48 hours of appropriate medical therapy. A high-resolution computed tomography (HRCT) chest reveals the following:

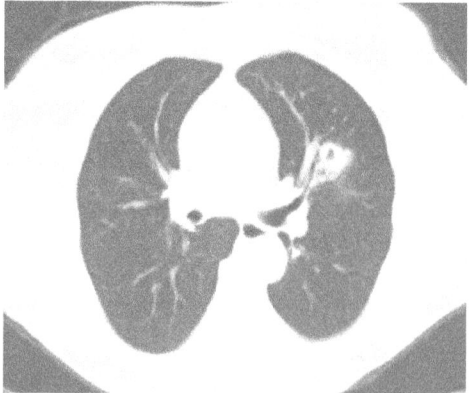

What is the next appropriate step?
a. Serum galactomannan and IV voriconazole
b. Beta-D-glucan and IV echinocandins
c. To plan for fiber-optic bronchoscopy and biopsy
d. Continue IV antibiotics and observe for 48 hours

Ans. a

Explanation: Initiation of antifungal therapy on the basis of typical CT findings for invasive aspergillosis, which include halo sign, cavitation, or macronodules, is associated with better response to treatment and improved outcomes.

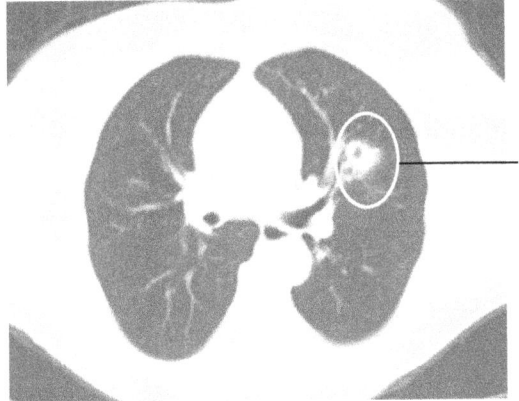

HRCT chest showing macronodule with cavitation and halo sign suggestive of invasive aspergillosis

Suggested Reading
1. Franquet T, Muller NL, Giménez A, Guembe P, de la Torre J, Bagué S. Spectrum of pulmonary aspergillosis: histologic, clinical, and radiologic findings. Radiographics. 2001;21(4):825-37.

Q.6. A 62-year-old male visits the emergency department with history of abdominal pain and vomiting for last 72 hours. His abdomen is distended without any signs of peritonitis. He has been assessed by the emergency physician who has ordered a CT scan of his abdomen. His vital are as follows: heart rate (HR) 120 beats/min, blood pressure (BP) 100/60 mm Hg, respiratory rate (RR) 24 breaths/min, and oxygen saturation (SpO_2) 93% on room air. His CT abdomen shows the following picture:

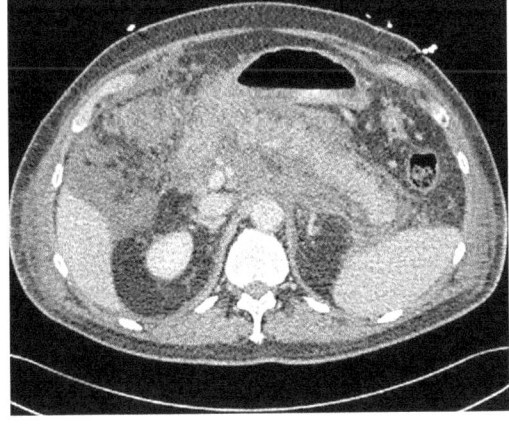

(a) Which features in the image are associated with increased severity of acute pancreatitis?
  a. Extensive fat stranding
  b. Peripancreatic fluid collection

c. Necrosis of the pancreas
d. All of the above
e. None of the above

After 3 weeks of getting discharged, the patient presents to the hospital with complaints of abdominal distention. He is asymptomatic otherwise. His CT abdomen shows the following:

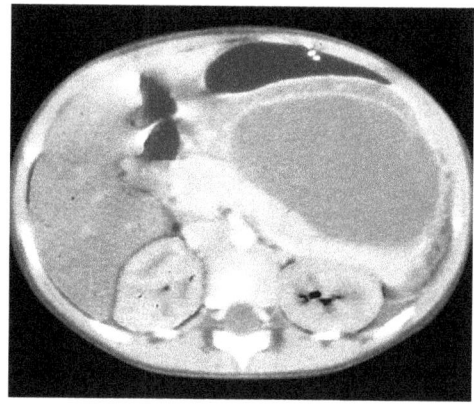

(b) What is the next best step?
a. CT-guided cyst aspiration
b. Exploratory laparotomy to excise the cyst
c. Observation only

Ans. (a). d.

Explanation: Features, if found on CT, associated with an increased severity of pancreatitis are:
- Extensive fat stranding
- Peripancreatic fluid collections
- Necrosis of the pancreas

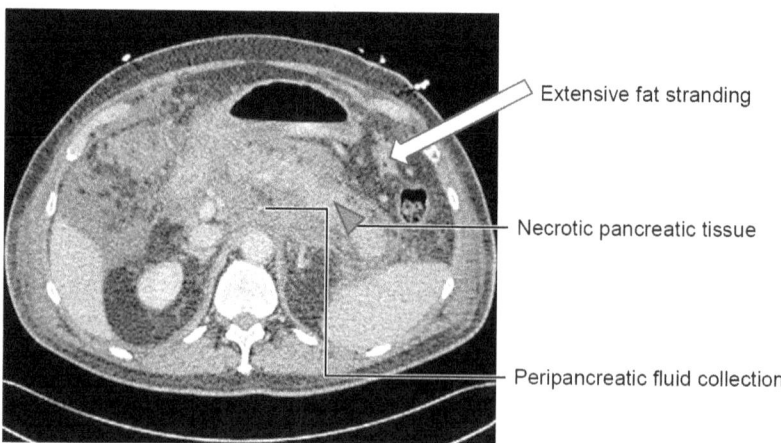

Ans. (b). c.

Explanation: Asymptomatic pancreatic and/or extrapancreatic necrosis and/or pseudocysts should not be treated regardless of their size, location, and/or extension. In asymptomatic patients who show signs of infection in the necrotic areas of the pancreas, interventions namely, surgical, endoscopic, and radiological should be delayed, as mortality is reduced. One should consider therapeutic antibiotics for worsening sepsis if this is indicated after cultures have been sent.

Suggested Reading
1. Raghuwanshi S, Gupta R, Vyas MM, Sharma R. CT evaluation of acute pancreatitis and its prognostic correlation with CT severity index. J Clin Diagn Res. 2016;10(6):TC06-11.

Q.7. Look at the computed tomography (CT) scan:

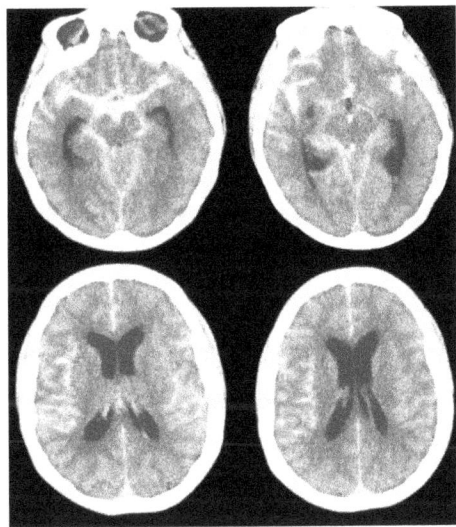

Which of the following scales can be used to predict worst outcomes in terms of delayed cerebral ischemia?
a. World Federation of Neurosurgeons (WFNS) grading
b. Hunt and Hess scale
c. Glasgow coma scale
d. VASOGRADE scale

Ans. d

Explanation: In a multiethnic cohort of patients with aneurysmal subarachnoid hemorrhage (aSAH), VASOGRADE-Green predicted the absence of delayed cerebral ischemia (DCI) and good clinical outcome at discharge with very high specificity, and patients in this category might be selected for early intensive care unit (ICU) discharge, minimizing costs and medical complications associated with prolonged hospital stay. On the other hand, patients categorized as VASOGRADE-Yellow and VASOGRADE-Red were at the highest risk for DCI. They should, therefore, be selected as a priority for care in high-volume aSAH centers, being aggressively monitored for DCI at the ICU.

Such stratification methods are crucial, especially in countries with low financial resources and high healthcare services demand.

VASOGRADE	WFNS	Modified Fisher scale
Green	1–2	1–2
Yellow	1–3	3–4
Red	4–5	Any

(WFNS: World Federation of Neurosurgical Societies)

Suggested Reading

1. de Oliveira Manoel AL, Jaja BN, Germans MR, Yan H, Qian W, Kouzmina E, et al. The VASOGRADE: a simple grading scale for prediction of delayed cerebral ischemia after subarachnoid hemorrhage. Stroke. 2015;46(7):1826-31.

Q.8. A 65-year-old female patient with diabetes was admitted to the emergency department, after experiencing fever and left back pain for 10 days. The following was discovered during a physical examination: temperature 100.2°F, HR 120 beats/min, and BP 154/83 mm Hg. Pain was elicited by percussion in the left flank region. Her laboratory findings were as below:

- *White blood cell (WBC) count:* 11.17×10^9/L
- *Absolute neutrophil count (ANC):* 10.69×10^9/L
- *Hemoglobin:* 81 g/L
- *Platelets:* 129×10^9/L
- *C-reactive protein (CRP):* 244.90 mg/L
- *Procalcitonin (PCT):* 4.5 ng/mL
- *Albumin:* 26.5 g/L
- *Serum creatinine:* 155 mmol/L
- *BSL:* 26.7 mmol/L
- *Fibrinogen:* 429.1 mg/dL

Her abdominal CT revealed the following:

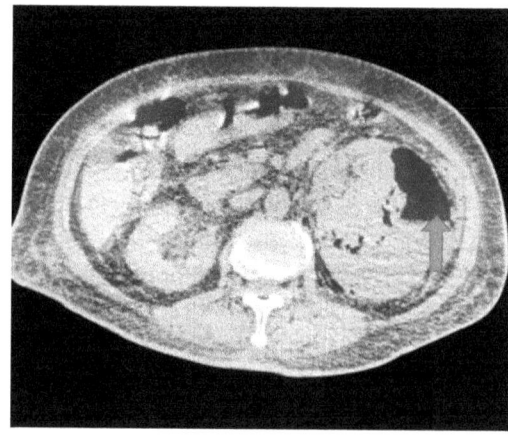

How would you like to manage this case?
a. IV antibiotics and IV hydration
b. IV antibiotics with hydration and percutaneous drainage (PCD)
c. Total nephrectomy
d. PCD followed by nephrectomy

Ans. b

Explanation: Radiological classification of emphysematous pyelonephritis (EPN):

Class	Radiological Findings
1	Gas in the collecting systems only (also known as emphysematous pyelitis)
2	Gas in the renal parenchyma without extension into the extrarenal space
3A	Extension of gas or abscess into the perinephric space
3B	Extension of gas or abscess into the pararenal space
4	Bilateral EPN or solitary kidney with EPN

Flowchart for management of EPN:

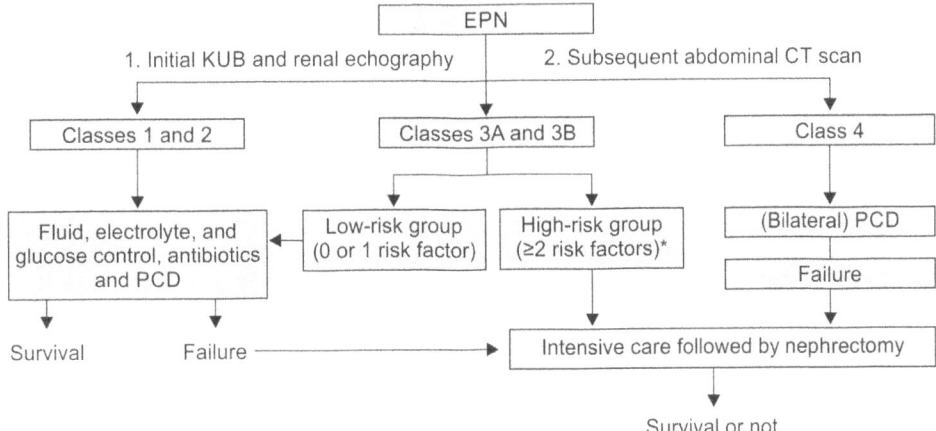

(CT: computed tomography; EPN: emphysematous pyelonephritis; KUB: Kidneys, Ureters, and Bladder; PCD: percutaneous drainage)

Asterisk (*) indicates the presence of two or more of the following risk factors:
1. Thrombocytopenia
2. Acute renal failure
3. Disturbance of consciousness
4. Shock

Suggested Reading
1. Huang JJ, Tseng CC. Emphysematous pyelonephritis: clinicoradiological classification, management, prognosis, and pathogenesis. Archives of internal medicine. 2000;160(6): 797-805.

Q.9. A 34-year-old male patient is shifted to your institution for progressive dyspnea followed by multiple episodes of GTCS for which he gets intubated and ventilated. The patient had suffered an injury 48 hours back secondary to a heavy object falling on his pelvis and lower extremity. His abdomen and pelvic CT revealed multiple fracture in his pelvis bone, no solid organ or hollow viscus injury to structures in the abdomen. He was diagnosed with fracture shaft of left femur which was immobilized before the patient was shifted to your hospital. Patients MRI brain and HRCT chest revealed the following:

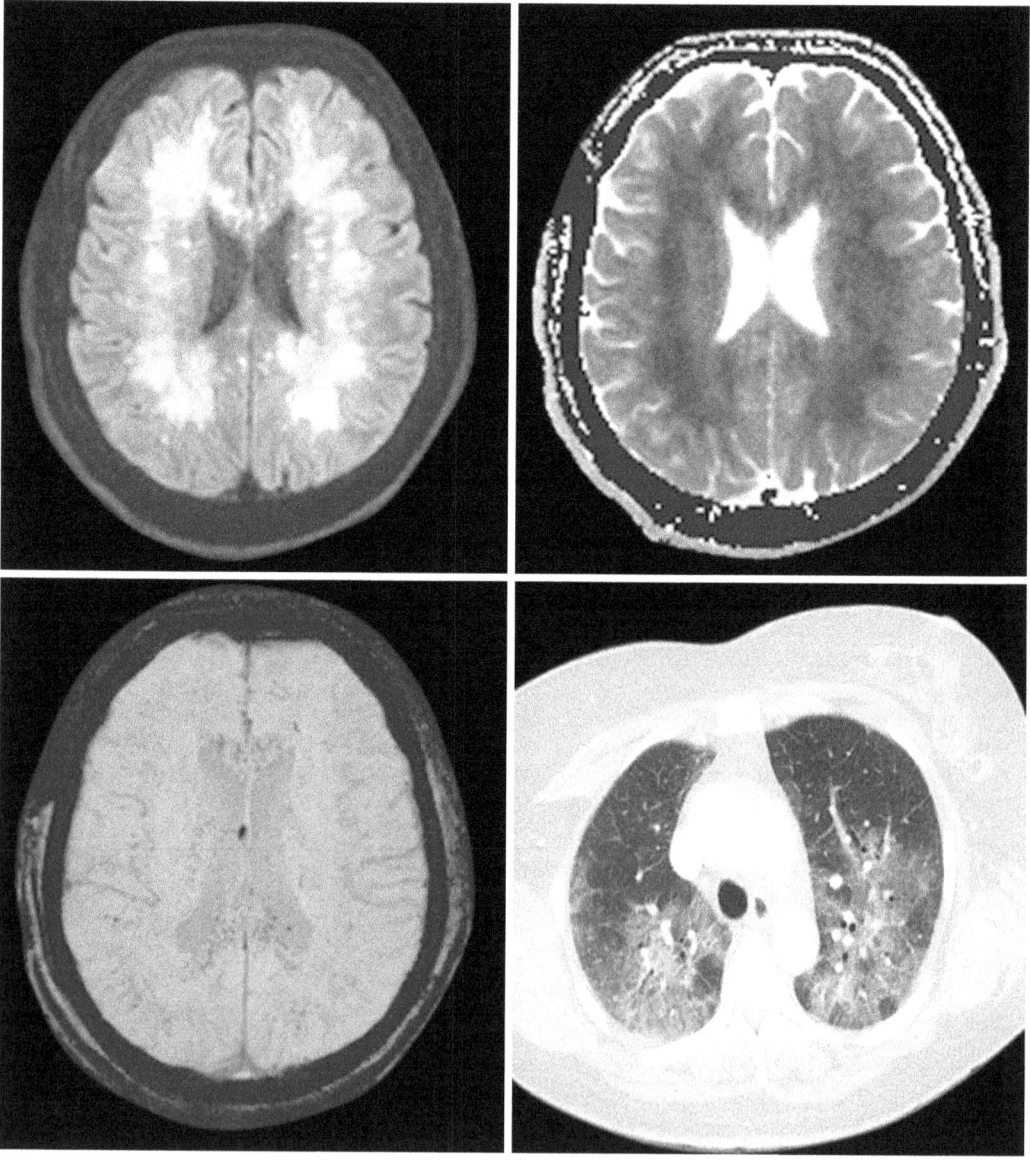

What is the diagnosis?
a. Diffuse axonal injury with lung contusion secondary to trauma
b. Fat embolism syndrome
c. Acute ischemic infarct
d. Infective endocarditis

Ans. b

Explanation: Fat embolism syndrome is a systemic manifestation of dissemination of fat molecules or globules in microcirculation. Traumatic causes of fat embolism syndrome are more common than nontraumatic causes. Trauma as a cause of fat embolism syndrome can occur from the fracture of the long bones, specifically:
- Femur
- Tibia
- Pelvis

Gurd et al. in 1970 and later Wilson in 1974 put forward the following diagnostic criterion requiring two major criteria or at least one major criteria and four minor criteria.

Major criteria:
- Petechial rash
- Respiratory insufficiency
- Cerebral involvement in nonhead injury patients

Minor criteria:
- Fever >38.5°C
- Tachycardia heart rate >110 beats/min
- Retinal involvement
- Jaundice
- Renal signs
- Anemia
- Thrombocytopenia
- High erythrocyte sedimentation rate
- Fat macroglobulinemia

Radiological findings:
- *HRCT chest:* Commonly reported findings include:
  - May show areas of consolidation
  - *Ground-glass opacities:* With or without interlobular septal thickening, occasionally appearing as a geographic pattern 7
  - *Small (<1 cm) nodules (can sometimes be ground glass-like) of various sizes:* Presumed to represent alveolar edema, inflamed intrapulmonary lymph nodes, or hemorrhage secondary to the fat embolism syndrome
  - *Fat-attenuating filling defects in pulmonary arteries:* Rarely described in nonfulminant fat embolism syndrome

- *MRI brain:* The distribution of changes in the brain is bilaterally symmetric and predominantly in the subcortical and deep white matter, including subcortical U-fibers, corpus callosum, and internal capsule. Susceptibility-weighted image (SWI) and diffusion-weighted imaging (DWI) are the most sensitive sequences. The distribution and pattern are variable and depend on how extensive embolization is, but often has an external watershed distribution (similar to other microembolisms).
  - DWI:
    - *Early (most common at 1-4 days):* Scattered punctate foci of cytotoxic edema (starfield pattern)
    - *Later (most common at 5-14 days):* Confluent areas of cytotoxic edema in the white matter
  - SWI: Profuse microhemorrhages in the white matter (walnut kernel pattern):
    - T2/FLAIR—may show small areas of high signal intensity indicating vasogenic edema.
    - T1—corresponding focal regions may show low T1 signal.
    - T1 C+—some of the areas of vasogenic may enhance.

Suggested Reading
1. Adeyinka A, Pierre L. Fat embolism.

Q.10. A 58-year-old female, with history of diabetes, hypertension, post-return of spontaneous circulation (ROSC) status, after 48 hours of optimization in the intensive care unit was seen to not follow commands once she was weaned off the sedation. An urgent MRI brain was done for the lady which showed the following:

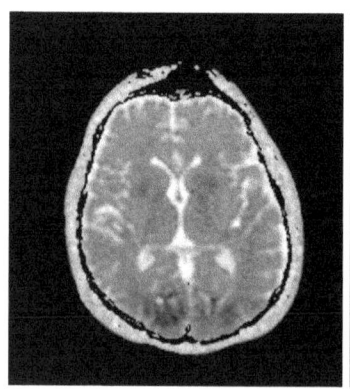
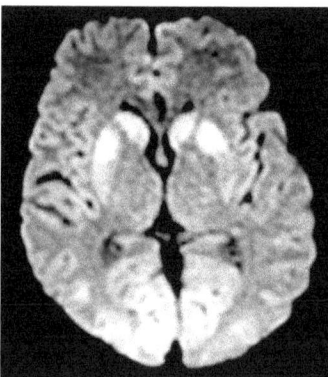
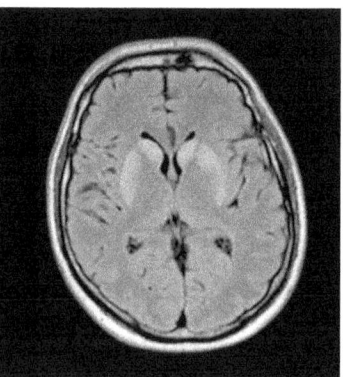

What is the diagnosis?
a. Diffuse axonal injury
b. Multi-infarct state
c. Hypoxic–ischemic encephalopathy
d. Nontraumatic fat embolism

Ans. c

Explanation: *Hypoxic–ischemic encephalopathy* is seen in the following conditions:
- *Children*: Asphyxiation or drowning
- *Adults*: Secondary to cardiac arrest or cerebrovascular disease

Affects the gray matter first which are highly susceptible to hypoxia due to higher metabolic oxygen and glucose demands. Structures involved are as follows:
- Basal ganglia
- Thalami
- Cerebral cortex
- Cerebellum
- Hippocampus

Diffusion-weighted MR imaging is the earliest imaging modality to become positive, usually within the first few hours after a hypoxic–ischemic event due to early cytotoxic edema. During the first 24 hours, there may be restricted diffusion in the cerebellar hemispheres, basal ganglia, or cerebral cortex (in particular, the peri-rolandic and occipital cortices). The thalami, brainstem, or hippocampi may also be involved. Diffusion-weighted imaging abnormalities usually pseudonormalize by the end of the first week.

In the early subacute period (24 hours to 2 weeks), conventional T2-weighted images typically become positive and show increased signal intensity and swelling of the injured gray matter structures.

Suggested Reading
1. Tabban HA, Hassan IA, ABHS-R, Salem KY, Salem TA, Ibrahim S, et al. Hypoxic Ischemic Encephalopathy MRI Findings and Patterns Review, Revisited. OMICS J Radiol 2022;11(12): 415.

Q.11. **A 39-year-old male patient with history of severe headache, dull aching in nature on the left side of the hemisphere for last 5 days, was brought to the emergency department. He had associated history of intermittent confusion and drowsiness for last 24 hours. No significant history of fever with meningismus was elicited. His MRI brain showed the following:**

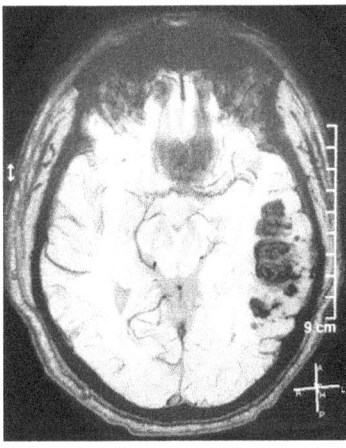
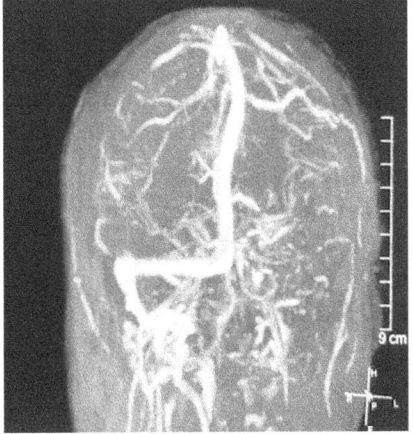

What is the next best immediate step of management?
a. Mechanical thrombectomy
b. LMWH
c. Unfractionated heparin
d. Intravenous thrombolysis
e. NOAC

Ans. b

Explanation: The 2017 European Stroke Organization guidelines for the diagnosis and treatment of cerebral venous sinus thrombosis (CVST), endorsed by the European Academy of Neurology, recommend heparin at therapeutic dosage to treat adult patients with CVST, including those with an intracerebral hemorrhage at baseline. The guidelines suggest use of low-molecular-weight heparin (LMWH) instead of unfractionated heparin (UFH).

No recommendation was made for intravenous thrombolysis. The guidelines recommend not exposing patients who have a low pretreatment poor risk of outcome to aggressive therapies such as thrombolysis.

For selected patients with progressive thrombosis despite therapeutic anticoagulation, mechanical thrombectomy may be a treatment options at center experienced with these methods. A randomized controlled trial (RCT) named thrombolysis or anticoagulation for cerebral venous thrombosis (TO-ACT) failed to show benefit of endovascular treatment over anticoagulation in patients with acute CVT and at least one clinical factor for acute deterioration which involves coma, mental status disturbances, CVT involving the deep venous system, and intracerebral hemorrhage.

Suggested Reading
1. Ulivi L, Squitieri M, Cohen H, Cowley P, Werring DJ. Cerebral venous thrombosis: a practical guide. Pract Neurol. 2020;20(5):356-67.

Q.12. A 67-year-old male, chronic smoker, attended the pulmonology clinic with complaints of increased fatigue. He stated, "I become short of breath when I bend over. It lasts about 60 seconds, with some dizziness and head pain." Review of systems is positive for neck swelling noted in the morning, hoarseness of voice during the past week, purplish discoloration across his chest (as shown in below Figure), thick vessels under his tongue, increased dyspnea on exertion, difficulty swallowing, and a dry cough lasting over a week. Pertinent physical findings are as follows—blood pressure = 124/64 mm Hg, respirations = 20 breaths/min, pulse = 72 beats/min regular, and temperature = 97.8°C; diffuse edema in the neck; dilated, engorged blood vessels on the chest and under the tongue; and edema in the right arm and hand. He underwent a CT chest with contrast which revealed the following:

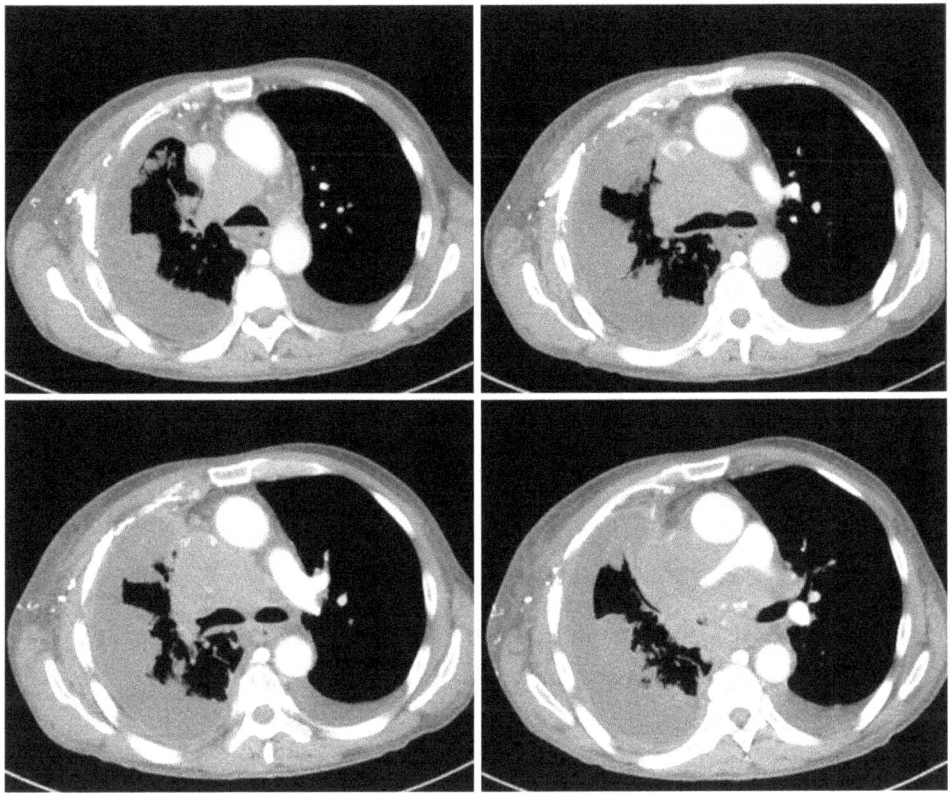

What is the patient suffering from?
a. SVC syndrome
b. Pulmonary thromboembolism
c. Parapneumonic pleural effusion with underlying consolidation

Ans. a

Explanation: Superior vena cava syndrome (SVC) comprises a collection of clinical signs and symptoms secondary to obstruction of blood flow through the SVC. Malignancy being the most common cause accounts for approximately 70% of cases. Recently, however, the incidence of SVC syndrome secondary to central venous catheters and pacemaker or defibrillator leads has been on the rise. Symptoms include facial and neck edema, distended neck and chest veins, and dizziness, especially when bending forward. Patients may also present with neurological symptoms (blurred vision, headache, and decreased consciousness), laryngopharyngeal symptoms (dyspnea, swelling of the tongue), upper extremity edema, and facial edema. Patients describe worsening of their symptoms in the supine position. In rare cases, proximal esophageal varices may be observed.

In this case, the patient has a right-sided mediastinal mass that is compressing the right main bronchus, right pulmonary artery, and SVC leading to the patient's symptoms and findings on the CT scan.

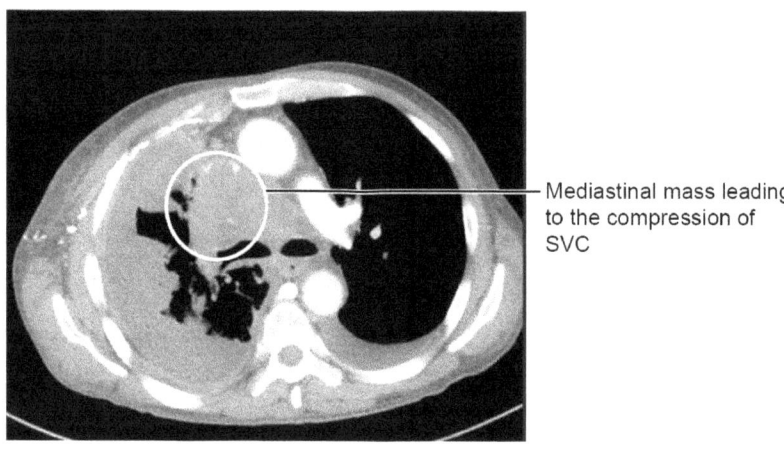

Mediastinal mass leading to the compression of SVC

Classification of SVC obstruction based on location and severity:

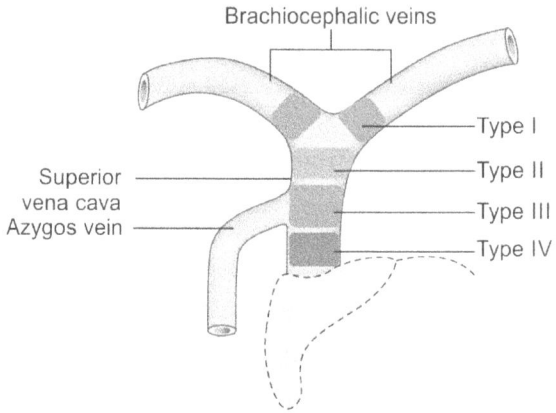

Lesion location	Grade A severity	Grade B severity	Grade C severity
Type I: Bilateral brachiocephalic vein occlusion with or without supra-azygos SVC	Moderate-to-severe (50–90%)	Pre-occlusive (>90%)	Totally occluded (100%)
Type II: Supra-azygos SVC without brachiocephalic involvement	Moderate-to-severe (50–90%)	Pre-occlusive (>90%)	Totally occluded (100%)
Type III: Azygos SVC	Moderate-to-severe (50–90%)	Pre-occlusive (>90%)	Totally occluded (100%)
Type IV: Infra-azygos SVC	Moderate-to-severe (50–90%)	Pre-occlusive (90%)	Totally occluded (100%)

Management algorithm of SVC syndrome:

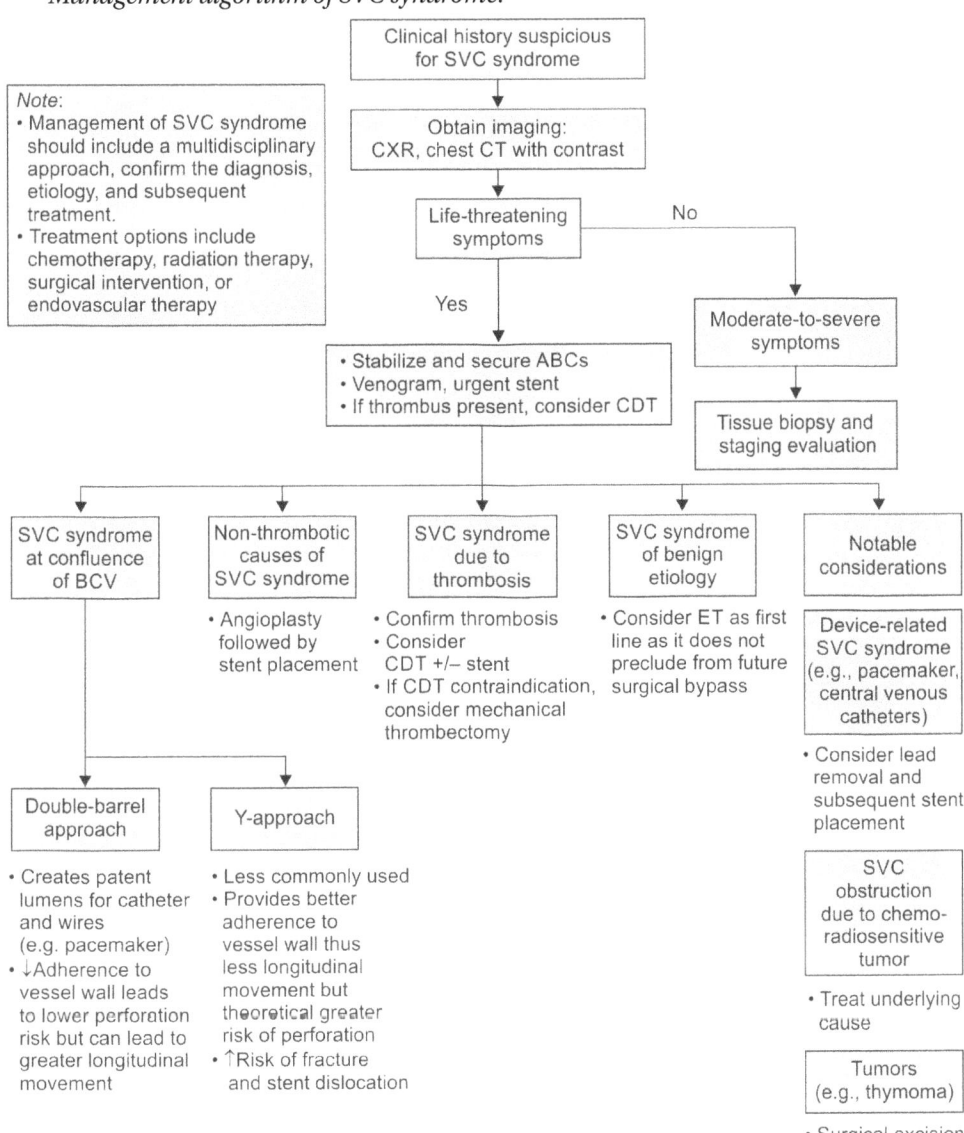

(BCV: brachiocephalic vein; CT: computed tomography; CDT: catheter-directed thrombolysis; CXR: chest X-ray; SVC: superior vena cava)

Suggested Reading
1. Azizi AH, Shafi I, Shah N, Rosenfield K, Schainfeld R, Sista A, et al. Superior Vena Cava Syndrome. JACC Cardiovasc Interv. 2020;13(24):2896-910.

Q.13. A 17-year-old female attended ER with an alleged history of RTA secondary to skid and fall from two-wheeler. On arrival her clinical parameters were as HR 170 beats/min, BP 70/40 mm Hg, RR 34 breaths/min, GCS 12/15, and BSL 272 mg/dL. On examination, the following findings were elicited:

- Abrasions over:
  - Epigastric region
  - Right thigh
- Bluish discoloration and swelling over left forearm
- Swelling and puncture wound over the left knee

Patient is intubated and ventilated, vasopressors are started, and massive transfusion protocol is initiated. Patient is shifted to the CT gantry which reveals the following:

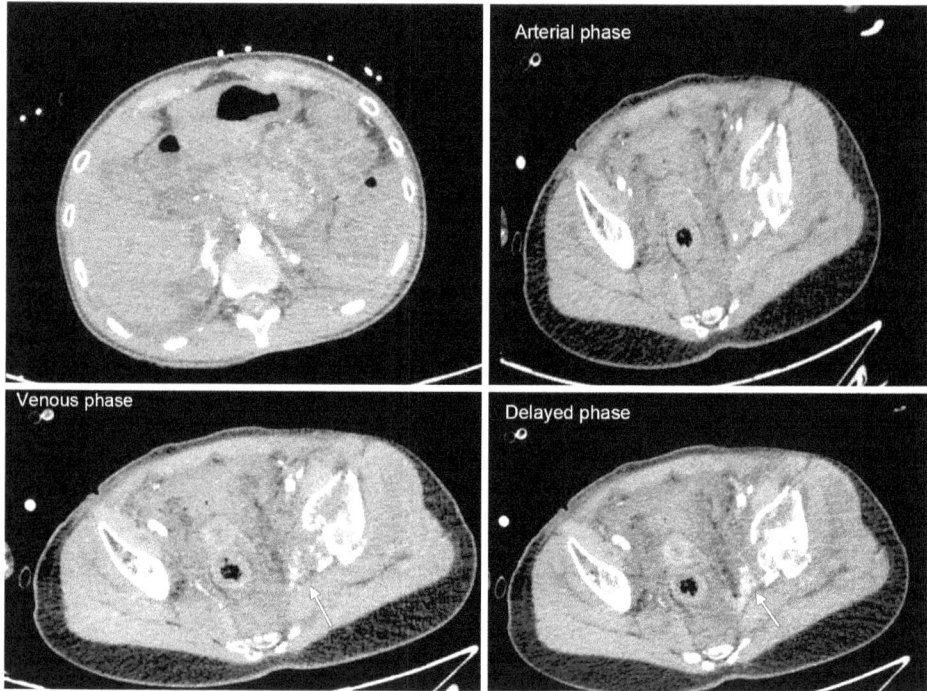

How would you proceed with the management of the patient?
a. Exploratory laparotomy for bleeding control
b. Angioembolization for bleeding control
c. Stabilization in ICU followed by definitive surgery
d. Correction of coagulopathy and close observation

Ans. b

Explanation: *World Society of Emergency Surgery (WSES) gradation of pelvic injuries*:
- *Minor pelvic injuries: WSES grade I (should be formatted in bold and cursive as the other grade of classification)* includes anteroposterior compression I (APC I), lateral compression I (LC I) hemodynamically stable pelvic ring injuries.
- *Moderate pelvic injuries:*
  - *WSES grade II* includes APC II–III and LC II–III, hemodynamically stable pelvic ring injuries.
  - *WSES grade III* includes VS and CM, hemodynamically stable pelvic ring injuries.

- *Severe pelvic injuries*: WSES grade IV includes any hemodynamically unstable pelvic ring injuries.

WSES algorithm for management of pelvic injuries:

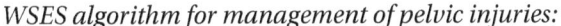

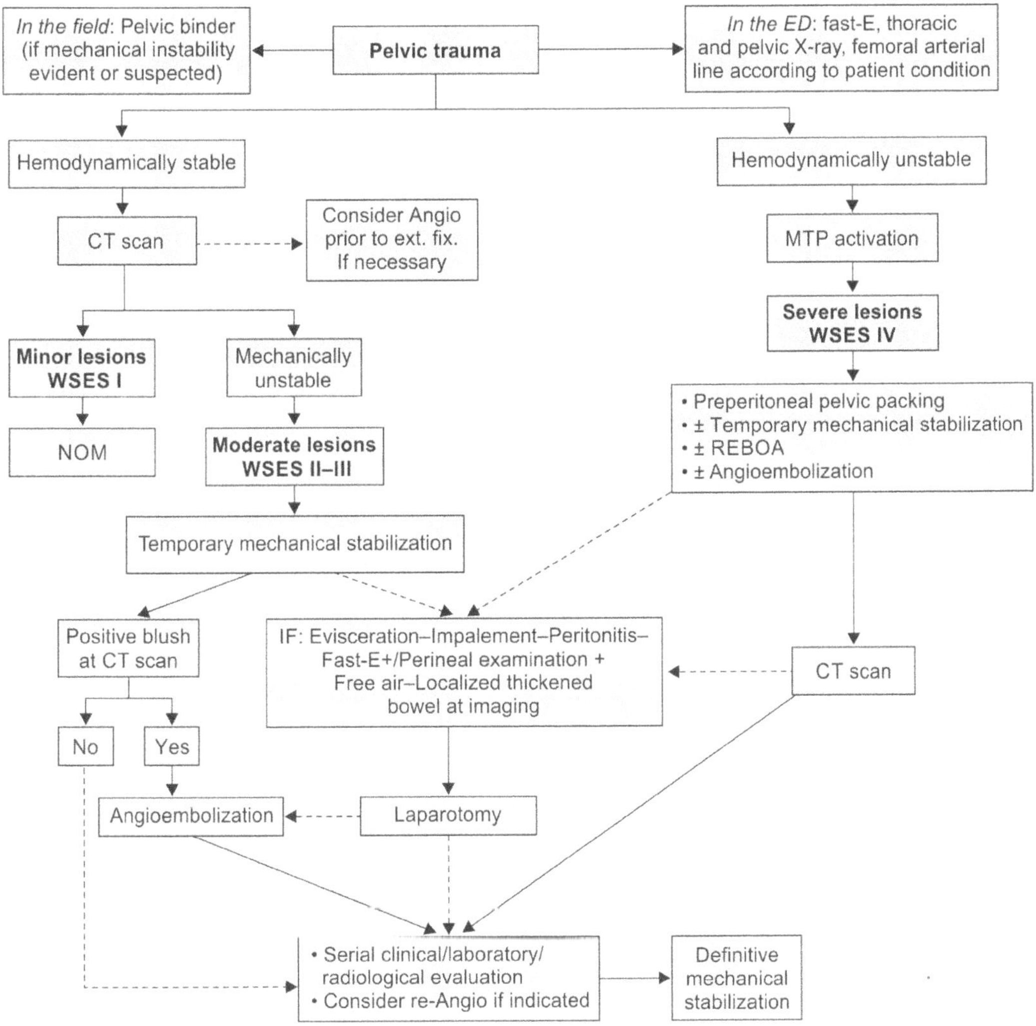

(CT: computed tomography; FAST-E: extended focused assessment with sonography for trauma; REBOA: resuscitative endovascular balloon occlusion of the Aorta; WSES: World Society of Emergency Surgery)

Suggested Reading

1. Coccolini F, Stahel PF, Montori G, Biffl W, Horer TM, Catena F, et al. Pelvic trauma: WSES classification and guidelines. World J Emerg Surg. 2017;12:5.

Q.14. A 50-year-old man, known hypertensive presents with a history of acute-onset back pain radiating to the chest, severe in nature which came on whilst playing squash. His vitals are HR 120 beats/min, BP 120/60 mm Hg, RR 24 breaths/min, and SpO$_2$ 94% on RA. On clinical examination, patient is seen to have unequal pulses in the upper extremity associated with right upper limb hemiparesis. You are informed that the ADD-RS score for the patient is >1. A CT aortogram is done for the patient which reveals the following:

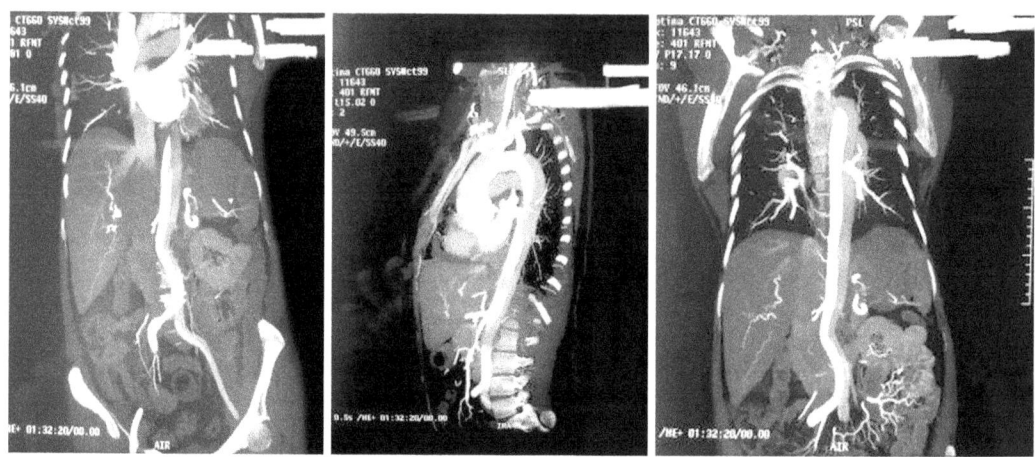

What is the next best management strategy for the patient?
a. Target HR < 70 beats/min and SBP <110 mm Hg
b. Urgent CVTS call for repair of aortic dissection
c. ICU stabilization followed by repair of aortic dissection
d. To counsel relatives for initiating palliative care for the patient

Ans. b

Explanation:

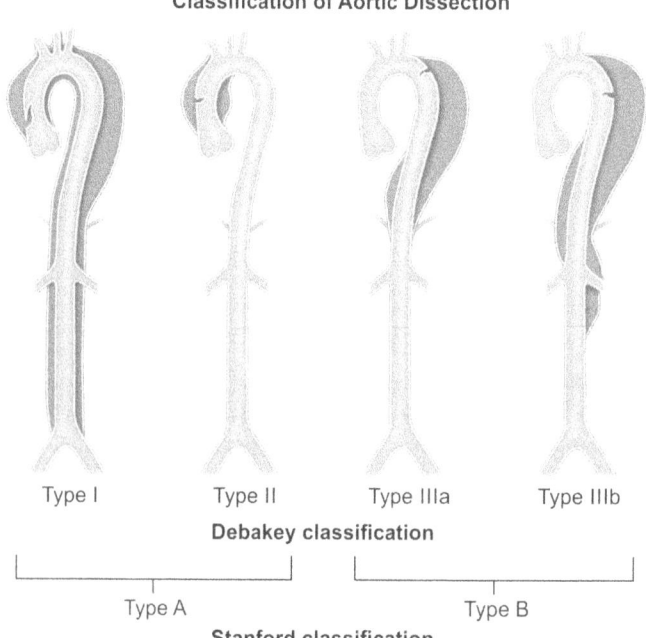

Classification of Aortic Dissection

Management protocol for acute aortic dissection with malperfusion:

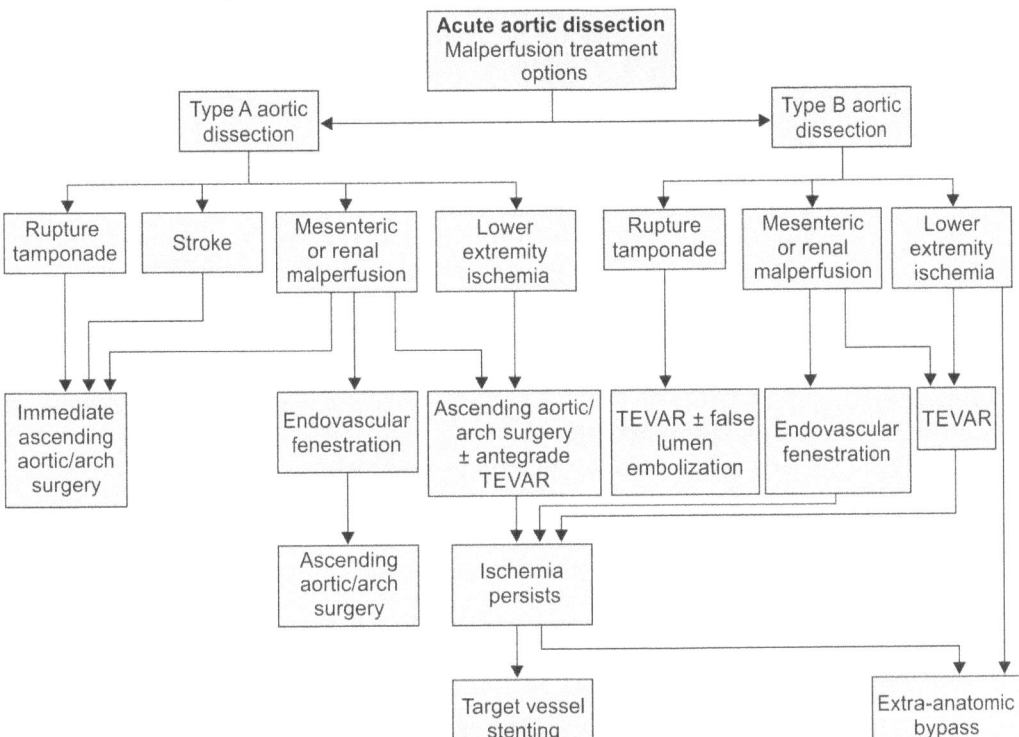

(TEVAR: thoracic endovascular aortic repair)

Suggested Reading

1. Writing Committee Members; Isselbacher EM, Preventza O, Hamilton Black III J, Augoustides JG, Beck AW, Bolen MA, et al. 2022 ACC/AHA Guideline for the diagnosis and management of aortic disease: A report of the American Heart Association/American College of Cardiology Joint Committee on Clinical Practice Guidelines. J Am Coll Cardiol. 2022;80(24):e223-393.

Q.15. An 84-year-old confused man complained of abdominal pain, nausea, and breathlessness. Past medical history was noteworthy for chronic obstructive pulmonary disease with atrial fibrillation on rate control therapy. Examination revealed abdominal distension and periumbilical guarding, associated with mottled appearing legs. Mean blood pressure was >65 mm Hg, SpO_2 was >90% with oxygen therapy, heart rate, and temperature normal. A CT abdomen was performed for the patient which revealed the following:

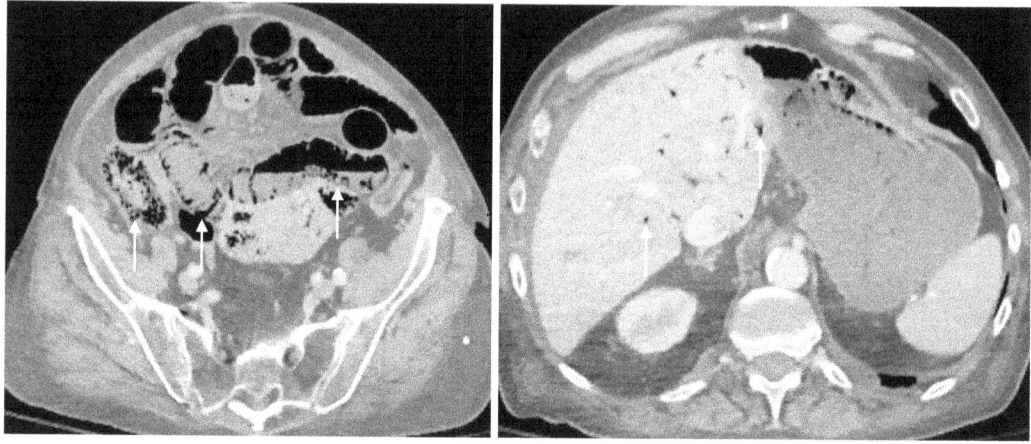

Name the signs and the diagnosis
a. Pneumatosis intestinalis, acute mesenteric ischemia
b. Pneumatosis hepatis, acute mesenteric ischemia
c. Pneumatosis portalis, pneumatosis intestinalis and acute mesenteric ischemia
d. Pneumatosis portalis, pneumatosis hepatis and acute mesenteric ischemia

Ans. c

Explanation:

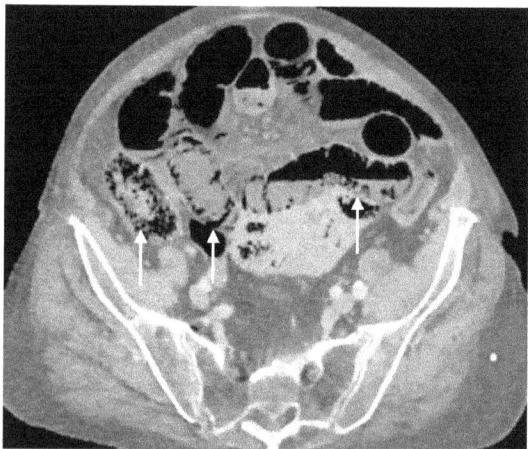

Axial image of contrast-enhanced abdominal CT (CECT) scan shows multiple locations of intramural bowel air in small bowel loops (arrows), a finding referred to as *pneumatosis intestinalis*.

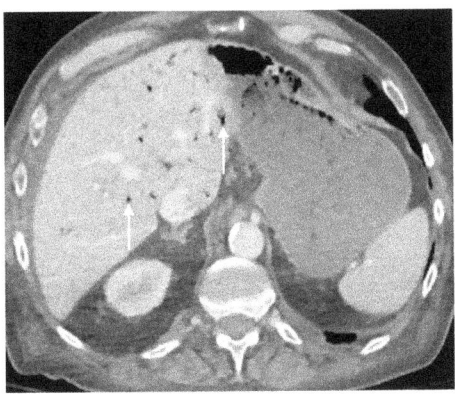

Computed tomography image of the same patient at the level of the liver. Multiple small bubbles of portal venous gas (arrows) are present. This finding is also called *pneumatosis portalis*.

Suggested Reading
1. Fitzpatrick LA, Rivers-Bowerman MD, Thipphavong S, Clarke SE, Rowe JA, Costa AF. Pearls, pitfalls, and conditions that mimic mesenteric ischemia at CT. Radiographics. 2020;40(2):545-61.

Q.16. A 50-year-old male got admitted in the intensive care unit with new-onset blurring of vision, diplopia, headache, and dizziness, 24 hours after being discharged from her local hospital. He was previously admitted for hypertensive urgency with a blood pressure of 230/120 mm Hg, requiring administration of IV enalaprilat. The recent set of symptoms as described above started shortly after discharge and worsened over 24 hours. On arrival in the emergency department, he was afebrile, in sinus rhythm with a BP of 170/100 mm Hg. On examination, no focal neurologic deficits could be elicited, and there was no observation of exophthalmos, ptosis, or nystagmus. He received metoclopramide 10 mg by mouth once keeping in mind a diagnosis of primary headache syndrome namely migraine. The noncontrast CT (NCCT) brain showed no evidence of intracranial hemorrhage. An MRI of the head with and without contrast was performed which was suggestive of the following:

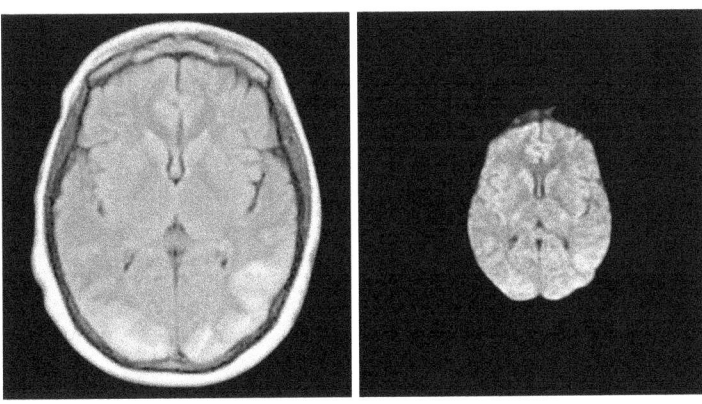

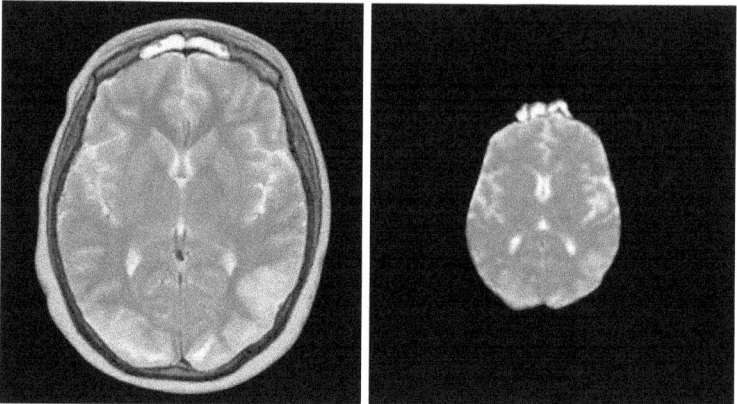

Which of the following drugs is not implicated in the precipitation of this condition?

a. Bevacizumab
b. Tacrolimus
c. Cyclosporine
d. Infliximab

Ans. d

Explanation: Posterior reversible encephalopathy syndrome (PRES) is a clinicoradiological syndrome characterized by symptoms including a headache, seizures, altered consciousness, and visual disturbances. It is commonly but not always associated with acute hypertension. This clinical syndrome is increasingly recognized, commonly because of improvement and availability of brain imaging.

MRI findings: Signal characteristics of affected areas usually reflect vasogenic edema with some exceptions:

- *T1:* Hypointense in affected regions
- *T1 C+ (Gd):* Patchy variable enhancement can be seen in ~35% of patients, in either a leptomeningeal or cortical pattern.
- *T2:* Hyperintense in affected regions
- *DWI:* Usually normal, sometimes hyperintense due to edema (T2 shine-through) or true restricted diffusion
- *ADC:* Usually increased signal due to increased diffusion, but restricted diffusion is present in a quarter of cases.
- *GRE/SWI:* It may show hemorrhages (including microhemorrhages) in 9–50%.

Medical conditions associated with reversible posterior leukoencephalopathy syndrome:

- Hypertensive encephalopathy and acute fluctuations of blood pressure
- Acute or chronic renal disease
- Thrombotic thrombocytopenic purpura
- Hemolytic and uremic syndrome
- Eclampsia
- *Vasculitis:*
  - SLE
  - Polyarteritis nodosa
  - Granulomatosis with polyangiitis
  - Cryoglobulinemia
- *Immunosuppressive, immunomodulatory, and chemotherapeutic drugs:*
  - Bevacizumab and other VEGF inhibitors
  - Cisplatin and other platinum-based drugs
  - Combination therapy
  - Cytarabine
  - Cyclosporine A
  - Gemcitabine
  - Interferon
  - Intravenous immunoglobulin
  - Ipilimumab
  - Methotrexate
  - Rituximab
  - Tacrolimus and sirolimus
  - Vincristine
  - Tyrosine kinase inhibitors
- Porphyrias
- Hypocalcemia and hypomagnesemia
- Sepsis
- Transplantation, i.e., solid organ, bone marrow, and stem cells

Suggested Reading

1. Bartynski WS. Posterior reversible encephalopathy syndrome, part 1: fundamental imaging and clinical features. Am J Neuroradiol. 2008;29(6):1036-42.

Q.17. A contrast CT brain scan of a 50-year-old man with history of sinusitis with and high-grade fever for last 7–10 days associated with running nose and frontal headache, now presenting with **seizures** reveals the following:

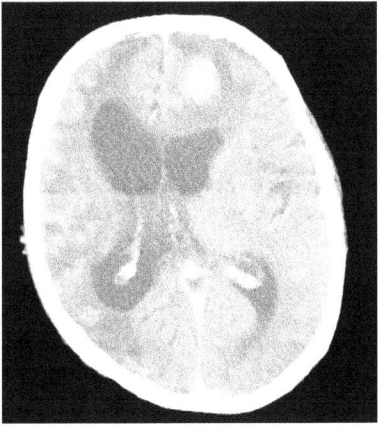

What is the diagnosis?
a. Cerebral abscess
b. Intracerebral hemorrhage
c. Intracranial SOL
d. Aneurysmal ICH

Ans. a

Explanation: Image reveals a left-sided enhancing mass (white) with surrounding gray edema in the frontal lobe of the brain. Sulcal effacement (squashing) is noted on both sides with midline deviation to the right. Lateral ventricles appear large, suggestive of hydrocephalus, although the left is marginally effaced by the mass. In contention with the clinical history, the patient has a cerebral abscess secondary to extension of infection from the frontal sinus.

Suggested Reading
1. Bhargava R. CT Imaging in neurocritical care. Indian J Crit Care Med. 2019;23 (Suppl 2):S98-S103.

Q.18. A NCCT brain scan from a female with no history of background illness presenting with a severe headache and sudden collapse. What is the diagnosis?

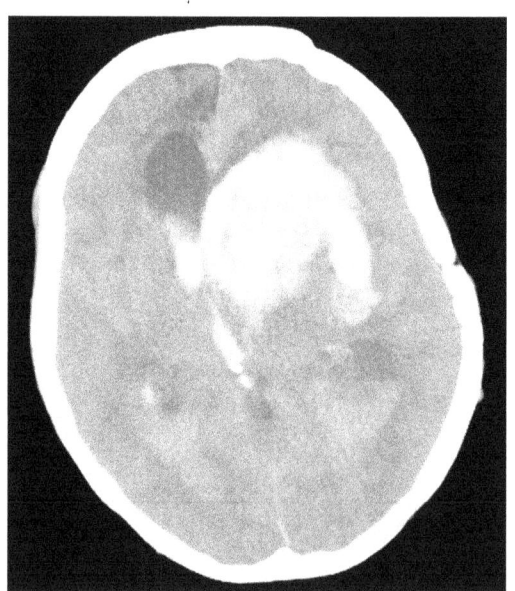

a. Hypertensive ICH
b. Aneurysmal ICH
c. Traumatic ICH
d. CVST related ICH

Ans. b

Explanation: The NCCT brain shows a large intracranial hemorrhage (white) in the left frontoparietal region. There is perilesional edema, associated with effacement of the ipsilateral sulci, and lateral ventricle with deviation of the midline to the right. History and CT findings are suggestive of a posterior communicating artery aneurysm rupture.

Suggested Reading
1. Bhargava R. CT Imaging in neurocritical care. Indian J Crit Care Med. 2019;23 (Suppl 2):S98-S103.

Q.19. A 62-year-old male driver involved in a high-speed road traffic accident undergoes an MRI cervical spine. What are the findings?

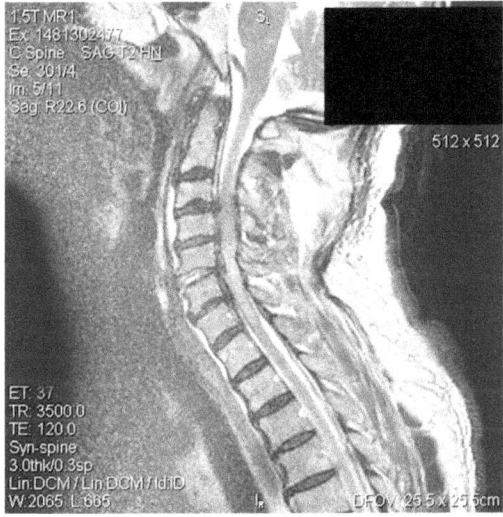

a. C3 vertebrae fracture with spinal cord edema
b. C6 vertebrae fracture with spinal cord edema
c. C4 vertebrae fracture with spinal cord edema
d. C5 vertebrae with fracture with spinal cord edema

Ans. b

Explanation: Sagittal MR slice through the cervical spine shows abnormality in C4, C5, and C6 with the body of C6 being fractured. There is evidence of anterior edema. The CSF space around the respective vertebrae has been obliterated and the cord itself appears to have sustained a contusion with the darker area visible around C4. This signifies a cervical spine fracture with cord involvement.

Suggested Reading
1. Mangrum W, Christianson K, Duncan S, et al. Duke Review of MRI Principles. Mosby, 2012

Q.20. NCCT brain of a 65-year-old female presenting with sudden-onset unilateral weakness and inability to articulate words as she would have liked is as follows:

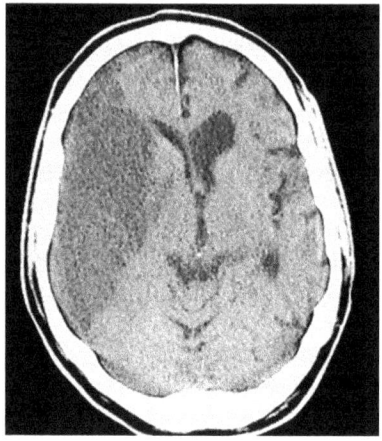

What is the diagnosis?
a. Chronic subdural hematoma
b. Intracranial SOL
c. Acute right MCA ischemic infarct
d. Extradural hematoma

Ans. c

Explanation: There is a wedge-shaped area of low density in the right parietal lobe with mass effect, evident by compression of ipsilateral lateral ventricle and midline shift to the opposite side. In context with the history given, this represents an acute middle cerebral artery infarct.

Suggested Reading:
1. Bhargava R. CT Imaging in neurocritical care. Indian J Crit Care Med. 2019;23 (Suppl 2):S98-S103.

Q.21. As you enter into the critical care area to start your shift as consultant on duty, your colleague asks, what needs to be done about the bleeding chest drain that was inserted at an outside hospital to treat a simple pneumothorax that occurred on a ventilator. The patient has lost 1,000 mL of blood postinsertion of the implantable cardioverter defibrillator (ICD). The CT scan done at your center shows, the chest drain is clearly in the liver with some fresh bleeding. There is a residual pneumothorax.

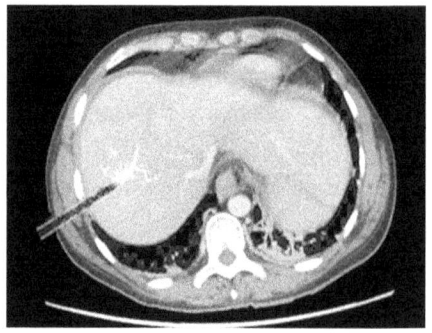

What is the next best step in the management of the patient?
a. Remove the drain and place a new drain
b. Keep the drain and observe
c. Place another ICD to drain the pneumothorax
d. Resuscitate and seek expert advice in considering laparotomy versus interventional radiology.

Ans. d

Explanation: In view of the given clinical scenario, following steps need to be taken for the management of the patient:
- Avoid pulling the chest drain out.
- Resuscitate and keep massive transfusion in mind.
- Expert advice in considering interventional radiology versus laparotomy.
- Transferring the patient to theatre or even to another specialist center.

Suggested Reading
1. Kesieme EB, Dongo A, Ezemba N, Irekpita E, Jebbin N, Kesieme C. Tube thoracostomy: complications and its management. Pulm Med. 2012;2012:256878.

Q.22. A 25-year-old male arrived at the emergency room with an alleged history of blunt trauma over the right side of his chest, post which the patient became progressively breathless. On auscultation in the ER, breath sounds were not audible on the right side of the thoracic cavity. An urgent HRCT chest was done which revealed the following:

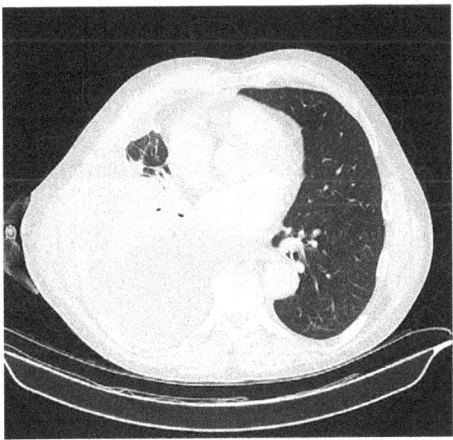

What is the pathology?
a. Massive pleural effusion
b. Empyema thoracis
c. Hemothorax
d. Hemopneumothorax

Ans. c

Explanation: The CT scan shows a large collection in the right hemithorax which is somewhat dependent and is associated with compressive atelectasis. Given the clinical context, this collection represents blood in the thoracic cavity, i.e., hemothorax. The same can be confirmed by calculating the Hounsfield units of the collection in the right hemithorax.

Suggested Reading
1. Lewis BT, Herr KD, Hamlin SA, Henry T, Little BP, Naeger DM, et al. Imaging manifestations of chest trauma. Radiographics. 2021;41(5):1321-34.
2. Naeem M, Hoegger MJ, Petraglia III FW, Ballard DH, Zulfiqar M, Patlas MN, et al. CT of penetrating abdominopelvic trauma. Radiographics. 2021;41(4):1064-81.

Q.23. Which of the following features is not present in the image?

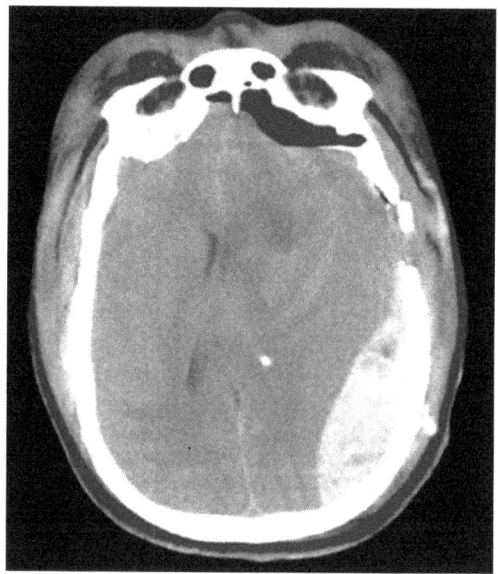

a. Acute left parieto-occipital EDH
b. Pneumocranium
c. Midline shift with subfalcine herniation
d. Basifrontal contusion

Ans. d

Explanation: The NCCT head shows the following:
- Large left-sided occipitoparietal extradural hematoma
- Fractured skull in the temporoparietal region
- Midline shift with subfalcine herniation
- Pneumocranium

Suggested Reading
1. Bhargava R. CT Imaging in neurocritical care. Indian J Crit Care Med. 2019;23 (Suppl 2):S98-S103.

Q.24. What does the NCCT brain depict?

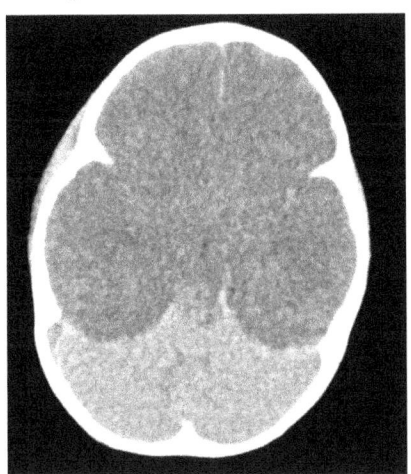

a. Cerebellar contusion
b. Irreversible anoxic brain injury
c. Normal CT brain
d. Acute cerebral infarct

Ans. b

Explanation: *White cerebellar sign:* Markedly hyperdense appearance of the infratentorial structure than that of the supratentorial structure, which is a sign of poor prognosis in head injury. It is associated with diffuse effacement of the gray-white interface of the cerebral cortex and loss of sulci-gyri. This sign is associated with traumatic brain injury, child abuse, central nervous system (CNS) infections, and postpartum seizures.

Suggested Reading
1. Krishnan P, Chowdhury SR. "White cerebellum" sign—A dark prognosticator. J Neurosci Rural Pract. 2014;5(4):433.

Q.25. Identify the MRI sequence:

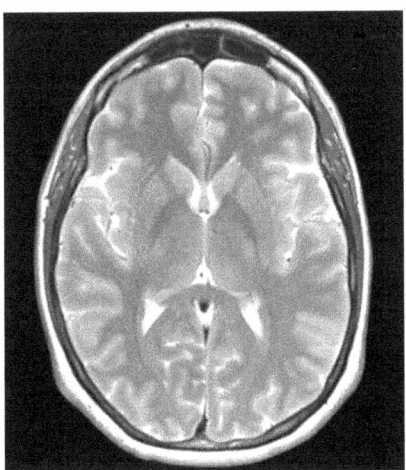

a. T1W sequence
b. T2W sequence
c. FLAIR sequence
d. SWI sequence

Ans. b

Explanation:

Tissue	T1-weighted	T2-weighted	FLAIR
CSF	Dark	Bright	Dark
White Matter	Light	Dark gray	Dark gray
Cortex	Gray	Light gray	Light gray
Fat (within bone marrow)	Bright	Light	Light
Inflammation (infection, demyelination)	Dark	Bright	Bright

(CSF: cerebrospinal fluid; FLAIR: fluid-attenuated inversion recovery)

Suggested Reading
1. Chen MYM, Pope TL, Ott DJ. Basic Radiology, 2nd edition. Philadelphia, PA: Lippincott Williams & Wilkins, 2011.
2. Mangrum W, Christianson K, Duncan S, et al. Duke Review of MRI Principles. Mosby, 2012.

Q.26. Identify the components of basal ganglia on the MRI sequence given.

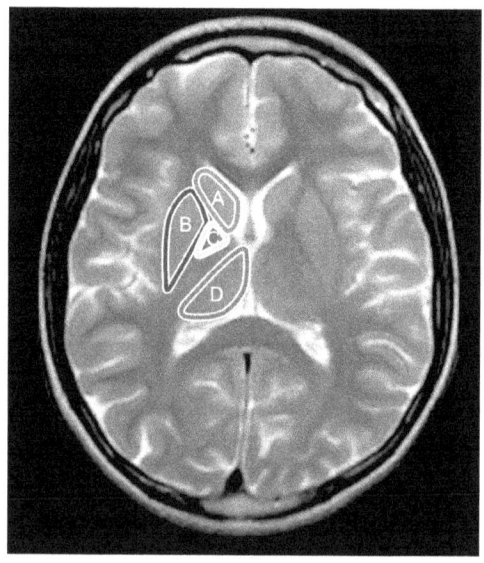

Ans.
a. Caudate nucleus
b. Putamen
c. Globus pallidus
d. Thalamus

Suggested Reading
1. Chen MYM, Pope TL, Ott DJ. Basic Radiology, 2nd edition. Philadelphia, PA: Lippincott Williams & Wilkins, 2011.
2. Mangrum W, Christianson K, Duncan S, et al. Duke Review of MRI Principles. Mosby, 2012.

Q.27. A 75-year-old female gets admitted to the critical care unit with progressive yellowish discoloration of the sclera and the body for the last 14 days associated with itching and decreased appetite. Her hemodynamics are maintained and the patient gives no history suggestive of cholangitis. The patient had undergone interval laparoscopic cholecystectomy 3 months back in view of cholecystitis, recovery from which was unremarkable. On admission, the following investigation was performed for evaluation of jaundice.

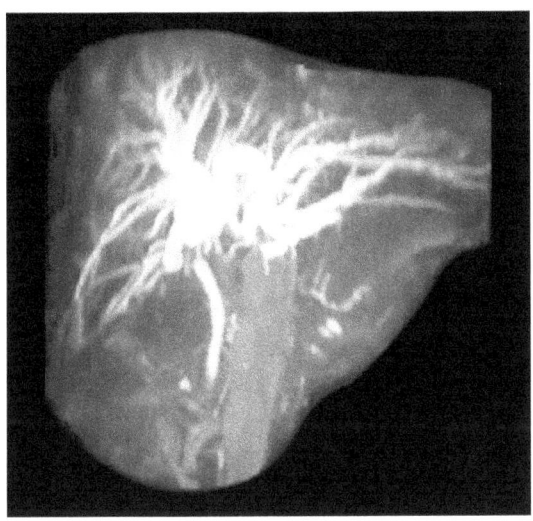

Identify the investigational modality by looking at the image provided?
a. Cholangiogram b. ERCP
c. MRCP d. CECT abdomen

Ans. c

Explanation: *Magnetic resonance cholangiopancreatography (MRCP)* is a noninvasive imaging technique to visualize the intra- and extrahepatic biliary tree and pancreatic ductal system.

It can provide diagnostically-equivalent images to ERCP and is a useful technique in high-risk patients to avoid significant morbidity.

Suggested Reading
1. Griffin N, Charles-Edwards G, Grant LA. Magnetic resonance cholangiopancreatography: the ABC of MRCP. Insights Imaging. 2012;3(1):11-21.

Q.28. A 35-year-old male patient is brought to the hospital with an alleged history of assault by an iron rod on the left side of the chest. On arrival patient's HR 100 beats/min, BP 110/50 mm Hg, RR 30 breaths/min, and SpO$_2$ 84% on RA. Inspection revealed bluish color discoloration on the left side of the chest wall. Air entry on the left side was markedly reduced. A CT abdomen is done for the patient, which reveals the following:

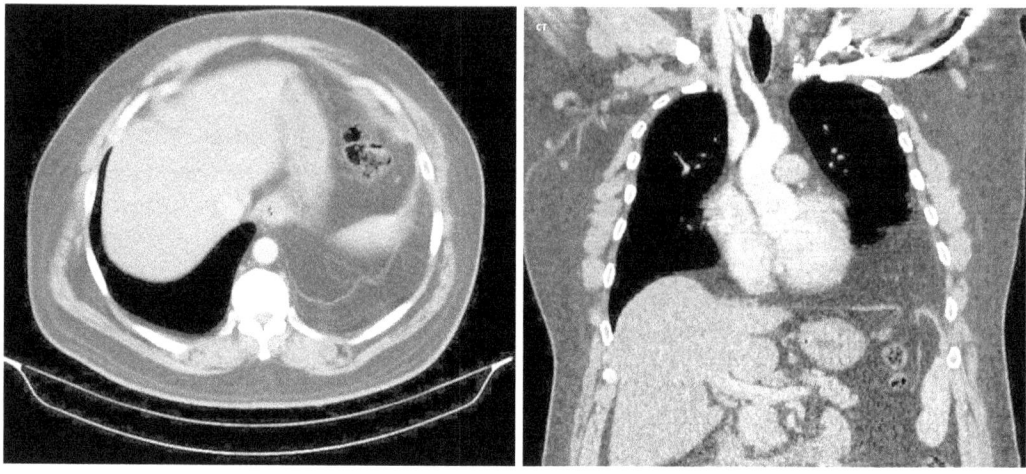

What is the cause of patient's breathlessness?
a. Left-sided hemothorax
b. Traumatic diaphragmatic rupture
c. Left lower lobe collapse
d. Left-sided pneumothorax

Ans. b

Explanation: Traumatic diaphragmatic rupture (TDR) occurs in approximately 5% of patients with major blunt thoracoabdominal trauma, most of them on the left side and an early correct diagnosis is made in <50% of cases. The difficulty of the diagnosis and the high mortality and morbidity rates of the untreated cases make this clinical entity more important. A 30% mortality rate has been found in cases with bowel strangulation associated with diaphragmatic hernia.

The axial and coronal CT cuts of this patient reveal a tear in the left diaphragm leading to herniation of the abdominal contents into the thoracic cavity, causing decreased air entry on the left side of the chest and breathlessness.

Suggested Reading
1. Turhan K, Makay O, Cakan A, Samancilar O, First O, Icoz G, et al. Traumatic diaphragmatic rupture: Look to see. Euro J Cardiothorac Surg. 2008;33(6):1082-5.

Q.29. A 38-year-old man, with no comorbidities, is rushed into the emergency department with history of sudden-onset severe headache and central chest pain, radiating to the back. His BP is 180/110 mm Hg, HR is 105 beats/min, temperature is 99.4°F, SpO$_2$ is 98% on room air, and RR 28 breaths/min on arrival. His ECG showed sinus rhythm with slight ST-depressions in the leads V4–6. 2D echo revealed regional wall motion abnormality (RWMA) in the lateral wall of the left ventricle, and a left ventricular ejection fraction (LVEF) of 20–30%. His troponin T is 300 ng/L. A CT aortogram with CECT abdomen was done, which revealed the following:

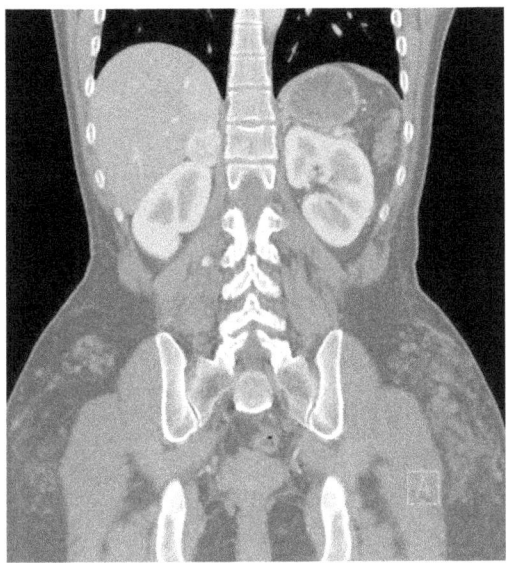

Which of the following investigations should be carried out to confirm the diagnosis?

a. Urinary metanephrines
b. Urinary norepinephrine
c. Plasma norepinephrine
d. Plasma free and urine fractional metanephrines

Ans. d

Explanation: The CECT abdomen reveals a right-sided suprarenal contrast-enhancing mass making the diagnosis of pheochromocytoma a possibility. Urinary fractional metanephrines or plasma-free metanephrines are used to confirm the diagnosis along with the imaging findings.

Biochemical approach to diagnosis of pheochromocytoma:

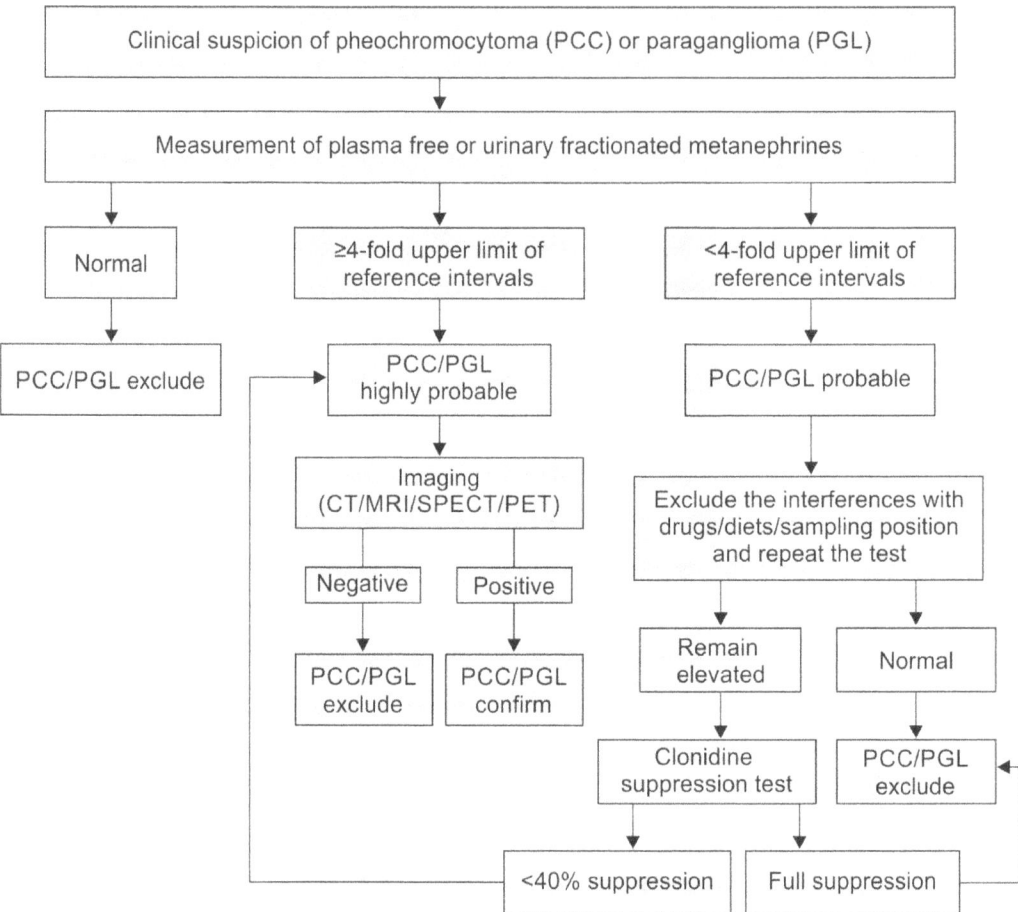

(CT: computed tomography; MRI: magnetic resonance imaging; PET: positron emission tomography; SPECT: single photon emission computed tomography)

Suggested Reading

1. Shen Y, Cheng L. Biochemical Diagnosis of Pheochromocytoma and Paraganglioma. In: Mariani-Costantini R (Ed). Paraganglioma: a multidisciplinary approach. Brisbane (AU): Codon Publications; 2019.

Q.30. An 81-year-old man visited the emergency department with a 3-day history of productive cough with yellowish sputum, dyspnea, and pain during inspiration. He reported a 50-pack-year history of cigarette smoking and a medical history of hypertension but not of diabetes. Patient gives history of suffering from pulmonary tuberculosis 20 years back for which he completed the treatment as per the government guidelines. His vitals are HR 100 beats/min, SpO_2 86% on RA, RR 32 breaths/min, and BP 120/70 mm Hg. Auscultation revealed decreased air entry in the left upper quadrant of the thoracic cavity. HRCT chest was done keeping in mind the history of tuberculosis which revealed the following:

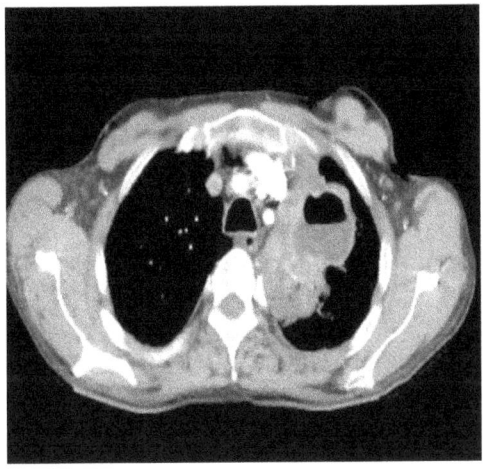

What is the diagnosis?
a. Lung abscess
b. Hydropneumothorax
c. Empyema thoracis
d. Pneumatocele

Ans. a

Explanation: HRCT chest shows cavitary lesion in the left upper lobe of the lung with air-fluid levels, which on the background of the given clinical scenario is suggestive of lung abscess.

Suggested Reading
1. Stark DD, Federle MP, Goodman PC, Podrasky AE, Webb WR. Differentiating lung abscess and empyema: radiography and computed tomography. Am J Roentgenol. 1983; 141(1):163-7.

CHAPTER

27

X-rays (Chest/Abdomen)

Khalid Ismail Khatib, Abhijit Deshmukh

Q.1. A 40-year-old man was involved in a high-speed road traffic accident. He was in the front passenger side seat when the car hit a tree. He was wearing a seat belt. He developed acute shortness of breath. This is his chest X-ray. What is the diagnosis?

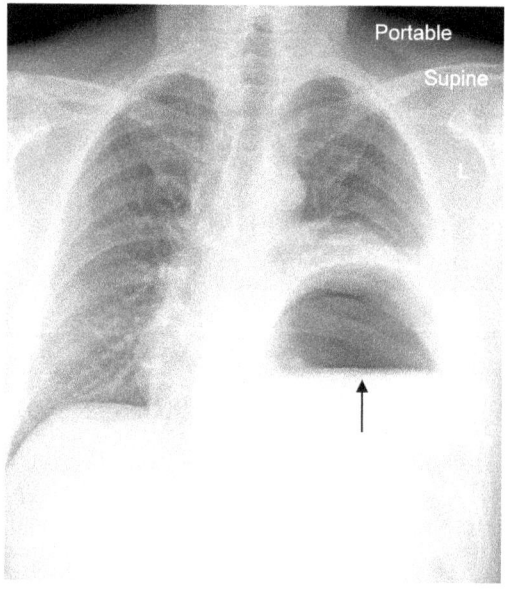

a. Pneumoperitoneum
b. Left traumatic diaphragmatic hernia
c. Left pneumatocele
d. Left lung abscess

Ans. b

Explanation: Rather than continuous dome-shaped course, free edge of torn diaphragm moves upward in axial image. Herniation of abdominal content (air-fluid level stomach) is seen on left side with shift of mediastinum on right side.

Given the clinical scenario, patient is likely to have a traumatic diaphragmatic tear leading to acute herniation of the stomach into the thoracic cavity leading to shortness of breath. The confirmatory study for the same would be a computed tomography (CT) abdomen.

Suggested Reading
1. McDonald AA, Robinson BRH, Alarcon L, Bosarge PL, Dorion H, Haut ER, et al. Evaluation and management of traumatic diaphragmatic injuries: A Practice Management Guideline from the Eastern Association for the Surgery of Trauma. J Trauma Acute Care Surg. 2018;85(1):198-207.

Q.2. A 33-year-old male, postappendicectomy status, develops fever on postoperative day 3 associated with shortness of breath and cough with expectoration. His oxygen saturation (SpO$_2$) on room air is 89%. A chest X-ray (CXR) is ordered for the patient, which is as follows:

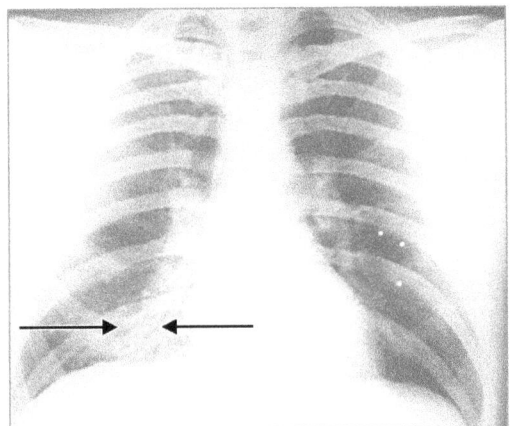

What are the findings on the CXR?
a. Right lower lobe consolidation
b. Right lower lobe pulmonary infarct
c. Right lower lobe pleural thickening
d. Right lower lobe collapse

Ans. a

Explanation: This X-ray demonstrates an inhomogeneous opacity in the right lower lobe, which is associated with visible air bronchogram suggestive of right lower lobe consolidation. As the opacity is not homogeneous and there is no evidence of volume loss, mediastinal shift, shifting of the fissures, or pleural fluid, the likelihood of the patient having a collapse or pleural thickening is highly unlikely.

Suggested Reading
1. Yang CK, Teng A, Lee DY, Rose K. Pulmonary complications after major abdominal surgery: National Surgical Quality Improvement Program analysis. J Surg Res. 2015;198(2):441-9.

Q.3. An 88-year-old female presents to the emergency department with complaints of progressive dyspnea and cough. On examination, she has oxygen saturation of 85% on room air and is afebrile. There is reduced air entry in the left lower zone. A chest X-ray is done, which reveals the following:

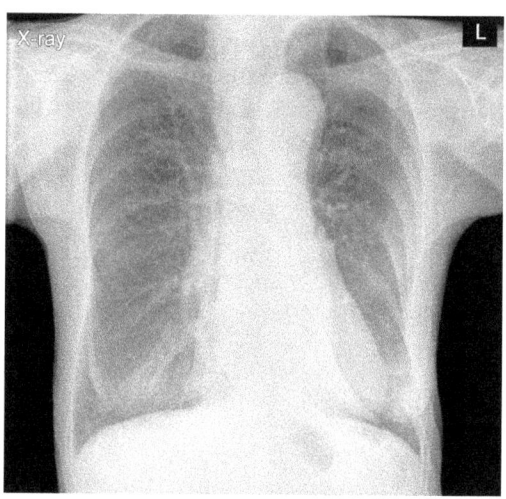

What are the findings on the X-ray?
a. Left lower lobe consolidation
b. Left lower lobe collapse
c. Left lower lobe pulmonary infarct
d. Left lower lobe pulmonary thickening

Ans. b

Explanation: This X-ray shows a left lower lobe collapse (sail sign, apparent double left heart border and loss of descending aortic outline). Resultant volume loss in the left hemithorax is depicted by depression of left hilum and mediastinal shift.

Suggested Reading
1. Radiology Masterclass. Chest X-ray—Airways and lung collapse—Left lower lobe collapse. [online] Available from https://www.radiologymasterclass.co.uk/gallery/chest/airways/airways_h. [Last accessed June, 2023].

Q.4. A 40-year-old male is admitted with complaints of high-grade fever with chills and rigors for last 7 days, which is associated with progressive breathlessness. On examination, his heart rate (HR) is 122 beats/min, oxygen saturation is 88% on room air, and blood pressure (BP) is 120/70 mm Hg. Auscultation reveals decreased breath sounds over the left side of his lungs. His X-ray is as follows:

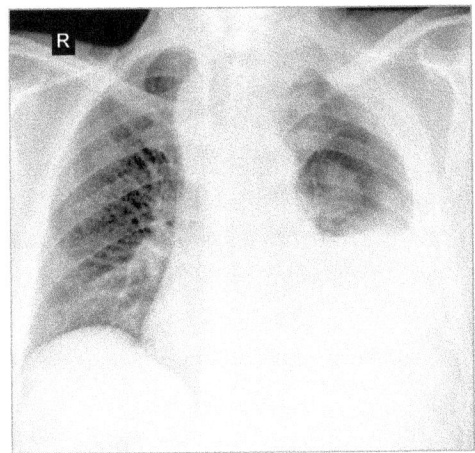

What does the X-ray show?
a. Left lower lobe consolidation
b. Left lower lobe collapse
c. Left lung pleural thickening
d. Left-sided hydropneumothorax

Ans. d

Explanation: There is opacification of the left lower hemithorax due to a pleural effusion which is associated with an air-fluid level which is not associated with major mediastinal shift. In the given clinical context, the patient is likely to have a left-sided hydropneumothorax.

Suggested Reading
1. Kasargod V, Awad NT. Clinical profile, etiology, and management of hydropneumothorax: An Indian experience. Lung India. 2016;33(3):278-80.

Q.5. A 70-year-old male, known case of chronic obstructive pulmonary disease (COPD), is admitted with sudden-onset breathlessness which was preceded by fever and increased secretions over the last 5–6 days. His oxygen saturation on room air is 82%. His chest X-ray showed the following:

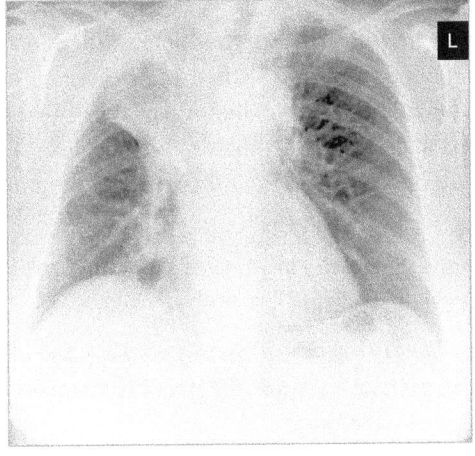

What is the abnormality?
a. Right upper lobe fibrosis
b. Right lower lobe consolidation
c. Right upper lobe collapse
d. Right upper lobe mass lesion

Ans. c

Explanation: There is volume loss of the right upper lobe. The right upper zone has become dense due to lobar collapse. The volume loss has displaced the trachea, which is *pulled* to the right, and the horizontal fissure has been *pulled* upward. Absence of air bronchogram rules out consolidation.

Suggested Reading
1. Kattan KR. The various faces of right upper lobe atelectasis. Crit Rev Diagn Imaging. 1991;32(2):119-63.

Q.6. Identify the pathology on the chest X-ray.

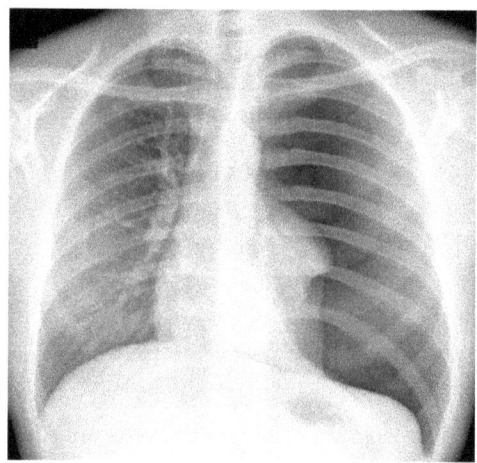

a. Left-sided pneumothorax
b. Left-sided emphysematous bullae
c. Left-sided lung cyst
d. Hyperinflation of the left lung

Ans. a

Explanation: The left hemithorax is hyperlucent due to air in the pleural cavity. The left lung is completely compressed with shift of mediastinum to right side. The left hemidiaphragm is depressed (double diaphragm sign). To diagnose bulla or cavity, one should be able to mark at least two-thirds of its margins. In hyperinflation, rest of the lung markings should be visualized near the hyperlucent lung area.

Suggested Reading
1. McKnight CL, Burns B. (2023). Pneumothorax. [online] Available from https://www.ncbi.nlm.nih.gov/books/NBK441885/. [Last accessed June, 2023]

Q.7. A 74-year-old man is extubated following surgery for an ankle fracture. He was a known case of bronchial asthma on regular treatment and is now coughing persistently. His X-ray is shown:

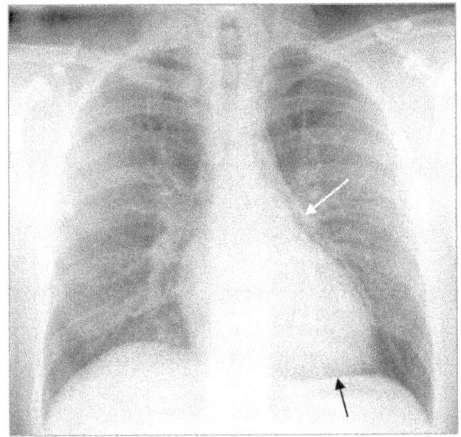

What can you see on the CXR?
a. Left hydropneumopericardium
b. Pneumomediastinum
c. Left hydropneumomediastinum
d. Left side pneumothorax

Ans. b

Explanation: A thin layer of air without fluid level can be seen over the left heart border along with air level under the inferior surface of the heart suggesting pneumomediastinum. No left lung hyperlucency noted which rules out pneumothorax.

Suggested Reading
1. Kouritas VK, Papagiannopoulos K, Lazaridis G, Baka S, Mpoukovinas I, Karavasilis V, et al. Pneumomediastinum. J Thorac Di. 2015;7(Suppl 1):S44-9.

Q.8. A young male with a history of peptic ulcer disease presents to the ER with complaints of severe abdominal pain not getting relieved with antacids. He admits to having recurrent episodes of abdominal pain, which subsides after intake of antacids. On examination, patient is tachycardic and diaphoretic. His abdomen is distended and he winces in pain on palpation of his abdomen. His abdominal X-ray is as follows:

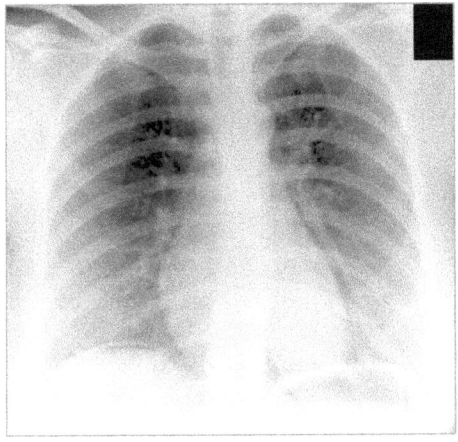

Identify the cause of his abdominal pain by looking at his X-ray.
a. Chilaiditi syndrome
b. Bowel perforation
c. Subdiaphragmatic abscess
d. Subpulmonary abscess

Ans. b

Explanation: Free gas under subdiaphragmatic area on right side is well appreciated with well-diaphragmatic counter noted on right side. Absence of febrile illness and localized collection below diaphragm with air-fluid level rules out subdiaphragmatic abscess.

Suggested Reading
1. Mori PA, Barrett HA. A sign of intestinal perforation. Radiology. 1962;79:654-9.

Q.9. A 43-year-old male was admitted with history of progressive dyspnea associated with hypotension and muffled heart sounds. An urgent CXR revealed a globular enlarged cardiac shadow, which was confirmed as pericardial tamponade with the help of an urgent 2D-echo. Urgent pericardiocentesis was performed and the sheath was left in situ. The sheath was removed after 3 days of draining the pericardial fluid. The patient was discharged a day later. 3 days postdischarge, the patient attended the ER with complaints of progressive dyspnea and hypotension. An urgent X-ray chest was done which revealed the following:

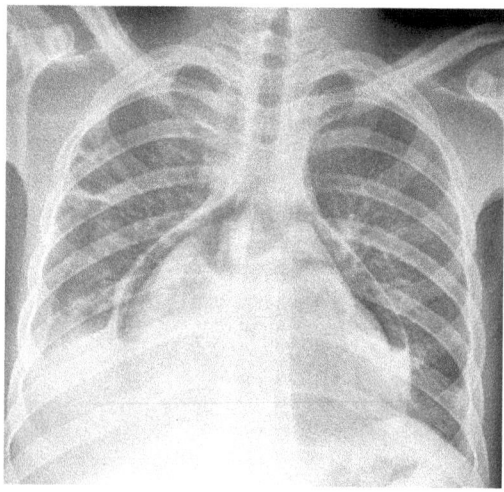

What is the diagnosis?
a. Pneumopericardium
b. Pneumomediastinum
c. Hydropneumopericardium
d. Bilateral pneumothorax

Ans. c

Explanation: The chest X-ray depicts air-fluid level inside the pericardium suggestive of hydropneumopericardium. Given the clinical scenario, the air would have been inadvertently introduced into the pericardial sac during pericardiocentesis at the time of admission for pericardial tamponade.

Suggested Reading

1. Brander L, Ramsay D, Dreier D, Peter M, Graeni R. Continuous left hemidiaphragm sign revisited: a case of spontaneous pneumopericardium and literature review. Heart. 2002;88(4):e5.

Q.10. A 50-year-old male patient presents with upper abdominal pain, vomiting, and not passed gas or stools for 2 days. His X-ray abdomen is given below. Choose the correct diagnosis.

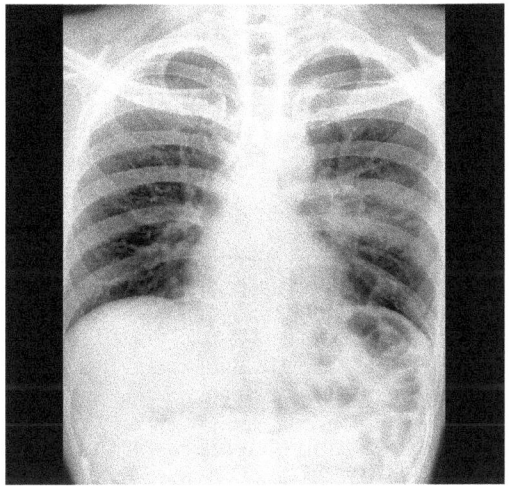

a. Chilaiditi sign
b. Chilaiditi syndrome
c. Megacolon
d. Colonic perforation

Ans. a

Explanation: A radiologic finding depicting interposition of the colon between the liver and diaphragm, either on the right or left is called Chilaiditi sign. It is rarely seen incidentally on CXR or abdominal X-rays, with an incidence of 0.025–0.28%. Chilaiditi syndrome refers to the disease in which a Chilaiditi sign is accompanied by clinical symptoms such as abdominal pain, vomiting, and constipation. As there is absence of gas under diaphragm and colon is normal in size, the last two options are incorrect.

Suggested Reading

1. Weng WH, Liu DR, Feng CC, Que RS. Colonic interposition between the liver and left diaphragm—management of Chilaiditi syndrome: A case report and literature review. Oncol Lett. 2014;7(5):1657-60.

Q.11. A 25-year-old male patient presents with history of fever, cough with expectoration, and breathlessness for 3 days. He has tachycardia (HR = 118 beats/min), tachypnea

(RR = 28 breaths/min), and his temperature is 102°F. His CXR is shown below. What is most likely diagnosis?

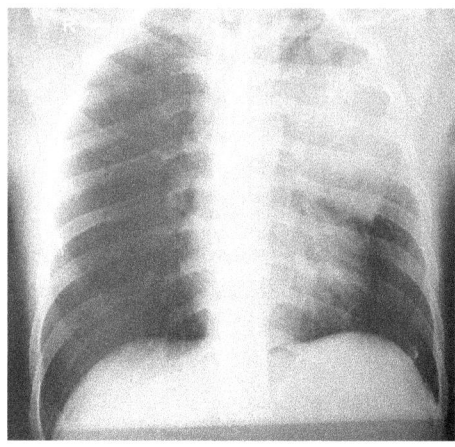

a. Pleural effusion
b. *Klebsiella* pneumonia
c. Wegener's granulomatosis
d. Bronchogenic carcinoma

Ans. b

Explanation: *Klebsiella* pneumonia usually presents with lobar pneumonia, bulging fissures of the lung on the X-ray, and early cavitation.

Suggested Reading
1. Hansell DM, Lynch DA, McAdams HP, Bankier AA. Imaging of Diseases of the Chest, 5th edition. Maryland Heights: Mosby; 2010.

Q.12. According to the Berlin definition of acute respiratory distress syndrome (ARDS), in addition to the below CXR, which of the following is not correct in the diagnosis of ARDS?

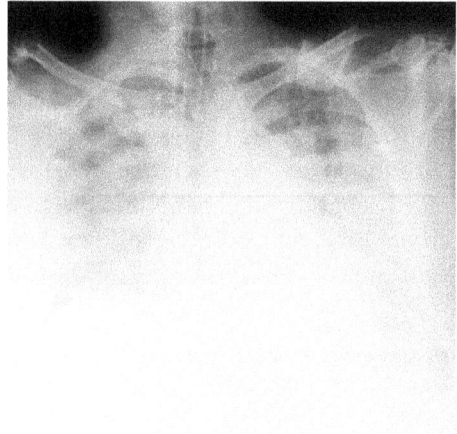

a. Respiratory failure develops within 15 days of known clinical insult.
b. Respiratory failure not fully explained by cardiac failure.

c. Partial pressure of oxygen (PaO$_2$)/fraction of inspired oxygen (FiO$_2$) < 300
d. Respiratory failure develops within 7 days of known clinical insult.

Ans. a

Explanation: The Berlin definition of ARDS specifies the following criteria for the diagnosis of ARDS: (1) respiratory failure should have developed within 1 week of a known clinical insult, like pneumonia, pancreatitis, etc., (2) respiratory failure should not be fully explained by cardiac failure. If required, additional testing such as 2D-echocardiography may be done to rule out hydrostatic edema, (3) CXR findings should include bilateral opacities not fully explained by effusions, atelectasis, or nodules.

Suggested Reading
1. ARDS Definition Task Force; Ranieri VM, Rubenfeld GD, Thompson BT, Ferguson ND, Caldwell E, et al. Acute respiratory distress syndrome: the Berlin Definition. JAMA. 2012;307(23):2526-33.

Q.13. **A 55-year-old male, known case of ulcerative colitis, noncompliant to treatment, came with complaints of severe abdominal pain and distension, vomiting, and constipation for 36 hours. His X-ray is shown below. What is the diagnosis?**

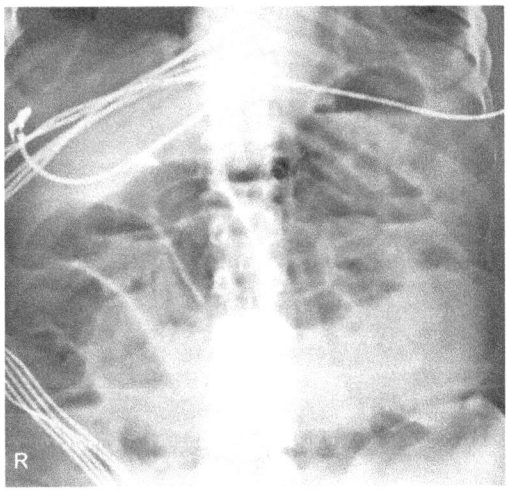

a. Intestinal perforation
b. Diverticulitis
c. Colitis
d. Toxic megacolon

Ans. d

Explanation: Toxic megacolon (TM) is a potentially fatal complication of severe ulcerative colitis (UC). It is defined as a segmental or total colonic distension of >6 cm in the presence of acute colitis and signs of systemic toxicity. TM may be seen in up to 10% of all UC admission.

Suggested Reading
1. Ong SCL, Mohaidin N. Imaging features of toxic megacolon. BMJ Case Rep. 2018;2018: bcr2018227121.

Q.14. A 53-year-old male patient presents with history of breathlessness, cough with occasional expectoration, and low-grade fever for last 15 days. His X-ray is shown below. As per Silhouette sign, in which lobe of the lung is the lesion?

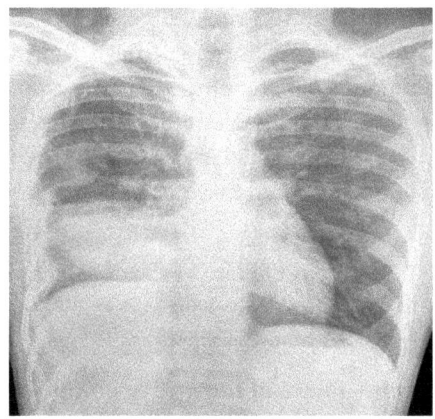

a. Right upper lobe collapse
b. Right lower lobe collapse
c. Right middle lobe collapse
d. Right posterior lobe collapse

Ans. c

Explanation: The right heart border is merged with the lesion while the lower border of the diaphragm can be clearly seen suggestive of right middle lobe involvement. This is indicated by the silhouette sign.

Suggested Reading
1. Felson B, Felson H. Localization of intrathoracic lesions by means of the postero-anterior roentgenogram; the silhouette sign. Radiology. 1950;55:363-74.

Q.15. The continuous diaphragm sign, as shown in the X-ray, is seen in which of the following condition?

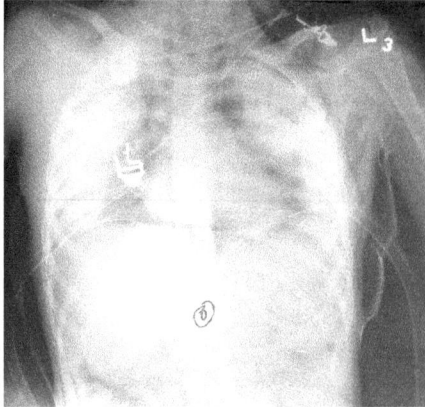

a. Pneumothorax
b. Pleural effusion
c. Pericardial effusion
d. Pneumomediastinum

Ans. d

Explanation: The continuous diaphragm is seen in pneumomediastinum. Due to interposition of air between the diaphragm and the mediastinum, the diaphragm is seen as a continuous entity in the chest X-ray. Occasionally, the sign may be visible in pneumopericardium.

Suggested Reading
1. Kumaresh A, Kumar M, Dev B, Gorantla R, Sai PV, Thanasekaraan V. Back to Basics—'Must Know' Classical Signs in Thoracic Radiology. J Clin Imaging Sci. 2015;5:43.

Q.16. A 60-year-old male with a history of cigarette smoking for 20 years presents with fever and cough for 3 days. He also has history of worsening dyspnea for last 3 years. He is diagnosed to have COPD with acute infective exacerbation. His CXR is given below. Which classic radiologic sign is present?

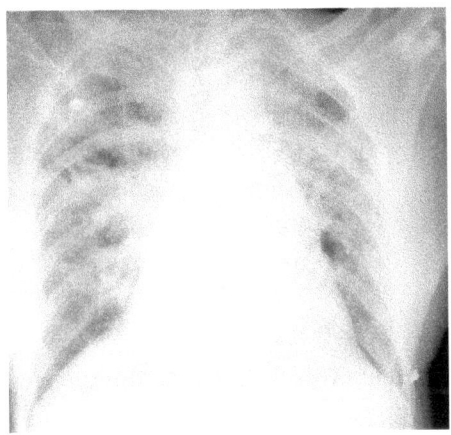

a. Deep sulcus sign
b. False deep sulcus sign
c. Continuous diaphragm sign
d. Comet tail sign

Ans. b

Explanation: The deep sulcus sign is seen in supine CXR in pneumothorax, in which air is collected in the dependent part of the lung. In the supine position, this is the lateral aspect of the costophrenic angle, which appears radiolucent. The false deep sulcus sign is sometimes seen in COPD, as shown in the CXR on the right side.

Suggested Reading
1. Gordon R. The deep sulcus sign. Radiology. 1980;136:25-7.

Q.17. All of the following are signs of pulmonary thromboembolism, except:
a. Hampton's hump
b. Westermark sign
c. Fleischner sign
d. Signet ring sign

Ans. d

Explanation: Signet ring sign is seen on computerized tomography and represents a pulmonary artery lying adjacent to the dilated bronchi, and is seen in cases of bronchiectasis. All the other signs are seen in pulmonary thromboembolism.

Suggested Reading
1. Worsley DF, Alavi A, Aronchick JM, Chen JT, Greenspan RH, Ravin CE. Chest radiographic findings in patients with acute pulmonary embolism: observations from the PIOPED Study. Radiology. 1993;189(1):133-6.

Q.18. A 35-year-old male presented with long-standing history of dyspnea and palpitations. He had irregularly irregular pulse and a mid-diastolic murmur. His X-ray is given below. All are radiological signs found in mitral stenosis, except:
   a. Double-density sign
   b. Carinal widening
   c. Straightening of left heart border
   d. Polo mint sign

Ans. d

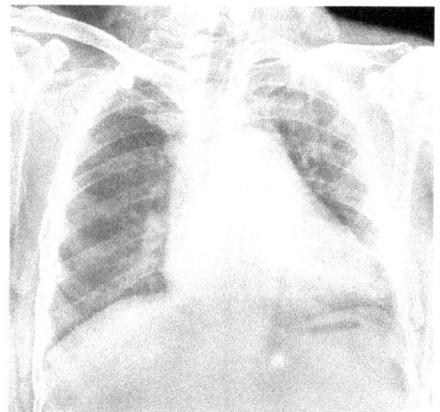

Explanation: Enlargement of the left atrium and the left atrial appendage in mitral stenosis leads to the double-density sign, widening of angle of the carina, and straightening of the left border of the heart. The Polo mint sign is seen on contrast-enhanced CT scan in pulmonary thromboembolism.

Suggested Reading
1. Higgins CB, Reinke RT, Jones NE, Broderick T. Left atrial dimension on the frontal thoracic radiograph: A method for assessing left atrial enlargement. Am J Roentgenol. 1978;130:251-5.

Q.19. A 44-year-old male presented with history of severe dyspnea for 1 day. He had pulsus paradoxus, elevated jugular venous pressure (JVP), and faint heart sounds. His CXR is given below. The classical Beck's triad found in this condition includes all of the following, except:

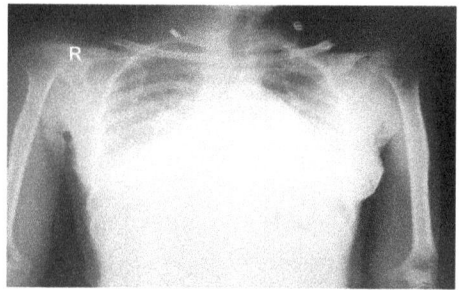

a. Elevation of JVP
b. Hypotension
c. Muffled or distant heart sounds
d. Pulsus paradoxus

Ans. d

Explanation: Beck's triad consists of elevated jugular venous pressure, hypotension, and muffled or distant heart sounds. Though pulsus paradoxus is a sign of cardiac tamponade, it is not a part of the classic Beck's triad.

Suggested Reading
1. Sternbach G. Claude Beck: Cardiac compression triads. J Emerg Med. 1988;6(5):417-9.

Q.20. A 32-year-old male was admitted with severe abdominal pain following a night of partying. His laboratory investigations revealed elevated serum amylase and lipase. After 5 days, he developed dyspnea. CXR done is given below. All are true about pleural effusion in pancreatitis, except:

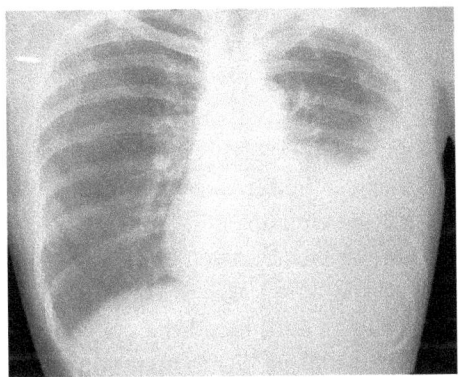

a. Usually left sided
b. Usually mild to moderate
c. Usually resolves without any interventions
d. Usually right sided

Ans. d

Explanation: Usually, pleural effusions associated with pancreatitis are mild to moderate and left sided. Ultrasonography is the most sensitive method for detecting even a mild pleural effusion in the intensive care setting and has the advantage of being easily available at the bedside. The pleural effusion usually resolves on its own without any intervention, once the inflammation subsides. If the effusion persists for >2 weeks duration, it is right-sided or it is massive, the possibility of a pancreatic pseudocyst or pancreaticopleural fistula should be considered.

Suggested Reading
1. Kumar P, Gupta P, Rana S. Thoracic complications of pancreatitis. JGH Open. 2018;3(1): 71-9.

CHAPTER 28

Approach for Acid–Base Disorders and Blood Gas Analysis

Balkrishna Nimavat

Q.1. Bicarbonate-based approach in acid–base analysis also known as:
a. Copenhagen approach
b. Boston approach
c. Stewart approach
d. Singer approach

Ans. b

Explanation: Bicarbonate-centered approach is also known as Boston approach. Importance of bicarbonate as buffer was emphasized by Henderson. Henderson-Hasselbalch equation provides relationship among the respiratory parameter (pCO_2), the nonrespiratory parameter bicarbonate (HCO_3^-), and the overall acidity parameter (pH). Base excess (BE) or standard base excess (SBE) is also known as Copenhagen approach. Singer and Hastings introduced the concept of the buffer base. Siggaard-Andersen et al. measured the plasma bicarbonate concentration at a fixed temperature and partial pCO_2 and compared the difference between their results that helped to standardized base excess formula. In Stewart approach, three independent variables responsible for maintaining electrical neutrality; (1) strong ion difference (SID); (2) total concentration of weak acids (ATOT); and (3) partial pCO_2 of the solution.

Suggested Reading
1. Kimura S, Shabsigh M, Morimatsu H. Traditional approach versus Stewart approach for acid–base disorders: Inconsistent evidence. SAGE Open Med. 2018;6:2050312118801255.

Q.2. Identify false statement regarding definitions of acid–base.
a. According to Arrhenius theory, acid is the substance that dissociates to produce H^+ in aqueous solution.
b. According to Bronsted-Lowry theory, base is an acceptor of hydrogen ions.
c. Lewis proposed base as a potential donor of a pair of electrons.
d. Usanovich theory defined acid as donor of anions or an acceptor of cations.

Ans. d

Explanation: Definitions of acid–base evolved overtime. Most recent, Usanovich theory defined acid as donor of cations and acceptor of anions. Rest of statements are true.

Suggested Reading
1. Hasan A. Handbook of Blood Gas/Acid-Base Interpretation, 2nd Edition. London: Springer; 2013. pp. 1-332.

Q.3. All are true statement, except:
   a. Standard base excess (SBE) standardizes effect of Hb on CO_2 in vivo compared to BE.
   b. SBE is still slightly subject to pCO_2 change.
   c. BE and SBE methods are unable to detect complicated acid–base disorders or identify different types of metabolic acidosis.
   d. Decrease in albumin or phosphate does not affect SBE.

Ans. d

Explanation: Base excess equation was modified to "standardize" the effect of hemoglobin on CO_2 titration known as standard base excess equation. Standard base excess (SBE) is still slightly subjected to pCO_2 change and equation of SBE assumes normal nonbuffer ion levels. While in intensive care unit (ICU) decrease in albumin or phosphate is quite common, results in biased SBE. Because of above-mentioned limitations, BE and SBE are unable to detect complicated acid–base disorders or identify different types of metabolic acidosis.

Suggested Reading
1. Kimura S, Shabsigh M, Morimatsu H. Traditional approach versus Stewart approach for acid–base disorders: Inconsistent evidence. SAGE Open Med. 2018;6:2050312118801255

Q.4. All are true statement, except:
   a. The anion gap (AG), the difference between measured plasma anions and the measured plasma cations
   b. For each 10 g/L decrement in the serum albumin concentration, the AG is expected to decrease by 2.5 mmol/L and needs to be corrected to compensate for abnormality of serum albumin concentration.
   c. Corrected AG (AGc) ignores the phosphate contribution to all of the weak acids.
   d. Albumin and phosphate, one of the circulatory proteins, mainly account for the AG under normal conditions.

Ans. a

Explanation: The anion gap (AG) is the difference between unmeasured plasma anions and the unmeasured plasma cations. Albumin and phosphate are mainly accounted for the AG under normal conditions. The rest of molecules are urate, lactate, ketone bodies, sulphate, salicylates, penicillins, citrate, pyruvate, and acetate. For each 10 g/L decrement in the serum albumin concentration, the AG is expected to decrease by 2.5 mmol/L, this value considered as corrected anion gap (AGc).

Suggested Reading
1. Kimura S, Shabsigh M, Morimatsu H. Traditional approach versus Stewart approach for acid–base disorders: Inconsistent evidence. SAGE Open Med. 2018;6:2050312118801255

Q.5. All are true, except:
a. Strong ion gap (SIG), the difference of SIDa and SIDe, quantifies *[unmeasured anions] - [unmeasured cations]* of both strong and weak ions.
b. One of the theoretical advantages of AG over SIG is the pure representation of unmeasured ions.
c. Normal AG ranges from 7 to 17 mEq/L when using (K^+) for the calculation, SIG is close to zero in normal situations.
d. "Unmeasured" ions derived from AG are composed of (Mg^{2+}), (Ca^{2+}), (A^-) (mainly albumin and phosphate), (lactate$^-$), and (other ions) clinicians do not routinely measure, whereas the unmeasured ions expressed by the SIG are composed of just (other ions).

Ans. b

Explanation: Apparent SID (SIDa) represents the difference between measured strong cations and strong anions. SID calculated to account for electrical neutrality is viewed as the effective SID (SIDe). The SIDe can be calculated as the sum of bicarbonate and weak acids (A^-), mainly albumin and phosphate. One of the theoretical advantages of SIG over AG is the pure representation of unmeasured ions. Normal AG ranges from 7 to 17 mEq/L [when using (K^+) for the calculation], SIG is close to zero in normal situations.

Suggested Reading
1. Kimura S, Shabsigh M, Morimatsu H. Traditional approach versus Stewart approach for acid-base disorders: Inconsistent evidence. SAGE Open Med. 2018;6:2050312118801255

Q.6. All are true, except:
a. ATOT, representing all nonbicarbonate buffers, is made up of mainly serum albumin and other minor charges such as phosphate and globulin.
b. In the Stewart approach, a decrease in ATOT would result in metabolic acidosis and an increase would result in metabolic alkalosis.
c. SID (SIDa) represents the difference between measured strong cations and strong anions.
d. SIDe can be calculated as the sum of bicarbonate and weak acids (A^-), mainly albumin and phosphate.

Ans. b

Explanation: Total concentration of weak acid, representing all nonbicarbonate buffers, is made up of mainly serum albumin and other minor charges such as phosphate and globulins. An increase in ATOT would result in metabolic acidosis and a decrease would result in metabolic alkalosis.

Suggested Reading
1. Kimura S, Shabsigh M, Morimatsu H. Traditional approach versus Stewart approach for acid-base disorders: Inconsistent evidence. SAGE Open Med. 2018;6:2050312118801255

Q.7. Identify the true statement about laws related to diffusion of gases.
a. Fick's law states that the volume of a gas that will dissolve in a given volume of liquid is directly proportional to the partial pressure of the gas above it.

b. Henry's law states that the quantity of gas that can pass through a sheet of tissue is *proportional to* the area (A), the diffusion constant (D), and the difference in partial pressure (P1–P2); inversely proportional to the thickness of the tissue slice (T).
c. Graham's law states that the rate of diffusion of a gas is directly proportional to the square root of its molecular weight.
d. The diffusion constant (D) is related to the solubility (Sol) and the molecular weight (MW) of the gas.

Ans. d

Explanation: Henry's law states that the volume of a gas that will dissolve in a given volume of liquid is directly proportional to the partial pressure of the gas above it. Fick's law states that the quantity of gas that can pass through a sheet of tissue is *proportional to* the area (A), the diffusion constant (D), and the difference in partial pressure (P1–P2); inversely proportional to the thickness of the tissue slice (T). Graham's law states that the rate of diffusion of a gas is inversely proportional to the square root of its molecular weight. The diffusion constant (D) is related to the solubility (Sol) and the molecular weight (MW) of the gas.

Suggested Reading
1. Hasan A. Handbook of Blood Gas/Acid-Base Interpretation, 2nd Edition. London: Springer; 2013. pp. 1-332.

Q.8. In O_2 cascade, which one of the following statements is false?
a. Partial pressure of oxygen at sea level is 160 mm Hg.
b. Alveolar partial pressure of oxygen depends on respiratory quotient.
c. One oxygen enters respiratory tract, water vapor pressure reduces partial pressure of oxygen to 95 mm Hg
d. Due to significant diffusion barriers, the amount of oxygen reached mitochondrion is a relatively tiny amount of inspired oxygen.

Ans. c

Explanation: Explanation: At sea level, the partial pressure of O_2 (PaO_2) is 760 mm Hg × 0.21 = 160 mm Hg. As the air enters into the respiratory tract due to addition of water vapor, PaO_2 is dropped by 0.21 × (760 − 47) = 149 mm Hg. At alveolar level, the PaO_2 is 149 − (40/0.8) = 99 mm Hg, where 0.8 is the respiratory quotient. "Shunt fraction" (which around 2–5% of the cardiac output) causes the systemic arterial oxygen from 100 mm Hg to 95 mm Hg. It is very important to note that only small fraction of oxygen reached at mitochondrial cell level due to multiple diffusion barriers.

Suggested Reading
1. Hasan A. Handbook of Blood Gas/Acid-Base Interpretation, 2nd Edition. London: Springer; 2013. pp. 1-332.

Q.9. Which of the following statement is false?
a. Increased $PaCO_2$ production seen in fever and hypercatabolic state.
b. Decreased CO_2 production seen in hypothermia.

c. Pain and chronic liver disease lead to decreased $PaCO_2$.
d. Hyperoxia hypoventilation and myxedema lead to decrease $PaCO_2$ level.

Ans. d

Explanation: Fever, rigors, and hypercatabolic states are etiologies for high CO_2 production and thus increased $PaCO_2$. Hypothermia reduces CO_2 production and thus reduces $PaCO_2$. Pain, anxiety, and chronic liver disease lead to hyperventilation and thus washout of CO_2, which leads to decrease $PaCO_2$. Hyperoxia hypoventilation, myxedema, metabolic alkalosis, and severe central sleep apnea lead to CNS depression and responsible for hypoventilation. This leads to higher $PaCO_2$ level.

Suggested Reading
1. Hasan A. Handbook of Blood Gas/Acid-Base Interpretation, 2nd Edition. London: Springer; 2013. pp. 1-332.

Q.10. All are true, except:
1. Low V/Q mismatch is the most common mechanism of hypoxemia.
2. V/Q mismatch is characterized by ventilation reduced relative to perfusion.
3. Shunt is defined as area where there is no ventilation but intact perfusion.
4. In low V/Q mismatch, PaO_2 does not rise with oxygen supplementation while in shunt PaO_2 rises with oxygen support.

Ans. d

Explanation: Low V/Q mismatch is the most common mechanism of hypoxemia. V/Q mismatch is characterized by ventilation reduced relative to perfusion while shunt is defined as area where there is no ventilation but intact perfusion. The administration of 100% O_2 enables differentiation between a low V/Q mismatch and shunt. PaO_2 rises with V/Q mismatch but not with shunt.

Suggested Reading
1. Hasan A. Handbook of Blood Gas/Acid-Base Interpretation, 2nd Edition. London: Springer; 2013. pp. 1-332.

Q.11. Which of the following statement pertaining to oxygen dissociation curve is wrong?
a. The Bohr effect is the CO_2 produced rightward shift of the oxygen dissociation curve.
b. O_2 unloading favors CO_2 uptake by hemoglobin by the Haldane effect.
c. In oxygen dissociation curve between 20 and 60 mm Hg PaO_2, rise in PaO_2 does not affect SpO_2 much as it is flat part of curve.
d. In normal condition of oxygen dissociation curve (ODC), PaO_2 of 70 mm Hg corresponds to SpO_2 of 92%.

Ans. c

Explanation: The Bohr effect is the CO_2 produced rightward shift of the oxygen dissociation curve. O_2 unloading favors CO_2 uptake by hemoglobin by the Haldane effect. In oxygen dissociation curve between 20 and 60 mm Hg PaO_2, rise in PaO_2 significantly affect oxygen saturation (SpO_2) much while value <20 or >60 mm Hg represents flat part of curve. In normal condition of oxygen dissociation curve (ODC), PaO_2 of 70 mm Hg corresponds to SpO_2 of 92% (PaO_2 100 with SpO_2 97 and PaO_2 40 with SpO_2 75, respectively).

Suggested Reading
1. Hasan A. Handbook of Blood Gas/Acid-Base Interpretation, 2nd Edition. London: Springer; 2013. pp. 1-332.

Q.12. All are true statement, except:
a. When the difference between SaO_2 and SpO_2 is >5%, it is labeled as saturation gap.
b. Saturation gap is a clue about presence of abnormal hemoglobins in the blood.
c. Modern pulse oximetry works on spectrophotometry and optical plethysmography.
d. Normal value of P_{50} is 50 mm Hg and value more than that suggestive of left shift of oxygen dissociation curve.

Ans. d

Explanation: Oxygen saturation is the Hb saturation of O_2 measured by pulse oximetry. Arterial oxygen saturation (SaO_2) is the Hb saturation of O_2 calculated by the arterial blood gas (ABG) machine. Difference in SaO_2 and SpO_2 is >5%, is known as saturation gap that seen in presence of abnormal hemoglobins in blood. Principle of spectrophotometry is based on the Beer–Lambert law which states that "the concentration of light-absorbing species within a sample is a logarithmic function of the amount of light absorbed by that sample." Standard pulse oximetry cannot differentiate carboxyhemoglobin from oxyhemoglobin. CO-oximeters measure absorption at several wavelengths. The normal P_{50} is 26.6 mm Hg. Value less than that suggestive of left shift and value more than that suggestive of right shift of oxygen dissociation curve.

Suggested Reading
1. Hasan A. Handbook of Blood Gas/Acid-Base Interpretation, 2nd Edition. London: Springer; 2013. pp. 1-332.

Q.13. Leftward shift of the oxygen dissociation curve occurs in the following conditions, except:
a. Hypothermia
b. Abnormal hemoglobins, e.g., *carboxyhemoglobin*
c. Myxedema
d. Steroid therapy

Ans. d

Explanation: Leftward shift of the oxygen dissociation curve occurs in alkalemia, hypothermia, abnormal hemoglobins (e.g., carboxyhemoglobin, methemoglobin, and fetal hemoglobin), myxedema, low inorganic phosphates, and acute pancreatitis. In such scenario, SpO_2 overestimates the oxygenation (i.e., PaO_2). Rightward shift of the ODC occurs in acidemia, fever, and abnormal hemoglobins, e.g., Hb Kansas, thyrotoxicosis, raised inorganic phosphate, anemia, and steroid therapy. In rightward shift of ODC, SpO_2 underestimates the PaO_2.

Suggested Reading
1. Hasan A. Handbook of Blood Gas/Acid-Base Interpretation, 2nd Edition. London: Springer; 2013. pp. 1-332.

Q.14. Rightward shift of the oxygen dissociation curve occurs in the following conditions, except:
a. Acidemia
b. Abnormal hemoglobins, e.g., *Hb Kansas*
c. Anemia
d. Acute pancreatitis

Ans. d

Explanation: Leftward shift of the oxygen dissociation curve occurs in alkalemia, hypothermia, abnormal hemoglobins (e.g., carboxyhemoglobin, methemoglobin, and fetal hemoglobin), myxedema, low inorganic phosphates, and acute pancreatitis. In such scenario, SpO_2 overestimates the oxygenation (i.e., PaO_2). Rightward shift of the ODC occurs in acidemia, fever, and abnormal hemoglobins, e.g., Hb Kansas, thyrotoxicosis, raised inorganic phosphate, anemia, and steroid therapy. In rightward shift of ODC, SpO_2 underestimates the PaO_2.

Suggested Reading
1. Hasan A. Handbook of Blood Gas/Acid-Base Interpretation, 2nd Edition. London: Springer; 2013. pp. 1-332.

Q.15. Which of the following statement pertaining to Stewart's determinants of the acid-base status is wrong?
a. Based on Stewart's principle of acid–base balance, it depends primarily on $PaCO_2$, strong ion difference (SID) and ATOT.
b. Based on Stewart's principle, six primary acid–base disturbances are possible.
c. Strong ion defined as dissociate almost completely in solution while weak electrolytes having dissociation constants normally range between 10^{-4} mEq/L and 10^{-12} mEq/L.
d. An increase in the strong ion difference will decrease blood pH, whereas a decrease in the strong ion difference will increase it.

Ans. d

Explanation: Stewart's principle of acid–base balance, it depends primarily on $PaCO_2$, strong ion difference (SID) and ATOT. Based on Stewart's principle, six primary acid–base disturbances are possible: (1) respiratory acidosis; (2) respiratory alkalosis; (3) strong ion acidosis; (4) strong ion alkalosis; (5) nonvolatile buffer acidosis; and (6) nonvolatile buffer alkalosis. Normal strong ion gap 0 mEq/L. An increase in the strong ion difference will increase blood pH, whereas a decrease in the strong ion difference will decrease it. Strong ion dissociate completely in solution with dissociative constants range excess of 10^{-4} mEq/L, while weak ions dissociate partly in solution with range of 10^{-4} mEq/L and 10^{-12} mEq/L. Examples of strong anions are sodium, potassium, magnesium, and calcium while example of strong cations are chloride.

Suggested Reading
1. Hasan A. Handbook of Blood Gas/Acid-Base Interpretation, 2nd Edition. London: Springer; 2013. pp. 1-332.

Q.16. Decrease in anion gap seen in all, except:
 a. Hypocalcemia
 b. Hypermagnesemia
 c. Lithium intoxication
 d. Paraproteinemia

Ans. a

Explanation: Hypocalcemia, hypomagnesemia, and hypoalbuminemia are associated with increase in anion gap. Hyper-albuminemia, hypermagnesemia, hyperkalemia, lithium intoxication, paraproteinemia are associated with decrease anion gap.

Suggested Reading
1. Hasan A. Handbook of Blood Gas/Acid-Base Interpretation, 2nd Edition. London: Springer; 2013. pp. 1-332.

Q.17. Negative anion gap is seen in all except:
 a. Hyponatremia
 b. Hyperchloremia
 c. Pseudohypochloremia
 d. Chronic pyridostigmine bromide therapy

Ans. c

Explanation: Anion gap is calculated by $[Na^+] - [Cl^-] - [HCO_3^-]$. Chronic pyridostigmine bromide therapy for myasthenia gravis results in high serum bromide levels and most laboratories report the bromide as chloride. This finding gives rise to false high-chloride level (pseudo-hyperchloremia) and negative anion gap on calculation. Hyponatremia and hyperchloremia value make anion gap negative.

Suggested Reading
1. Hasan A. Handbook of Blood Gas/Acid-Base Interpretation, 2nd Edition. London: Springer; 2013. pp. 1-332.

Q.18. Which one is true statement?
 a. In metabolic disorders, both actual bicarbonate (ABC) and standard bicarbonate (SBC) are altered in the different directions.
 b. In respiratory disorders, ABC and SBC are altered in same direction.
 c. The SBC is unaffected by metabolic disturbances.
 d. Standard base excess is calculated as for blood with a hemoglobin concentration of 5 g/dL.

Ans. d

Explanation: Standard bicarbonate (SBC) is a measure of plasma HCO_3 under standard conditions of PO_2, PCO_2, and temperature. Actual bicarbonate (ABC) affected by both respiratory and metabolic disorders, while standard bicarbonate. ABC < SBC suggestive of respiratory acidosis while ABC > SBC seen in respiratory alkalosis. Pure metabolic acidosis leads to fall in both ABC and SBC. In summary, in metabolic disorder both ABC and SBC altered in same directions, while in respiratory disorders they altered in different directions.

Suggested Reading
1. Hasan A. Handbook of Blood Gas/Acid-Base Interpretation, 2nd Edition. London: Springer; 2013. pp. 1-332.

Q.19. All are true about renal tubular acidosis (RTA), except:
a. Type 1 RTA characterized by preserved ability to acidify urine and it also known as classical RTA.
b. Type 2 RTA characterized by preserved property of acidification of urine but bicarbonate loss is significant.
c. Type 3 RTA characterized by loss of urine acidify property plus bicarbonate loss.
d. Type 4 and 5 RTA characterized by hyperkalemia with negligible bicarbonate loss.

Ans. a

Explanation: Type 1/distal/classical RTA characterized by loss of ability to acidify urine and negligible bicarbonate wastage. Type 2 RTA known as proximal RTA where there is significant bicarbonate wastage with preserved ability of acidify urine. Type 3 having both like wastage of bicarb with loss of acidify ability. Type 4 RTA having hyperkalemia with aldosterone deficiency.

Suggested Reading
1. Hasan A. Handbook of Blood Gas/Acid-Base Interpretation, 2nd Edition. London: Springer; 2013. pp. 1-332.

Q.20. *Urinary anion gap:* **UAG = UA − UC or ($Na^+ + K^+ - Cl^-$) all true statements, except:**
a. UAG helps distinguish between the principal causes of hyperchloremic acidosis.
b. Negative urinary anion gap seen in diarrhea.
c. Positive urinary gap seen in type 2 RTA.
d. Urinary anion gap value misleading in case of ketoacidosis.

Ans. c

Explanation: Urinary anion gap (UAG) serves as a useful estimate of urine NH_4^+. A positive UAG in a hyperchloremic metabolic acidosis suggests renal loss of bicarbonate. Similarly, negative UAG is seen in bowel loss of bicarbonate, i.e., diarrhea or type 2 RTA. In ketoacidosis, due to high value of ketone bodies excretion in urine (those are unmeasured anion), there is simultaneous loss of Na^+ and K^+ also. This affects urinary anion gap value.

Suggested Reading
1. Hasan A. Handbook of Blood Gas/Acid-Base Interpretation, 2nd Edition. London: Springer; 2013. pp. 1-332.

Q.21. **Which of the following statement is false about buffering system?**
a. Physicochemical buffering is the pivotal buffering responsible for intracellular pH management.
b. Intracellular protein and phosphate are important contributors of intracellular buffering.
c. Ammonia and phosphate are major buffer for urine.
d. Bicarbonate is the strongest buffering responsible for intracellular fluid pH.
e. Extracellular nonbicarbonate buffer system responds to acid loading immediately.

Ans. d

Explanation: Physicochemical buffering is the strongest buffering system responsible for intracellular pH management. Intracellular protein and phosphate are main component of this buffering system. Role of bicarbonate is pivotal for extracellular pH management not for intracellular. Hemoglobin and bicarbonate are important buffer for blood. Ammonia and phosphate are important major buffer for urine. Extracellular nonbicarbonate buffer system works immediately to acid load. Then comes respiratory compensation (2-4 hours), intracellular buffer mechanism, and renal (hours to days).

Suggested Reading
1. Hasan A. Handbook of Blood Gas/Acid-Base Interpretation, 2nd Edition. London: Springer; 2013. pp. 1-332.

Q.22. **All are true, except:**
a. Kassirer and Bleich's rule and the Henderson-Hasselbalch equation can be used to confirm whether ABG obtained are reliable.
b. Bicarbonate gap that is $\Delta AG - \Delta HCO_3$, if value >6 mEq/L suggestive of presence of metabolic alkalosis.
c. If bicarbonate gap is < +6 mEq/L, it is suggestive of hidden presence of high anion gap metabolic acidosis.
d. Colloid gap is also known as osmolar gap that is measured osmolality minus calculated osmolality.

Ans. c

Explanation: The modified Henderson-Hasselbalch equation: $H^+ = (24 \times CO_2)/HCO_3$. This formula is used for validity of ABG. The difference between the increase in the anion gap (ΔAG) and the decrease in the bicarbonate (ΔHCO_3^-) is termed the bicarbonate gap. If bicarbonate gap is >6, it suggests metabolic alkalosis while <6 suggest hidden presence of narrow anion gap metabolic acidosis. Colloid gap or osmolar gap defined as difference between measured osmolality and calculated osmolality. Methanol, ethylene glycol, mannitol, isopropyl alcohol, and IV immune globulin given in maltose are some of examples who create osmolar gap.

Suggested Reading
1. Hasan A. Handbook of Blood Gas/Acid-Base Interpretation, 2nd Edition. London: Springer; 2013. pp. 1-332.

Q.23. All are true, except:
a. O_2 electrode is also known as Clark electrode and it is work on principle of polarography.
b. pH electrode is known as the Sanz electrode.
c. CO_2 electrode, the Severinghaus electrode, is immersed in bicarbonate buffer solution.
d. Most blood gas machines measure pH, PCO_2, and HCO_3^- while rest of values are calculated from it.

Ans. d

Explanation: Point-of-care blood gas analysis machine measures pH, PaO_2, $PaCO_2$ while HCO_3^-, tCO_2, base excess, and SpO_2 are derived parameters.

Suggested Reading
1. Hasan A. Handbook of Blood Gas/Acid-Base Interpretation, 2nd Edition. London: Springer; 2013. pp. 1-332.

Q.24. All are true, except:
a. If the syringe is not iced immediately, the PaO_2 will come false low.
b. Abnormally high number of leukocytes or thrombocytes leads to pseudohypoxemia.
c. O_2 can diffuse out of plastic syringes, especially at high PaO_2 leads to false high PaO_2.
d. PaO_2 will be more or less unaltered for couple of hours in an iced sample of blood contained within a glass syringe.

Ans. c

Explanation: Abnormally high value of WBCs and platelets can consume a large amount of O_2 that leads to fall in PaO_2. O_2 can diffuse out of plastic syringes, especially at high PaO_2 value, this leads to spuriously low value of PaO_2. Glass syringes are less permeable to O_2 and thus PaO_2 will not be altered for up to 3 hours if icing is done well. Icing is needed if sample not analyzed within 15 minutes. If the syringe is not iced immediately, the PaO_2 is consumed by the blood cells in the sample.

Suggested Reading
1. Hasan A. Handbook of Blood Gas/Acid-Base Interpretation, 2nd Edition. London: Springer; 2013. pp. 1-332.

Q.25. What is false regarding statements on factors affecting SpO_2?
a. Fetal Hb has no special impact on SpO_2.
b. In presence of CO-Hb, SpO_2 can be displayed normal value even in severe hypoxia.
c. When Met-Hb levels >30%, SpO_2 tends to drift toward 85%, which leads to overestimation of SaO_2.
d. Red color nail polish and hyperbilirubinemia having significant effect on SpO_2.

Ans. d

Explanation: CO-Hb having almost identical absorption spectrum to Oxy-Hb. So, in presence of CO-Hb SpO_2 shows false high value, in presence of hypoxemia. This can be picked up by CO-oximeter. Hb-S having variable effect on SpO_2 while fetal-Hb having negligible to nil impact on SpO_2. Skin pigmentation, hyperbilirubinemia, and red color nail polish having negligible effect on SpO_2. Other nail color can drop SpO_2 by 3–6%.

Suggested Reading
1. Hasan A. Handbook of Blood Gas/Acid-Base Interpretation, 2nd Edition. London: Springer; 2013. pp. 1-332.

CASE-BASED MULTIPLE CHOICE QUESTIONS

Q.26. A 56-year-old COPD patient was brought to the emergency department. During transport, he had been given partial rebreathing mask at 12 L/min. At ICU, he found drowsy and was breathing with rate of 5–6 breaths/min. An ABG done, shows pH 7.30, PaO_2 65 mm Hg, HCO_3^- 30 mEq/L and $PaCO_2$ 60 mm Hg. Which one is best treatment strategy?
   a. Administering FiO_2 at 4 liters by Ventimask
   b. Making the patient breathe room air to activate hypoxic ventilatory drive
   c. Apply noninvasive ventilation with minimum oxygen support
   d. Intubation and mechanical ventilation

Ans. c

Explanation: It seems that by giving high oxygen support by partial rebreathing mask, blunt the respiratory drive and leads to worsening of respiratory acidosis in COPD patient. Applying noninvasive ventilation (NIV) in COPD patient is highly recommended in such scenario with minimum oxygen support. This is one of the few conditions where NIV is applied despite drowsiness.

Suggested Reading
1. Ahmed SM, Athar M. Mechanical ventilation in patients with chronic obstructive pulmonary disease and bronchial asthma. Indian J Anaesth. 2015;59(9):589-98.

Q.27. An 80-year-old man on having known case of diabetes mellitus (DM), hypertension (HTN), and ischemic heart disease (IHD) with poor ejection fraction (EF). Patient is on maintenance dose of diuretic therapy for EF of 20%. Patient presented to the ICU with lethargy and generalized weakness. On evaluation ABG shows pH 7.61, $PaCO_2$ 51 mm Hg, HCO_3^- 45 mEq/L, Na^+ 145 mEq/L, K^+ 1.8 mEq/L, and Cl^-: 95 mEq/L. While urinary spot chloride shows value of 70 mEq/L. What is likely acid–base disorder in this clinical scenario?
   a. High anion gap metabolic acidosis with metabolic alkalosis
   b. Metabolic alkalosis with chloride resistance
   c. Metabolic alkalosis with respiratory compensation
   d. Metabolic alkalosis with chloride responsive

Ans. b

Explanation: Clinical context is very important with ABG interpretation. Here, patient having multiple comorbidities with poor EF for which on diuretic therapy. Overzealous use of diuretic therapy leads to metabolic alkalosis (volume contraction and low potassium) and hypokalemia (due to urinary potassium loss).

- Validity of ABG checked by H^+ 24($PaCO_2/HCO_3$) = 27, correlated with pH around 7.6.
- pH is alkalosis. This alkalosis is contributed by high bicarbonate value (rather than respiratory etiology), so this is metabolic alkalosis.
- *As it is metabolic problem, it is important to do anion gap:* AG = Na^+ - (Cl^- + HCO_3^-) = 145 - (95 + 45) = 145 - 140 = 5. This normal anion gap rules out metabolic acidosis component.
- *Is any respiratory disorder:* Predicted CO_2 = [(0.7 × HCO_3^-) + 21] ±2 (as primary pathology here is metabolic alkalosis) = [(0.7 × 45) + 21] ± 5 = 31.5 + 21 ± 2 = 52.5 ± 2. Here $PaCO_2$ 51 mm Hg, so no respiratory disorder.
- Urine chloride >40 (here value 70), suggestive of chloride resistant alkalosis. Cushing's disease, diuretics, bicarbonate therapy, and low magnesium level are example of chloride resistant alkalosis.

Suggested Reading

1. Kimura S, Shabsigh M, Morimatsu H. Traditional approach versus Stewart approach for acid-base disorders: Inconsistent evidence. SAGE Open Med. 2018;6:2050312118801255

Q.28. A 35-year-old man is admitted with dehydration due to gastroenteritis. pH is 7.39, $PaCO_2$ is 38 mm Hg, HCO_3 is 22 mEq/L, Na^+ is 144 mEq/L, K^+ is 3.3 mEq/L, and Cl^- is 95 mEq/L. What is the best appropriate answer in this clinical scenario?
a. Normal ABG
b. High anion gap metabolic acidosis
c. Normal anion gap metabolic acidosis
d. High anion gap metabolic acidosis with metabolic alkalosis

Ans. d

Explanation:
1. *Validity of ABG:* H^+: 24($PaCO_2/HCO_3$) = 24(38/22) = 41 that correlate with pH of around 7.4.
2. *Patient having <7.4 pH contributed to low bicarbonate:* Metabolic acidosis primary pathology
3. *Anion gap:* 144 - (95 + 22) = 27
4. *Bicarbonate gap or delta gap:* ΔAG - ΔHCO_3^- = (27 - 10) - (24 - 22) = 17 - 2 = 15 that is higher than 6: Suggestive of metabolic alkalosis present.
5. *To find out any associated respiratory component:* Winter's formula: Predicted $PaCO_2$ = (1.5 × HCO_3^-) + 8 ± 2 = 1.5 × 22 + 8 ± 2 = 33 + 8 ± 2 = 41 ± 2 = 39: Here, $PaCO_2$ around 38.

Suggested Reading

1. Kimura S, Shabsigh M, Morimatsu H. Traditional approach versus Stewart approach for acid-base disorders: Inconsistent evidence. SAGE Open Med. 2018;6:2050312118801255

Q.29. A 42-year-old male was brought to ER after he was found lying in bed with liquor bottle, on examination, vitals are BP 110/70 mm Hg, HR: 118 beats/min, RR 28 breath/min, and temperature 37°C. He was unresponsive, pupils minimally reactive, basilar crackles with deep tendon reflex were brisk. Laboratory investigations sent which shows pH 7.25, PaCO$_2$ 34, PaO$_2$ 90, Na$^+$ 144, K$^+$ 5, Cl 98 HCO$_3^-$ 14, BUN 30, creatinine 1.5, glucose 110, lactate 1, and ketones: negative. Identify acid–base abnormality with this clinical background.

a. High anion gap metabolic acidosis
b. High anion gap metabolic acidosis with metabolic alkalosis
c. High anion gap metabolic acidosis, metabolic alkalosis with respiratory acidosis
d. Normal anion gap metabolic acidosis, metabolic alkalosis with respiratory acidosis

Ans. c

Explanation:
- *Validity of ABG checked:* H$^+$ 58 correlate with pH of 7.25
- *Acidotic pH likely due to low bicarbonate:* Metabolic acidosis
- *Anion gap:* 144 − (14 + 98) = 32: High anion gap metabolic acidosis
- *Bicarbonate gap or delta gap = 12:* Suggestive of presence of metabolic alkalosis
- *To find out respiratory component:* Winter's formula = 29 ± 2 = 31: Here value of PaCO$_2$ is 34 suggestive of presence of respiratory acidosis component also.

Suggested Reading
1. Kimura S, Shabsigh M, Morimatsu H. Traditional approach versus Stewart approach for acid–base disorders: Inconsistent evidence. SAGE Open Med. 2018;6:2050312118801255

Q.30. A 42-year-old woman presents to ICU with history of nausea and recurrent vomiting for 2 days. She also gives a history of having taken several tablets of aspirin for relief of joint pains before experiencing nausea. Her blood gas analysis shows pH 7.61, PaCO$_2$ 34, HCO$_3^-$ 34 mEq/L, and electrolyte values are Na$^+$ 135, K$^+$ 4, and Cl$^-$ 101. Which one of the following is the best suitable answer?

a. Metabolic alkalosis with respiratory alkalosis
b. Metabolic alkalosis with respiratory acidosis
c. Metabolic alkalosis with high anion gap metabolic acidosis
d. Metabolic alkalosis, respiratory acidosis, and normal anion gap metabolic acidosis

Ans. a

Explanation:
- *Validity of ABG:* H$^+$ = 24 that correlate with pH of 7.6.
- *Alkalotic pH likely due to increased bicarbonate value:* Metabolic alkalosis
- *Anion gap should be done to rule out hidden metabolic acidosis:* AG = 0, no metabolic acidosis component present.
- *For respiratory component:* PaCO$_2$ = [(0.7 × HCO$_3^-$) + 21] ± 2 = 44.8 ± 2, respiratory alkalosis present (as here PaCO$_2$ value is 34).

Suggested Reading
1. Kimura S, Shabsigh M, Morimatsu H. Traditional approach versus Stewart approach for acid–base disorders: Inconsistent evidence. SAGE Open Med. 2018;6:2050312118801255.

CHAPTER 29

Ultrasonography

Shrikanth Srinivasan, Balaji Kannamani, Ankit Purohit

Q.1. When ultrasound waves encounter air/gas, they are:
   a. Immediately reflected 100% back to the probe
   b. Deflected in all directions
   c. Pass through easily
   d. None of the above

Ans. a

Explanation
- Ultrasound waves are produced by stimulation of piezoelectric crystals located in the probe (piezoelectric effect). When the ultrasound waves are transmitted into the biological tissue, some of them are reflected back and some are absorbed by the tissue (depend on acoustic impedance of the tissue). Reflected waves are analyzed by probe and producing the image (pulse echo principle).
- Fluid and soft tissue allow the ultrasound waves to pass through and provide clear media for imaging.
- Bone and air are poor conductor, almost all of the sound waves are reflected back at soft tissue-air or soft tissue—bone interface.
- The resistance to passage of ultrasound beams is called acoustic impedance (Z), dense structures like bone have high-acoustic impedance and hence reflect back 100% of the ultrasound beams from its surface itself leading to appearance of a bright hyperechoic line representing the surface of the bone and a dark acoustic shadow beneath as there is no penetration through the surface.
- Also, the higher the acoustic impedance (product of density and velocity of the sound) difference between materials, the more reflection occurs at their boundary.
- Air has very low-acoustic impedance and due to the extreme difference in the acoustic impedance between air and the surrounding structures, air acts as a barrier to ultrasound producing hyperechoic artifacts without any acoustic shadowing. Due to the reflections of ultrasound beams from the air interphase, air acts as an enemy for ultrasound.

Suggested Reading
1. Abu-Zidan FM, Hefny AF, Corr P. Clinical ultrasound physics. J Emerg Trauma Shock. 2011;4(4):501-3.

2. Powles AEJ, Martin DJ, Wells ITP, Goodwin CR. Physics of ultrasound. Anaesth Intensive Care Med. 2018;19(4):202-5.

Q.2. As the ultrasound probe frequency increases, ultrasound penetration proportionately:
   a. Decreases
   b. Increases
   c. Remains unaffected
   d. None of the above

Ans. a

Explanation
- Ultrasound frequencies (f) inversely proportional to wavelength and directly proportional to velocity in particular tissue (C).
- $(\lambda = \frac{C}{f})$
- Low-frequency probes provide better access to deep tissue examination but lacks resolution.

    Axial resolution = ½ (spatial pulse length)
- Higher frequency probe has less depth penetration but provide better detail and spatial resolution (sharpness).

Suggested Reading
1. Abu-Zidan FM, Hefny AF, Corr P. Clinical ultrasound physics. J Emerg Trauma Shock. 2011;4(4):501-3.
2. Powles AEJ, Martin DJ, Wells ITP, Goodwin CR. Physics of ultrasound. Anaesth Intensive Care Med. 201819(4):202-5.

Q.3. If an image displayed on the monitor is too dark, how can it be optimized?
   a. Increases gain
   b. Decrease gain
   c. Apply less ultrasound gel
   d. Increases depth

Ans. a

Explanation
- When the ultrasound wave passes through biological tissue some of them gets absorbed, so reflected waves from deeper structures have less amplitude. It is known as attenuation.
- So, one might expect late echoes from deeper layers to have smaller amplitudes than early echoes (superficial tissue) even if those layers have same echogenicity. So, the image becomes darker from superficial to deep.
- Gain compensation allows us to overcome this artifact. Time gain compensation (TGC) and lateral gain compensation (LGC) allow to increase resolution in along the beam and perpendicular to beam respectively.

Suggested Reading
1. Abu-Zidan FM, Hefny AF, Corr P. Clinical ultrasound physics. J Emerg Trauma Shock. 2011;4(4):501-3.
2. Powles AEJ, Martin DJ, Wells ITP, Goodwin CR. Physics of ultrasound. Anaesth Intensive Care Med. 2018;19(4):202-5.

Q.4. Which of the following conditions is not consistent with this sonographic finding?

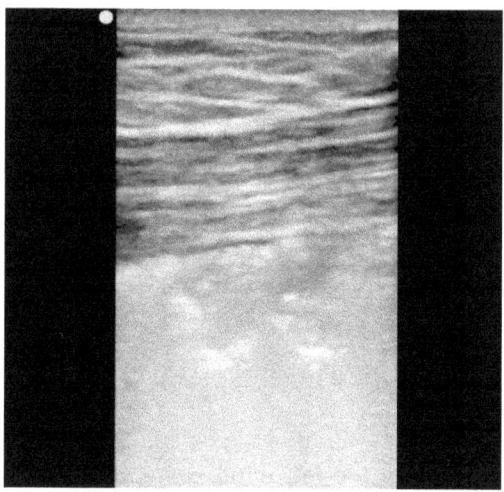

a. Pneumonia
b. Cardiogenic pulmonary edema
c. Infarcted lung parenchyma
d. Lung Cancer

Ans. b

Explanation
- Cardiogenic pulmonary edema causes accumulation of fluid in extravascular space starting from alveolar interstitium to interlobular septum.
- Thickened interlobular septum among air-filled alveoli causes reverberation of ultrasound waves and creates reverberation artifact known as B-lines.
- B-lines (lung rockets) are vertical lines originating at the pleural line extending to deepest part of image.
- More than 3 B-lines in any single view is pathological.
- Although B-lines or B-profile is pathognomonic of pulmonary edema, it won't differentiate cardiogenic from noncardiogenic pulmonary edema.

Suggested Reading
1. Soldati G, Demi M, Demi L. Ultrasound patterns of pulmonary edema. Ann Transl Med. 2019;7(Suppl 1):S16.
2. Soldati G, Demi M, Smargiassi A, Inchingolo R, Demi L. The role of ultrasound lung artifacts in the diagnosis of respiratory diseases. Expert Rev Respir Med. 2019;13:163-72.

Q.5. The IVC's diameter should be measured:
a. At the 1-cm point distal to the right atrium—IVC junction
b. 2-cm point distal to IVC-RA junction
c. At the diaphragmatic junction
d. At the IVC—right atrial junction

Ans. b

Explanation
- Inferior vena cava (IVC) measurement and caval index are being used frequently to assess the volume status of the patients.
- The IVC collapses nonuniformly.
- Most studies measure the IVC at or around the confluence with the hepatic veins.
- Wallace et al. warned against measuring at the junction with the right atrium (RA) since this produces high collapsibility not correlating with actual volume status of the patient.
- Most practiced approaches are measurement of diameter 2-3 cm from right atrium IVC junction or just distal to IVC—hepatic vein junction.

Suggested Reading
1. Finnerty NM, Panchal AR, Boulger C, Vira A, Bischof JJ, Amick C, et al. Inferior vena cava measurement with ultrasound: What is the best view and best mode? West J Emerg Med. 2017;18(3):496-501.
2. Wallace DJ, Allison M, Stone MB. Inferior vena cava percentage collapse during respiration is affected by the sampling location: an ultrasound study in healthy volunteers. Acad Emerg Med. 2010;17(1):96-9.

Q.6. In the parasternal long-axis view of the heart, a fluid collection posterior to the left ventricle that is seen between the descending thoracic aorta and left atrium is likely to be located in which of the following spaces?
   a. Left pleural cavity
   b. Abdominal cavity
   c. Pericardial space
   d. Bilateral pleural spaces

Ans. c

Explanation
- Pericardial effusion—anechoic (black) space noted between walls of the heart and hyperechoic (bright) pericardium layer.
- Pericardial effusion can be visualized in subxiphoid view as part of extended focused assessment with sonography in trauma (e-FAST) in trauma patients. Parasternal short-axis view is necessary to rule out localized effusion from circumferential one.
- Parasternal long-axis view—anechoic visualized between left chamber and pericardial layer and descending thoracic aorta (DTA).
- DTA marks the boundary to differentiate pericardial effusion from left pleural effusion. Anechoic space below DTA usually indicates pleural effusion on the left side.

Suggested Reading
1. Pérez-Casares A, Cesar S, Brunet-Garcia L, Sanchez-de-Toledo J. Echocardiographic evaluation of pericardial effusion and cardiac tamponade. Front Pediatr. 2017;5:79.

Q.7. Regarding inferior vena cava, the best way to confirm whether the vessel being imaged is the inferior vena cava is:
   a. The vessel wall is thin
   b. Nonpulsatility

c. Color Doppler revealing triphasic waves
d. By visualizing the hepatic vein joining the vessel

Ans. d

Explanation
- IVC can be differentiated from aorta by its thin wall, collapsibility, nonpulsatility, and triphasic flow in Doppler study.
- Gold standard to differentiate IVC is identification of hepatic vein and its confluence with IVC.
- IVC diameter and caval index can be measured distal to IVC—hepatic vein confluence or 2–3 cm distal to RA—IVC junction.

Suggested Reading
1. Akkaya A, Yesilaras M, Aksay E, Sever M, Atilla OD. The interrater reliability of ultrasound imaging of the inferior vena cava performed by emergency residents. Am J Emerg Med. 2013;31(10):1509-11.
2. Charron C, Caille V, Jardin F, Viellard-Baron A. Echocardiographic measurement of fluid responsiveness. Curr Op Crit Care. 2006;12(3):249-54.

Q.8. A pericardial effusion is considered as large when the pericardial space is:
a. >2 cm during diastole
b. >2 cm during systole
c. 1–2 cm during diastole
d. 1–2 cm during systole

Ans. a

Explanation
- Pericardial effusion is classified into mild, moderate, and severe based on its volume. Volume is indirectly measured based on distance between pericardial layer and heart chamber during diastole (smallest at fluid-tissue interface).
- Effusion seen only during systole is trivial, mild <10 mm, moderate 10–20 mm, and considered as severe if distance is >20 mm.
- Size of the effusion is always measured in parasternal long-axis view.
- Localized effusion and any amount of effusion causing RV free wall collapse need immediate attention.

Suggested Reading
1. Pérez-Casares A, Cesar S, Brunet-Garcia L, Sanchez-de-Toledo J. Echocardiographic evaluation of pericardial effusion and cardiac tamponade. Front Pediatr. 2017;5:79.

Q.9. Earliest sign of pericardial tamponade is:
a. Mid-diastolic collapse of right atrium
b. Mid-systolic collapse of right atrium
c. Mid-diastolic collapse of right ventricle
d. Mid-systolic collapse of right ventricle

Ans. b

Explanation
- Right atrial collapse precedes the clinical signs of pericardial tamponade. Right atrium collapse starts from late diastole but it has poor sensitivity.

Chamber collapse when the intrachamber pressure is low compared to pericardial pressure.
- For atrium, it happened during ventricular systole, because apart from atrial systole, atrium spends its time for chamber filling in cardiac cycle. During RV systole, atrium chambers tend to have low pressures.
- If the right atrial collapse exceeds >30% of cardiac cycle, it predicts tamponade.
- RV mid-diastolic collapse is classic sign of evident pericardial tamponade which needs immediate attention.

Suggested Reading
1. Alerhand S, Carter JM. What echocardiographic findings suggest a pericardial effusion is causing tamponade? Am J Emerg Med. 2019;37(2):321-6.

Q.10. Identify the structures seen in the image:

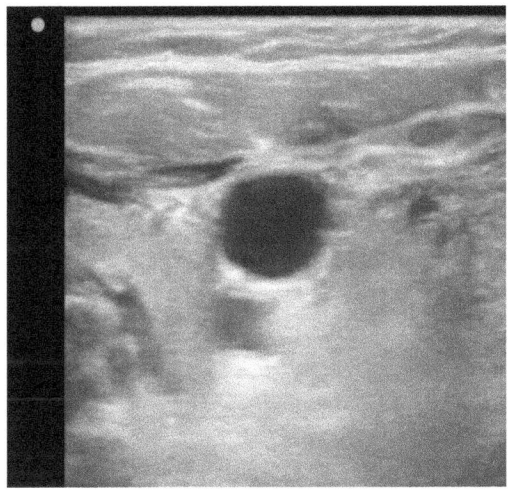

a. Internal jugular vein and carotid
b. Subclavian vein and artery
c. External and internal carotid artery
d. Brachial vein and artery

Ans. a

Explanation
- Image shows the internal jugular vein (IJV) and carotid artery.
- It can be identified based on its relation to trachea—sternocleidomastoid muscle
- Overlapping nature of vessels also indicates the possibility of IJV, carotid.

Suggested Reading
1. Solanki SL, Doctor JR, Kapila SJ, Jain A, Joshi M, Patil VP. Ultrasonographic assessment of internal jugular vein diameter and its relationship with the carotid artery at the apex, middle, and base of the triangle formed by two heads of sternocleidomastoid muscle: a pilot study in healthy volunteers. Saudi J Anaesth. 2018;12(4):578-83.
2. Turker G, Kaya FN, Gurbet A, Aksu H, Erdogan C, Atlas A. Internal jugular vein cannulation: an ultrasound-guided technique versus a landmark-guided technique. Clinics (Sao Paulo). 2009;64(10):989-92.

Q.11. **With regards to safety of cannulation, based on the above image, which of the following statement is correct?**
 a. Venous cannulation is technically easy as vein and artery are separate and not overlapped.
 b. Venous cannulation at this point may be avoided due to risk of injury to surrounding structures, however, there is no arterial puncture.
 c. Venous cannulation at this point may be avoided due to risk of arterial puncture.
 d. Venous cannulation at this point may be avoided due to presence of thrombus.

Ans. c

Explanation
- Overlapping nature of the vein and artery increases the risk of inadvertent carotid puncture and hematoma. Choosing the appropriate window for venous cannulation is crucial for successful venous cannulation.
- Various studies compared the longitudinal and short axis cannulation techniques, it revealed that long axis cannulation techniques had less carotid puncture compared to other technique. Longitudinal cannulation techniques needs expertise to get appropriate window and differentiating artery and vein is crucial before cannulation.

Suggested Reading
 1. Saugel B, Scheeren TWL, Teboul, JL. Ultrasound-guided central venous catheter placement: a structured review and recommendations for clinical practice. Crit Care. 2017;21(1); 225. https://doi.org/10.1186/s13054-017-1814-y

Q.12. **What does the ultrasound image show?**

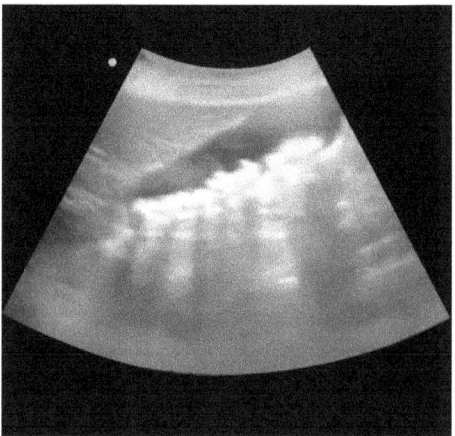

 a. Multiple gallstones
 b. Multiple renal calculi
 c. Gallbladder sludge
 d. Acalculous cholecystitis

Ans. a

Explanation: Multiple bright echogenic focus inside the gallbladder indicates the possibility of multiple gallstones. Hypoechoic shadowing posterior to the bright foci confirms the possibility of gallstones.

Suggested Reading

1. Bortoff G, Chen M, Ott D, Wolfman N, Routh W. Gallbladder stones: imaging and intervention. Radiographics. 2000;20(3):751-66.

Q.13. What type of artifact does the above image show?
a. Mirror image artifact
b. Posterior acoustic shadowing
c. Acoustic enhancement
d. Reverberation artifacts

Ans. b

Explanation
- Posterior acoustic shadowing is pathognomonic of stones irrespective of their composition.
- It is formed by high-acoustic impedance of stones which reflected all the ultrasonic beam and did not allow it pass through. It creates shadowing behind the stones.

Suggested Reading

1. Bortoff G, Chen M, Ott D, Wolfman N, Routh W. Gallbladder stones: imaging and intervention. Radiographics. 2000;20(3):751-66.

A young lady on treatment for infertility presents with dyspnea and hypoxia, the ultrasound scan of the chest and abdomen showed the following findings:

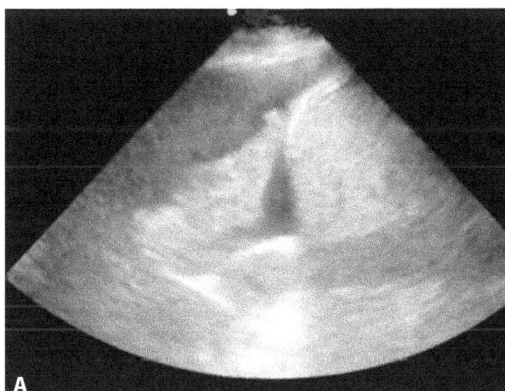
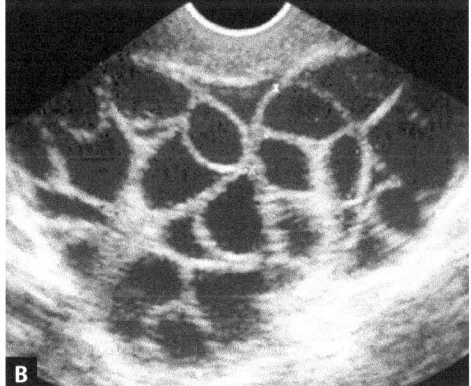

Q.14. The thoracic scan (Figure A) is suggestive of:
a. Consolidation of lung
b. Pleural fluid with consolidation
c. Pleural fluid, ascites, and consolidation
d. Pleural fluid with hepatomegaly

Ans. c

Explanation
- Ultrasound image shows massive right pleural effusion with underlying lung collapse/consolidation with ascites. USG has high sensitivity to detect even small amount of effusion (5-10mL) that cannot be detected by radiograph.

- Thoracic spine sign appears to due to excellent acoustic medium (fluid) in pleural cavity and it indicates moderate to massive collection. Mild effusion can be detected by quad sign, it is quadrangle space between parietal, visceral pleura and aerated lung margins. Large pleural effusion causes compression atelectasis of lung.
- USG also helps to differentiate exudate from transudate based on echogenicity of fluids. Plankton sign is hyperechoic spots in the middle of homogeneous collection which indicates the possibility of exudates.

Suggested Reading
1. Soni NJ, Franco R, Velez MI, Schnobrich D, Dancel R, Restrepo MI, et al. Ultrasound in the diagnosis and management of pleural effusions. J Hosp Med. 2015;10(12):811-6.

Q.15. What is seen in the pelvic window (Figure B)?
a. Loculated ascites
b. Hydatid cyst with ascites
c. Dilated bowel loops with ascites
d. Polycystic ovaries

Ans. d

Explanation: Figure B shows multiple loculated thin-walled cysts, which increase the possibility of polycystic ovaries with ovarian hyperstimulation syndrome (OHSS). Multiple cysts of varying sizes cause the reflection of spoke-wheel appearance. Clear liquids within cyst, absence of calcifications and thin walls increases the possibility of ovarian cysts.

Suggested Reading
1. Nastri CO, Teixeira DM, Moroni RM, Leitão VM, Martins WP. Ovarian hyperstimulation syndrome: pathophysiology, staging, prediction and prevention. Ultrasound Obstet Gynecol. 2015;45(4):377-93.

Q.16. What is the most likely clinical picture?
a. Disseminated tuberculosis
b. Hydatid cyst with peritonitis
c. Paralytic ileus with peritonitis
d. Ovarian hyperstimulation syndrome

Ans. d

Explanation: Prior history of infertility treatment increases the possibility of ovarian hyperstimulation syndrome. It is complication of controlled ovarian induction during assisted reproductive techniques. It increases the vasoactive mediators release and causes water retention which leads to accumulation of fluids in peritoneal, pericardial, pleural cavity. Young females usually presents with dyspnea and abdominal distension. Prior history of PCOD, hypothyroidism, low BMI increases the risk of OHSS.

Suggested Reading
1. Bortoff G, Chen M, Ott D, Wolfman N, Routh W. Gallbladder stones: imaging and intervention. Radiographics. 2000;20(3):751-66.
2. Nastri CO, Teixeira DM, Moroni RM, Leitão VM, Martins WP. Ovarian hyperstimulation syndrome: pathophysiology, staging, prediction and prevention. Ultrasound Obstet Gynecol. 2015;45(4):377-93.

Q.17. The correct order of increasing acoustic impedance in different media is:
a. Air < fat < soft tissue < bone
b. Air < bone < fat < soft tissue
c. Bone < fat < soft tissue < air
d. Soft tissue < fat < air < bone

Ans. a

Explanation
- Acoustic impedance (Z) is resistance encountered by ultrasound waves when entering the biological tissues.
- It depends on density of tissue (d) and velocity (c) of sound waves in that tissue (Z = d × c).
- Impedance increases depend on density of tissues.
- The ability of an ultrasound wave to transfer from one tissue type to another depends on the difference in impedance of the two tissues.
- If the difference is large, then the sound is reflected completely like bone.
- Air has least impedance followed by fat, water, soft tissue, muscle, and bone.

Suggested Reading
1. Abu-Zidan FM, Hefny AF, Corr P. Clinical ultrasound physics. J Emerg Trauma Shock. 2011;4(4):501-3
2. Powles AEJ, Martin DJ, Wells ITP, Goodwin CR. Physics of ultrasound. Anaesth Intensive Care Med. 2018;19(4):202-5.

Q.18. A 53-year-old male presented with complaints of polytrauma with diffuse grade-IV subarachnoid hemorrhage (SAH) with cerebral edema with shock. A transcranial Doppler (TCD) performed on day 2 is suggestive of:

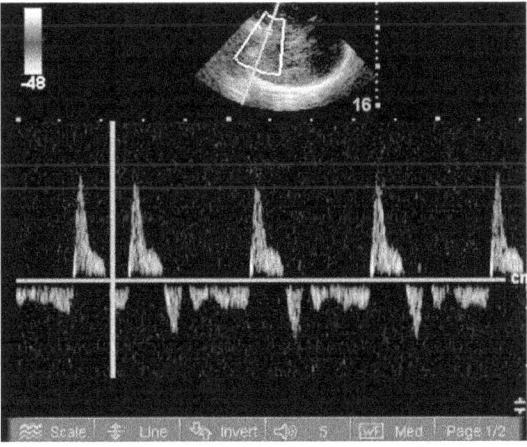

a. Vasospasm
b. Impending brain death
c. Anemia due to blood loss
d. hypercarbia

Ans. b

Explanation
- TCD shows sharp spike systolic flow with reversed diastolic flow.

- Early stage of intracranial pressure (ICP) rise, TCD shows decreased diastolic flow. It needs immediate attention.
- Forward systolic and backward diastolic flow is known as "oscillating flow".
- When the forward flow current meets equal backward flow current, it indicates zero blood flow. That means the ICP has crossed the cerebral perfusion pressure and blood flow stopped.
- When ICP approaches systolic pressures, diastolic reverse flow disappears, it is evident of brain dead. Absent diastolic flow is considered as an irreversible sign of neural recovery.

Suggested Reading
1. Kasapoğlu US, Haliloğlu M, Bilgili B, Cinel I. The role of transcranial Doppler ultrasonography in the diagnosis of brain death. Turk J Anaesthesiol Reanim. 2019;47(5):367-74.
2. Lampl Y, Gilad R, Eschel Y, Boaz M, Rapoport A, Sadeh M. Diagnosing brain death using the transcranial Doppler with a transorbital approach. Arch Neurol. 2002;59(1): 58-60.

Q.19. FAST examination view of right upper quadrant in a young patient with history of assault has the finding shown. He is not in shock.

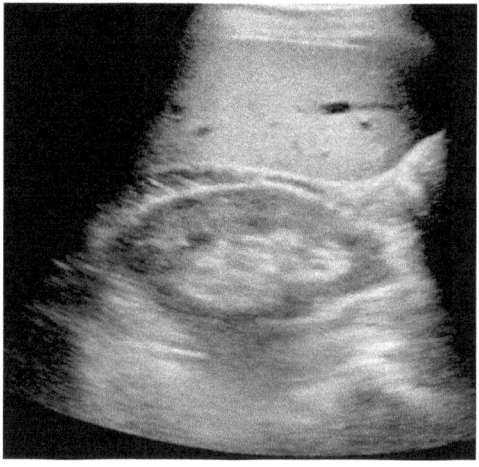

What will be your next action?
a. Diagnostic peritoneal lavage
b. Urgent laparotomy
c. CT abdomen with contrast
d. Percutaneous drainage and culture. Empiric antibiotics

Ans. c

Explanation
- Ultrasonography (USG) image shows free fluid in hepatorenal pouch, possibility of hemoperitoneum. Since the patient is not in shock, computed tomography (CT) abdomen with contrast should be advised to evaluate the extent and site of injury.

- Diagnostic peritoneal lavage indicated only when patient presented with free fluid and compromised hemodynamics. It is indicated in hemodynamically unstable patient with blunt trauma/penetrating trauma where the option of CT/e-FAST is not available.
- Emergency laparotomy indicated as resuscitative measure to stop the bleeding in hemodynamically unstable patient.

Suggested Reading
1. Bloom BA, Gibbons RC. Focused assessment with sonography for trauma. Treasure Island (FL): StatPearls Publishing; 2023.

Q.20. Which of the following is not typically inspected during an e-FAST examination?
a. Pericardium
b. Right costophrenic angle
c. Pelvis
d. Right paracolic gutter

Ans. d

Explanation
- Focused assessment with sonography for trauma includes examination of abdominal and pelvic injuries to identify life-threatening bleeding.
- Extended fast included thoracic cavity and pericardium assessment.
- Classic views include:
  - Subxiphoid view/PLAX
  - Right upper quadrant view
  - Left upper quadrant view
  - Pelvic view
  - Right and left lung view

Suggested Reading
1. Richards J, McGahan J. Focused assessment with sonography in trauma (FAST) in 2017: What radiologists can learn. Radiology. 2017;283(1):30-48.

Q.21. Identify the pathology.

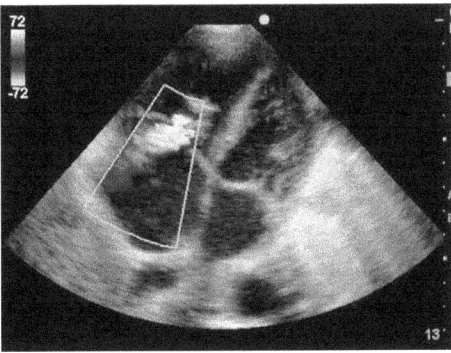

a. Dilated RA, RV, and tricuspid regurgitation
b. Dilated LA, LV, and mitral regurgitation

c. Ventricular septal rupture
d. Pericardial tamponade

Ans. a

Explanation
- Apical four-chamber view shows dilated right ventricular (RV), RA chambers and color Doppler show sever tricuspid regurgitation.
- It indicates RV dysfunction. Common causes of acute cor pulmonale include pulmonary embolism, severe acute respiratory distress syndrome (ARDS), and postcardiac surgery.
- RV assessment includes measurement of tricuspid regurgitation velocity (TRV), tricuspid annular plane systolic excursion (TAPSE), RV fractional area change, and Tei index.
- TRV >2.4 m/s and TAPSE <1.7 cm indicate severe RV dysfunction.

Suggested Reading
1. Schneider M, Aschauer S, Mascherbauer J, Ran H, Binder C, Lang I, et al. Echocardiographic assessment of right ventricular function: current clinical practice. Int J Cardiovasc Imaging. 2019;35(1):49-56.

Q.22. **The reflection coefficient of ultrasound waves between air and water is:**
a. 90%
b. 1%
c. Nearly 100%
d. 50%

Ans. c

Explanation
- Reflection coefficient is the ratio of amplitude of reflected wave to the incident wave. R value ranges from −1 to +1.
- It depends on the density and velocity of two different medium.
- R value is −1 from water to air, it means nearly 100% of energy is reflected back.
- R value −0.5 from water to solid.

Suggested Reading
1. Bushberg JT, Seibert JA, Leidholdt EM Jr, Boone JM. The Essential Physics of Medical Imaging. Philadelphia: Lippincott Williams & Wilkins; 2011.
2. Powles AEJ, Martin DJ, Wells ITP, Goodwin CR. Physics of ultrasound. Anaesth Intensive Care Med. 2018;19(4):202-5.

Q.23. **Regarding the frequency of ultrasound waves in tissues. The correct statement is:**
a. Lower frequency waves are better the resolution.
b. Increasing frequency will increase tissue penetration.
c. Frequency is inversely proportionate to wavelength.
d. Increasing frequency will increase velocity of the sound wave.

Ans. c

Explanation
- Frequency is inversely related to wavelength. Higher the frequency lesser the depth penetration but better resolution.

- Lower frequency probes give access to examine deeper structures such as abdominal cavity, thoracic examination but at the cost of low resolution.
- Velocity equals frequency times wavelength.

Suggested Reading
1. Abu-Zidan FM, Hefny AF, Corr P. Clinical ultrasound physics. J Emerg Trauma Shock. 2011;4(4):501-3.
2. Powles AEJ, Martin DJ, Wells ITP, Goodwin CR. Physics of ultrasound. Anaesth Intensive Care Med. 2018;19(4):202-5.

Q.24. The time gain compensation (TGC) control compensates for:
a. The time taken to undertake the scan
b. Attenuation deficits
c. The difference in ultrasound speed in different body tissues
d. The video image displays lag time

Ans. b

Explanation
- The amplitude of waves decreases as they pass through biological tissues, it is known as attenuation.
- Attenuation causes decreased resolution. Superficial images look brighter and deeper one becomes black.
- Conversion of energy (heat) when passes through tissues causes the attenuation. Bone and lung have highest attenuation coefficient.
- Time gain compensation helps to overcome this attenuation artifact.

Suggested Reading
1. Abu-Zidan FM, Hefny AF, Corr P. Clinical ultrasound physics. J Emerg Trauma Shock. 2011;4(4):501-3.
2. Powles AEJ, Martin DJ, Wells ITP, Goodwin CR. Physics of ultrasound. Anaesth Intensive Care Med. 2018;19(4):202-5.

Q.25. The following M-mode lung ultrasound shows:

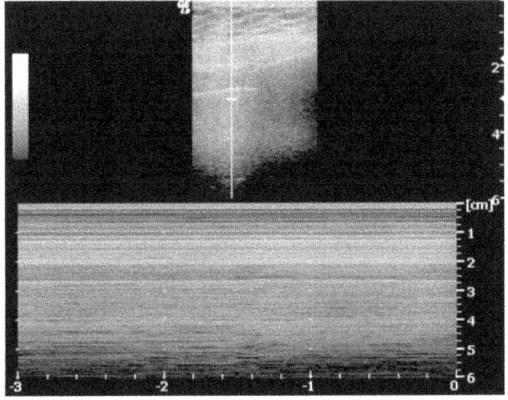

a. The "seashore" sign, which indicates a pneumothorax.
b. The "stratosphere" sign, which indicates a pneumothorax.
c. The "seashore" sign, which indicates normal lung and no pneumothorax.
d. The "stratosphere" sign, which indicates normal lung and no pneumothorax.

Ans. b

Explanation
- Normal lung interface with pleura produces lung sliding sign. In M-mode, it is visualized as seashore sign, because of movement of lung and pleura.
- Absence of seashore sign denotes absence of lung movement with pleura. It produces barcode sign or stratosphere sign in M-mode. It indicates pneumothorax. Conditions such as active lung collapse, endobronchial intubation also can produce stratosphere sign.
- Identification of lung point (point between moving lung and collapsed one) confirms the pneumothorax with sensitivity and specificity of almost 100%.

Suggested Reading
1. Lichtenstein DA. Lung ultrasound in the critically ill. Ann Intensive Care. 2014;4:1.

Q.26. **With regards EFAST examination in trauma, the appropriate statement is:**
a. It is possible to distinguish free blood from ascites or urine in the peritoneal cavity.
b. Ultrasound of the lungs is less reliable than a supine CXR to detect a pneumothorax.
c. An empty bladder does not affect the ability to detect pelvic free fluid.
d. Depending on operator, up to 10% of scans may be indeterminate.

Ans. c

Explanation: An empty bladder does not affect the ability to detect pelvic free fluid. "A full bladder is preferable, however, if the bladder is decompressed aim the probe caudally. Increase the depth to visualize posterior to the bladder where free fluid collects. Sweep caudally and cephalad to obtain complete views of the rectovesical space in men and the rectouterine and vesicouterine pouches in women. These pouches are the most dependent recesses of the intraperitoneal cavity. In order to achieve greater sensitivity, rotate the probe 90° clockwise into the sagittal orientation to best assess the pouch of Douglas and vesicouterine pouch in women."

Suggested Reading
1. Bloom BA, Gibbons RC. Focused assessment with sonography for trauma. Treasure Island (FL): StatPearls Publishing; 2023.

Q.27. In the following transverse ultrasound view of the mid abdominal aorta, aortic diameter is:

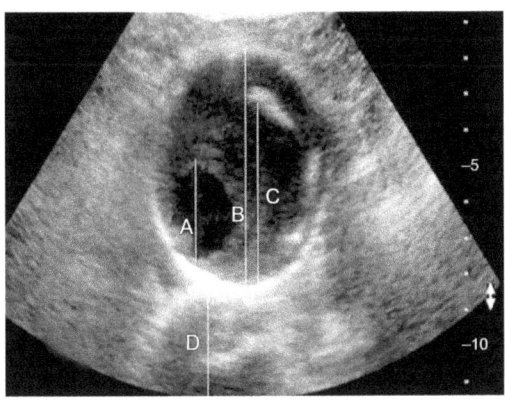

a. A
b. B
c. C
d. D

Ans. a

Explanation: This is an image of aortic dissection. The true diameter is A as with complete continuity of the intima A is true diameter.

B indicates the diameter of the false lumen which is the gap between intima and externa.

Further the color Doppler application and difference between the flow of the velocities help to differentiate true from false lumen.

Suggested Reading
1. Williams J, Heiner JD, Perreault MD, McArthur TJ. Aortic dissection diagnosed by ultrasound. West J Emerg Med. 2010;11(1):98-9.

Q.28. What does the liver ultrasound image show?

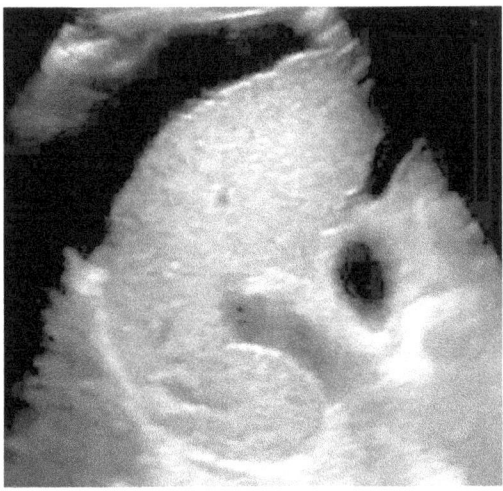

a. Hepatomegaly with fatty infiltration
b. Small shrunken liver with surface granularity
c. Multiple liver space-occupying lesions
d. Thickened gallbladder with normal liver parenchyma

Ans. b

Explanation: USG has high sensitivity to find early changes of liver cirrhosis. Echotexture of liver and surface nodularity detects the severity of liver cirrhosis. Early changes include caudate lobe hypertrophy followed by right posterior segments atrophy. Liver span less than 12 cm denotes shrunken liver. Changes in portal venous flow and diameter can denotes the associated portal hypertension.

Suggested Reading
1. John P. McGahan, Barry B. Goldberg. Diagnostic Ultrasound. (2008) ISBN: 9781420069785

Q.29. What is the likely diagnosis as per the previous image?
a. Acute hepatitis b. Early cirrhosis
c. Advanced cirrhosis with free fluid d. Acute cholecystitis

Ans. c

Explanation: Liver cirrhosis is characterized by changes in liver volume distribution, surface nodularity, accentuation of the fissure, heterogeneity, bright and coarsening of the hepatic architecture, cirrhotic nodules including regenerative and dysplastic nodules, and signs of portal hypertension. Studies showed an overall sensitivity to chronic liver disease of 65–95%, with a positive predictive value of 98%. The most indicative finding of liver cirrhosis was nodular surface, which was more sensitive on the undersurface of the liver than the superior surface (86% vs. 53%).

The black shadow on the upper border of the liver signifies collection or ascites. It is in the Morrison pouch (right paracolic gutter).

Suggested Reading
1. Yeom SK, Lee CH, Cha SH, Park CM. Prediction of liver cirrhosis, using diagnostic imaging tools. World J Hepatol. 2015;7(17):2069-79.

Q.30. What is the application of this view and mode selection?

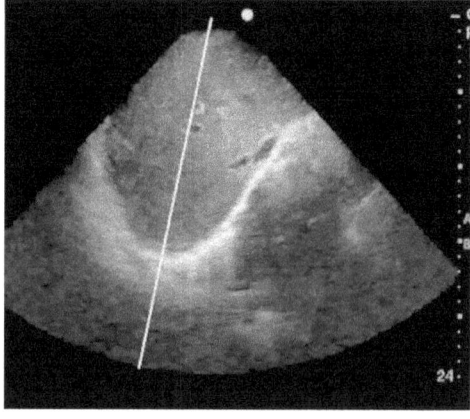

a. IVC respiratory variation measurement
b. Diaphragm excursion measurement
c. Diaphragm thickness fraction measurement
d. Myocardial fractional shortening

Ans. b

Explanation: The diaphragm is the main muscle of respiration. The assessment of diaphragmatic motion by ultrasound could be a useful indicator for the diagnosis and follow-up of respiratory diseases. Diaphragmatic excursion imaging is important for the diagnosis of diaphragmatic dysfunction or paralysis.

Diaphragmatic excursion is 1–2 cm during tidal breathing and 7–11 cm during deep inspiration. Age, sex, and body mass index (BMI) significantly affect diaphragmatic motion with variable extents during different types of breathing (quiet, deep, and sniffing).

An excursion >12 mm during a spontaneous breathing, trail can be used as a surrogate for extubation success.

With regards to diaphragmatic strength, it is a relatively less sensitive marker than diaphragmatic thickening fraction.

Suggested Reading
1. Boussuges A, Rives S, Finance J, Brégeon F. Assessment of diaphragmatic function by ultrasonography: current approach and perspectives. World J Clinl Cases. 2020;8:2408-24.
2. Le Neindre A, Philippart F, Luperto M, Wormser J, Morel-Sapene J, Aho SL. Diagnostic accuracy of diaphragm ultrasound to predict weaning outcome: a systematic review and meta-analysis. Int J Nurs Stud. 2021;117:103890.
3. Lloyd T, Tang YM, Benson MD, King S. Diaphragmatic paralysis: the use of M-mode ultrasound for diagnosis in adults. Spinal Cord. 2006;44:505-8.

CHAPTER 30

Electrocardiogram

Syed Nabeel Muzaffar, Saumitra Misra

Q.1. A 70-year-old female, known case of type 2 diabetes mellitus (DM), hypertension (HTN), and hypothyroidism, presented to emergency room (ER) with shortness of breath for 6 months and pedal edema for 2 weeks. She was on inhaled bronchodilators intermittently for last 12 months for chronic obstructive pulmonary disease (COPD) and was also on antitubercular treatment (ATT) for last 3 months for recently diagnosed sputum-positive pulmonary tuberculosis. At admission, she was febrile, conscious but disoriented, heart rate 102 beats/min, blood pressure 110/60 mm Hg, and peripheral oxygen saturation 89% on room air. Arterial blood gas (ABG) revealed pH 7.30, PaO_2 55 mm Hg, $PaCO_2$ 75 mm Hg, HCO_3 36, BE+1, and lactates 1.6 mmol/L. Electrocardiogram (ECG) done at bedside showed following changes:

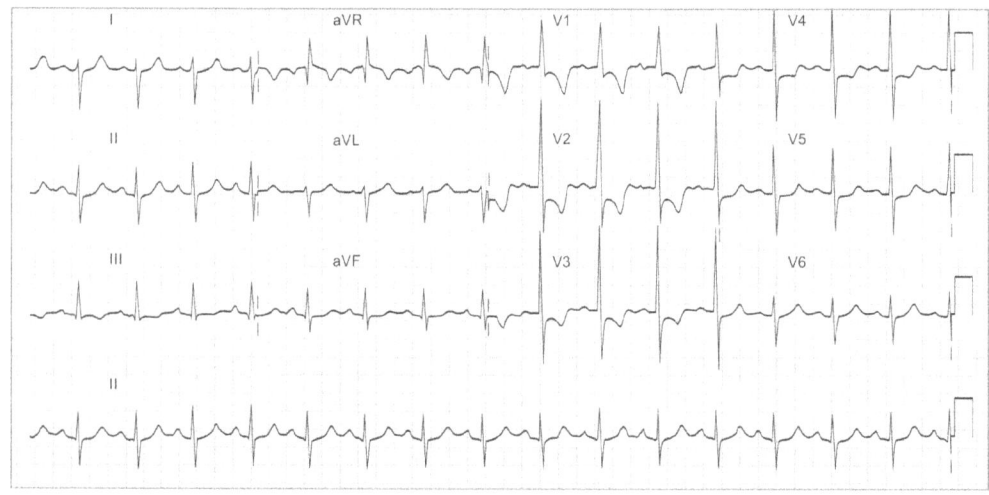

What is the most likely abnormality in ECG?
a. Left bundle branch block (LBBB)
b. Trifascicular block
c. Right ventricular hypertrophy (RVH) with strain pattern
d. Left ventricular hypertrophy (LVH) with strain pattern

Ans. c

Explanation: ECG depicts changes of right ventricular overload secondary to COPD (COPD with cor pulmonale). Lead V1 shows features of RVH [tall R (R > S) waves due to rightward shift of QRS vector] with strain pattern (T-wave inversion). Right axis deviation is also seen (QRS downward in lead 1 and upright in leads II and III). Peaked and tall P waves [> 2.5 mm; 1 mm = 0.1 millivolts (mV)] may also be seen in lead II due to right atrial enlargement.

Suggested Reading
1. Bhattacharya PT, Ellison MB. Right Ventricular Hypertrophy. [Treasure Island (FL): Stat Pearls Publishing; 2023.

Q.2. What are the ECG findings?

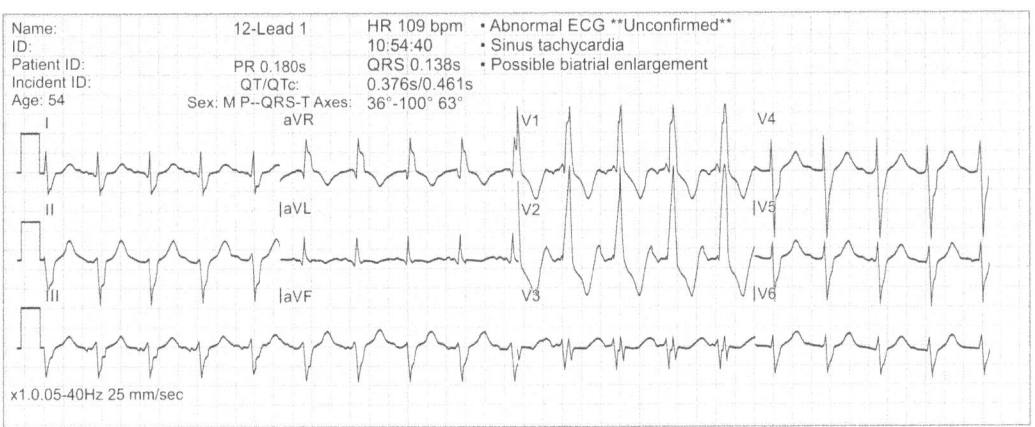

a. Right bundle branch block (RBBB)
b. Bifascicular block
c. Trifascicular block
d. Left bundle branch block (LBBB)

Ans. b

Explanation: ECG depicts broad QRS complexes (>3 small squares or > 140 ms; 1 small square = 40 ms) in right chest leads (V1-2) suggestive of ventricular conduction defect. Right bundle branch block (RBBB) is seen as rSR pattern in lead V1. Left axis deviation (LAD) is also seen (QRS upright in lead 1 and downward in leads II and III), which may be due to left anterior fascicular block (LAFB). This finding of RBBB + LAFB points toward a bifascicular block in ECG. Trifascicular block involves RBBB + LAFB + first-degree AV block (prolonged PR interval).

Suggested Reading
1. Goldberger AL, Goldberger ZD, Shvilkin A. Ventricular conduction disturbances. In: Goldberger's Clinical Electrocardiography, 9th edition. Netherlands: Elsevier; 2018.

Q.3. A 50-year-old male with severe community-acquired pneumonia (CAP) presented to ICU with respiratory failure and shock. Which of the following drugs should be avoided based on ECG findings?

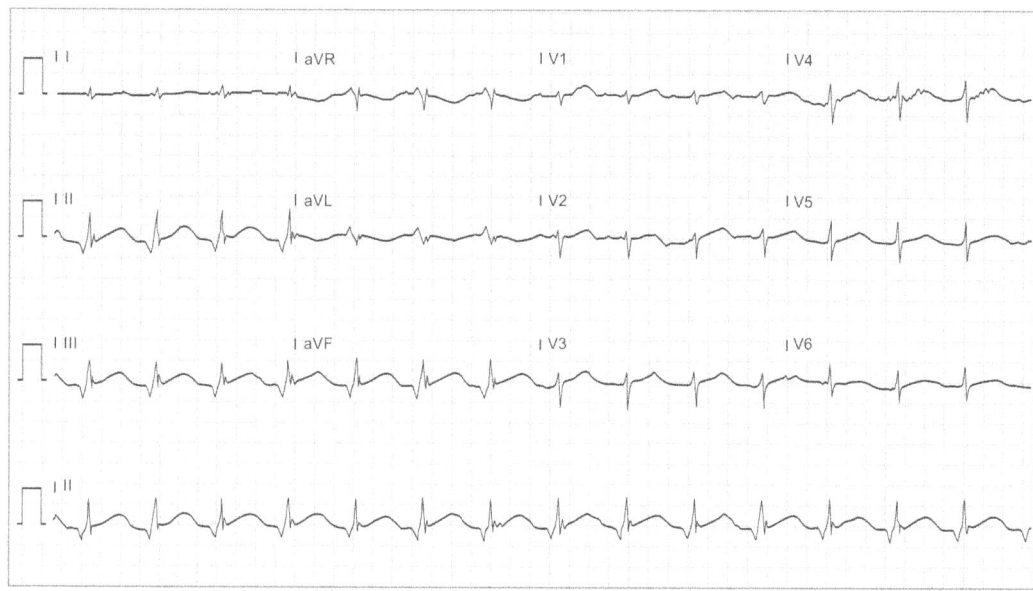

a. Amoxicillin
b. Ceftriaxone
c. Azithromycin
d. Piperacillin + tazobactam

Ans. c

Explanation: Macrolides (e.g., azithromycin) are commonly prescribed for the treatment. But, in patients with prolonged QT interval [corrected QT interval (QTc) > 440 ms in males and > 460 ms in females], azithromycin may trigger life-threatening ventricular arrhythmias like Torsades de Pointes. The learning point is to not miss the baseline ECG findings before prescribing any drug, besides ruling out history of allergy or any other contraindication to that drug.

Suggested Reading
1. Goldstein EJC, Owens RC Jr, Nolin TD. Antimicrobial-associated QT interval prolongation: Pointes of interest. Clin Infect Dis. 2006;43(12):1603-11.

Q.4. A 60-year-old male with no prior medical history presents to the emergency room (ER) with crushing central chest pain. On examination, the findings are– alert patient, respiratory rate 22 breaths/min, oxygen saturations 96% on room air, chest clear, pulse 118 beats/min, blood pressure 92/61 mm Hg, jugular venous pressure (JVP) elevated 5 cm above sternal angle and abdominal distension. ECG shows 3-mm ST-segment elevation in leads II, III, and aVF. 2D echocardiogram (2D ECHO) is performed. What do you expect to see?
a. Regional wall motion abnormality (RWMA) in the inferior wall of LV
b. RWMA in inferior wall of LV with dilated and impaired RV

c. Normal biventricular function
d. RWMA in inferior wall of LV with mitral regurgitation

Ans. b

Explanation: *Inferior and right ventricular (RV) myocardial infarction (MI):* Acute myocardial infarction presents with ST-T changes depending upon time course of MI.

- In initial minutes of onset, ECG shows hyperacute and tall T waves with ST elevation.
  - Leads V2, V3: ≥ 2 mm in males and ≥ 1.5 mm in females
  - ≥ 1 mm in other leads
- Subsequently, in next few hours, pathological Q waves (>40 ms width and > 2-mm depth) appear along with normalization of ST segment and T wave inversion.
- Within next few days of MI, Q waves persist and ST-T changes return to baseline.

Similarly, ST-T changes also point toward the site of MI depending upon the contiguous leads involved, as shown in **Table 1**.

TABLE 1: Contiguous leads and site of myocardial infarction (MI) along with its corresponding blood supply.

Lead	Site of MI	Blood vessel
V1–V2	Septal	Left anterior descending (LAD)
V3–V4	Anterior wall of LV	LAD
I, aVL, V5–6	Lateral wall of LV	Left circumflex (LCx)
I, aVL, V3–6	Anterolateral wall	LAD (proximal)
II, III, aVF	Inferior wall of LV	• *Right coronary artery (RCA):* 80% cases • *LCx:* 18% cases • *LAD:* 2% cases
V4R–V6R	Right ventricle	RCA
V7–9	Posterior wall of LV	RCA and LCx

In this case, 3-mm ST-segment elevation in leads II, III, and aVF suggests inferior wall MI.

- Inferior wall MI may also be associated with right ventricular infarction in 30–40% patients (due to a common blood supply of from right coronary artery in majority of cases). Diagnosis of right ventricular (RV) infarction is confirmed by the presence of ST elevation in the right-sided leads (V4R–V6R). Patients with RV infarction are preload-sensitive and require adequate RV filling pressures. Preload reducing agents (such as nitrates, diuretics, and morphine) should not be given in RV infarction to avoid hypotension.
- Similarly, inferior wall MI may coexist with posterior wall MI (ST-depression V1-V3, Prominent R in V1-V2, Upright T in V1-V3, and ST elevation in V7-9).

Suggested Reading
1. Namana V, Gupta SS, Abbasi AA, Raheja H, Shani J, Hollander G. Right ventricular infarction. Cardiovasc Revasc Med. 2018;19(1 Pt A):43-50.

Q.5. A 58-year-old man presents with chest pain for the past 2 hours. He is tachycardic, vomiting, and sweating with blood pressure of 136/80 mm Hg.

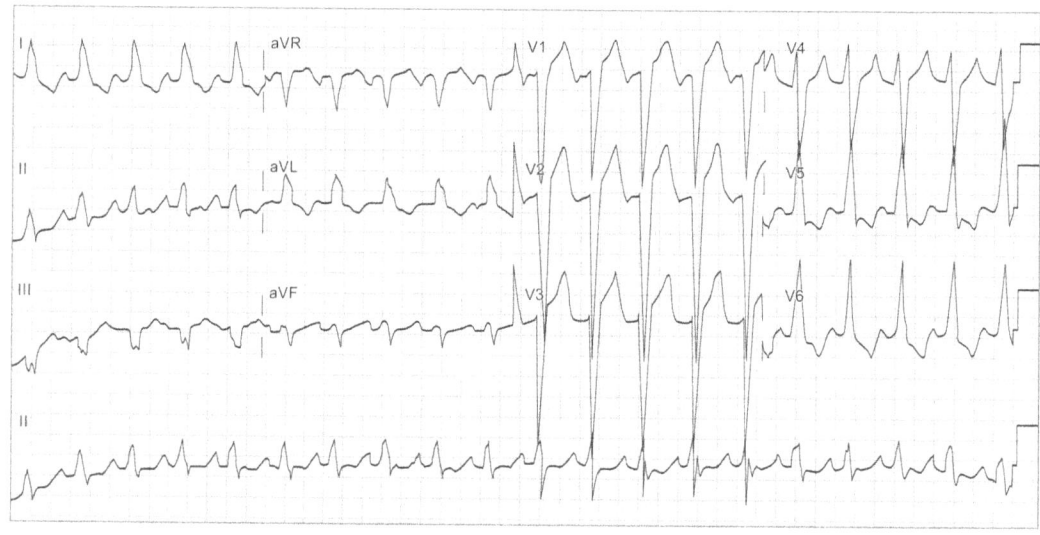

What does the ECG show?
a. Narrow complex tachycardia with ST elevation
b. Left bundle branch block with ST elevation
c. Right bundle branch block with ST elevation
d. Ventricular tachycardia

Ans. b

Explanation: ECG depicts broad QRS complexes (>3 small squares or >140 ms; 1 small square = 40 ms] with tall R waves in lateral leads (I, aVL, and V5-6) and deep S waves in right precordial leads (V1-3) indicating spread of depolarization vector from right to left side, suggestive of left bundle branch block (LBBB). LBBB often indicates an underlying heart disease, e.g., myocardial ischemia and aortic stenosis.

Presence of LBBB makes interpretation of ECG difficult in patients with MI. In this regard, Sgarbossa criteria defined certain ECG criteria to improve the diagnosis of MI in background of LBBB. In this case, as per Sgarbossa criteria, excessively discordant ST elevation (with respect to QRS complex) is seen in leads V1-3 qualifying for LBBB with ST elevation.

Suggested Reading
1. Smith SW, Dodd KW, Henry TD, Dvorak DM, Pearce LA. Diagnosis of ST-elevation myocardial infarction in the presence of left bundle branch block with the ST-elevation to S-wave ratio in a modified Sgarbossa rule. Ann Emerg Med. 2012;60(6):766-76.

Q.6. **A 65-year-old man presents to ER with crushing central chest pain with onset around 25 minutes ago. The nearest center offering primary coronary angioplasty is >180 minutes away. Cardiac enzymes are elevated. There is no contraindication to thrombolysis. ECG shows the following findings:**

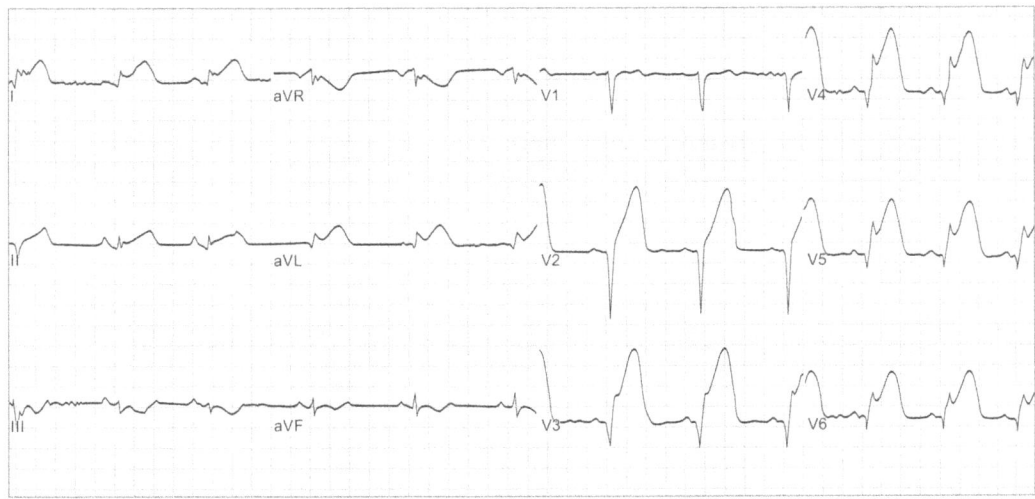

In addition to standard acute coronary syndrome treatment (analgesia, antiplatelets, and heparin), what would be the most appropriate management plan for this patient?
a. Immediate transfer for acute angioplasty
b. Nonurgent angioplasty
c. Thrombolysis and immediate transfer for acute angioplasty
d. Thrombolysis

Ans. c

Explanation: ECG reveals changes suggestive of acute anterolateral MI. The patient requires urgent revascularization of involved coronaries to salvage the myocardium.
- *Primary percutaneous coronary intervention (PCI)—capable center*: Primary PCI is the treatment of choice, if door to balloon (D2B) time (i.e., time from presentation to ER till crossing of catheter guidewire across the culprit-coronary lesion) is <90 minutes.
- *Non-PCI center*: Transfer to PCI center should be done if anticipated time for PCI is <120 minutes. Otherwise, fibrinolysis should be considered (if no contraindications) and the patient transferred to the nearby PCI center.

In this case, as patient is in non-PCI center and the transfer time to nearby PCI center is > 120 minutes, the most suitable treatment option would be thrombolysis followed by referral to PCI-capable center for angiography/PCI within 24 hours of fibrinolysis, also known as pharmacoinvasive approach).

Suggested Reading
1. Bergmark BA, Mathenge N, Merlini PA, Lawrence-Wright MB, Giugliano RP. Acute coronary syndromes. Lancet. 2022;399(10332):1347-58.
2. Naples RM, Harris JW, Ghaemmaghami CA. Critical care aspects in the management of patients with acute coronary syndromes. Emerg Med Clin North Am. 2008;26(3):685-702.

Q.7. A 75-year-old gentleman presents to ER with crushing central chest pain. He has a past medical history of angina and hypertension. He is transferred for immediate PCI to nearby PCI-capable center within 1 hour of onset of pain. At admission, he is dizzy, heart rate was 55 beats/min, BP 80/60 mm Hg, and is having ongoing chest pain. ECG shows the following findings:

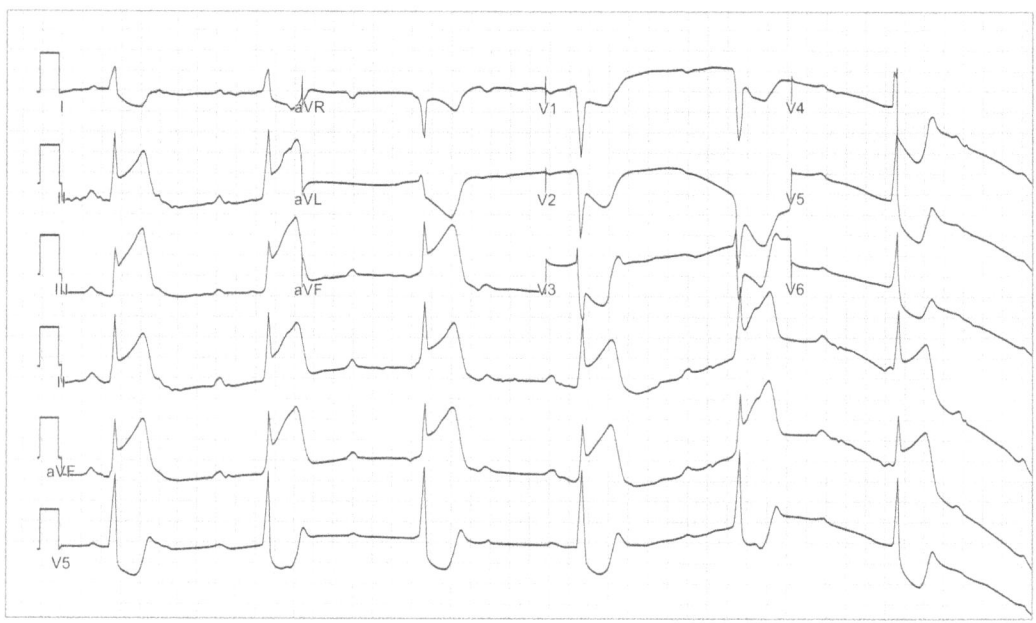

What is the most appropriate management?
a. IV atropine + primary percutaneous coronary intervention (PCI)
b. Synchronized DC cardioversion + primary PCI
c. IV dobutamine infusion + primary PCI
d. Insertion of temporary pacemaker + primary PCI

Ans. d

Explanation: ECG depicts ST-segment elevation in leads II, III, and aVF suggestive of acute inferior wall MI. In addition, atrial rate (P-P interval) is faster than the ventricular rate (R-R interval) and atria are beating independent of ventricles. ECG pattern and ventricular rate are maintained by a junctional escape rhythm, which is characteristic of third-degree AV block, also known as complete heart block. Acute inferior wall MI is prone to high-degree AV blocks due to AV nodal ischemia from occlusion of right coronary artery (RCA).

In view of ongoing inferior wall MI and symptomatic bradyarrhythmia, the patient needs urgent coronary revascularization and pacing. Till the time, patient is being stabilized in ER, IV adrenaline infusion (2–10 μg/min) and/or urgent transcutaneous cardiac pacing should be initiated to improve tissue perfusion (if not responding to adrenaline) along with antiplatelet therapy. Simultaneously, preparation for transvenous pacing should also be kept ready. Atropine acts at the SA and AV nodes by blocking vagal nerve and is either not effective or may even worsen infranodal blocks such as Mobitz type II and complete heart blocks.

Suggested Reading
1. Berger PB, Ryan TJ. Inferior myocardial infarction: High-risk subgroups. Circulation. 1990;81(2):401-11.

Q.8. A 67-year-old female, known case of rheumatoid arthritis (RA) for 35 years (not on treatment) with RA-induced interstitial lung disease, presented to ER with left hemiparesis and facial deviation since waking up in the morning. She also had a history of bilateral lower limb digital amputation due to gangrene 6 years ago. Noncontrast computed tomography (NCCT) head was suggestive of right middle cerebral artery (MCA) infarct. ECG done bedside revealed the following findings:

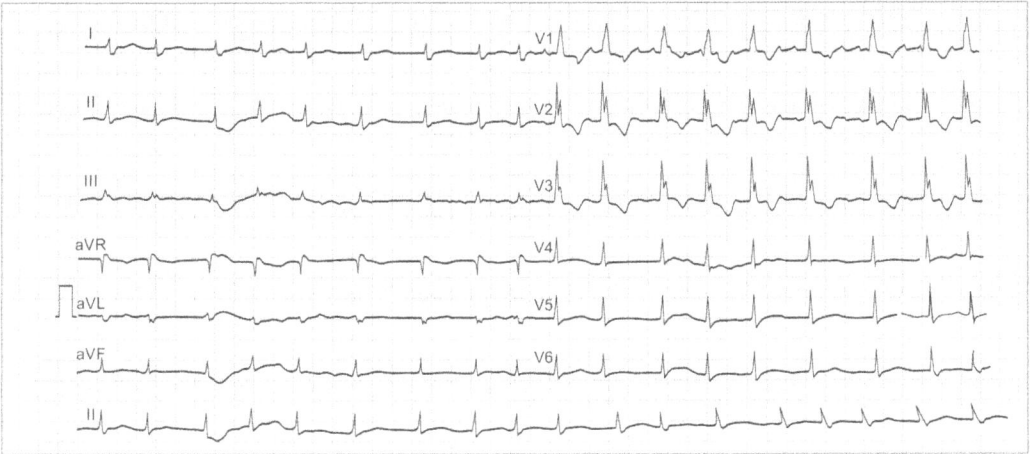

What is the most likely finding in ECG?
a. Ventricular tachycardia (VT)
b. Atrial fibrillation (AF)
c. Atrioventricular nodal reentry tachycardia (AVNRT)
d. Atrioventricular dissociation

Ans. b

Explanation: ECG depicts narrow complex tachyarrhythmia (<3 small squares or 120 ms) suggestive of supraventricular tachyarrhythmia, with irregular rhythm with absent P waves characteristic of atrial fibrillation (AF). Patients with chronic AF (>48 hours) are prone to clot formation in left atrial (LA) appendage due to dilated LA and chaotic LA activity, which predisposes them to cardioembolic stroke. Thus, anticoagulation based on the risk stratification scores is essential in patients with chronic AF to prevent stroke.

Suggested Reading
1. Migdady I, Russman A, Buletko AB. Atrial fibrillation and ischemic stroke: A clinical review. Semin Neurol. 2021;41(4):348-64.

Q.9. While on ER duty overnight, 62-year-old man gets admitted with palpitations. He describes palpitations in the chest for last 48 hours. He is a known case of type 2 diabetes mellitus (adequately controlled on oral hypoglycemics). Glasgow Coma Scale (GCS) is 15/15 but the patient complained of light-headedness, heart rate 150–170 beats/min, blood pressure 78/60 mm Hg, and chest is clear to auscultation. ECG shows atrial fibrillation with fast ventricular rate of 150–170 beats/min.

What is the most appropriate next step in management?
a. Give 5 mg intravenous metoprolol as a slow bolus
b. Load with 300 mg intravenous amiodarone
c. DC cardioversion
d. Attempt vagal maneuvers

Ans. c

Explanation: As per American Heart Association (AHA) guidelines, in unstable patients (altered mentation, chest pain, and shortness of breath) of tachyarrhythmia with pulse, the treatment of choice is synchronized direct current (DC) cardioversion. In synchronized cardioversion, low-energy DC shock is delivered in synchrony with R wave of QRS complex to avoid shock delivery during repolarization phase of cardiac action potential ("R on T" phenomenon). This prevents precipitation of ventricular fibrillation (VF) during shock delivery. Anticoagulation should also be started in patients with chronic AF (>48 hours) undergoing cardioversion to prevent thromboembolization.

Dose of shock in synchronized cardioversion depends upon underlying rhythm:
- Narrow (<120 ms) and irregular [e.g., atrial fibrillation (AF)]: 120–200 Joules (J) biphasic or 200 J monophasic
- Narrow and regular [e.g., supraventricular tachycardia (SVT) and atrial flutter]: 50–100 J
- Wide (>120 ms) and regular [e.g., ventricular tachycardia (VT)]: 100 J

Suggested Reading
1. Panchal AR, Bartos JA, Cabañas JG, Donnino MW, Drennan IR, Hirsch KG, et al; Adult Basic and Advanced Life Support Writing Group. Part 3: Adult Basic and Advanced Life Support: 2020 American Heart Association Guidelines for Cardiopulmonary Resuscitation and Emergency Cardiovascular Care. Circulation. 2020;142(16_suppl_2):S366-S468.

Q.10. A 68-year-old male is admitted with confusion and an ataxic gait. His past medical history includes heart failure and atrial fibrillation (AF). His drug history includes dabigatran, bisoprolol, and ramipril.

Noncontrast CT (NCCT) head	Large acute right-sided frontotemporal subdural hematoma with ventricular effacement and midline shift

How will you manage this patient besides stopping the anticoagulant?
a. Fresh frozen plasma
b. Platelet transfusion
c. Tranexamic acid
d. Idarucizumab

Ans. d

Explanation: Patients with AF are prone to cardioembolic stroke, for which risk stratification scores are also used. Hence, anticoagulants are prescribed for patients with chronic AF to avoid this complication of thromboembolism. Dabigatran is a nonvitamin K oral anticoagulant (NOAC), which belongs to the group of direct thrombin inhibitor. In patients who bleed secondary to dabigatran, idarucizumab acts as an antidote for reversing the effect of dabigatran. Other management strategies include factor VII, oral charcoal (if recently ingested), and hemodialysis (as dabigatran is dialyzable). Besides controlling the bleed, institution of cerebral protective strategies and timely neurosurgical intervention are also quintessential. The learning point is to not miss drug history and ECG findings of AF in patients who present with stroke (ischemic or hemorrhagic).

Suggested Reading
1. Kuramatsu JB, Sembill JA, Huttner HB. Reversal of oral anticoagulation in patients with acute intracerebral hemorrhage. Crit Care. 2019;23(1):206.

Q.11. 15-year-old female presented to ER with acute febrile illness and status epilepticus, for which stabilization of airway, breathing, and circulation was done and antiepileptic drugs initiated. In subsequent workups, NCCT head was suggestive of multiple tuberculomas and CSF revealed pleocytosis with lymphocytic predominance and high protein levels. In view of poor venous access, central venous catheter (CVC) insertion was planned. But postguidewire insertion, the patient developed palpitations with heart rate 220–230 beats/min, cold peripheries, feeble pulse, and BP 70/60 mm Hg. The intensivist immediately repositioned the guidewire and administered shock, after which hemodynamic stability was restored.

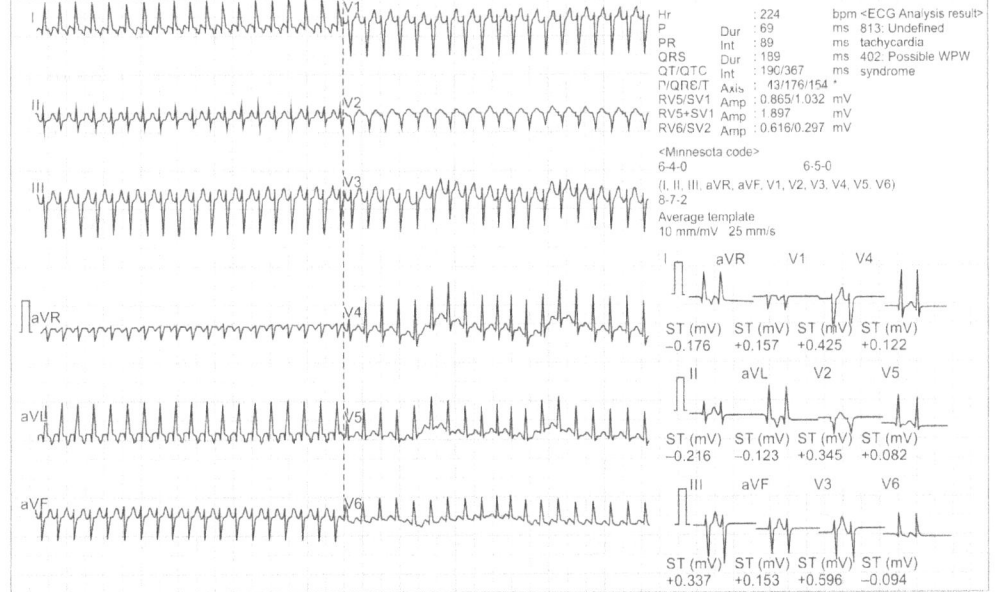

Identify the ECG abnormality and its most appropriate treatment:
a. Ventricular tachycardia (VT); synchronized DC cardioversion + withdrawing guidewire
b. Paroxysmal supraventricular tachycardia (PSVT); intravenous (IV) adenosine + withdrawing guidewire
c. PSVT; synchronized DC cardioversion + withdrawing guidewire
d. Atrial fibrillation (AF); IV amiodarone + withdrawing guidewire

Ans. c

Explanation: ECG depicts narrow complex tachycardia (<120 ms) with regular R-R interval suggestive of supraventricular tachyarrhythmia (SVT). SVT that appears and terminates suddenly is known as paroxysmal supraventricular tachycardia (PSVT).

In SVT, reentry circuit is formed between adjacent myocytes with disparate electrophysiological properties (conduction velocity and refractory period) allowing impulse propagation in a closed-loop circuit. SVT is of two types:

1. *Atrioventricular (AV) nodal reentry tachycardia (AVNRT)*: AVNRT is the most common type of SVT, where reentry circuit is formed in AV node between slow and fast AV nodal pathways.
2. *AV reentry tachycardia (AVRT)*: Reentry circuit is formed between atria and ventricles via accessory tracts.

As patient is hemodynamically unstable, urgent synchronized DC cardioversion is required along with guidewire repositioning (precipitating factor). IV adenosine is the drug of choice for stable patients with SVT, if not responding to vagal maneuvers. Always rule out preexcitation syndromes in baseline ECG before administering IV Adenosine.

Suggested Reading
1. Panchal AR, Bartos JA, Cabañas JG, Donnino MW, Drennan IR, Hirsch KG, et al; Adult Basic and Advanced Life Support Writing Group. Part 3: Adult Basic and Advanced Life Support: 2020 American Heart Association Guidelines for Cardiopulmonary Resuscitation and Emergency Cardiovascular Care. Circulation. 2020;142(16_suppl_2): S366-S468.

Q.12. A 50-year-old man, known case of coronary artery disease (CAD), presented with palpitations to ER. ECG showed broad QRS complex tachyarrhythmia at 180 beats/min, suggestive of ventricular tachycardia. Blood pressure was 134/80 mm Hg. Intravenous (IV) 300 mg bolus of amiodarone was given and IV amiodarone infusion initiated with 900 mg total dose administered over next 24 hours. The heart rate transiently settled down with normal QT interval in sinus rhythm but on the next day of admission, he again developed VT. Blood pressure was 120/70 mm Hg. Beta-blockers were then added and IV magnesium sulfate infusion initiated but the patient continued to have recurrent VT. Electrical cardioversion was then attempted but without much benefit.

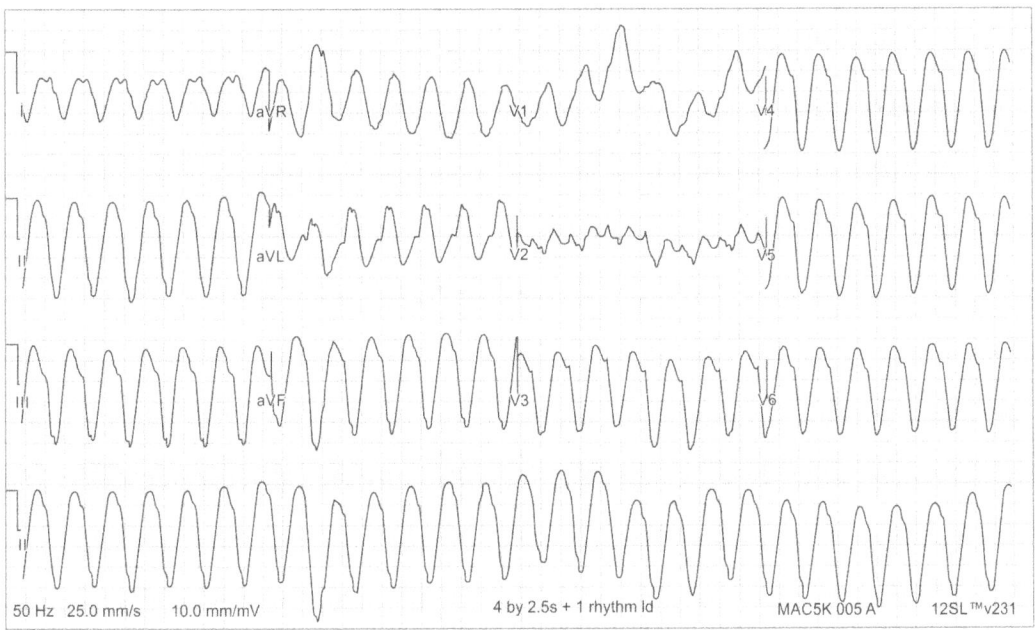

What would be the next most appropriate treatment plan?
a. Intravenous (IV) adenosine
b. Repeat bolus of amiodarone 300 mg
c. IV quinidine
d. IV lidocaine infusion

Ans. d

Explanation: Electrical storm (VT or VF storm) is defined as ≥ 3 sustained VT (>30 seconds)/VF in 24-hour period, which usually occurs in the setting of myocardial ischemia, structural heart disease, implantable cardioverter–defibrillator (ICD), or inherited arrhythmic syndromes (e.g., Brugada syndrome and long QT syndrome). In this case, the patient has developed refractory monomorphic VT.

Precipitating factors include myocardial ischemia, acute decompensated heart failure, inherited arrhythmic syndromes, dyselectrolytemias, metabolic parameters, drugs (including alcohol), thyroid disorders, etc. Management approach includes correction of triggering factors, pharmacological agents (such as amiodarone and beta-blockers), reprogramming of ICD, radiofrequency catheter ablation, intra-aortic balloon pump (IABP), LV assist device (LVAD), etc. In some cases, IV lidocaine (sodium-channel blocker) infusion may be useful in recurrent VT, especially if precipitated by ischemic myocardium.

Suggested Reading
1. Eifling M, Razavi M, Massumi A. The evaluation and management of electrical storm. Tex Heart Inst J. 2011;38(2):111-21.

Q.13. A 64-year-old male presents to the emergency department with dyspnea. He had been feeling intermittently dizzy and dyspneic for the past 1–2 weeks. On examination, his pulse is 180 beats/min, blood pressure 120/66 mm Hg, and oxygen saturations 98% on room air. On auscultation, chest is clear and he appears well perfused. ECG is obtained:

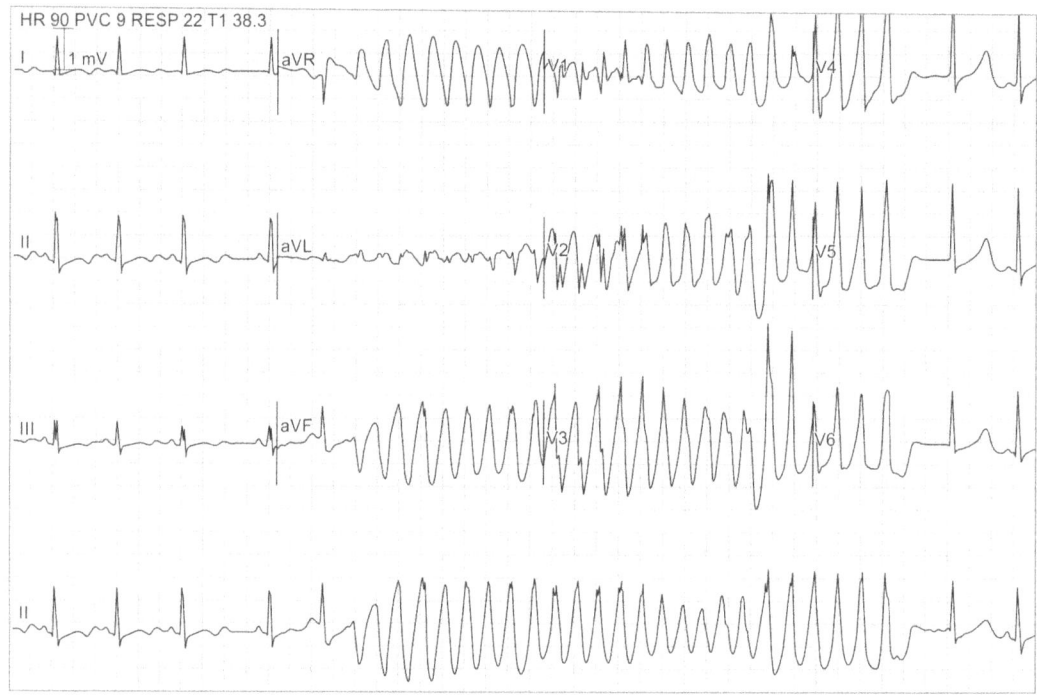

What is the most appropriate treatment?
a. Intravenous (IV) amiodarone
b. IV adenosine
c. Unsynchronized DC shock
d. IV magnesium sulfate

Ans. d

Explanation: ECG depicts tachyarrhythmia with broad QRS complexes of varying morphology/amplitude in precordial chest leads, suggestive of polymorphic ventricular tachycardia (VT). In baseline ECG, QT interval is also prolonged. ECG picture thus shows polymorphic VT with long QT interval, characteristic of Torsades de Pointes (TdP).

Intravenous (IV) magnesium sulfate is the drug of choice for stable patients with TdP. Unstable patients require immediate defibrillation with 200 J biphasic shock.

Suggested Reading
1. Panchal AR, Bartos JA, Cabañas JG, Donnino MW, Drennan IR, Hirsch KG, et al; Adult Basic and Advanced Life Support Writing Group. Part 3: Adult Basic and Advanced Life Support:

2020 American Heart Association Guidelines for Cardiopulmonary Resuscitation and Emergency Cardiovascular Care. Circulation. 2020;142(16_suppl_2):S366-S468.

Q.14. A 65-year-old male collapses in a nearby shopping complex and is rushed to the ER. At admission, he is unconscious and pulseless. ECG reveals the following abnormality:

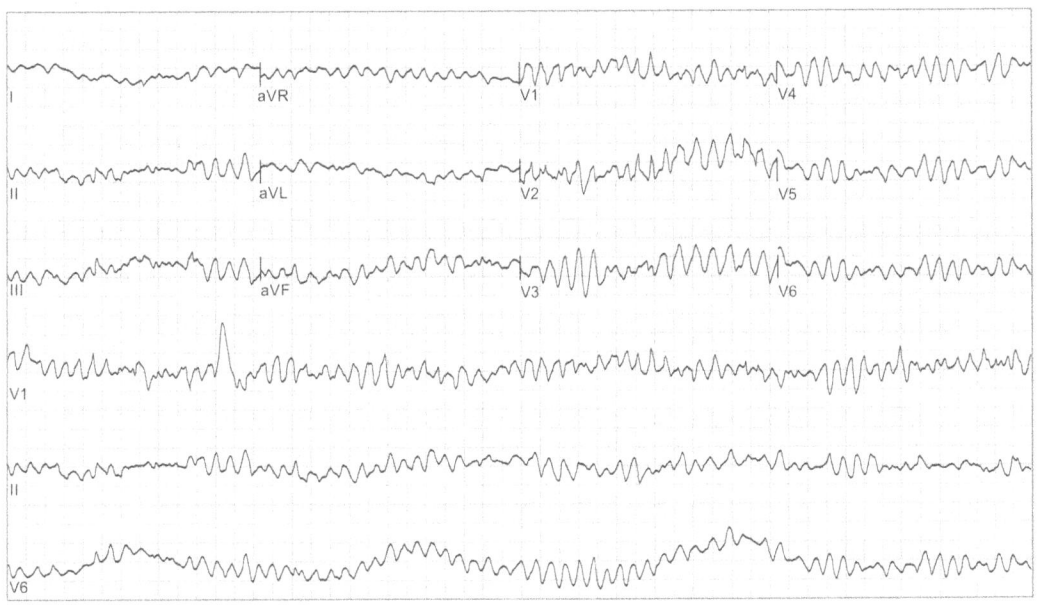

What is the most appropriate treatment?
a. Cardiopulmonary resuscitation (CPR) + synchronized DC cardioversion 200 J shock
b. CPR + defibrillation with biphasic 200 J shock
c. CPR + defibrillation with monophasic 200 J shock
d. CPR + defibrillation with biphasic 100 J shock

Ans. b

Explanation: ECG depicts disorganized electrical activity with no identifiable P, QRS, and T waves, characteristic of ventricular fibrillation (VF), in which heart pumps in a very rapid and uncoordinated fashion resulting in immediate loss of cardiac output. As per American Heart Association 2020 guidelines, pulseless shockable rhythms [such as pulseless ventricular tachycardia (VT) and VF] require immediate defibrillation with 200 joules (J) biphasic shock. To improve defibrillation success, high-quality CPR with minimal interruption in chest compressions should be ensured. Pharmacological agents given along with CPR and defibrillation to facilitate return of spontaneous circulation (ROSC) include adrenaline and amiodarone/lidocaine.

Often, VF is precipitated by acute coronary syndrome (ACS) in adult population which needs urgent coronary revascularization. Besides ACS, other precipitating factors include "6Hs 5Ts": hypoxia, hypercapnia, hypovolemia, hypokalemia/hyperkalemia, hydrogen ion (acidosis), hypoglycemia, tension pneumothorax, thrombosis (pulmonary, cardiac), temperature (hypothermia), tamponade, toxins, and trauma.

Suggested Reading
1. Panchal AR, Bartos JA, Cabañas JG, Donnino MW, Drennan IR, Hirsch KG, et al; Adult Basic and Advanced Life Support Writing Group. Part 3: Adult Basic and Advanced Life Support: 2020 American Heart Association Guidelines for Cardiopulmonary Resuscitation and Emergency Cardiovascular Care. Circulation. 2020;142(16_suppl_2):S366-S468.

Q.15. To differentiate supraventricular tachycardia (SVT) with aberrancy from ventricular tachycardia (VT) as per Brugada criteria, all of the following favor VT, except:
   a. Morphology criteria present for VT in precordial leads (V1/V2 and V6)
   b. R-S interval >100 ms
   c. A-V dissociation
   d. Presence of RS complex in all precordial leads

Ans. d

Explanation: The Brugada criteria is applied for wide complex tachycardias with regular rhythm to differentiate between SVT with aberrant conduction and VT, in which four criteria are included:
1. A-V dissociation
2. Absence of RS complex in all precordial leads
3. R-S interval > 100 ms
4. Morphology criteria present for VT in precordial leads (V1/V2 and V6)

If any one of the above points is present, diagnosis goes in favor of VT. SVT with aberrant conduction is considered if none of the above points are present.

Suggested Reading
1. Salim Rezaie. (2013). SVT with Aberrancy Versus VT, REBEL EM blog. [online] Available from https://rebelem.com/svt-aberrancy-versus-vt/ [Last accessed June, 2023].

Q.16. A 56-year-old man is brought to the emergency department. He works as an electrician. His brother gives a history of his suddenly fainting from stool at work. On admission, he is conscious with heart rate of around 35 beats/min. His blood pressure is 90/60 mm Hg and is well perfused with no signs of heart failure. ECG is taken for his bradycardia. A prior ECG 4 months ago was normal. What is the most likely diagnosis?

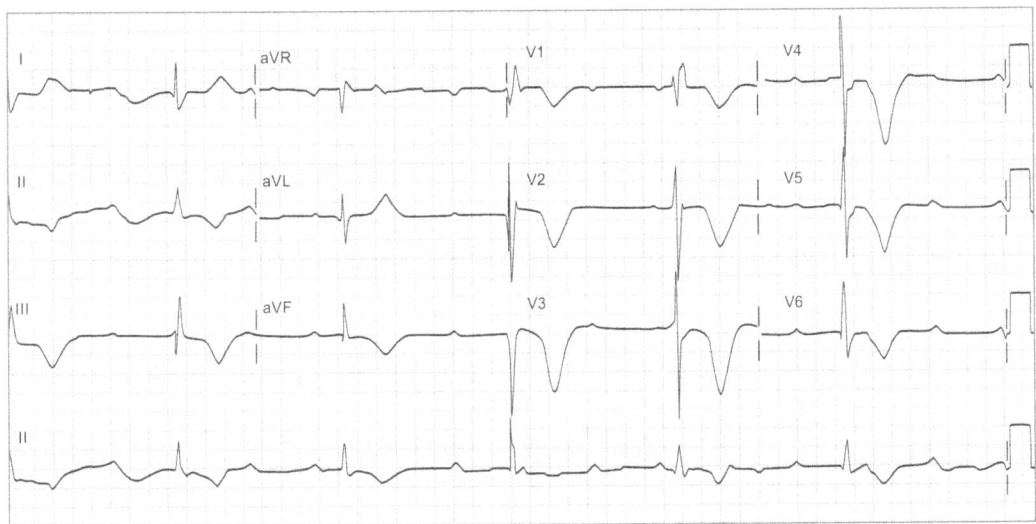

a. Sick sinus syndrome (tachycardia-bradycardia syndrome)
b. Myocardial infarction with new left bundle branch block
c. Stokes–Adams attack with complete heart block
d. Second-degree atrioventricular block (Mobitz II)

Ans. c

Explanation: Stokes–Adams attack includes syncopal spells without warning, due to reduced cardiac output to brain, which may be associated with bradycardia, hypotension, and seizures if prolonged. Previous history of sudden fainting spells is present. Commonly, high-degree AV blocks (Mobitz type II second degree or complete heart block) are present during the attack but sinoatrial disease, supraventricular and ventricular arrhythmias may also be seen during the attack. Between attacks, patients generally remain in sinus rhythm with broad QRS complex. Pacemaker insertion is often required.

Suggested Reading
1. Nikolic G. Stokes-Adams attack. Pediatr Cardiol. 1989;10(3):177.

Q.17. A 30-year-old man is admitted to ICU after suffering a "blackout" at work. His colleagues reported him fainting without warning while waiting in the washroom. This has never happened before and he is normally fit and well. On examination, blood pressure is 100/68 mm Hg, pulse 85 beats/min, oxygen saturations 97% on room air, and respiratory rate 18 breaths/min. ECG revealed the following findings:

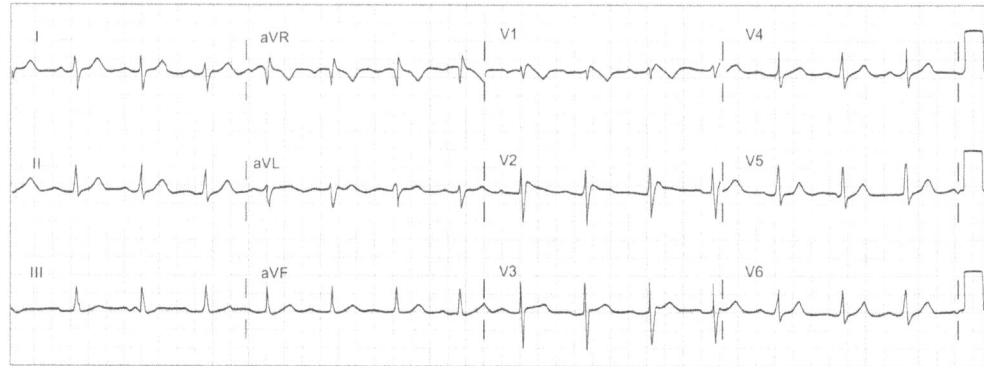

What is the most likely diagnosis?
a. Hypertrophic obstructive cardiomyopathy
b. Long QT syndrome
c. Arrhythmogenic right ventricular dysplasia
d. Brugada syndrome

Ans. d

Explanation: ECG shows most marked in V1: Incomplete RBBB, coved-type ST elevation, and inverted T wave, suggestive of Brugada syndrome. Brugada syndrome is an inherited cardiac sodium channelopathy. Symptoms range from syncope, seizures, palpitations, and sudden cardiac death in structurally normal hearts from fatal ventricular arrhythmias during sleep. Implantable cardioverter–defibrillator (ICD) is the only proven therapy.

Suggested Reading
1. Brugada P, Brugada J, Mont L, Smeets J, Andries EW. A new approach to the differential diagnosis of a regular tachycardia with a wide QRS complex. Circulation. 1991;83(5):1649-59.

Q.18. **A 48-year-old female presents with sudden palpitations and dyspnea. Her blood pressure is 140/90 mm Hg, pulse is 196 beats/min, respiratory rate is 24 breaths/min, and oxygen saturation is 98% on air. ECG is obtained which shows following changes:**

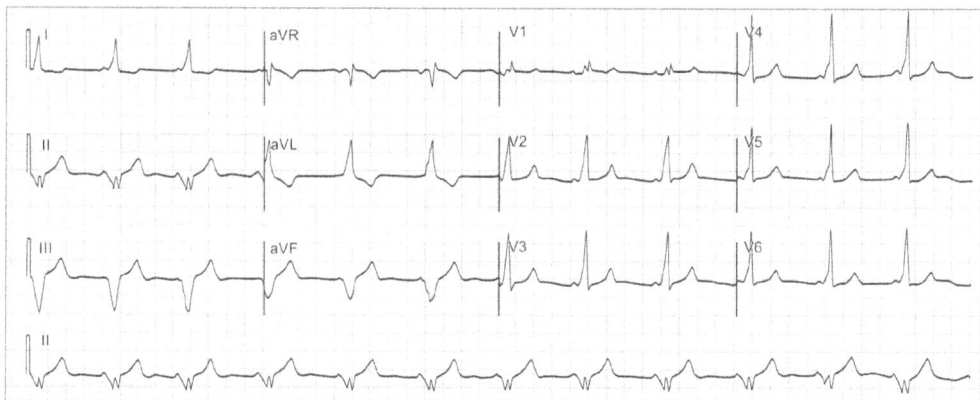

Which of the following drugs should be used to control heart rate in this case?
a. Flecainide
b. Diltiazem
c. Digoxin
d. Verapamil

Ans. a

Explanation: ECG depicts changes of preexcitation syndrome, e.g., Wolff–Parkinson–White (WPW) syndrome, wherein an accessory pathway (bundle of Kent) is present between the atria and ventricles depolarization wave from the atria reaches the ventricles early without having to face the delay seen in AV node conduction. This results in shortening of PR interval and slurring of early part of QRS upstroke (delta wave), also known as "preexcitation". The clinical significance of these preexcitation syndromes is their potential to trigger tachyarrhythmias such as atrial fibrillation or flutter and AV reentry tachycardia. (AVRT). However, AV nodal blocking agents (such as digoxin, diltiazem, verapamil, beta-blockers, and adenosine) should not be used in the management of tachyarrhythmias in such preexcitation syndromes to avoid precipitation of life-threatening arrhythmias such as ventricular fibrillation (VF). Thus, it is essential to pick up the baseline ECG changes of "preexcitation" in any patient.

Suggested Reading
1. Leong KM, Kelland NF. Pre-excitation on the electrocardiogram: what next? Br J Hosp Med (Lond). 2013;74(11):636-40.

Q.19. A 20-year-old boy with history of chronic epilepsy (since childhood) presented to ED with sudden-onset palpitations after taking some medication for a flu-like illness. Shortly after admission, he had recurrent cardiac arrest. ECG prior to the arrest showed following trace:

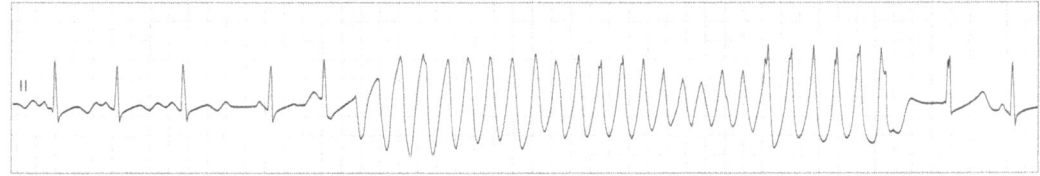

Despite timely resuscitation, he sustained recurrent episodes of cardiac arrest in ED. The family members give a similar family history also. What could be the probable diagnosis?
a. Myotonia congenita
b. Congenital long QT syndrome
c. Brugada syndrome
d. Short QT syndrome

Ans. b

Explanation: Congenital long QT syndrome (cardiac channelopathy) with a drug precipitating Torsade de Pointes is discussed in this case (please refer to the discussion in questions 3 and 14 also).

Suggested Reading
1. Moss AJ. Long QT syndrome. JAMA. 2003;289:2041-4.

Q.20. A 27-year-old female presented to ER with complaints of fever with chills and rigors for last 1 week followed by shortness of breath and generalized edema for last 3 days. At admission, she was agitated, bradycardic (heart rate 30–35 beats/min), hemodynamically unstable with feeble pulses and cold peripheries, peripheral oxygen saturation 85% (on oxygen mask @ 10 L/min), and oliguric. Chest X-ray (CXR) was suggestive of cardiogenic pulmonary edema. Routine laboratories were sent. Urine pregnancy test (UPT) was negative. In prior workups, Weil–Felix test was positive and serum ammonia was raised. Cardiac enzymes depicted troponin T (normal value: 0–0.04 ng/mL): 8 ng/mL and B-type natriuretic peptide (BNP) (normal value < 100 pg/mL): 35,000 pg/mL with progressively rising trend. 2D ECHO revealed global LV hypokinesia. ECG showed the following findings:

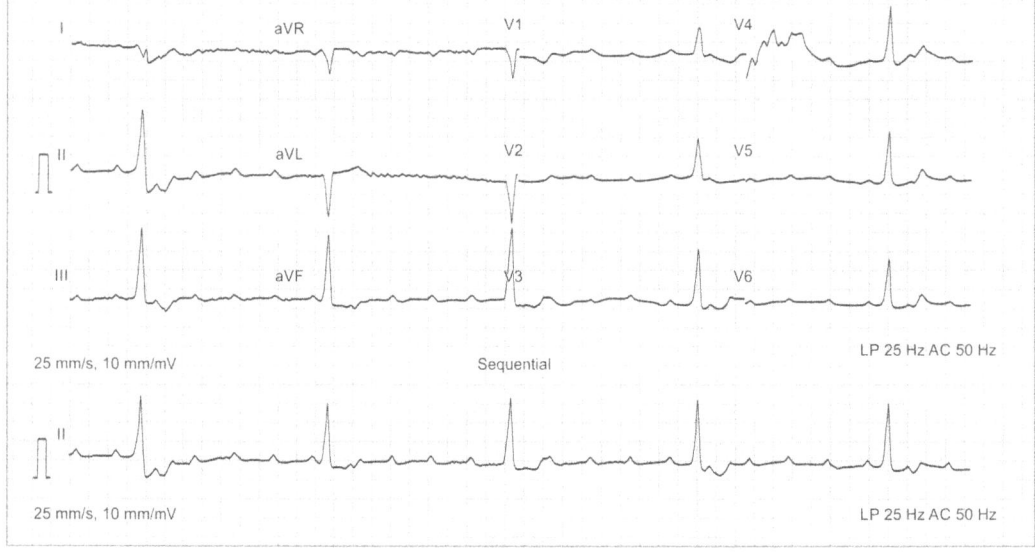

Consultants were sent to cardiology, neurology, nephrology, and rheumatology. Tracheal intubation was done, invasive mechanical ventilation initiated and central venous catheterization (CVC) in right internal jugular vein done. The patient did not respond to intravenous (IV) adrenaline infusion through CVC. What would be the next management plan based on ECG findings?

a. Urgent pacing
b. IV dobutamine infusion
c. DC unsynchronized cardioversion
d. IV amiodarone infusion

Ans. a

Explanation: ECG is suggestive of complete heart block (CHB) with ventricular escape rhythm, which requires urgent pacing. In view of the clinical presentation of acute febrile illness and myocardial involvement presenting as CHB with cardiogenic shock and pulmonary edema, the patient appears to be having fulminant myocarditis secondary

to rickettsial infection. Myocarditis commonly occurs secondary to autoimmune, toxic, and infectious causes, as mentioned below:
- *Autoimmune*: Connective tissue disease, giant cell myocarditis, Kawasaki disease, inflammatory bowel disease, sarcoidosis, hypereosinophilic syndrome, hypersensitivity myocarditis, and endomyocardial fibrosis
- *Toxic*: Cyclophosphamide, arsenic, cocaine, checkpoint inhibitors, and bites (spider/wasp/scorpion)
- *Infectious*: Bacterial, viral, parasitic, protozoal, and fungal

Besides shock, most patients are present with chest pain, dyspnea, and tachy- or bradyarrhythmias. ECG abnormalities include ST elevation (most common), broad QRS, AV block, VT, and VF. Serum cardiac troponins and inflammatory markers (C-reactive protein, ESR) are raised. 2D ECHO is one of the mainstays of diagnosis revealing regional wall motion abnormalities (without typical coronary pattern), wall thickening and mottling, RV dysfunction, and pericardial effusion. Coronary angiography is often needed to rule out ACS. Other useful tests are cardiac magnetic resonance imaging (CMR) and endomyocardial biopsy. Management approach includes supportive care, immunosuppressive therapy (such as cyclosporine, prednisolone, and azathioprine) for certain cases of myocarditis, namely eosinophilic myocarditis, GCM, cardiac sarcoidosis, and as specific therapy for underlying collagen vascular disease. Mechanical circulatory support including venoarterial ECMO, ventricular assist devices (VADs) may also be required in certain fulminant cases. Cardiac transplantation may also be required in some patients.

Suggested Reading
1. Sagar S, Liu PP, Cooper LT Jr. Myocarditis. Lancet. 2012;379(9817):738-47.

Q.21. A 25-year-old female with no comorbidities presented to ER with complaints of flu-like symptoms around 2 weeks ago followed by continuous high-grade fever > 39°C, chest pain, nonproductive cough, and dyspnea for last 6–7 days. At admission, she was conscious but restless, tachycardic up to 100–110 beats/min, blood pressure 130/80 mm Hg, and peripheral oxygen saturation 95% (room air). On auscultation, pericardial rub was present. Cardiac enzymes revealed elevated troponin T and BNP. On workup, inflammatory markers (ESR, CRP) were elevated. 2D ECHO revealed mild pericardial effusion.

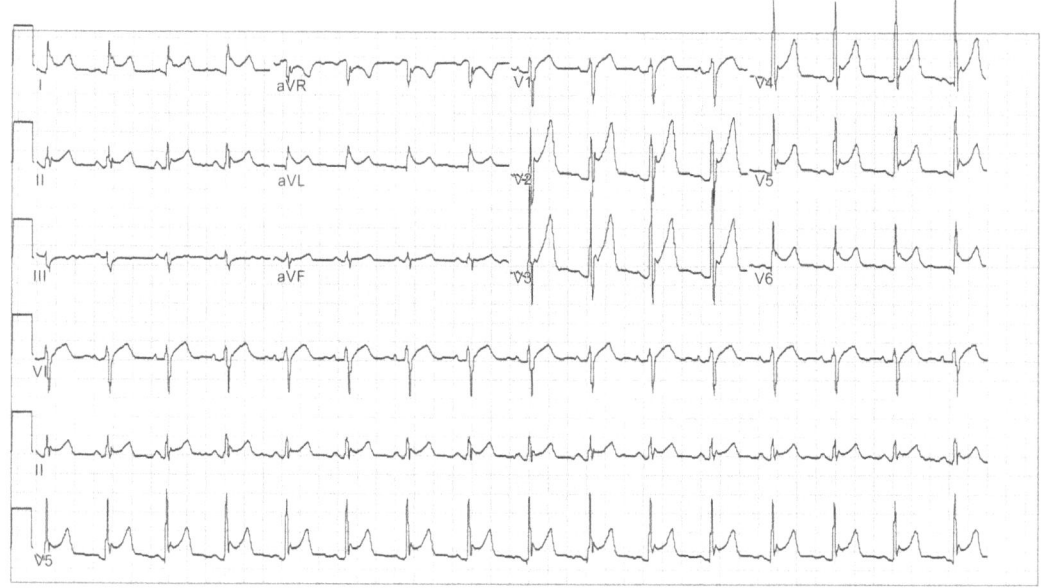

What would be the most appropriate management of this condition?
a. Conservative management only
b. Nonsteroidal anti-inflammatory drugs (NSAIDS) ± colchicine ± corticosteroids
c. Thrombolysis
d. Pericardiocentesis

Ans. b

Explanation: ECG shows widespread concave ST-segment elevation and PR segment depression in most of the limb leads (I, II, III, aVL, and aVF) and in all precordial leads (V1-6), which is characteristic of pericarditis, which in this case could be acute pericarditis (inflammation of pericardium), possibly secondary to a viral infection. Sinus tachycardia is also present, may be secondary to chest pain and fever.

Major etiologies of acute pericarditis include infection [viral, bacterial, and tubercular (TB)], autoimmune diseases, uremia, neoplastic pericardial invasion, previous acute MI, aortic dissection, thoracic trauma, previous cardiotomy/thoracic surgery, etc. The patients generally present with chest pain, pericardial friction rub, ECG changes of pericarditis, and new/worsening pericardial effusion. In some patients, myocardium may also be involved. Workup includes laboratories for inflammatory markers and/or myocarditis workup, pericardial fluid workup (purulent/TB/neoplastic etiologies), ECG, 2D ECHO for pericardial effusion/tamponade, and cardiac CT/MRI (pericardial thickening and pericardial effusion. Management approach includes NSAIDS (idiopathic/viral myocarditis), colchicine, steroids, and/or pericardiocentesis.

Suggested Reading
1. Lazarou E, Tsioufis P, Vlachopoulos C, Tsioufis C, Lazaros G. Acute pericarditis: Update. Curr Cardiol Rep. 2022;24(8):905-13.

Q.22. A 41-year-old male, known case of uncontrolled hypertension, presented to ER with sudden-onset "severe tearing" chest pain, spreading across the neck after lifting weights in a nearby gym. At admission, he was conscious and agitated, tachycardic (heart rate 110 beats/min), BP 160/90 mm Hg, but BP readings in both arms were different. CXR was suggestive of mediastinal widening. ECG revealed >1-mm ST elevation in anterior leads. Cardiac enzymes and D-dimer levels were elevated although the subsequent cardiac markers did not rise dynamically. Urgent thrombolysis was planned in view of anterior wall myocardial infarction (MI) and no absolute contraindications for thrombolysis. However, the patient immediately collapsed post-thrombolysis and could not be revived. What could have been the underlying problem in this case?

a. Anterior wall MI
b. Thoracic aortic dissection
c. Pulmonary embolism
d. Tension pneumothorax

Ans. b

Explanation: The patient had thoracic aortic dissection at the level of origin of coronary arteries, and thus impeding the supply of coronaries to the heart leading to ST elevation. However, the underlying cause was aortic dissection and the false lumen created by blood flowing into the aortic wall was actually compressing the true arterial lumen. Administration of thrombolytics worsened the aortic dissection further and proved fatal. Both acute coronary syndrome (ACS) and thoracic aortic dissection present with sudden onset chest pain. These conditions can be easily missed in emergency settings. As misdiagnosis can be fatal, it is essential to have a checklist for differentiating these similar but life-threatening conditions, which have different treatments. Careful clinical evaluation (history, chest pain characteristic, pulse deficits, and difference in BP readings between limbs), CXR (mediastinal widening), bedside echocardiography (to look for intimal flap formation between true and false lumens), and CT chest can be useful tools for the same.

Suggested Reading
1. Jackson E, Stewart M. Thoracic aortic dissection presenting as acute coronary syndrome. BMJ Case Rep. 2013;2013:bcr2013201904.

Q.23. A 42-year-old lady, a known case of hypertension, presented with complaints of cough for 2 months, and breathlessness for 1 month. 1 month after admission, the patient developed shortness of breath and loss of consciousness and was admitted to ICU. She was intubated, Glasgow Coma Scale (GCS) score was E4VTM4, pupils were reactive to light. Patient had a history of right-sided hemiparesis 9 years back, although power had improved gradually. At admission, the patient was in altered sensorium, tachycardic and hypotensive with raised JVP.

General blood picture (GBP) showed normocytic and normochromic RBCs with mild anisocytosis, WBC count was 6,800 cells/cu mm, differential leukocyte count (DLC) showed 75% neutrophils, 15% lymphocytes, 5% monocytes, 1% eosinophils, and no basophils, platelet count was 50,000 cells/cu mm and no atypical cells were seen. Anti-Leptospira IgM enzyme-linked immunosorbent assay (ELISA) was positive, serum antiscrub typhus IgM ELISA negative, and *Salmonella typhi*

IgM negative. Magnetic resonance imaging (MRI) brain showed small chronic infarcts in bilateral corona radiata and basal ganglia with basilar top aneurysm which was an incidental finding.

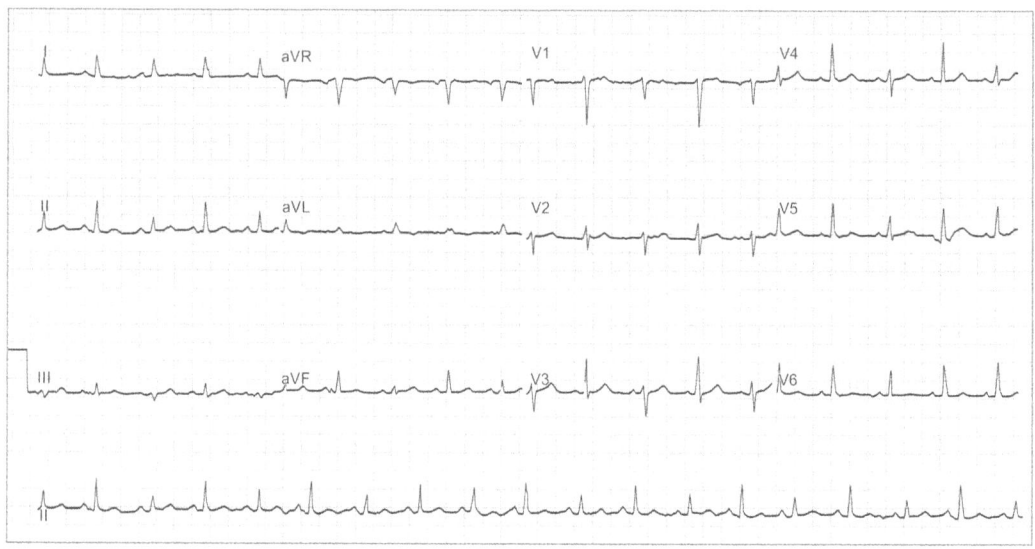

What is the most likely abnormality?
a. Pericardial tamponade
b. Pulmonary embolism
c. Pulmonary hypertension
d. Aortic dissection

Ans. a

Explanation: ECG depicts QRS complex of varying amplitudes without any conduction abnormality, known as electrical alternans. Electrical alternans is seen in large pericardial effusion and pericardial tamponade, due to swinging motion of heart in pericardial cavity. Other ECG abnormalities in pericardial tamponade include sinus tachycardia and low-voltage QRS complexes (<0.5 mV in limb leads). Underlying findings of acute pericarditis may also be seen.

2D echocardiography (including Doppler studies) is the main diagnostic tool for pericardial tamponade. Typical echocardiographic findings are pericardial effusion, late diastolic collapse of RA and early diastolic collapse of RV, sonographic pulsus paradoxus (ventricular interdependence), and dilated inferior vena cava (IVC) with < 50% collapse.

Patients with pericardial tamponade require urgent pericardiocentesis. 2D ECHO is also helpful in ruling out life-threatening conditions such as aortic dissection and LV free wall rupture leading to tamponade, which require urgent surgical intervention.

Suggested Reading
1. Niarchos AP. Electrical alternans in cardiac tamponade. Thorax. 1975;30(2):228-33.

Q.24. A 30-year-old female is admitted to ER with complaints of pleuritic chest pain and shortness of breath for last 24 hours. She has recently undergone an emergency cesarean section 2 weeks ago at 37 weeks of gestation in view of fetal bradycardia. She also complains of swelling and redness in right leg for last 7 days. CXR is normal. On examination, she is conscious, heart rate is 110 beats/min, blood pressure 100/70 mm Hg, peripheral oxygen saturation 95% (spontaneous respiration without oxygen supplementation). Baseline routine laboratories are normal.

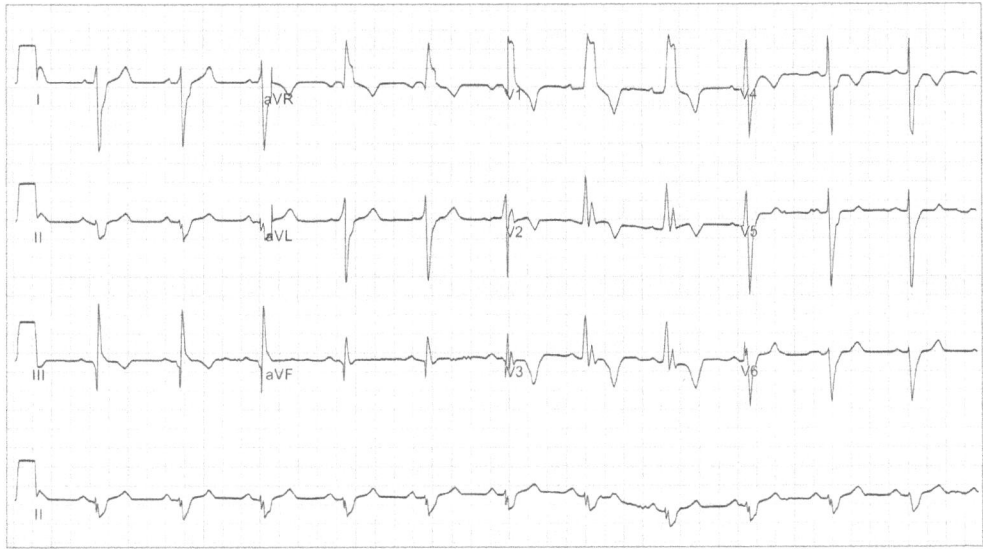

What is the next most suitable diagnostic approach for this patient?
a. Ventilation/perfusion (V/Q) scan
b. High sensitivity D-dimer assay
c. Multidetector CT pulmonary angiogram (CTPA)
d. Cardiac catheterization to assess right-sided pressures

Ans. c

Explanation: ECG shows S1Q3T3 pattern, suggestive of pulmonary embolism. Other ECG findings in pulmonary embolism include sinus tachycardia (most common), signs of right-sided heart failure (RAD, RBBB, right ventricular strain pattern, dominant R in V1, and P pulmonale), atrial tachyarrhythmias, and nonspecific ST-T changes.

D-dimer has a high negative predictive value in patients with low clinical probability. Clinical probability score for pulmonary embolism is high (Wells score > 6) in this case. In patients with high clinical probability, multidetector CTPA is the diagnostic modality of choice, if no contraindications for IV contrast administration exist. 2D ECHO (direct and indirect signs of pulmonary embolism) is useful for patients in shock or if CT scan is unavailable. V/Q scan is done when CTPA is contraindicated or inconclusive, or if additional testing is required.

Anticoagulation therapy with heparin should be started without delay in patients with confirmed or high clinical probability for pulmonary embolism. Systemic thrombolysis is required for massive pulmonary embolism presenting with hemodynamic instability.

Suggested Reading
1. Bahloul M, Chaari A, Kallel H, Abid L, Hamida CB, Dammak H, et al. Pulmonary embolism in intensive care unit: Predictive factors, clinical manifestations and outcome. Ann Thorac Med. 2010;5(2):97-103.

Q.25. A 25-year-old male, while on a boating trip with his friends in Nainital in December, met with an accident and suffered from near drowning for around 4–5 minutes. Lifeguards, who had witnessed the accident, came to his rescue immediately and shifted him to the ER of a nearby hospital. At admission, he was cold to touch (90°F), drowsy, bradycardic (heart rate 45 beats/min), blood pressure 80/60 mm Hg. Peripheral oxygen saturation was unable to record SpO$_2$ correctly. Arterial blood gas (ABG) was awaited. Meanwhile, ECG done at bedside revealed the following changes:

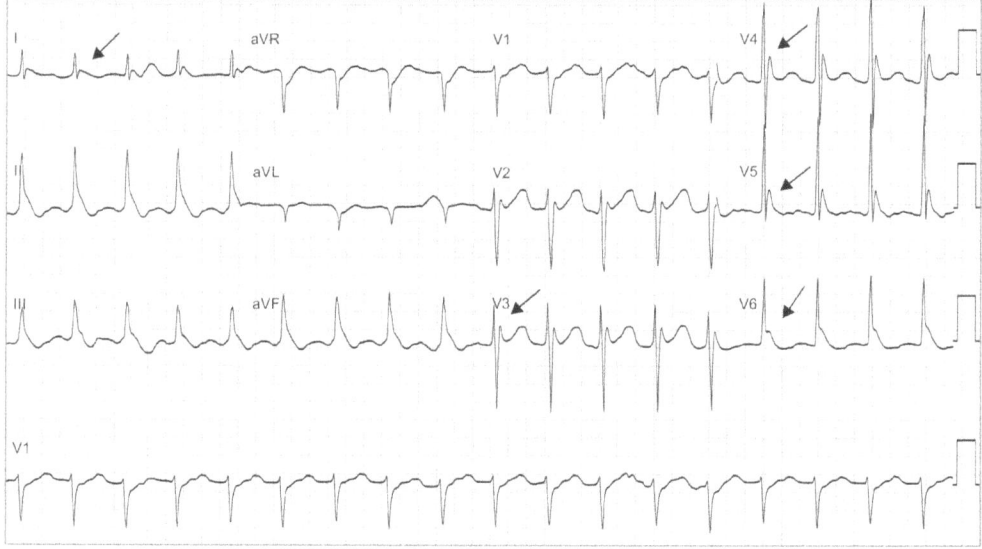

What is the most likely reason behind the abnormality in ECG in this patient?
a. Hyperkalemia
b. Acute coronary syndrome (ACS)
c. Hypothermia
d. Right bundle branch block (RBBB)

Ans. c

Explanation: ECG depicts J waves, also known as Osborn's waves, which is seen as deflection at the J point (J point is the junction between QRS complex and ST segment).

Hypothermia is an important cause of Osborn's waves caused by increase in outward cardiac potassium current (I$_{to}$ current) secondary to low temperature leading to repolarization abnormality. Osborn's waves can also be seen in other pathological conditions such as hypercalcemia, Takotsubo cardiomyopathy, acute myocardial ischemia, severe myocarditis, neurological insults like head injury and subarachnoid hemorrhage, early repolarization, and Brugada syndromes. Other ECG changes of hypothermia include artifacts due to shivering, interval prolongation (PR, QRS, and QT intervals), trial, and ventricular arrhythmias.

Suggested Reading
1. Ram P, George G. Osborn waves of hypothermia. Postgrad Med J. 2017;93(1100):366.

Q.26. A 70-year-old female, from a nursing home was transferred to hospital because of profound weakness and areflexia. Her oral intake had been poor for a few days. Current medication was a thiazide diuretic for heart failure. ABG report was as mentioned below:

> pH: 7.54
> $PaCO_2$: 59 mm Hg
> PaO_2: 65 mm Hg
> HCO_3: 44.4 mmol/L

Admission biochemistry (in mmol/L) is awaited. ECG was done at admission, which is mentioned below:

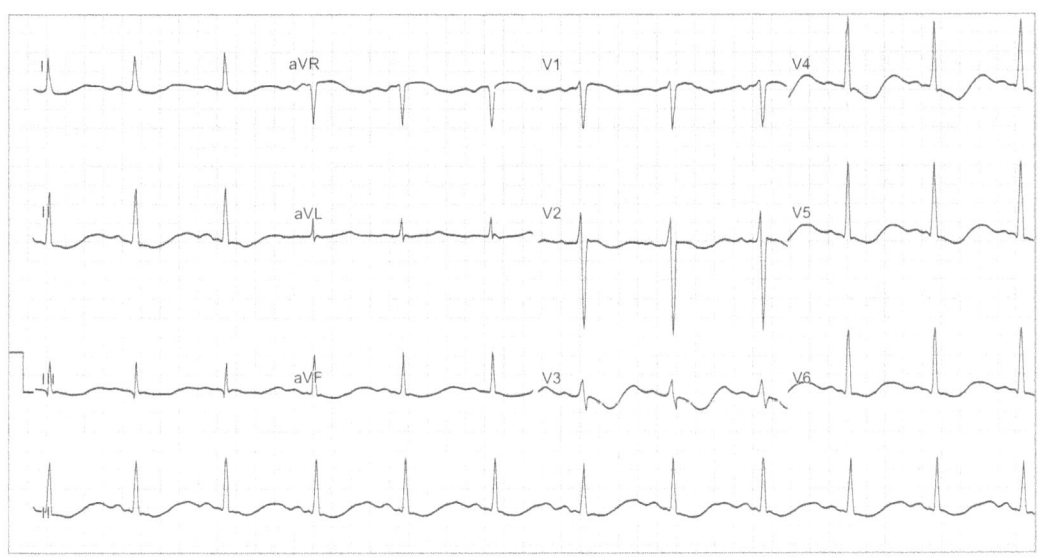

What would be the most likely electrolyte abnormality?
a. Hyperkalemia   b. Hypocalcemia
c. Hypokalemia   d. Hyponatremia

Ans. c

Explanation: Table 2 shows ECG changes in various common dyselectrolytemias:

TABLE 2: ECG changes in various dyselectrolytemias.

Dyselectrolytemia	ECG changes
Hypokalemia	Increased P wave amplitude → PR prolongation → ST depression and T-wave inversion prominent U waves → prolonged QU interval or pseudoprolonged QT (Fusion of T and U waves)
Hyperkalemia	Tall, narrow, and peaked T waves → prolonged PR → reduced P wave amplitude → broad QRS → P waves absent → sine wave pattern
Hypocalcemia	Prolonged ST segment, long QT interval, and T-wave spared
Hypercalcemia	Short ST segment, short QT interval, Osborn's waves, and wide T waves
Hypomagnesemia	Similar to that of hypokalemia (prolonged PR, depressed ST, and flat T wave) (In hypomagnesemia, always look for coexisting hypokalemia and hypocalcemia)

Suggested Reading

1. Wang X, Han D, Li G. Electrocardiographic manifestations in severe hypokalemia. J Int Med Res. 2020;48(1):300060518811058.

Q.27. A 75-year-old male, known case of uncontrolled hypertension, coronary artery disease (CAD) and chronic kidney disease (CKD) presented to ER with sudden-onset generalized seizures and loss of consciousness. At admission, his GCS after intubation for airway protection was E1VTM2 with right hemiparesis, heart rate 92 beats/min (sinus rhythm), BP 190/100 mm Hg (IV labetalol infusion started) and SpO_2 95% on spontaneous respiration without oxygen supplementation. He was on regular oral antiplatelets for last 6–7 months for CAD. Noncontrast computed tomography (NCCT) brain revealed acute left-sided frontotemporal subdural hematoma (SDH) with midline shift. The patient was anuric and gradually developed gasping respiration with bradycardia up to 55 beats/min. ECG revealed following changes:

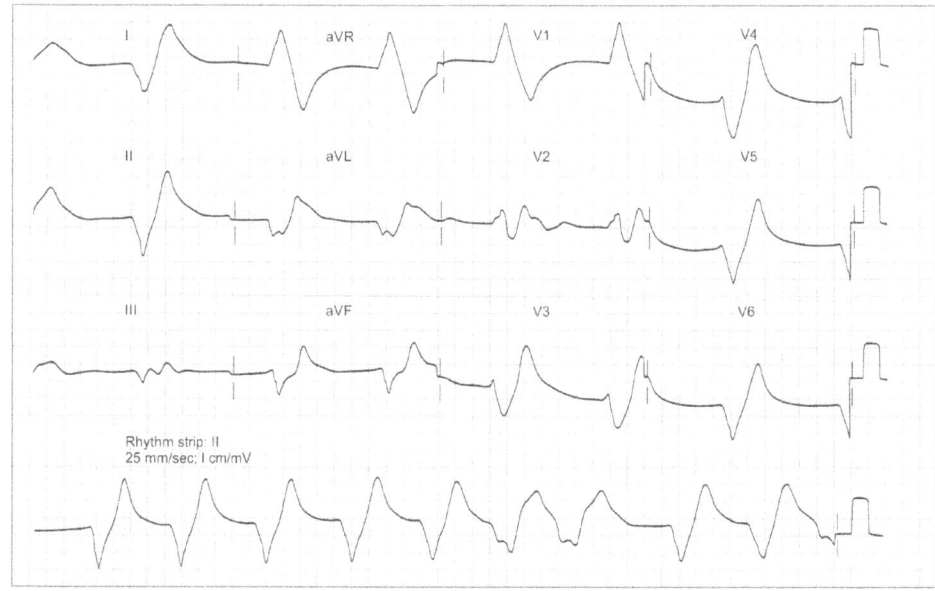

What is the most likely electrolyte abnormality in ECG?
a. Hypocalcemia
b. Hyperkalemia
c. Hypokalemia
d. Hypercalcemia

Ans. b

Explanation: ECG is suggestive of features of hyperkalemia. Refer to **Table 2** in discussion of question 26.

Suggested Reading
1. Littmann L, Gibbs MA. Electrocardiographic manifestations of severe hyperkalemia. J Electrocardiol. 2018;51(5):814-7.

Q.28. A 25-year-old female, P2L1+0 was admitted in ICU from OT with history of cardiac arrest intraoperatively due to high spinal anesthesia during cesarean section around 6 hours ago. At admission, she was received in intubated condition and was having generalized seizures, which were controlled with intravenous (IV) midazolam and IV phenytoin infusions. Vitals at admission were heart rate 55 beats/min, peripheral oxygen saturation (SpO$_2$) 98% at volume control mode, fraction of inspired oxygen (FiO$_2$) 0.30, positive end-expiratory pressure (PEEP) 6, respiratory rate (RR) 20 breaths/min, and set tidal volume (Vt) 6 mL/kg ideal body weight. On examination, she had a scar mark at neck suggestive of prior surgery and was having facial twitches. ECG done at admission showed the following changes:

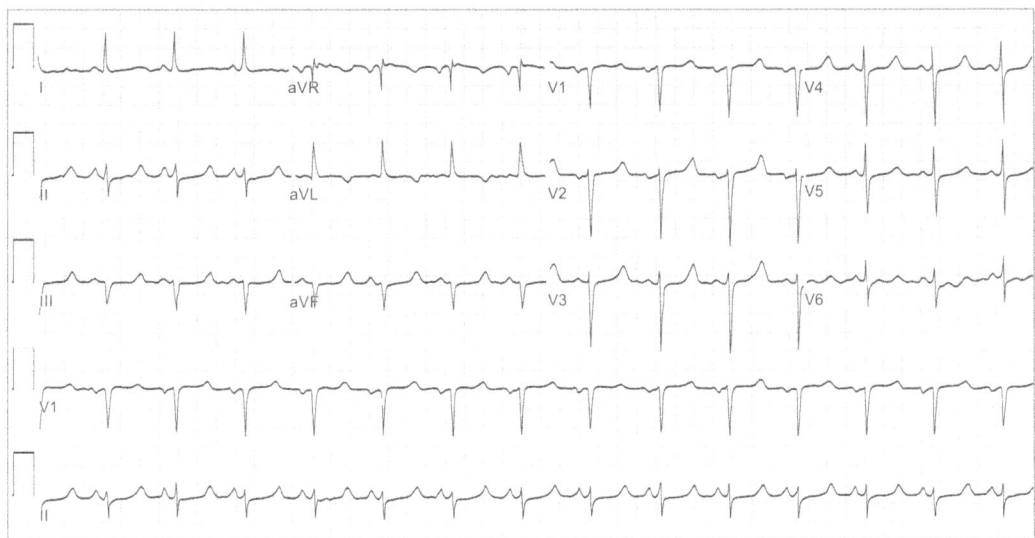

What is the most likely electrolyte abnormality in ECG?
a. Hypocalcemia
b. Hypermagnesemia
c. Hyperkalemia
d. Hypercalcemia

Ans. a

Explanation: Refer to **Table 2** in discussion of question 26.

Suggested Reading
1. RuDusky BM. ECG abnormalities associated with hypocalcemia. Chest. 2001;119(2):668-9.

Q.29. In a patient with digoxin toxicity, which of the following arrhythmias are not seen?
a. Atrial tachyarrhythmias with fast ventricular rate
b. Ventricular premature complexes (VPCs)
c. AV blocks
d. Ventricular tachycardia (VT)

Ans. a

Explanation: Both digoxin effect and digoxin toxicity are different entities. Digoxin effect suggests that patient is simply receiving digoxin and is manifested by a "reverse tick" or "Salvador Dali Sagging" appearance in ST segment. However, digoxin toxicity represents digoxin overdose and can present with sinus bradycardia, atrial/junctional tachycardia with AV block, ventricular premature complexes (VPCs), and in severe toxicity with bidirectional VT or VF. Atrial tachyarrhythmias with fast ventricular rate are typically absent (due to digoxin-induced AV nodal blockade).

Besides cardiac toxicity, other signs and symptoms include:
- *Gastrointestinal symptoms (most common symptom of digoxin toxicity)*: Anorexia, nausea/vomiting, and diarrhea
- Visual disturbance, lethargy, confusion, and dyspnea

Precipitating factors for digoxin toxicity:
- Hypercalcemia, hypokalemia, and hypomagnesemia
- Renal failure
- Avoid cardioversion as cardioversion precipitates life-threatening arrhythmias in digoxin toxicity
- Avoid IV calcium administration and beta-agonists in the treatment of hyperkalemia in digoxin toxicity

Treatment approach includes activated charcoal (early phase), supportive care, brady- and tachyarrhythmia management, and digoxin-specific (Fab) antibody fragments (especially if hyperkalemia > 5 mEq/L, life-threatening arrhythmia, and cardiac arrest).

Suggested Reading
1. Bauman JL, Didomenico RJ, Galanter WL. Mechanisms, manifestations, and management of digoxin toxicity in the modern era. Am J Cardiovasc Drugs. 2006;6(2):77-86.

Q.30. A 60-year-old female presented to ER with alleged history of intake of approximately 80 tablets of some unknown drug (50 mg each). Upon arrival in ER, she was febrile up to 102°F, unconscious, pupils were dilated but reactive to light, BP 80/60 mm Hg, HR 145 beats/min, RR 26 breaths/min, and she was unable to pass urine. ECG done at bedside revealed the following findings:

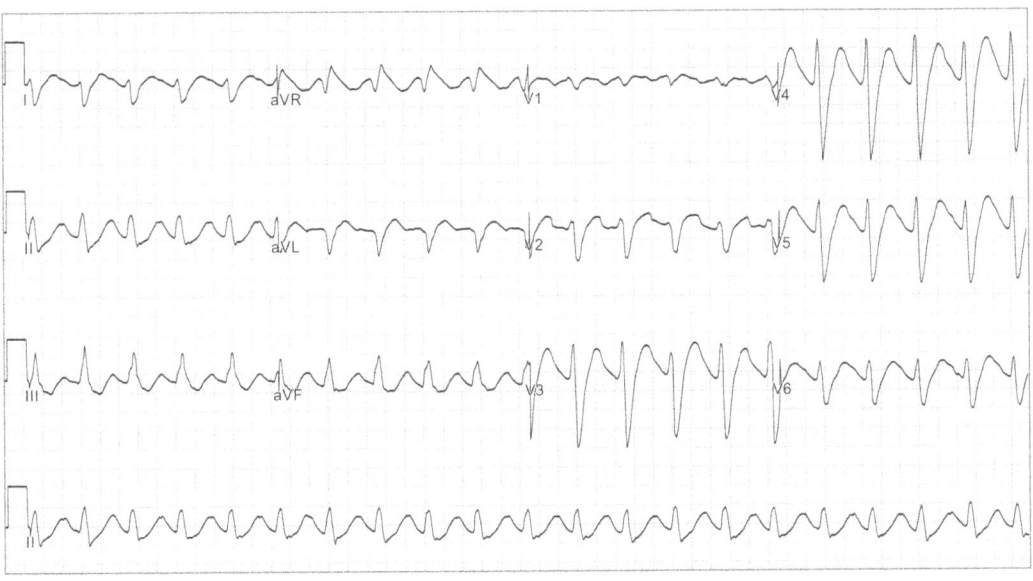

What could be the probable drug ingested as per clinical presentation and ECG findings ?

a. Diazepam
b. Calcium channel blocker
c. Tricyclic antidepressant
d. Beta-blocker

Ans. c

Explanation: ECG depicts sinus rhythm with broad QRS, terminal R wave in aVR, and long QT interval suggestive of tricyclic antidepressant overdose (sodium channel blockade).

Features of TCA overdose are as mentioned below:
- *Cardiac toxicity*:
  - *QRS prolongation (blockade of fast sodium channels phase "0" of action potential prolongation):* QRS > 100 ms → predictive of seizures; QRS > 160 ms → predictive of arrhythmias
  - *QT prolongation (potassium channel blockade):* Torsades de Pointes
- *Blockade of alpha-receptors*: Hypotension
- *Blockade of muscarinic receptors*: Altered mentation, dilated pupils, tachycardia, fever, dry mouth, dry skin, decreased bowel sounds, and urinary retention
- *Blockade of histamine receptors*: Altered mentation

Management approach includes supportive therapy, charcoal gastrointestinal decontamination (early phase), controlling seizures, IV sodium bicarbonate, vasopressors, and/or pacing for refractory bradyarrhythmias.

Suggested Reading
1. Kerr GW, McGuffie AC, Wilkie S. Tricyclic antidepressant overdose: A review. Emerg Med J. 2001;18(4):236-41.

CHAPTER

Quality, Medication Errors, and Research

Anuj Clerk, Nandita Divekar, PL Gautam

MULTIPLE CHOICE QUESTIONS ON QUALITY

A 77-year-old man was admitted to the accident and emergency department of the hospital with severe abdominal pain and diarrhea for 3 days. He had a history of type II diabetes mellitus, hypertension, chronic obstructive pulmonary disease, body mass index (BMI) of 40 (weight 120 kg), and very poor exercise tolerance.

The patient was transferred to the intensive care unit (ICU) at midnight post a prolonged emergency laparotomy with division of adhesions and resection of a small segment of ischemic-looking large bowel. A decision was made to leave him intubated overnight. The intensive care and the hospital were very busy on that night.

He had three large cannulas in his arms and a right radial arterial line on arrival from the operating theaters. The anesthetist handed over that the patient had been very stable throughout the procedure. However, the blood pressure was 80/50 mm Hg after arrival in the unit. He was sedated and ventilated and given more fluids. Despite that, the blood pressure continued to remain low. A five-lumen central venous line was inserted by a trainee under ultrasound guidance. The procedure was slightly difficult but successful. A chest X-ray was requested. Noradrenaline was commenced. One lumen was left unused for total parenteral nutrition (TPN).

At 6 AM the relatives came to the ICU entrance complaining that they were waiting for so long and no one had spoken to them. The doctors were still busy and so the wife had to wait for another hour. The doctors apologized for keeping them waiting and the relatives settled.

One of the nurses pointed out that there was high-pressure alarm in the central infusion pump. On reviewing the line it was found that the guidewire was still remaining in one of the lumens. It was removed immediately and a DATIX (incident reporting form) was filled out. A duty of candour was performed (the mistake was explained to the relatives and a verbal and written apology was given). It was a *never event* and had to be reported nationally. "*Never events*" are defined as serious, largely preventable patient safety incidents that should not occur if relevant preventive measures have been put in place. A root cause analysis was done. A Plan-do-Study-Act cycle was planned. An audit conducted into the documentation of checklists for invasive procedures in intensive care found that documentation for invasive procedures was poor at times. The standard required was 100% documentation but the compliance was only 60%. The findings were presented to the department. Changes implemented were—(i) the documentation came up as mandatory on the electronic systems, (ii) educational sessions for doctors and nurses during their induction and team meetings, and (iii) good communication, immediate documentation, and teamwork were emphasized to improve patient safety. This quality improvement project had a significant impact. The repeat audit showed that the documentation was complete in 99.9% of invasive procedures. There was no *never event* related to invasive procedures for the next 3 years.

The patient was extubated 2 days later. He was given an explanation and apology for the wire remaining in the body for some time. He did not come to any harm and was discharged a day later to the ward.

Q.1. Which of the following is the correct abbreviation for QIP?
   a. Quality innovation process
   b. Quality innovation project
   c. Quality improvement project
   d. Quality initiation process
   e. Quantity initiation procedure

Ans. c

Explanation: Quality improvement projects in NHS UK, allow clinicians working within a team, to identify an issue and implement interventions that can result in true improvements in quality. It aims to make a difference to patients by improving safety, effectiveness, and experience of care.

Quality improvement projects are now part of training of various healthcare organizations.

Suggested Reading
1. Jones B, Vaux E, Olsson-Brown A. How to get started in quality improvement. BMJ. 2019;364:k5408.

Q.2. Select two correct options for clinical audit from the following:
   a. Is completely unrelated to clinical governance
   b. Can answer whether we are doing the right thing in the right way
   c. Is regulated by hospital management
   d. Seeks to improve patient care and outcomes through a systematic review of care against explicit criteria
   e. Is just a data-collection exercise

Ans. b and d

Explanation: Clinical audit forms part of clinical governance, which aims to ensure that patients receive the best quality of care. It answers whether we are doing the right thing in the right way. It is a quality improvement process that seeks to improve patient care and outcomes through a systematic review of care against explicit criteria.

Suggested Reading
1. Limb C, Fowler A, Gundogan B, Koshy K, Agha R. How to conduct a clinical audit and quality improvement project. Int J Surg Oncol (N Y). 2017;2(6):e24.
2. National Institute for Clinical Excellence. Principles for Best Practice in Clinical Audit. United Kingdom: Radcliffe Medical Press Ltd; 2002.

Q.3. Audit includes which of the following?
   a. Selecting topic
   b. Agreeing standards
   c. Collecting and analyzing data
   d. Implementing changes and repeating cycle
   e. All of the above

Ans. e

Explanation: One of the first clinical audits ever undertaken was during the Crimean War of 1853-1855 by Florence Nightingale.

The National Institute for Health and Clinical Excellence (NICE), published "The Principles for Best Practice in Clinical Audit in 2002, which defined clinical audit as, "a quality improvement process that seeks to improve patient care and outcomes through a systematic review against explicit criteria and the implementation of change."

Clinical audit plays an important part in the drive to improve the quality of patient care.

The audit cycle is made of six stages namely—(1) choosing a topic, (2) agreeing on target standards, (3) collecting and analyzing data, (4) comparing performance with targets, (5) implementing change and planning care, and (6) finally repeating the audit cycle.

Suggested Reading
1. Benjamin A. Audit: how to do it in practice. BMJ. 2008;336(7655):1241-5.
2. Gnanalingham J, Gnanalingham MG, Gnanalingham KK. An audit of audits: are we completing the cycle? 2001;94(6):288-9.

Q.4. PDSA cycle stands for which of the following?
   a. Procedure demonstrate study act
   b. Procedure do study action
   c. Plan demonstrate strategies action
   d. Plan do study act

Ans. d

Explanation: PDSA cycle stands for Plan-Do-Study-Act (PDSA) cycle. The PDSA cycle started out as the plan, do, check, and act cycle and was introduced by Walter Shewhart in the 1920s.

The model for improvement provides a framework for developing, testing, and implementing changes leading to improvement. It is based in scientific method and moderates the impulse to take immediate action with the wisdom of careful study.

Changes are tested on a small scale first, building on the learning from these test cycles in a structured way one can bring major changes. This gives stakeholders the opportunity to see if the proposed change will succeed and is a powerful tool for learning from ideas that do and do not work.

It provides a structure for iterative testing of changes to improve the quality of systems.

Suggested Reading
1. National Health Service. (2022). Quality, Service Improvement and Redesign Tools: Plan, Do, Study, Act (PDSA) cycles and the model for improvement. [online] Available from https://www.england.nhs.uk/wp-content/uploads/2022/01/qsir-pdsa-cycles-model-for-improvement.pdf [Last accessed June, 2023].
2. Taylor MJ, McNicholas C, Nicolay C, Darzi A, Bell D, Reed JE. Systematic review of the application of the Plan–Do–Study–Act method to improve quality in healthcare. BMJ Qual Saf. 2014;23(4):290-8.

Q.5. Choose three correct options for *never events* from the following:
a. Will never occur again
b. Will occur repeatedly even if measures are in place
c. Should not occur if preventable measures are in place
d. Are serious and preventable
e. Any investigation after a *never event* should primarily focus on systemic failings rather than putting blame on individuals

Ans. c, d, and e

Explanation: *Never events* are serious, largely preventable patient safety incidents that should not occur if relevant preventive measures have been put in place. They have potential to cause serious patient harm or death (whether or not harm actually happened). These incidents have to be reported nationally in UK. They are deemed unacceptable. *Never events* may act as surrogates of the patient safety culture within a healthcare organization. Repeated occurrence of *never events* may be interpreted as a failure of implementation or adherence to guidelines and protocols. When a *never event* occurs the primary focus should be on the reasons behind such failures rather than on the actions of the individuals involved.

Suggested Reading
1. Adyanthaya S, Patil V. Never events: an anaesthetic perspective. Contin Educ Anaesth, Crit Care Pain. 2014;14:197-201.
2. Zaslow J, Fortier J, Bowman C, de Gorter R, Tsai E, Desai D, et al. Defining healthcare never events to effect system change: a protocol for systematic review. PLoS ONE. 2022;17(12):e0279113.

Q.6. Which of the following are true about duty of candour?
a. The healthcare professional must be open and honest
b. Only done when a patient raises concern
c. Apologize to the patient or carer when something has gone wrong
d. It has to be done by the junior most member of the team
e. A verbal apology followed by a written apology may be required

Ans. a, c, and e

Explanation: Every health and care professional must be open and honest with patients and people in their care when something that goes wrong with their treatment or care causes, or has the potential to cause, harm or distress. They must tell the person (or, where appropriate, their advocate, carer or family) when something has gone wrong, apologize, offer an appropriate remedy or support to put matters right (if possible) explain fully the short- and long-term effects of what has happened.

Suggested Reading
1. The General Medical Council. Openness and honesty when things go wrong: the professional duty of candour. [online] Available from https://www.gmc-uk.org/ethical-guidance/ethical-guidance-for-doctors/candour—openness-and-honesty-when-things-go-wrong/the-professional-duty-of-candour#:~:text=Every%20health%20and%20care%20professional,to%20cause%2C%20harm%20or%20distress [Last accessed June, 2023].

Q.7. Choose 2 correct options for root cause analysis (RCA) from the following:
a. Can emphasize on individual action lapses so that the right person causing the error can be identified.
b. Emphasizes on lapses in system-level processes.
c. Always leads to immediate changes in processes.
d. The head of the ICU team should carry out the RCA.
e. Can be used to improve patient safety.

Ans. b and e

Explanation: Root cause analysis (RCA) is a process for identifying the factors causing variations in performance which can cause an adverse event. It can help an institution to develop strategies and prevent further errors. It aims to assess lapses in system level processes and not blame individuals. Although early studies suggested that RCAs are effective in promoting ideas for preventing recurrence of events, more recent studies do not confirm these findings.

It aims to look at lapses in system-level processes and issues which led to the event and not individual human errors. The goal is to improve patient safety. There are various stages: Identify adverse event, organize a team, develop an initial flow map, develop an event story map, develop a cause and effect diagram, identify root cause contributing factors, develop corrective actions, measure outcomes and communicate results.

Suggested Reading
1. Charles R, Hood B, Derosier JM, Gosbee JW, Li Y, Caird MS, et al. How to perform a root cause analysis for workup and future prevention of medical errors: a review. Patient Saf Surg. 2016;10:20.
2. Martin-Delgado J, Martínez-García A, Aranaz JM, Valencia-Martín JL, Mira JJ. How much of root cause analysis translates into improved patient safety: a Systematic review. Med Princ Pract. 2020;29(6):524-31.
3. Singh G, Patel RH, Boster J. Root Cause Analysis and Medical Error Prevention. STAT Pearls May 2023. https://www.ncbi.nlm.nih.gov/books/NBK570638/

Q.8. Challenges to performing quality improvement projects include:
a. A supportive leader for the department.
b. Lack of motivation and knowledge gaps in members of the department.
c. Well developed protocols in the department.
d. Good relations with other professions in the hospital.
e. Choosing projects that align with the department's or hospital's long-term change agenda

Ans. b

Explanation: Though quality improvement in healthcare have been introduced since 19th century, it has now become mandatory for many healthcare professions. However there are real life challenges in conducting these Quality Improvement Projects.

Some of them include organizational rigidity, inter professional friction, inadequate support, poor resources, lack of motivation and team work and knowledge gaps.

Suggested Reading
1. Hines K, Mouchtouris N, Knightly JJ, Harrop J. A brief history of quality improvement in health care and spinal surgery. Global Spine J. 2020; 10(Suppl 1): 5S–9S.
2. Madu A. Challenges in conducting quality improvement projects: reflections of a junior doctor. Future Healthc J. 2022; 9(3): 333-4.

Q.9. Aims of Quality Improvement Projects should be (Choose the most appropriate option):
   a. Measurable
   b. Timely
   c. Specific
   d. Realistic
   e. All of the above.

Ans. e

Explanation: Quality Improvement Projects are fraught with challenges at times. It can be helpful if one develops the aims using the SMART framework: Specific (S), Measurable (M), Achievable (A), Realistic (R), and Timely (T). This allows to assess the scale of the intervention and to pare it down if the original idea is too ambitious.

Suggested Reading
1. Jones B, Vaux E, Olsson-Brown A. How to get started in quality improvement. BMJ. 2019; 364: k5408.
2. Improvement NHS. (NHSI) Quality, Service Improvement and Redesign Tools: Developing your aims statement. January 2018. https://improvement.nhs.uk/resources/aims-statement-development/.
3. SMART GUIDELINES: World Health Organization, https://www.who.int › digital-health-and-innovation.

Q.10. Regarding incident reporting in hospitals the following is true:
   a. It is compulsory.
   b. It should include names of the personnel involved.
   c. It should be done by the doctor or nurse in charge on the day.
   d. Reflects the organizational transparency and the drive toward patient safety and quality improvement in healthcare.
   e. Feedback should only be given to the person who has reported it.

Ans. d

Explanation: Incident reporting is an effective strategy used to enhance patient safety and quality improvement in healthcare. Incident is an event which could eventually result in harm to a patient. Good incident reporting by hospital staff reflects the organizational transparency and the driving forces behind patient safety and quality improvement in healthcare. Reasons for not reporting are unawareness, no recognition of the incident, lack of clear incident definition, time pressure, fear of punitive measures, lack of feedback and lack of belief that reporting results in future improvement. Incident reporting should be voluntary, anonymous, and confidential and feedback should be given. Incident reporting can be done by any member of staff.

Suggested Reading
1. Brunsveld-Reinders AH, Arbous MS, Vos RD, Jonge ED. Incident and error reporting systems in intensive care: a systematic review of the literature. Int J Qual Health Care. 2016;28(1):2-13.
2. Fukami T, Uemura M, Nagao Y. Significance of incident reports by medical doctors for organizational transparency and driving forces for patient safety. Patient Saf Surg. 2020;16:14:13.

MULTIPLE CHOICE QUESTIONS ON MEDICATION ERRORS

Q.1. Medical errors are a common cause of death in the USA. How common it is?
a. Tenth common cause of death
b. Third common cause of death
c. Fifth common cause of death
d. Second common cause of death
e. Seventh common cause of death

Ans. b

Explanation: Medical errors are considered the third common cause accounting for over 2.51 lac deaths annually in the USA as per John Hopkins University group publication in the BMJ. As per an old study done by Donchin Yoel in 1995, errors in medications account for 78% of total errors in medical field. Thus, one needs to study and pay attention to prevention of medication errors as much as learning about any disease. With each passing years, the complexity in critical care is going to increase so is the probability of errors in medications.

Suggested Reading
1. Donchin Y, Gopher D, Olin M, Badihi Y, Biesky CL, Sprung CL, et al. A look into the nature and causes of human errors in the intensive care unit. Crit Care Med. 1995;23(2): 294-300.
2. Makary MA, Daniel M. Medical error—the third leading cause of death in the US. BMJ. 2016;353:i2139.

Q.2. Which of the following is the correct way of prescribing?
a. Tab Rocaltorl.25 mcg BID
b. Tab Rocaltrol 0.25 microgram Two times a day
c. Tab Rocaltrol .25 mcg BID
d. Tab Rocaltrol0.25 mics BD

Ans. b

Explanation: Syntax error is one of the common errors of prescription. As per Institute For Safe Medication Practices (ISMP) guidelines and recommendations issued by National Coordination Council for Medication Error Reporting and Prevention (*www.nccmerp.org*), certain short forms must be avoided as they are prone to errors. Typing in capital, keep space between name and dose strength, keep prevailing zero in front of decimal, writing microgram in place of MCG or Mics, and full syntax "two times a day" are few examples included in the question above. Readers are advised to visit these web pages to get full details.

Suggested Reading
1. Institute of Safe Medication Practices. (2021). List of error-prone abbreviations, symbols, and dose designations. [online] Available from https://www.ismp.org/recommendations/error-prone-abbreviations-list [Last accessed June, 2023].
2. National Coordination Council for Medication Error Reporting and Prevention. (2014). Recommendations to enhance accuracy of prescription/medication order writing. [online] Available from https://www.nccmerp.org/recommendations-enhance-accuracy-prescription-writing [Last accessed June, 2023].

Q.3. The correct way of preventing errors in prescribing cycloserine from cyclosporine is cycloSERINE and cycloSPORINE. This method is called?
   a. Capital lettering
   b. Tall lettering
   c. Differential lettering
   d. Tall man lettering

Ans. d

Explanation: This method recommended by ISMP as well as many quality organizations such as Joint Commission International (JCI) and National Accreditation Board for Hospitals and Healthcare Providers (NABH), is a good way to differentiate "LOOK ALIKE, SOUND ALIKE" medications. International norm is to type the name of the drugs in capital, but to avoid errors this unique system of typing the confusing LASA component of the name in CAPITAL. This seemingly odd way of prescription not only catches attention but also prevents the misinterpretation of the errors.

Suggested Reading
1. Institute for Safe Medicine Practices. (2008). Use of Tall Man Letters Is Gaining Wide Acceptance. [online] Available from https://www.ismp.org/resources/use-tall-man-letters-gaining-wide-acceptance [Last accessed June, 2023].
2. Institute of Safe Medication Practices. (2021). List of error-prone abbreviations, symbols, and dose designations. [online] Available from https://www.ismp.org/recommendations/error-prone-abbreviations-list [Last accessed June, 2023].

Q.4. Patient developed a sudden loss of responsiveness with the rhythm shown as in the diagram here. He was admitted with pneumonia and developed drug allergies. His medications were injection ceftriaxone, tablet azithromycin, and tablet hydroxyzine. Treating team added a tablet of voriconazole as his sputum showed hypha of *Aspergillus spp*. What do you think has happened?

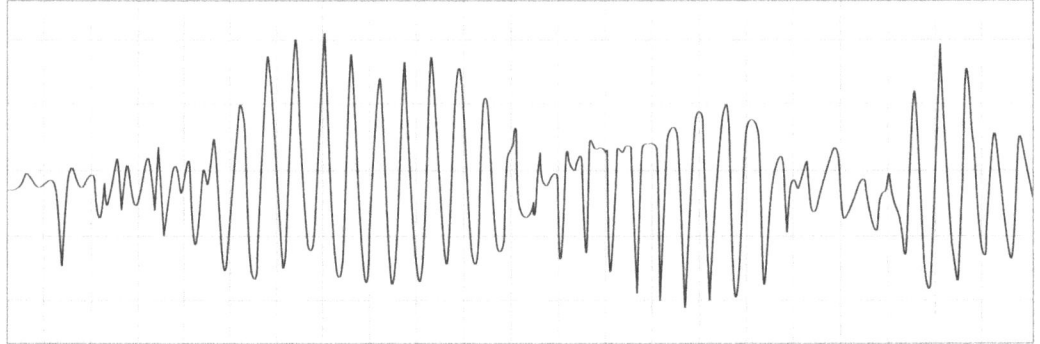

a. Ventricular tachycardia due to myocarditis
b. Ventricular tachycardia due to infection and hypoxia
c. Ventricular tachycardia due to QT-prolongation
d. Ventricular tachycardia due to new myocardial ischemia

Ans. c

Explanation: Patient developed torsades de pointes variety of multifocal ventricular tachycardia. This is due to many QT-prolonging drugs on patient's medication chart namely azithromycin, hydroxyzine, and voriconazole. Concomitant hypokalemia and hypomagnesemia which is very common in ICU can further prolong QT interval. Patient are often on long-term medicines such as amiodarone and itopride need to be looked at when a new drug with the potential to prolong QT is added to the chart. This error can result in fatal outcomes in otherwise nonfatal illness and thus need utmost importance.

Suggested Reading
1. Crediblemeds.org. QTdrugs List for a drug. [online] Available from https://crediblemeds.org/ [Last accessed June, 2023].
2. Khatib R, Sabir FRN, Omari C, Pepper C, Tayebjee MH. Managing drug-induced QT prolongation in clinical practice. Postgrad Med J. 2021;97(1149):452-8.

Q.5. **An 80-year-old male is admitted to intensive care with atrial fibrillation with a fast ventricular rate and is not responding to amiodarone infusion. Amiodarone was infused by dilution of 300 mg in 500 mL of normal saline at the rate of 1 mg/min for 6 hours. Despite doubling the dose the drug seems to have minimal effect. Venous access site was checked, potassium and calcium levels optimized, and no β-stimulants were on board. What from the following seems to be a pharmacological cause?**
a. Drug infusion rate is too slow
b. Drug concentration is too high
c. Drug dilution (solvent and concentration) is wrong
d. Inappropriate choice of drug for the patient

Ans. c

Explanation: Amiodarone is incompatible with saline and should be administered solely in a 5% dextrose solution. Amiodarone diluted with 5% dextrose solution to a concentration of <0.6 mg/mL is unstable. Solutions containing <2 ampoules of amiodarone in 500 mL dextrose 5% are unstable and should not be used. This drug is incompatible with many commonly drugs coinfused in clinical practice. Furosemide, piperacillin-tazobactam, ceftazidime, sodium bicarbonate, potassium phosphate, cefazoline, etc.

Suggested Reading
1. Fresenius-Kabi. (2020). Amiodarone prescribing information. [online] Available from http://editor.fresenius-kabi.us/PIs/US-PH-Amiodarone_HCl_FK-45887J_May_2020-PI.pdf [Last accessed June, 2023].
2. Medicines.org. Amiodarone on electronic Medical Compedium. [online] Available from https://www.medicines.org.uk/emc/product/8739/smpc [Last accessed June, 2023].

Q.6. A 76-year-old male patient was on dobutamine and frusemide infusion for the treatment of congestive heart failure. He was on an intravenous potassium supplement. Staff nurse tapered off dobutamine. Staff nurse connected antibiotic infusion in the line of potassium infusion. Within minutes; he developed bradycardia with a broad complexed rhythm. His vitals at this time were temperature—97.6°C, HR—-38/min, BP—80/60 mm Hg, RR—24/min, and SpO$_2$—92%. What is the most likely cause of this symptomatic bradycardia?
a. Cessation of dobutamine infusion
b. Worsening heart failure
c. Unintentional potassium bolus
d. Anaphylaxis due to antibiotics

Ans. c

Explanation: Medical errors are common with high risk medications. High risk medications like Inotropes, Vasopressors, Potassium, insulin Chemotherapeutic agents must be controlled by a standardized dilution and infusion protocol endorsed by clinical and pharmacy team. Piggy back incompatibilities as well as inadvertent boluses of the medication in the tubings (like in this case, potassium bloused) can prove fatal if nor prevented. Safety measures like adequate lumens for IV access is must when more than one of these high risk medications are used.

Suggested Reading
1. Kane-Gill SL, Dasta JF, Buckley MS, Devabhakthuni S, Liu M, Cohen H, et al. Clinical Practice Guideline: Safe Medication Use in the ICU. Crit Care Med. 2017;45(9):e877-915.
2. Makary MA, Daniel M. Medical error—the third leading cause of death in the US. BMJ. 2016;353:i2139.
3. Rothschild JM, Landrigan CP, Cronin JW, Kaushal R, Lockley SW, Burdick E, et al. The Critical Care Safety Study: The incidence and nature of adverse events and serious medical errors in intensive care. Critical Care Med. 2005;33(8):1694-700.

Q.7. A 73-year-old male developed severe body ache and was unable to walk after he received clarithromycin for his acute bronchitis episode. He was a case of ischemic heart disease and recurrent stroke for which he was on dual antiplatelets (aspirin

+ clopidogrel) + atorvastatin 80 mg once daily. He feels his legs are sore and tender on touching. Recently diltiazem was added by a family physician a week ago. What seems to cause of his condition? His laboratories were complete blood count (CBC: Hb 12.5 g%, total leukocytes count (TLC) 14,500, platelets 220,000, creatinine 1.8 mg%, and creatine phosphokinase test (CPK) 6,500 U/L.
   a. Infection-associated myositis
   b. Occult fall-associated muscle injury
   c. Myocarditis
   d. Statin associated rhabdomyolysis

Ans. d

Explanation: Clarithromycin is a strong cytochrome p450 3A4 inhibitor. Diltiazem is known to inhibit the same enzyme as well. Once both come on board the metabolism of atorvastatin is reduced causing increased system exposure. This when occurs in patients with renal insufficiency can lead to severe rhabdomyolysis. The muscle soreness and weakness, in this case, is due to these drug-drug interactions based on cytochrome p450 enzyme inhibition. CYP p450 3A4 is responsible for >60% of drugs metabolized via cytochrome pathway, keeping these interactions in mind while prescribing cannot be overemphasized.

Suggested Reading
1. Flockhart DA. Drug Interactions Flockhart TableTM. [online] Available from https://drug-interactions.medicine.iu.edu/MainTable.aspx [Last accessed June, 2023].
2. Mann HJ. Drug-Associated Disease: Cytochrome P450 Interactions. Crit Care Clin. 2006;22(2):329-45.
3. Ogu CC, Maxa JL. Drug interactions due to cytochrome P450. Proc (Bayl Univ Med Cent). 2000;13(4):421-3.

Q.8. Medical error includes all the following except for
   a. Wrong plan of treatment
   b. Wrong implementation
   c. Complications of the treatment (wrong act, an act of commission)
   d. Not doing the desired action
   e. Failure of plan to work

Ans. e

Explanation: Medical science is an incomplete ever progressive science. As per World Health Organization (WHO) definition an error is the failure of a planned action to be completed as intended (i.e., error of execution), or the use of a wrong plan to achieve an aim (i.e., error of planning). Errors may be errors of commission or omission and usually reflect deficiencies in the systems of care. Whether a therapeutic plan works or not depends on many factors beyond the control of medical team. So failure of treatment does not amount to be called a *medical error*.

Suggested Reading
1. World Health Organization. WHO Draft Guidelines for Adverse Event Reporting and Learning Systems. Geneva: World Health Organization; 2005.

Q.9. A 55-year-old female was started on tablet levofloxacin 750 mg once daily for her sinusitis. She was on calcium supplements for osteoporosis and iron supplements for anemia. Due to her dyspepsia, she takes all the medication with milk. She took all the medication at night time. Despite 3 days after commencement of the regime her infection seems worsening. Her nasal discharge culture grew streptococci sensitive to levofloxacin. Possible cause of failure of antibiotic regime in this case is?
   a. Inadequate dose
   b. Wrong time of dosing
   c. Inadequate absorption from bowel
   d. Inadequate drug concentration in sinuses

   Ans. c

   Explanation: Fluoroquinolones are known to get chelated when taken with elements such as calcium and iron in the intestine. When taken with milk the bioavailability drops further. This has led to inadequate absorption of levofloxacin in this case leading to failure of the antibiotic regime.

   Suggested Reading
   1. USA Food and Drug Administration. Levofloxacin prescribing information. [online] Available from https://www.accessdata.fda.gov/drugsatfda_docs/label/2013/020634s065,0 20635s071,021721s032lbl.pdf [Last accessed June, 2023].

Q.10. A 28-year-old male patient developed multiple furuncles on the limbs. He develops scalds on the skin and hypotension. So he was started in linezolid 600 mg twice daily after the dressing of the skin lesions. He was in high-dose sertraline and clonazepam for his depression. His fever increased to 103°F and developed marked tremulousness along with flushing all over the body. His inflammatory markers showed a downtrend but his fever was worsening. The cause seems to be which of the following?
   a. Allergic reaction to an antibiotic
   b. Linezolid resistance and occult abscess
   c. Linezolid a bacteriostatic drug
   d. Drug interaction

   Ans. d

   Explanation: Linezolid or any other monoamine oxidase inhibitor must be used with caution in patients on serotonin inhibitors (e.g., sertraline in this case). It can lead to serotonin syndrome due to combined SSRI and MAO inhibition and consequent serotonin excess.

   Drug-drug interactions are very crucial in intensive care as physiological reserves of ICU patients are very poor. Readers are advised to refer to partnership to prevent drug-drug interaction project which revealed most common and clinically relevant 25 interactions in ambulatory outpatients. Drug-drug interactions included in the article is of special interest as many of these medications are frequently used in ICU patients.

   Suggested Reading
   1. Malone DC, Abarca J, Hansten PD, Grizzle AJ, Armstrong EP, Van Bergen RC, et al. Identification of serious drug-drug interactions: results of the partnership to prevent drug-drug interactions. J Am Pharm Assoc (Wash). 2004;44(2):142-51.

2. USA Food and Drug Administration. Highlights of prescribing information. [online] Available from https://www.accessdata.fda.gov/drugsatfda_docs/label/2018/206473s002lbl.pdf [Last accessed June, 2023].

MULTIPLE CHOICE QUESTIONS ON RESEARCH

Q.1. Which statement is the most correct about reliability?
  a. Consistency of an instrument/measurement
  b. Accuracy of an instrument/measurement
  c. It is of two types internal and external reliability
  d. It is the degree to which you are measuring what you claim to

Ans. a

Explanation: In statistics, reliability is the consistency a measure or any equipment performance. Measurement is considered reliable if you measure the same thing many times, and the measurements are consistent, falling in the same range. A highly reliable measure is more consistent than a measure with low reliability. It may need not be valid or accurate.

Suggested Reading
1. Betz JM, Brown PN, Roman MC. Accuracy, precision, and reliability of chemical measurements in natural products research. Fitoterapia. 2011;82(1):44-52.
2. Frost J. Reliability. [online] Available from https://statisticsbyjim.com/glossary/reliability/ [Last accessed June, 2023].

Q.2. Accuracy in research methodology is?
  a. The extent to which the study measures what it is intended to measure.
  b. The degree of resemblance among study results, were the study to be repeated under similar circumstances
  c. The degree to which a measurement represents the true value of something
  d. Consistency of an instrument or measurement
  e. It is the degree to which you are measuring what you claim to

Ans. c

Explanation: Accuracy refers to how close a measurement is to the true or correct value. Accuracy assesses whether a series of measurements are correct on average in an acceptable range. In statistical terms, accuracy is an absence of bias. It may not have high reliability but is close to the correct value. In other words, measurements are not systematically too high or too low. However, accuracy tells you nothing about the distance from the target.

Suggested Reading
1. Betz JM, Brown PN, Roman MC. Accuracy, precision, and reliability of chemical measurements in natural products research. Fitoterapia. 2011;82(1):44-52.
2. Frost J. Accuracy vs Precision: Differences & Examples. [online] Available from https://statisticsbyjim.com/basics/accuracy-vs-precision/ [Last accessed June, 2023].

Q.3. "PICO" in research methodology stands for which of the following?
   a. Patient/population, intervention, comparison, and outcome
   b. Prevalence, investigation, control, and operator
   c. Patient, intervention, computation, and outcome
   d. Purpose, intervention, calibration, and objections

Ans. a

Explanation: PICO in research methodology refers to population studied, intervention, comparison, and the outcome. Before you start any research, it is important to have a well-built and defined clear question. One way to construct a well-built question is to use the PICO model.

Suggested Reading
1. Aslam S, Emmanuel P. Formulating a researchable question: a critical step for facilitating good clinical research. Indian J Sex Transm Dis AIDS. 2010;31(1):47-50.
2. Medical College of Wisconsin Libraries. (2023). Evidence Based Medicine. [online] Available from https://mcw.libguides.com/EBM/PICO [Last accessed June, 2023].

Q.4. Which is true about the standardized mortality ratio (SMR) in quality?
   a. SMR is the ratio of the observed mortality versus predicted mortality for a specified time period.
   b. An ICU with healthy patients will have higher SMR values indicating better services.
   c. SMR is not affected by the tool used to calculate and predict mortality
   d. Absolute ICU mortality is a better indicator than SMR

Ans. a

Explanation: Standardized mortality ratio is the ratio of the observed or actual hospital mortality and the predicted (anticipated) hospital mortality for a specified time period. Requires an estimate of predicted mortality rate which can be calculated using a scoring system (e.g., APACHE II, ANZROD, SAPS, MPM,...). It is used to monitor quality standards of ICU. A value of one is considered normal or as expected, >1 worse than expected, and <1 better than expected.

Suggested Reading
1. Liddell FD. Simple exact analysis of the standardised mortality ratio. J Epidemiol Community Health. 1984;38(1):85-8.
2. Nickson C. (2015). Standardised Mortality Ratio. [online] Available from https://litfl.com/standardised-mortality-ratio/ [Last accessed June, 2023].

Q.5. What is the most appropriate statement about "Re-intubation rate" in quality control ICU?
   a. Reintubation means reintubation within 1 hour of extubation
   b. Reintubation means reintubation within 2 hours of extubation
   c. Reintubation means reintubation within 2 days of extubation
   d. Reintubation means reintubation within 1 day of extubation
   e. Reintubation rate should be targeted to zero

Ans. c

Explanation: Reintubation postfailed extubation is associated with a prolonged ICU stay and complications. Extubation failure or clinical judgment failure in a patient with anticipated successful extubation is quality indicator in ICU to monitor performance.

Suggested Reading
1. Jo YS, Lee YJ, Park JS, Yoon HI, Lee JH, Lee CT, et al. Readmission to medical intensive care units: risk factors and prediction. Yonsei Med J. 2015;56(2):543-9.
2. Whitmore D, Mahambray T. Reintubation following planned extubation: incidence, mortality and risk factors. Intensive Care Med Exp. 2015;3(Suppl 1):A684.

Q.6. What is ture about "Re-intubation rate" in quality control ICU?
   a. Zero reintubation rate means delayed extubation
   b. Zero reintubation rate means extraordinary care
   c. High reintubation rate means good standards as a team is very active in extubation
   d. Reintubation rate is used to calculate ventilator days by reintubation multiplied by a factor of seven

Ans. a

Explanation: Reintubation postfailed extubation is associated with a prolonged ICU stay and complications. Extubation failure or clinical judgment failure in a patient with anticipated successful extubation is quality indicator in ICU to monitor performance. If reintubation is high then it means we are extuabting to early. If rate is tending to zero that means are extubating late. Average reintubation or extubation failure of 10–15% is acceptable.

Suggested Reading
1. Jo YS, Lee YJ, Park JS, Yoon HI, Lee JH, Lee CT, et al. Readmission to medical intensive care units: risk factors and prediction. Yonsei Med J. 2015;56(2):543-9.
2. Whitmore D, Mahambray T. Reintubation following planned extubation: incidence, mortality and risk factors. Intensive Care Med Exp. 2015;3(Suppl 1):A684.

Q.7. Which of the following component is least beneficial in the prevention of ventilator-associated pneumonia (VAP)?
   a. Use of chlorhexidine solution for oral care
   b. Elevation of patient's head of bed to 30–45°
   c. Daily sedation vacation and daily assessment of readiness to extubation
   d. Regular subglottic suctioning

Ans. a

Explanation: In systematic reviews, oral care with chlorhexidine solution or gel reduces VAP risk by 25–40%, with uncertain or no additional benefit from augmenting oral care with tooth brushing. So it is the least recommended where as head end up, subglottic suction, and sedation vacation are very helpful and recommended.

Suggested Reading
1. Hellyer TP, Ewan V, Wilson P, Simpson AJ. The Intensive Care Society recommended bundle of interventions for the prevention of ventilator-associated pneumonia. J Intensive Care Soc. 2016;17(3):238-43.
2. Klompas M, Branson R, Cawcutt K, Crist M, Eichenwald EC, Greene LR, et al. Strategies to prevent ventilator-associated pneumonia, ventilator-associated events, and nonventilator hospital-acquired pneumonia in acute-care hospitals: 2022 Update. Infect Control Hosp Epidemiol. 2022;43(6):687-713.
3. Narang S. Use of ventilator bundle to prevent ventilator associated pneumonia. Oman Med J. 2008;23(2):96-9.

Q.8. What is *not* true about vacuum-assisted closure (VAC)?
a. Wound is thoroughly debrided, irrigated with normal saline, adequate hemostasis, and periwound skin is made dry
b. Sterile foams are used
c. Useful in malignant wounds, untreated osteomyelitis, and fistula
d. Useful in skin graft fixation

Ans. c

Explanation: Vacuum-assisted closure of a wound is a type of therapy to help wounds heal early. It is also known as wound VAC. A foam or gauze dressing is put directly on the wound. An adhesive film covers and seals the dressing and wound. A drainage tube leads from under the adhesive film and connects to a portable vacuum pump. This pump removes air pressure over the wound. It may do this either constantly or it may do it in cycles.

Suggested Reading
1. Johns Hopkins Medicine. Vacuum-Assisted Closure of a Wound. [online] Available from https://www.hopkinsmedicine.org/health/treatment-tests-and-therapies/vacuumassisted-closure-of-a-wound [Last accessed June, 2023].
2. Sheskin DJ. Handbook of Parametric and Nonparametric Statistical Procedures, 5th edition. Florida: CRC Press; 2011. p. 54.

Q.9. The rate of ICU readmission has been defined as a major performance indicator of the quality of intensive care medicine. Moreover, several studies also showed that patients with ICU readmission have higher mortality and longer hospital stays than patients without readmission. Readmission criteria is defined as return to ICU
a. Within 48 hours
b. Within 24 hours
c. Within 72 hours
d. Within 1 week

Ans. a

Explanation: The percentage of admitted patients who return to the hospital within 7 days of discharge will stay the same or decrease as changes are made to improve patient flow through the system.

Q.10. A central line-associated bloodstream infection (CLABSI) is a quality performance indicator. Which of the following statement is the *most* true?
   a. A CLABSI is a laboratory-confirmed bloodstream infection not related to an infection at another site that develops within 48 hours of central line placement.
   b. Antibiotic-coated central venous catheters are the most effective method to prevent CLABSI.
   c. The CLABSI rate is calculated by dividing the number of patients who have a CLABSI observed in the ICU by the number of central line placed during the reporting period.
   d. Femoral central venous catheters are associated with a lesser risk of CLABSI being larger vein as compared to internal jugular or subclavian catheters, but not preferred because of inconvenience, especially in female patients.

Ans. a

Explanation: A CLABSI is a laboratory-confirmed bloodstream with infection not related to an infection at another site that develops within 48 hours of central line placement. Most cases are preventable with proper aseptic techniques, surveillance, and management strategies. Centers for Disease Control (CDC), in collaboration with other organizations, has developed guidelines for the prevention of CLABSI and other types of healthcare-associated infections. Facilities can monitor the rates of CLABSI and assess the effectiveness of prevention efforts through the CDC's National Healthcare Safety Network (NHSN).

Suggested Reading
1. Haddadin Y, Annamaraju P, Regunath H. Central Line Associated Blood Stream Infections. StatPearls [Internet]. Treasure Island (FL): StatPearls Publishing; 2023.
2. O'Grady NP, Alexander M, Burns LA, Dellinger EP, Garland J, Heard SO, et al. Guidelines for the prevention of intravascular catheter-related infections, 2011 [online] Available from https://www.cdc.gov/hicpac/BSI/BSI-guidelines-2011.html [Last accessed June, 2023].

CHAPTER 32

Research Methodology

Harshal Tukaram Pandve, Sudha Bala, Khalid Ismail Khatib

Q.1. Which of the following sets correctly lists all the synonyms of reference population?
   a. Target population, source population or universe
   b. Target population, study population or universe
   c. Target population, study population or external population
   d. None of the above

Ans. a

Explanation: This is the total population of all subjects or units of study that the investigator keeps in mind while drawing the sample and further proposes to generalize the results (target population, universe, reference population or source population).

Suggested Reading
   1. Bhalwar R. Textbook of Community Medicine, 3rd edition. Gurugram: Wolters Kluwer India Pvt. Ltd.; 1019. p. 121.

Q.2. An organized collection of the values of the various variables which will be used for further analysis in an epidemiological study is known as:
   a. Data set
   b. Sample
   c. Statistics
   d. Population

Ans. a

Explanation: A chart duly completed with all the details for the required sample of subjects is the data set. Statistics is the branch of mathematics for collecting, analyzing, and interpreting data.

Suggested Reading
   1. Bhalwar R. Textbook of Community Medicine, 3rd edition. Gurugram: Wolters Kluwer India Pvt. Ltd.; 1019. p. 117.

Q.3. The requirements of the sample are:
   a. Should be adequately large
   b. Should be representative
   c. Both of the above
   d. None of the above

Ans. c

Explanation: Two important requirements of a sample are first, should be adequately large and second, it should be representative of the population in accordance with seasonality, day, and time of the week.

Suggested Reading
1. Bhalwar R. Textbook of Community Medicine, 3rd edition. Gurugram: Wolters Kluwer India Pvt. Ltd.; 1019. pp. 120-1.

Q.4. Numerical discrete scale belongs to which of the following measurement scales?
a. Qualitative
b. Quantitative
c. Both of the above
d. None of the above

Ans. b

Explanation: In a quantitative variable, information is recorded in terms of mathematical figures, whereas qualitative is recorded as per certain defined attributes.

Suggested Reading
1. Bhalwar R. Textbook of Community Medicine, 3rd edition. Gurugram: Wolters Kluwer India Pvt. Ltd.; 1019. p. 118.

Q.5. A quality, characteristic, or constituent of a subject which can be measured and which is likely to have a different value from one person to another is called:
a. Case definition
b. Variable
c. Epidemiology
d. Statistics

Ans. b

Explanation: Case definition is a set of standard criteria for classifying whether a person has a particular disease, syndrome, or other health condition. Epidemiology is the branch of medicine which deals with the incidence, distribution, and possible control of diseases and other factors relating to health. Statistics is the study and manipulation of data, including ways to gather, review, analyze, and draw conclusions from data.

Suggested Reading
1. Bhalwar R. Textbook of Community Medicine, 3rd edition. Gurugram: Wolters Kluwer India Pvt. Ltd.; 1019. p. 117.

Q.6. Objectives of the research should be:
a. Sensitive, meticulous, acceptable, rampant, and turn over
b. Specific, measurable, achievable, relevant, and time bound
c. Strong, meaningful, answerable, right, and tedious
d. Soft, measurable, acceptable, relevant, and tidy

Ans. b

Explanation: Specific—who and what; measurable—how much; achievable—how; relevant—why; and time bound—when. These format of objectives helps the research team to achieve the specific outcome in the given time period.

Suggested Reading
1. Kadri AM. IAPSM's Textbook of Community Medicine, 2nd edition. New Delhi: Jaypee Brothers Medical Publishers (P) Ltd; 2021. p. 194.

Q.7. What type of question is this for a data collection tool?
What are the conditions which significantly increase the risk of intensive care unit (ICU) delirium in a patient with dementia?
a. Open-ended
b. Close-ended

Ans. a

Explanation: Open-ended questions where the scope of answering is kept open for the respondent to decide. The respondent is given the freedom of length to provide the answer. Close-ended questions where the options are provided to enlist and these are the most common one used in the data collection tools.

Suggested Reading
1. Kadri AM. IAPSM's Textbook of Community Medicine, 2nd edition. New Delhi: Jaypee Brothers Medical Publishers (P) Ltd; 2021. p. 199.

Q.8. Frequency distribution of continuous variables is presented using:
a. Polygon
b. Histogram
c. Line diagram
d. Scatter diagram

Ans. b

Explanation: Continuous variables such as age, height, weight, etc. are represented on X-axis and frequency plotted on Y-axis for the histogram. Midpoints of the class interval of the variables are joined together at the height of their frequencies by straight lines. Line diagram is used to depict the trend of an event over a period of time. Scatter diagram is used to show the correlation between the two variables.

Suggested Reading
1. Kadri AM. IAPSM's Textbook of Community Medicine, 2nd edition. New Delhi: Jaypee Brothers Medical Publishers (P) Ltd; 2021. p. 202.

Q.9. In a drug trial a 50-year-old patient with coronary artery disease (CAD) is being interviewed about his dietary and smoking habits. The possible bias that might be introduced might be:
a. Selection bias
b. Berksonian bias
c. Recall bias
d. No possibility of bias

Ans. c

Explanation: Selection bias (susceptibility bias)—Groups to be compared are differentially susceptible to the outcome of interest, even before the experimental maneuver is performed. Berksonian bias (admission rate bias)—Bias due to hospital cases and controls being systematically different from each other. Recall bias—Cases are more likely to remember exposure more correctly than controls.

Suggested Reading
1. Park K. Park's Textbook of Preventive and Social Medicine, 26th edition. Jabalpur: Banarsidas Bhanot Publishers; 2021. p. 81.

Q.10. In study, first, hospitals are sampled, then intensive care units, and finally patients with hypertensive crises. This type of sampling is known as:
   a. Stratified sampling
   b. Simple random sampling
   c. Cluster sampling
   d. Multistage sampling

Ans. d

Explanation: Stratified sampling is to separately estimate the variable of interest in subgroups of the reference population. Simple random sampling is the simplest method where complete enumeration list to be available giving everyone an equal chance. Cluster sampling is aggregated in naturally occurring clusters, used in immunization coverage studies. Multistage sampling is used where large population has to be covered at different stages or units.

Suggested Reading
1. Kadri AM. IAPSM's Textbook of Community Medicine, 2nd edition. New Delhi: Jaypee Brothers Medical Publishers (P) Ltd; 2021. pp. 196-7.

Q.11. Not required for Chi-square test is:
   a. Mean and SD of the groups
   b. Each expected cell frequency >5
   c. Large sample
   d. Contingency table

Ans. a

Explanation: Chi-square test of association is applied to test the association between two categorical variables with prerequirements as large sample with at least 80% of expected cell values should be >5 and none should be less than one represented as 2 × 2 contingency table between the exposure and the disease.

Suggested Reading
1. Khanal AB. Mahajan's Methods in Biostatistics for Medical Students and Research Workers, 8th edition. New Delhi: Jaypee Brothers Medical Publishers (P) Ltd; 2016. pp. 154-69.

Q.12. The research results not generated from the study are called:
   a. Falsification
   b. Fabrication
   c. Duplication
   d. Plagiarism

Ans. b

Explanation: Falsification is the results generated by manipulating data; fabrication is the research results not generated from the study. Duplication is submitting the new manuscript with same hypothesis, data, results, and discussion. Plagiarism is the use of previously published manuscript by someone for his or her manuscript or unreferenced use of others published or unpublished ideas without consent, credit, or acknowledgement.

Suggested Reading
1. National Academy of Sciences, National Academy of Engineering (US) and Institute of Medicine (US) Committee on Science, Engineering, and Public Policy. On Being a Scientist: A Guide to Responsible Conduct in Research: Third Edition. Washington (DC): National Academies Press (US); 2009. RESEARCH MISCONDUCT.

Q.13. Sampling used in situations where occurrence of phenomenon is uncommon:
   a. Purposive
   b. Quota
   c. Snowball
   d. Judgmental

Ans. c

Explanation: In purposive sample people possessing specific characteristic of interest to the researcher are chosen. Quota sample is taken from different strata of accessible population. In Snowball method the researcher would get access to one person which would lead to next possible participant.

Suggested Reading
1. Kadri AM. IAPSM's Textbook of Community Medicine, 2nd edition. New Delhi: Jaypee Brothers Medical Publishers (P) Ltd; 2021. p. 218.

Q.14. Most common format of writing a research report is:
   a. IMRAD
   b. FINER
   c. SMART
   d. DIRECT

Ans. a

Explanation: IMRAD—**I**ntroduction tells why this topic is important and the rationale, **M**ethodology covers how the study was conducted in detail, **R**esults cover the findings of the study represented in tables and figures, **A**- and **D**-discussion which elaborates what does it mean.

Suggested Reading
1. Bhalwar RV, Vaidya R. Textbook of Public Health and Community Medicine, 2nd edition. World Health Organization, Pune: Department of Community Medicine, Armed Forces Medical College; 2009. p. 222.

Q.15. The STROBE guidelines are for:
   a. Observational studies
   b. Analytical studies
   c. Clinical trials
   d. Systematic reviews

Ans. a

Explanation: The Strengthening the Reporting of Observational studies in Epidemiology (STROBE) guidelines were created to aid the author in ensuring high-quality presentation of the conducted observational study consisting of 22 checklist items.

Suggested Reading
1. Cuschieri S. The STROBE guidelines. Saudi J Anaesth. 2019;13(Suppl 1):S31-4.

Q.16. All are the methods to deal with confounding at design stage except:
   a. Restriction
   b. Matching
   c. Randomization
   d. Multivariate analysis

Ans. d

Explanation: Confounder is a third factor, is a variable, which influences both the exposure and the outcome. At the design stage we can do restriction, matching, and randomization. Restriction—we can restrict our study participants to only those people who are in one stratum of the confounders, so that the confounders cannot play a role in the association between exposure and outcome. We can match our cases and controls on those particular confounders and which will negate the effect of the confounders. Randomization that actually automatically takes care of the confounders and makes sure that the two arms in a randomized trial are similar in all ways in terms of the confounding variable.

Suggested Reading
1. Gordis L. Chapter 15. More on causal inferences: Bias, confounding and interaction. In: Epidemiology: with STUDENT CONSULT Online Access, 5th edition. India: Saunders; 2014. p. 269.

Q.17. Logic of enquiry in qualitative research is deductive.
   a. True
   b. False

Ans. b

Explanation: Qualitative methods generally find their origin in the science of anthropology, sociology, and psychology, wherein which is more about dealing with human beings understanding their behaviors. In terms of the logic of inquiry, again, qualitative methods are more inductive and they are used in the way to understand the processes that are derived from the data compared to the quantitative methods, wherein which is more deductive and where we try to test our formal hypothesis using the data.

Suggested Reading
1. Bhalwar RV, Vaidya R. Textbook of Public Health and Community Medicine, 2nd edition. World Health Organization, Pune: Department of Community Medicine, Armed Forces Medical College; 2009. pp. 209-10.

Q.18. Which of the following statements is not true in case of pilot study?
   a. They are conducted for developing and testing adequacy of research instruments.
   b. They establish whether the sampling frame and technique are effective.
   c. Ethics committee approves the main study only after successful completion of the pilot study.
   d. They are small scale studies.

Ans. c

Explanation: Pilot studies are designed to explore a new research area to determine whether variables are measurable with sufficient precision as well as to check the logistics. And this does not require ethical committee approval to be conducted.

Suggested Reading
   1. Bhalwar RV, Vaidya R. Textbook of Public Health and Community Medicine, 2nd edition. World Health Organization, Pune: Department of Community Medicine, Armed Forces Medical College; 2009. p. 252.

Q.19. Which of the following is stated mainly for statistical purpose?
   a. Research question
   b. Objectives
   c. Research hypothesis
   d. All of the above

Ans. c

Explanation: Research hypothesis is a specific version of the research question that summarizes the main elements of the study that establishes the basis for statistical test of significance. So, it is stated for statistical purposes. This includes sample, the exposures, and outcomes.

Suggested Reading
   1. Bhalwar RV, Vaidya R. Textbook of public health and community medicine. 2nd edition. World Health Organization, Pune: Department of Community Medicine, Armed Forces Medical College; 2009. p. 218.

Q.20. Use of continuous intravenous anakinra infusion in multisystem inflammatory syndrome in children with critical coronavirus disease-2019 (COVID-19) infection is represented best with which study design?
   a. Case report
   b. Systematic review
   c. Narrative review
   d. Both b and c

Ans. a

Explanation: Case reports are the type of descriptive studies based on single or else series of cases of specific treated or untreated condition without any specific comparison group. This describes the signs, symptoms, and pathophysiological parameters.

Suggested Reading
1. Bhalwar RV, Vaidya R. Textbook of Public Health and Community Medicine, 2nd edition. World Health Organization, Pune: Department of Community Medicine, Armed Forces Medical College; 2009. p. 131.

Q.21. Which phase of a clinical trial is referred to as postmarketing surveillance?
   a. Phase 1
   b. Phase 2
   c. Phase 3
   d. Phase 4

Ans. d

Explanation: The phase I is the step 1 in clinical evaluation of any new intervention that comes in and here the trial is done in a very small number of individuals, to evaluate safety and acceptability. Phase II trial, which is generally done in larger number of individuals, generally 100–500 and who may have low risk of a particular disease to study the long-term safety, the dose, and schedule. A phase III design, essentially is a large trial, which looks at the efficacy of a particular intervention. Once, all these phases I, II, and III are completed, the product goes for licensures in the country, it gets a license and once it gets the license, it gets marketed in the country and then phase IV trials are undertaken, which are considered as postmarketing surveillance and they are done in again thousands of individuals.

Suggested Reading
1. Gordis L. Chapter 8-Randomized trials: Some further issues. In: Epidemiology: with STUDENT CONSULT Online Access, 5th edition. India: Saunders; 2014. p. 165.

Q.22. In a study on acute respiratory distress syndrome, patients are categorized based on their level of oxygen in the blood. What type of variable is this?
   a. Qualitative
   b. Descriptive
   c. Nominal
   d. Ordinal

Ans. d

Explanation: Ordinal scales only permit the ranking of items from highest to lowest. Ordinal measures have no absolute values, and the real differences between adjacent ranks may not be equal.

Suggested Reading
1. Kothari CR. Measurement and scaling techniques. In: Research Methodology Methods and Techniques, 2nd revised edition. KB Center; 2014. p. 71.

Q.23. The value of kappa <0.40 represents what level of agreement?
   a. Excellent
   b. Good
   c. Intermediate
   d. Poor

Ans. d

Explanation: Value of kappa >0.75 has an excellent agreement beyond chance, 0.40–0.75 represents intermediate to good agreement. Value <0.40 represents poor agreement.

Suggested Reading
1. Gordis L. Chapter 5: Assessing the validity and reliability of diagnostic and screening tests. In: Epidemiology: with STUDENT CONSULT Online Access, 5th edition. India: Saunders; 2014. p. 110.

Q.24. Drivers admitted to an emergency room after road traffic crashes in 2014 were interviewed about personal, vehicle, and crash characteristics as well as hourly patterns of driving, and alcohol and food intake in the 24 hours before the crash. Here the subject serves as his/her own control. What type of study is this?
 a. Prospective cohort
 b. Retrospective cohort
 c. Case-cohort
 d. Case-crossover
 e. Case control

Ans. d

Explanation: The case-crossover study design is a relatively new analytical epidemiological approach, and is unique in that the case serves as his/her own control and is used to investigate the transient effects of an intermittent exposure on the onset of acute outcomes.

Suggested Reading
1. Gordis L. Chapter 10: Case control and other study designs. In: Epidemiology: with STUDENT CONSULT Online Access, 5th edition. India: Saunders; 2014. pp. 206-7.

Q.25. An advertisement in a medical journal stated 2,000 subjects with sepsis were treated with new medicine. Within 3 days, 94% were asymptomatic. This claims that medicine is effective. Based on this, the claim is:
 a. Correct
 b. May be incorrect because conclusion is not based on a rate.
 c. May be incorrect because no statistical significance was used.
 d. May be incorrect because no control or comparison group was involved.

Ans. d

Explanation: Only the proportion is mentioned without any statistical significance test.

Suggested Reading
1. Gordis L. Chapter 8: Randomized trials: Some further issues. In: Epidemiology: with STUDENT CONSULT Online Access, 5th edition. India: Saunders; 2014. p. 175.

Q.26. Study subjects in a group may change their behavior when they come to know that they are being observed, called:
 a. Apprehension bias
 b. Attention bias (Hawthorne effect)
 c. Berksonian bias
 d. Recall bias

Ans. b

Explanation: Apprehension bias—Certain levels (pulse, blood pressure) may alter systematically from their usual levels when the subject is apprehensive. Attention bias (Hawthorne effect): Study subjects may systematically alter their behavior when they know they are being observed. Berksonian bias (admission rate bias): Bias due to hospital cases and controls being systematically different from each other. Recall bias—Cases are more likely to remember exposure more correctly than controls.

Suggested Reading
1. Bhalwar RV, Vaidya R. Textbook of Public Health and Community Medicine, 2nd edition. World Health Organization, Pune: Department of Community Medicine, Armed Forces Medical College; 2009. pp. 147-50.

Q.27. Which of the following is also called consensus method?
 a. Focus group discussions
 b. Delphi technique
 c. Projective method
 d. In-depth interview

Ans. b

Explanation: Delphi technique enables a large group of experts to be contacted usually by mail or questionnaire and are asked to rate the comments. Then summarized and sent back to experts to rethink on the subject. Re-rankings are analyzed for consensus. This repeated until consensus reached. Widely used in health research within the fields of technology assessment, education, training, priority setting, and information.

Suggested Reading
1. Mahajan BK, Roy RN, Saha I, Gupta MC. Textbook of Preventive and Social Medicine, 4th edition. New Delhi: Jaypee Brothers Medical Publishers (P) Ltd; 2013. p. 455.

Q.28. Population variance can be estimated from:
 a. A pilot study
 b. Reports of previous studies
 c. Guessing
 d. "a" and "b"

Ans. d

Explanation: Population variance can be obtained from a pilot survey. An estimate available from the pilot survey could be used or can use an estimate which is available from previous studies.

Suggested Reading
1. Ramakrishnan R. Calculating Sample Size and Power. In: Lecture-12: Basic course on biomedical research. 2020. p. 139.

Q.29. If we ask a patient attending OPD to evaluate his pain on a scale of 0 (no pain) to 5 (the worst pain), then this commonly applied scale is:
 a. Dichotomous
 b. Ratio scale
 c. Continuous
 d. Nominal

Ans. b

Explanation: Dichotomous is for categorical variable, Ratio scale is an interval scale with the additional property that its zero position indicates the absence of the quantity being measured. Nominal scale is simply a system of assigning number symbols to events in order to label them.

Suggested Reading
1. Bhalwar R. Textbook of Community Medicine, 3rd edition. Gurugram: Wolters Kluwer India Pvt. Ltd.; 1019. p. 237.

Q.30. Which of the following divides the group of ICU data into four subgroups?
  a. Quartiles
  b. Percentiles
  c. Standard deviation
  d. Median

Ans. a

Explanation: Quartiles divide a distribution into four equal parts. Percentiles divide a distribution into 100 equal parts, after arranging in an ascending order.

Suggested Reading
1. Bhalwar R. Textbook of Community Medicine, 3rd edition. Gurugram: Wolters Kluwer India Pvt. Ltd.; 1019. p. 238.

Q.31. The response which is graded by an observer on agree or disagree continuum is based on:
  a. Visual analog scale (VAS)
  b. Guttman scale
  c. Likert scale
  d. Adjectival scale

Ans. c

Explanation: Visual analog scale is a measurement instrument that tries to measure a characteristic that ranges across a continuum of values and cannot easily be directly measured; mostly used in anesthesia. Guttman scale also known as "cumulative scale", contains a "series of statements that expresses increasing intensity" of a characteristic and respondent is asked to agree or disagree to with each statement. Adjectival scale, a linguistic scale, is a set of words of the same grammatical category, which can be ordered by their semantic strength or degree of information. Likert scale also known as "summative scale" is a "type of ordinal scale" generally used to quantify attitudes and behavior. Responses are graded on a continuum.

Suggested Reading
1. Kishore J. A Dictionary of Public Health, 3rd edition. New Delhi: Century Publications; 2013. pp. 475-6.